Uniquest Series
BIOCHEMISTRY

Uniquest Series
BIOCHEMISTRY

A Compilation of All India University Questions 2003–2021

SECOND EDITION

Evangeline Jones MBBS MD (Biochemistry)
Formerly Professor and Head
Department of Biochemistry
Vinayaka Mission's Kirupananda Variyar Medical College, Salem
and
Government Mohan Kumaramangalam Medical College, Salem, Tamil Nadu, India

Co-author
Hariharan V MBBS MD (Biochemistry)
Associate Professor
Department of Biochemistry
Karpagam Faculty of Medical Sciences and Research
Coimbatore, Tamil Nadu, India

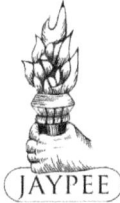

JAYPEE BROTHERS MEDICAL PUBLISHERS
The Health Sciences Publisher
New Delhi | London

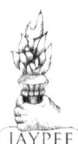
Jaypee Brothers Medical Publishers (P) Ltd

Headquarters
Jaypee Brothers Medical Publishers (P) Ltd
EMCA House, 23/23-B
Ansari Road, Daryaganj
New Delhi 110 002, India
Landline: +91-11-23272143, +91-11-23272703
+91-11-23282021, +91-11-23245672
Email: jaypee@jaypeebrothers.com

Corporate Office
Jaypee Brothers Medical Publishers (P) Ltd
4838/24, Ansari Road, Daryaganj
New Delhi 110 002, India
Phone: +91-11-43574357
Fax: +91-11-43574314
Email: jaypee@jaypeebrothers.com

Overseas Office
J.P. Medical Ltd
83 Victoria Street, London
SW1H 0HW (UK)
Phone: +44 20 3170 8910
Fax: +44 (0)20 3008 6180
Email: info@jpmedpub.com

Website: www.jaypeebrothers.com
Website: www.jaypeedigital.com

© 2023, Jaypee Brothers Medical Publishers

The views and opinions expressed in this book are solely those of the original contributor(s)/author(s) and do not necessarily represent those of editor(s) and publisher of the book.

All rights reserved. No part of this publication may be reproduced, stored or transmitted in any form or by any means, electronic, mechanical, photocopying, recording or otherwise, without the prior permission in writing of the publishers.

All brand names and product names used in this book are trade names, service marks, trademarks or registered trademarks of their respective owners. The publisher is not associated with any product or vendor mentioned in this book.

Medical knowledge and practice change constantly. This book is designed to provide accurate, authoritative information about the subject matter in question. However, readers are advised to check the most current information available on procedures included and check information from the manufacturer of each product to be administered, to verify the recommended dose, formula, method and duration of administration, adverse effects and contraindications. It is the responsibility of the practitioner to take all appropriate safety precautions. Neither the publisher nor the author(s)/editor(s) assume any liability for any injury and/or damage to persons or property arising from or related to use of material in this book.

This book is sold on the understanding that the publisher is not engaged in providing professional medical services. If such advice or services are required, the services of a competent medical professional should be sought.

Every effort has been made where necessary to contact holders of copyright to obtain permission to reproduce copyright material. If any have been inadvertently overlooked, the publisher will be pleased to make the necessary arrangements at the first opportunity.

Inquiries for bulk sales may be solicited at: jaypee@jaypeebrothers.com

Uniquest Series: Biochemistry

First Edition: 2019
Second Edition: **2023**
ISBN: 978-93-5465-521-0

Dedicated to

The Lord Almighty for giving me strength and health to compile this comprehensive question-answer series in biochemistry. I thank God. To HIM be all glory!

Preface to the Second Edition

Years ago, in the undergraduate medical course, the subject of Biochemistry was just a part of Physiology paper and the syllabus was simple with only carbohydrates, proteins, fats and vitamins. Hence, it was easy to read the subject, revise and get through in those days. Over the years the science of Biochemistry has exploded and is now established as the basis in causation and control of majority of disease processes, leading to Nobel prize winning research findings. The ever-increasing knowledge of molecular biology and intricacy of genetic engineering has made Biochemistry one of the tough subjects for the first year students of medicine.

The subject has expanded. The question formats have changed. The assessment has become stringent. Students are bewildered as to what to study in such a short period and how to answer the questions to the point. While contemplating on these, a spark kindled by a good physician friend, ignited a passion for compiling a comprehensive but compact University questions and answers book which will be useful for the present-day medical students.

This unique compilation has been done with utmost care and concern keeping in mind the medical student's need to make a rapid revision, orienting them to the nuances of answering the different formats of the questions crisply. The new formats of question patterns in the recent years as per the guidelines of NMC have been added, Multiple Choice Questions included and suitably updated in this second edition. Appropriate figures and tables have been appended, cycles and cascades have been attached then and there, making this self-explanatory and easy to understand. In addition, topic-wise questions and answers have been listed in the end to help the students to choose a topic and check the questions and answers pertaining to that chapter.

The subject of Biochemistry has been placed in the Questions and Answers format to help the medical students to revise and recheck their preparedness for the examination.

Wishing the students Good Luck.

Evangeline Jones
Hariharan V

Preface to the First Edition

Medical biochemistry is a vast subject which deals with the complex biological reactions that take place in human body under normal conditions and also under abnormal pathological states. There are standard textbooks of biochemistry to explain the subject in detail from which the medical student is expected to learn and enrich his knowledge. However, the students' need for a compilation of university questions and answers in the form of a book was felt by many and this book is born out of this idea. This book will help the medical students in preparing for the various tests during the preclinical course and will instill confidence while appearing for the university examinations. It will also help the medical students to revise the subject and plan the answers according to the formats of various universities. It covers university questions from 2003.

We hope and wish that this effort will be useful for the students in excelling in biochemistry examinations across the country.

Evangeline Jones
Hariharan V

Acknowledgments

The idea of compiling university examinations questions and answers in the form of a book was suggested by Dr TP Kalaniti MD, an eminent academician and a well wisher. We would like to thank him.

The encouragement given by our family has been very valuable, and special thanks to Dr Jones Ronald, for his guidance and advice in formatting this book.

We would like to express our gratitude to Shri Jitendar P Vij (Group Chairman), Mr Ankit Vij (Managing Director) and Mr MS Mani (Group President) of M/s Jaypee Brothers Medical Publishers (P) Ltd, New Delhi, India, for all their encouragement and efforts in bringing out this book.

Contents

MBBS Examination 2003	1
MBBS Examination 2004	35
MBBS Examination 2005	57
MBBS Examination 2006	103
MBBS Examination 2007	140
MBBS Examination 2008	175
MBBS Examination 2009	205
MBBS Examination 2010	243
MBBS Examination 2011	278
MBBS Examination 2012	307
MBBS Examination 2013	334
MBBS Examination 2014	376
MBBS Examination 2015	408
MBBS Examination 2016	436
MBBS Examination 2017	470
MBBS Examination 2018	499
MBBS Examination 2019	507
MBBS Examination 2020	523
MBBS Examination 2021	535
Topic-wise University Questions	559

General Instructions

- Answers for university questions in biochemistry are compiled from 2003 to 2021 for the essays, short notes and short answers separately.
- An index as per the topic is also given separately for easy reference.
- Answer details of the repeated questions are given in brackets.
- The reader is advised to study the standard textbooks in biochemistry before using this book for better understanding.

MBBS Examination 2003

ANSWER ALL QUESTIONS

I. Essay questions   **(10 Marks each)**

1. Write about the sources, activation, biochemical functions, deficiency disease and its detection of thiamine.
2. Write in detail about glucose homeostasis in the human organism and add a note on its biomedical importance.
3. Write detail about structural organization of proteins and briefly mention about various methods used in elucidation of primary structure.
4. Write how acid-base balances are maintained in the body. Mention causes and biochemical alteration of metabolic acidosis.

II. Short notes   **(5 Marks each)**

1. Biochemical function of vitamin D.
2. Absorption of lipids (TAG): (Bergstrom theory).
3. Excretion of bilirubin and clinical importance of bilirubin estimations.
4. Coupling of oxidative phosphorylation, uncouplers and their importance.
5. Clinical importance of isoenzymes with suitable example.
6. Biochemical changes in von Gierke disease and their relation to enzyme deficiency.
7. Role of LDL receptors in metabolism of LDL and the disease caused by its defect.
8. Definition, expression and significance of K_m value.
9. Role of liver in integration of metabolism during postprandial state.
10. Caloric requirement and its recommended distribution among nutrients in an adult male.
11. List various DNA repair mechanisms and give their biomedical importance.
12. Enzyme defects and biochemical consequences of two inborn errors of phenylalanine metabolism—Phenylketonuria and Alkaptonuria.
13. Name heavy metal poisons. Write biochemical consequences of any two.
14. Biochemical roles and nutritional importance of trace elements.
15. (a) List the different mechanisms involved in hormone action and (b) write about the mechanism of action of hormones using cAMP as second messenger.
16. List various thyroid function test and give the importance of free thyroid hormones in assessing thyroid function test.
17. Alternations in biochemical investigations in cirrhosis liver.
18. Metabolically important products formed from methionine.
19. Clinical application of DNA recombinant technology.
20. Biochemical application of tumor markers.

I. ESSAY QUESTIONS

1. Write about the sources, activation, biochemical functions, deficiency disease and its detection of thiamine.

Thiamine is vitamin B1. It is one of the water soluble vitamins.

Sources
- Plant sources like cereals (outer layer), pulses, oil seeds, nut and yeast
- Animal sources like organ meats, pork, milk, etc
- **RDA:** 1–1.5 mg/day
- **Chemistry:** Thiamine consists of a pyrimidine ring attached to a thiazole ring connected by methylene bridge.

Active form of Thiamine
- The co-enzyme form of vitamin is TPP (thiamine pyrophosphate)
- It is synthesized by phosphorylation of thiamine by kinase
- Thiamine + ATP ⟶ TPP + AMP.

Biochemical Functions
The thiamine pyrophosphate acts as codecarboxylase, and involved in oxidative decarboxylation reactions, and transketolase reactions.

Oxidative Decarboxylation
- Conversion of pyruvate to acetyl-CoA by pyruvate dehydrogenase complex:

Pyruvate →(PDH - Complex)→ Acetyl-CoA
TPP, NAD CO_2, NADH +H^+

- TCA cycle: alpha ketoglutarate dehydrogenase:

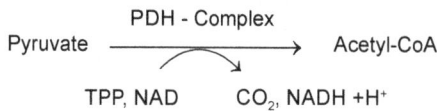

α-Ketoglutarate →(α-KG Dehydrogenase)→ Succinyl CoA
TPP, NAD CO_2, NADH +H^+

- Branched chain amino acid metabolism – alpha-ketoacid dehydrogenase

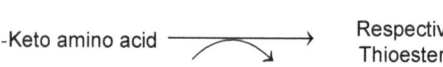

α-Keto amino acid →(α-KA dehydrogenase)→ Respective Thioesters
TPP, NAD CO_2, NADH +H

Transketolase Reaction – HMP Pathway

Involved in HMP pathway for the synthesis of pentoses and NADPH

Deficiency: Beriberi: The deficiency of thiamine leads to disease called beriberi, its features are depending on its type as follows:
- **Wet beriberi** affects cardiovascular system: It is related to edema of face, trunk, and serous cavities. Breathlessness, palpitation, swollen calf muscles, elevated systolic pressure, fast and bouncing pulse. Heart is weak
- **Dry beriberi:** Affects CNS
  - It is mostly related to degeneration of nervous system (peripheral neuritis)
  - Muscles are weak and unable to walk.
  - There will be peripheral neuritis and sensory disturbances leading to complete paralysis.
- **Infantile beriberi:** The child has symptoms like sleeplessness, restlessness, vomiting, convulsions, and death
- **Cerebral beriberi (Wernicke-Korsakoff syndrome):** There will be encephalopathy including ophthalmoplegia, nystagmus, cerebellar ataxia along with psychosis.

Polyneuritis: Seen in chronic alcoholic patients. Alcohol inhibits absorption of thiamine leading to thiamine deficiency. This causes impairment of conversion of pyruvate to acetyl CoA resulting in accumulation of lactate leading to lactic acidosis.

Assay
- Estimation of blood thiamine
- Estimation of pyruvate, alpha ketoglutarate and lactate
- Assessment of transketolase activity in RBC.

2. Write in detail about glucose homeostasis in the human organism and add a note on its biomedical importance.

- Normal fasting blood glucose - 70–110 mg/DL
- Normal postprandial blood glucose - 120–140 mg/dL.

Blood Glucose Homeostasis

Blood glucose is maintained at the normal range for optimal utilization of glucose by the body. In our body, certain tissues like brain, retina and testes are solely dependent on glucose for their energy at certain concentration.

Sources of Blood Glucose

- **Dietary sources:** Plant starch which is degraded to glucose in the intestine and absorbed in to blood
- **Gluconeogenesis:** Glucose is formed from noncarbohydrates sources like pyruvate, lactate, glycerol and glucogenic amino acids
- **Glycogenolysis:** The stored glycogen present in liver and muscle is broken down to glucose.

Utilization of Glucose

- Glycolysis and TCA cycle: Glucose is used as main energy source by all cells to produce ATP
- Glycogenesis: Excess glucose is converted to glycogen and stored in liver and muscle.
- Glucose is utilized for synthesis of non-essential amino acids and fat
- Glucose is utilized for synthesis of amino-sugars.

Excretion of Glucose

- The kidney is the major organ which regulates the glucose excretion. In normal healthy persons there is no excretion of glucose in urine
- Glucose is excreted through urine if blood glucose is more than 180 mg/dL. This is called as **renal threshold level**
- The maximum reabsorption of glucose by renal tubules is 350 mg/minute (tubular maximum).

Blood Glucose Regulation during Fed State

Following a meal, glucose level is increased in circulation. This high concentration of glucose is regulated via two processes:

1. **Action of glucokinase:** Glucokinase found only in liver and is having high K_m and low affinity to glucose. During postprandial conditions glucose level is high and so glucose binds with this enzyme. Hence, immediately after meals the glucose is acted upon by glucokinase in liver and utilized for energy production through glycolysis.
2. **Action of insulin:** High concentration of glucose in blood in the fed stage stimulates the production of insulin from pancreas. Uptake of glucose by most of extrahepatic tissues except brain is dependent on insulin.

Blood glucose regulation during fasting:

After meals, after about 2.5 hours the blood glucose level is regulated to the normal range. After another 3 hours, the glucose is supplied through glycogenolysis, and thereafter by gluconeogenesis.

Regulation of glucose by hormones:

The various hormones play significant role in regulation of blood glucose concentrations. They are as follows:

- **Hypoglycemic hormone-insulin:** It is 51 amino acid peptide hormone produced from β-cells of islets of Langerhans of pancreas. Insulin is a hypoglycemic hormone. Insulin lowers the blood glucose by means of following mechanisms:
    - Insulin stimulates glycolysis, glycogenesis, HMP shunt, fat synthesis
    - Insulin suppresses gluconeogenesis, glycogenolysis.
- **Hyperglycemic hormones**
    - **Glucagon:**
        - It is produced form α-cells of islets of Langerhans of pancreas
        - Its functions are agonist to the insulin actions – anti-insulin action

- It stimulates gluconeogenesis, glycogenolysis.
- **Epinephrine or adrenaline from adrenal medullary gland**
- **Thyroxine from thyroid gland**
- **Glucocorticoids from adrenal cortex.**
  - These hormones are hyperglycemic in nature
  - They stimulate gluconeogenesis, and glycogenolysis
  - Glucocorticoids stimulates protein metabolism.
- **Growth hormone:**
  - It inhibits the glucose utilization by cells
  - It stimulates protein synthesis.

3. **Write detail about structural organization of proteins and briefly mention about various methods used in elucidation of primary structure.**

Proteins have different levels of structural organization (**Fig. 1**). They are

- Primary structure
- Secondary structure
- Tertiary structure
- Quaternary structure.

Primary Structure (Fig. 2)

- It denotes the number and sequence of amino acids in the protein
- Primary structure is maintained by **peptide bond (CONH bond)**, e.g. **insulin.**

Secondary Structure

- It denotes the configurational relationship between residues which are about 3-4 amino acids apart in linear structure
- This structure is maintained by non-covalent forces or bonds like hydrogen bonds, electrostatic (ionic) bonds, hydrophobic bonds and van der Waals forces
- The types of secondary structure are: i) Alpha helix, e.g. alpha keratin, ii) Beta pleated sheet, beta bends (reverse turns,

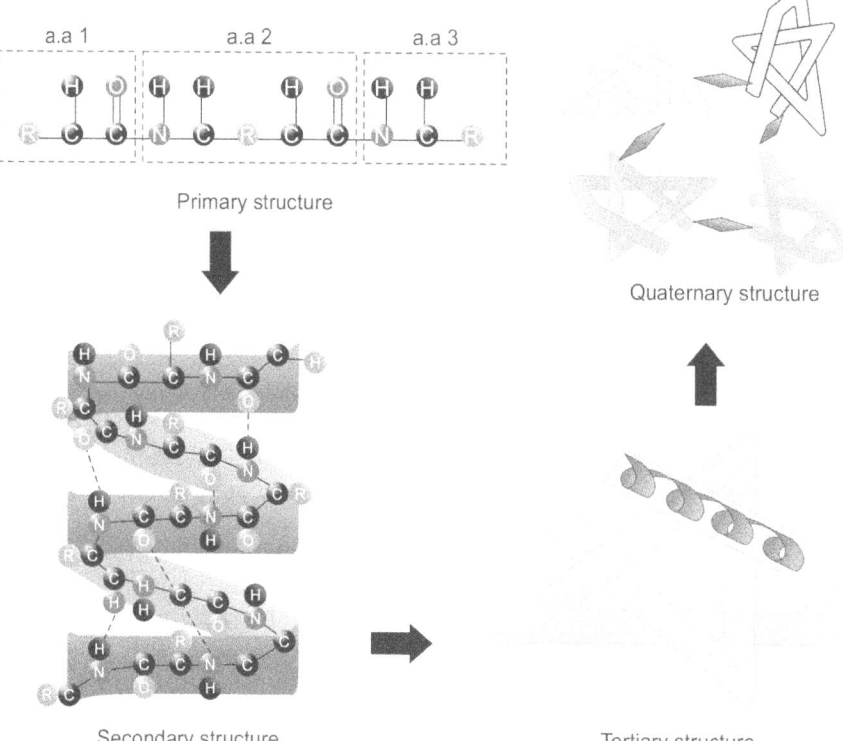

Fig. 1: Structural organizations of proteins.

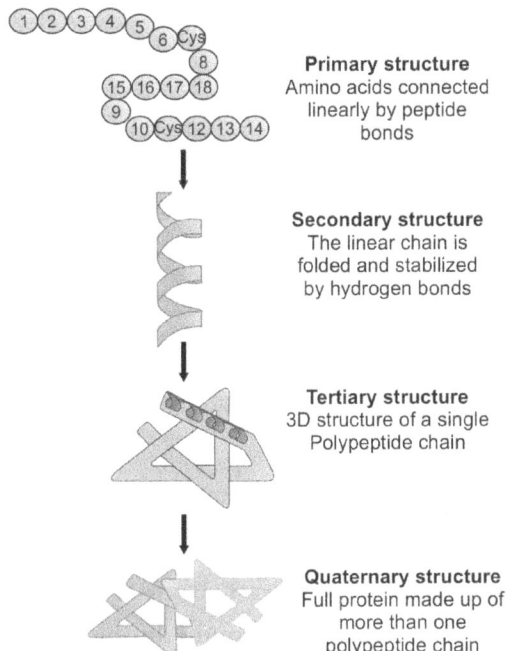

Fig. 2: Structures of proteins.

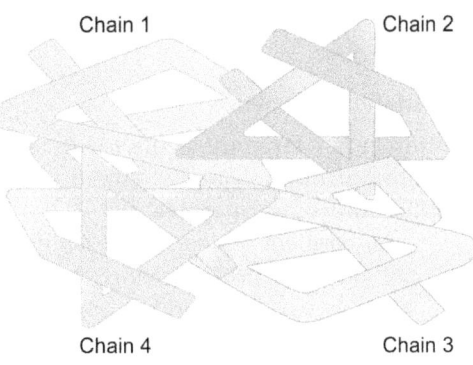

Fig. 3: Quaternary structure.

beta turns), non-repetitive secondary structure and super secondary motifs.

Tertiary Structure

- It denotes the 3 dimensional structure of whole protein by further folding, e.g. myoglobin
- It defines the stearic relationship of amino acids which are far apart from each other in linear structure, but are close in the 3 dimensional aspects
- Secondary, tertiary and quaternary structures are maintained by hydrogen bonds, electrostatic bonds, hydrophobic bonds and weak van der Waals forces
- Domains are the fundamental, functional and 3 dimensional structural units of polypeptides. The domains are connected with flexible areas of protein.

Quaternary Structure (Fig. 3)

- This occurs only in proteins which have more than one polypeptide chain—polymeric proteins
- These polypeptides aggregate to form quaternary structure to get one functional protein
- Each polypeptide chain is termed as sub-unit or monomer. Depending on the number of polypeptide chains, the proteins are dimer (2 chains), trimer (3 chains), and tetramer (4 chains) and so on
- If the protein has two copies of the same polypeptide chains they are termed as homodimer and if it has two different polypeptide chains they are called as heterodimer
- Example: Hemoglobin is a heterotetramer having 2 alpha chains and 2 beta chains
- Quaternary structures are maintained by hydrogen bonds, electrostatic bonds, hydrophobic bonds and weak van der Waals forces.

Elucidation of Primary Structure of Proteins

- Frederick Sanger was the first scientist to sequence a polypeptide. The first protein sequenced was insulin which has one A chain of 21 amino acid residues and one B chain of 30 amino acid residues
- Before analysing the structure of a protein it has to be extracted and isolated by various chromatographic techniques, like HPLC, etc.
- Then purity of the isolated protein is done by electrophoresis, like PAGE
- Molecular weight of the proteins is determined by mass spectroscopy
- Then the primary structure is determined by the following steps:
  - Degradation of protein or polypeptides- smaller fragments
  - Determination of amino acid sequence

- Determination of amino acid composition.

Degradation of Proteins

- Protein is a large molecule made up of more than one polypeptide chains
- **Liberation of polypeptides:**
  - Non-covalent bonds are broken down by treating proteins with urea or guanidine hydrochloride
  - Cleaving of disulfide bonds is done by treating with performic acid.
- **Identification of number of polypeptides (Fig. 4)**
  - This is done by treating the liberated polypeptide chains with dansyl chloride
  - Dansyl chloride binds with N terminal amino acid to form dansyl polypeptides
  - Hydrolysis of dansyl polypeptides by boiling with 6N HCl at 110°C for 18–36 hours produces N terminal dansyl amino acids which is equal to the number of polypeptide chains.
3. **Breakdown of polypeptides into fragments:**
  - Done by enzymatic or chemical cleavage
  - Enzymatic cleavage is done by treating with proteolytic enzymes like trypsin, chymotrypsin, pepsin, elastase which cleave the peptide bonds containing lysine or arginine residues on the C=O side
  - Chemical cleavage is done by treating with cyanogen bromide (CNBr) which is specific for methionine on the carbonyl side to split the polypeptides into smaller fragments.

Determination of Amino Acid Sequence

End group analysis to analyse the N terminal amino acid – By treating with Sanger's Reagent (Fig. 5)
- Polypeptides or their small fragments are treated with Sanger's reagent. Sanger's reagent (FDNB) is 1-Fluoro-2,4 dinitrobenzene. It binds specifically with the N terminal amino acid to form dinitrophenyl (DNP) derivative of peptide
- Hydrolysis of DNP peptide yields DNP-amino acid + free amino acids
- DNP amino acid is then identified by chromatography
- Sanger's reagent has limited use.

To analyse the N terminal amino acid – By treating with Edman reagent: Phenyl isothiocyanate (Fig. 6)
- N terminal amino acid binds with Edman reagent – Phenyl isothiocyanate to produce phenylthiocarbamyl derivative
- On treatment with mild acid-PTH – amino acid – Phenylthiohydantoin amino acid cyclic compounds are liberated
- This can be identified by chromatography
- Edman's reagent has an advantage as the peptide can be sequentially degraded
- Automated sequenator – based on Edman's degradation.

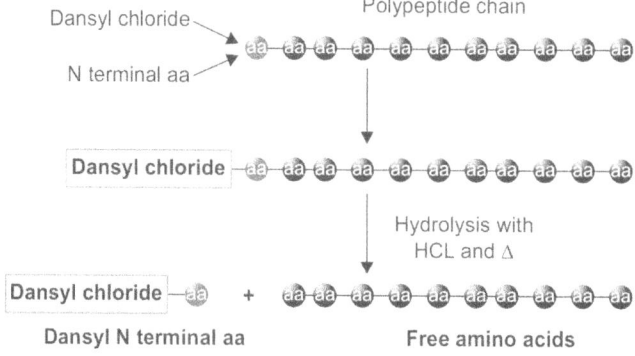

Fig. 4: Identification of number of polypeptides.

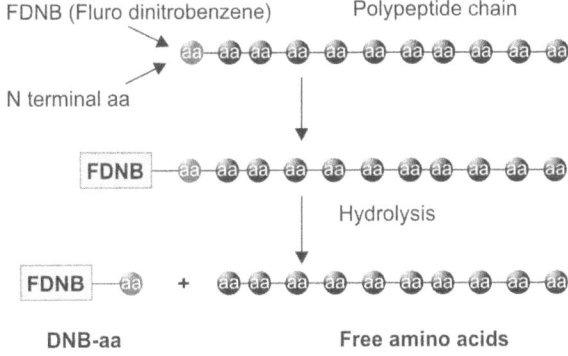

Fig. 5: Analysis of N-terminal amino acid with Sanger's reagent.

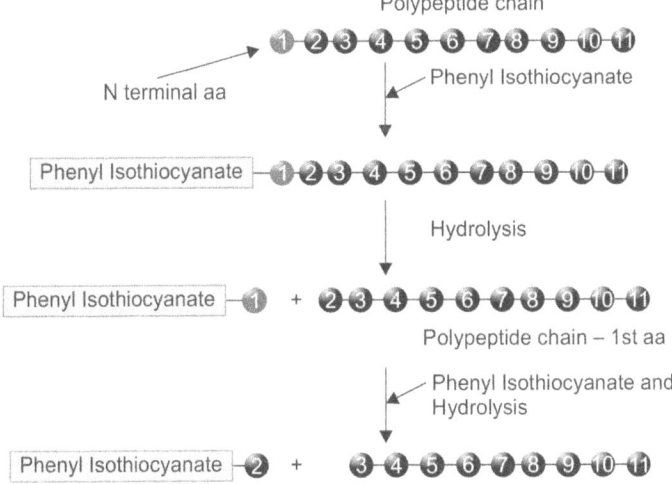

Fig. 6: Analysis of N-terminal amino acid with Edman reagent.

Determination of amino acid composition

- Hydrolysis of polypeptides or proteins into amino acids – by acid/alkali or enzymes- estimated quantitatively
- Pronase enzyme helps in complete hydrolysis
- Separation of mixture of amino acids - chromatography.

Reverse Sequencing Technique

- Sequencing the DNA – genetic material to find out the nucleotide sequence – by Frederick Sanger
- Translation of nucleotide sequence to form amino acid sequences
- Post translational modification – to form mature proteins.

4. Write how acid-base balances are maintained in the body. Mention causes and biochemical alteration of metabolic acidosis.

- Normal blood pH is between 7.38-7.42. (7.4)
- pH is the negative logarithm of hydrogen ion concentration
- As per Henderson-Hasselbalch equation, pH = pKa + log x [Base]/[Acid]

- If the concentration of base and acid are equal, pH = pKa.

Mechanisms of maintaining pH

- Buffers of body fluids – first line of defence
- Respiratory mechanism – second line of defence
- Renal mechanism – third line of defence.

Role of buffers in body fluids

Buffers resist changes in pH when small quantities of an acid or an alkali are added. Various buffers in blood are:

- **Bicarbonate buffer system**
- **Phosphate buffer system**
- **Protein buffer system.**

Bicarbonate buffer system: (Bicarbonate-Carbonic acid system) ($NaHCO_3/H_2CO_3$)

- It is the most important buffer in plasma and is formed by ($NaHCO_3/H_2CO_3$)
- It accounts for 40% in whole body and 65% in plasma
- The base HCO_3^- is the **metabolic component** and it is regulated by kidney and the carbonic acid (H_2CO_3) is called **respiratory component** since it is regulated by the lungs
- The **normal bicarbonate level** in plasma is 24 mmol/L
- The **normal pCO$_2$** of arterial blood is 40 mm of Hg
- The **normal carbonic acid concentration** in blood is 1.2 mmol/L
- Carbonic acid has a pKa of 6.1—so it is a poor buffer. But the high blood concentration and the ratio of base to salt is high (20:1), which makes it an effective buffer
- Under physiological conditions, with pH 7.4 the ratio of bicarbonate to carbonic acid is **20:1**
- When **strong acid such as HCl (H$^+$)** is added to the bicarbonate buffer
- $H^+ + HCO_3^- \rightarrow H_2CO_3 \rightarrow H_2O + CO_2$
- CO_2 stimulates respiratory center and it is excreted by lungs – respiratory compensation
- When **strong alkali like NaOH** is added to the bicarbonate buffer

- $NaOH + H_2CO_3 \rightarrow NaHCO_3 + H_2O$
- Level of H_2CO_3 decreases because it reacts with NaOH
- $H_2O + CO_2 \rightarrow H_2CO_3 \rightarrow H^+ + HCO_3^-$
- The rise in bicarbonate is compensated by increased excretion through kidney (renal compensation).

Phosphate buffer system: It is an intracellular buffer with low concentration in plasma.

- It is made of $NaHPO_4/NaH_2PO_4$. It has a pK_a of 6.8. It is an effective buffer system because its pKa value - 6.7 is nearer to physiological pH
- **The ratio of $HPO_4 : H_2PO_4 = 4:1$**
- In acidosis - $Na_2HPO_4 + H^+ \rightarrow NaH_2PO_4 \rightarrow$ excreted by the kidneys
- In alkalosis - $NaH_2PO_4 + NaOH \rightarrow Na_2HPO_4 + H^+ + H_2O$.

Protein buffer system

- Extracellular - (Na Protein/H protein)
  - Buffering capacity of proteins depend on the pKa value of ionisable side chains
  - The most effective buffer is imidazole group of **histidine** molecules with a pKa value of 6.1
  - Albumin contains 16 histidine residues and so albumin accounts for the non-bicarbonate buffer system
  - In acidosis $H^+ + Pr - HPr$
  - In alkalosis $HPr \rightarrow H^+ + Pr$.
- Intracellular – Hb buffer system (KHb/HHb) **(Fig. 7)**
  - Hb is the major blood buffer in RBCs and it acts along with bicarbonate system
  - It has 38 histidine residues
  - **In the lungs (Fig. 8):** OxyHb releases H$^+$ which is buffered by bicarbonate to form carbonic acid which is converted by carbonic anhydrase to CO_2 and water which get eliminated by ventilation.
  - **In the RBC:** CO_2 is converted to carbonic acid by carbonic anhydrase resulting in decrease in pH and the Hb becomes deoxy Hb

- DeoxyHb neutralizes carbonic acid to increase the pH and there will be increase in bicarbonate and decrease in pCO_2
- To maintain electroneutrality chloride ions enter into RBC for each bicarbonate leaves. This is called **chloride shift.**
- **In the tissue level (Fig. 9):** The oxyHb releases O_2 to the tissues which is facilitated by low pO_2, low pH and high pCO_2 and CO_2 produced is returned to the lungs, carried by Hb where CO_2 is eliminated in expired air

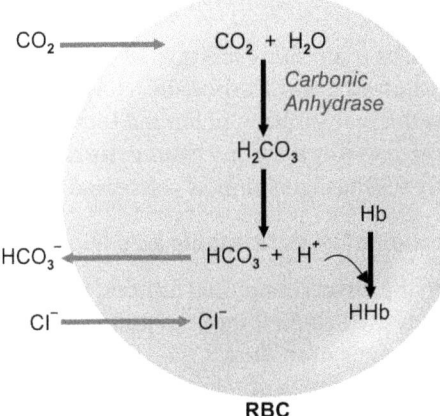

Fig. 7: Hemoglobin buffer system.

Role of respiratory system in acid base balance (second line of defence)

- When there is fall in pH (acidosis) the respiratory rate is stimulated resulting in hyperventilation. This would eliminate more CO_2 thereby lowering H_2CO_3
- In tissues pCO_2 is high and pH is low to the formation of acids by the cells like lactate and production of CO_2 by cells. CO_2 diffuses into RBC. It combines with water to form carbonic acid by carbonic anhydrase. And dissociates into H^+ and HCO_3^-. So RBC traps H^+ from the tissues. Some of the HCO_3^- diffuses out of the cell in exchange for chloride
- In the lungs H^+ combines with HCO_3^- to form H_2CO_3 which becomes H_2O and CO_2. This CO_2 is released into the lungs. So lungs reduce the acid load of H_2CO_3 by excretion of CO_2
- In metabolic acidosis lungs hyperventilate to excrete more acid. In metabolic alkalosis the reverse happens.

Renal Regulation of Acid Base Balance: (III Line of Defense)

- Kidneys regulate pH of extracellular fluid
- Normal urine has pH around 6. This pH is lower than that of ECF (7.4). This is called **acidification of urine.**

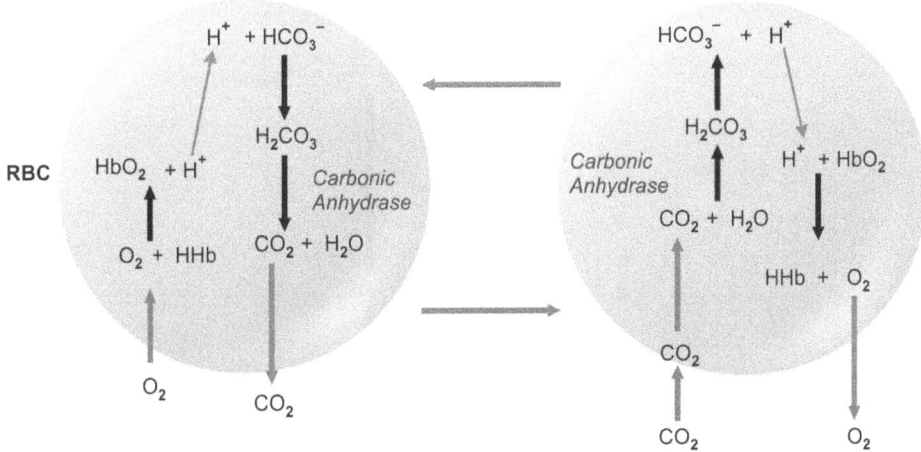

Fig. 8: Hemoglobin actions in lungs.   **Fig. 9:** Hemoglobin actions in tissues.

- The steps of this mechanism are:
  1. Excretion of H$^+$
  2. Reabsorption of bicarbonate
  3. Excretion of titratable acid
  4. Excretion of ammonia.

Excretion of H$^+$ (Fig. 10)

1. **Excretion of H$^+$** (generation of bicarbonate)-In proximal convoluted tubular cells, CO$_2$ combines with water to form carbonic acid using carbonic anhydrase.
   - Then it ionizes to H$^+$ and HCO$_3^-$ This H$^+$ is then secreted into the tubular lumen in exchange for Na$^+$

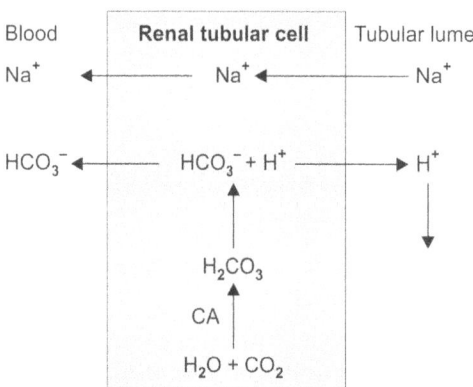

Fig. 10: Excretion of H$^+$.

- There is net excretion of hydrogen ions and net generation of bicarbonate. This increases the alkali reserve.

Reabsorption of HCO$_3^-$ (Fig. 11)

- Sodium bicarbonate in the lumen becomes sodium and bicarbonate
- Sodium is taken up by PCT cells in exchange of hydrogen ions. H$^+$ combines with HCO$_3^-$ in the tubular lumen to form carbonic acid, which forms CO$_2$ and water and both are diffused into the cell and converted back to carbonic acid
- In the cell, again it dissociates to H$^+$ and HCO$_3^-$. HCO$_3^-$ is taken into blood with sodium
- There is no net excretion of H$^+$ or generation of new bicarbonate. The net effect is the reabsorption of filtered bicarbonate mediated by sodium – hydrogen exchanger
- By this base reaction, is conserved.

Excretion of H$^+$ as titratable acid (Fig. 12)

- In the distal convoluted tubules, hydrogen ions are secreted into the tubular fluid in exchange of sodium
- This sodium is obtained from Na$_2$HPO$_4$ – disodium hydrogen phosphate which is a base

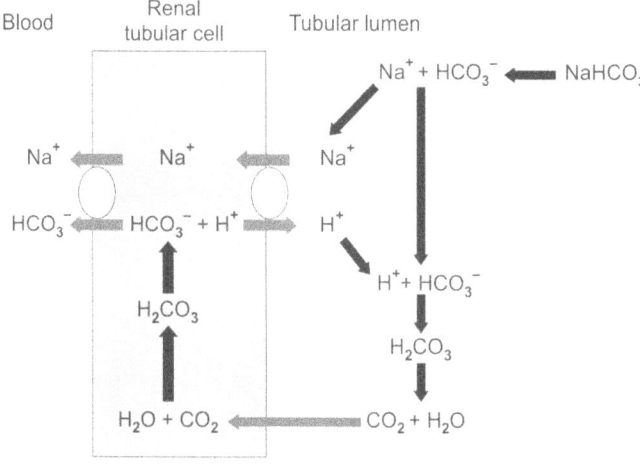

Fig. 11: Reabsorption of bicarbonate.

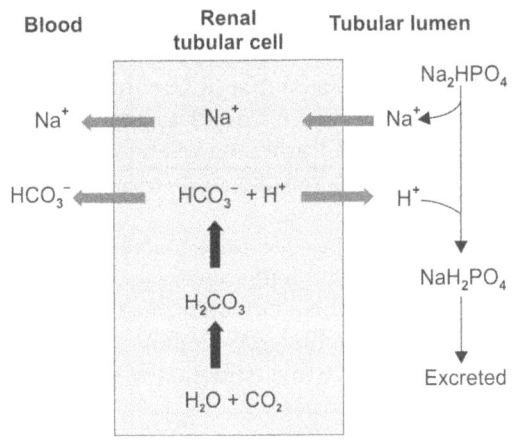

Fig. 12: Excretion of titratable acid as phosphate.

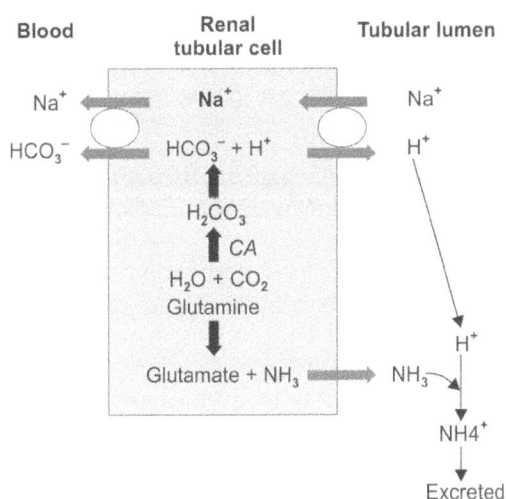

Fig. 13: Excretion of titratable acid as ammonium ions.

- Na_2HPO_4 combines with H^+ to form the acid NaH_2PO_4 which is the major form of titratable acid in urine
- Titratable acidity of urine refers to number of milliliters of N/10 NaOH required to titrate 1 litre of urine to pH 7.4. This is a measure of net acid excretion by kidney
- As the tubular fluid moves down the renal tubules, more H^+ ions are added causing more acidification of urine with fall in pH of urine up to pH 4.5
- The acid and basic phosphate pair is considered as urinary buffer.

Excretion of NH_4^+ (Fig. 13)

Occurs mostly at DCT. This helps to excrete H^+ and reabsorb HCO_3^-
- This is another mechanism to buffer H^+ ion into the tubular fluid
- H^+ ions combine with NH_3 to form ammonium ions (NH_4)
- The enzyme glutaminase deamidates glutamine in DCT becomes glutamate and ammonia
- This ammonia is secreted into the lumen which combines with hydrogen ions to become ammonium ions and get excreted in urine.

Disorders of Acid-base Balance

- **Acidosis:** Accumulation of acids and loss of bases causing fall of pH – 2 types.
  - **Metabolic acidosis:**
    - Primary change is decrease in plasma bicarbonate concentration which is compensated by ↓pCO_2 by hyperventilation
    - This occurs in diabetic ketoacidosis, lactic acidosis, renal failure, renal tubular acidosis, etc.
  - **Respiratory acidosis:**
    - Primary excess of carbonic acid with ↑pCO_2. This is compensated by increase in bicarbonate
    - This occurs in chronic obstructive airways diseases, asthma, emphysema, paralysis of respiratory muscles, respiratory depressant toxic drugs, etc.
- **Alkalosis:** Loss of acid or accumulation of bases causing increased pH – 2 types.
  - **Metabolic alkalosis:**
    - Primary change is excess of bicarbonate which is compensated by ↑pCO_2 by hypoventilation
    - This is seen in vomiting, hypokalemia, Cushing syndrome, diuretic therapy.
  - **Respiratory alkalosis:**
    - Primary change is deficit of pCO_2 (carbonic acid) which is compensated by decrease in bicarbonate

- This is seen in high altitude, hyperventilation, hysteria, septicemia, salicylate poisoning, etc.

Metabolic Acidosis

- Acidosis is reduction of pH less than 7.38. It is classified into metabolic and respiratory acidosis
- Metabolic acidosis is primarily due to base deficit. The bicarbonate deficit may occur due to excess acid production or depletion of bicarbonate
- **Anion gap:** It is difference between measured cations and measured anions. Usually it shows the unmeasured anions. **The normal value is 12 mmol/L**
- Anion gap is calculated as the difference between ($Na^+ + K^+$) and ($HCO_3^- + Cl^-$)
- Decreased anion gap is seen in hypoalbuminemia, multiple myeloma.

Metabolic Acidosis is Classified into

- **High anion gap metabolic acidosis (HAGMA)** accumulation of acid anions
  - Due to accumulation of acid anions - value between 15 and 20
  - **Causes:**
    - Renal failure-H^+ excretion is less.
    - Diabetic ketoacidosis - ketoacid production is more acetoacetate and beta hydroxybutyrate
    - Lactic acidosis- Hypoxia, circulatory failure, many drugs, and bacterial metabolism increase lactic acid. Methanol, ethanol also cause lactic acidosis.
- **Normal anion gap metabolic acidosis- (NAGMA)**
  - Loss of both anions and cations, the anion gap is normal, but acidosis may prevail
- **Causes:**
  - Diarrhea-loss of bicarbonate and cations – Na or K or both from intestinal secretions
  - Hyperchloremic metabolic acidosis in renal tubular acidosis, acetazolamide therapy and ureteric transplantation into large gut

- **Metabolic acidosis is compensated by**
  - Respiratory compensation—hyperventilation so that pCO_2 comes down. There will be Kussmaul respiration, low pH, bicarbonate will be low. pCO_2 starts decreasing due to respiratory compensation
  - Renal compensation—increased excretion of acid and conservation of base occurs. This sets within 2 to 4 days
  - Associated hyperkalemia is seen commonly due to distribution of K^+ and H^+.
- **Clinical features:**
  - Hyperventilation
  - Kussmaul respiration
  - Depressed myocardial contractility.
- **Treatment:**
  - To stop production of acid by giving IV fluids and insulin
  - Oxygen to be given to patients with lactic acidosis
  - Potassium level to be monitored
  - Required bicarbonate amount to be calculated from the base deficit
  - mEq of base needed = Body weight in Kg x 0.2 – base excess in mEq/L.

II. WRITE SHORT NOTES

1. Biochemical function of vitamin D.

Cholecalciferol or vitamin D is a derivative of cholesterol and the ultimate precursor for cholecalciferol is 7-dehydrocholesterol (7-DHC) in animals. Ergocalciferol is the precursor form of vitamin D in plants- vitamin D2.

Biosynthesis of active Vitamin D

$$7\text{-Dehydrocholesterol} \xrightarrow{\text{Light}} \text{Provitamin D}$$

$$\xrightarrow{\text{Thermal isomerization}} \text{Cholecalciferol}$$

1. 7-DHC is rich in malpighian layer of epidermis. The bond between 9 and 10 of 7-DHC is cleaved and converted into cholecalciferol by the action of UV light. That is why this is called as sunshine vitamin

2. Vitamin D is a prohormone. Activation of provitamin D (cholecalciferol) into active vitamin D (calcitriol) takes place at two different sites.

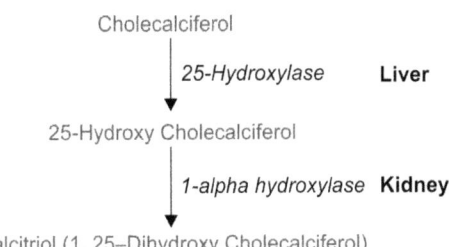

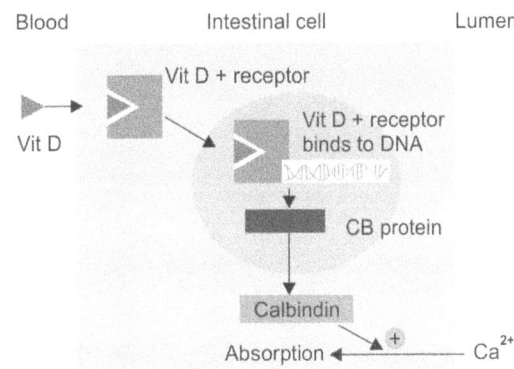

Fig. 14: Absorption of calcium by calcitriol.

- **25 hydroxylation of cholecalciferol in liver:** Cholecalciferol through blood reaches the liver cells and undergoes hydroxylation at 25th carbon. This reaction is catalysed by 25-hydroxylase to form 25 hydroxy cholecalciferol
- **In plasma** – 25 HCC is bound to vitamin D binding protein
- **1 hydroxylation in kidney:** The active form of vitamin D is synthesized at kidney. 25 hydroxy cholecalciferol is hydroxylated at 1st position and converted into 1, 25 dihydroxycholecalciferol/calcitriol. It is the **active form of vitamin D.**

Biochemical Functions of Calcitriol

The active form of vitamin D is calcitriol which is 1,25 dihydroxy cholecalciferol.

Calcitriol acts as steroid hormone. It binds to specific cytoplasmic receptors which interacts with DNA and induces the synthesis of mRNA for specific proteins called calbindin which is a calcium binding protein which will lead to biological actions.

- **Effect on intestine:** Calcitriol induces the synthesis of calbindin and helps in the absorption of calcium and phosphorus from the intestines **(Fig. 14)**
- **Effects on kidney:** Calcitriol increases the reabsorption of calcium and phosphorous from the renal tubules thereby conserving both the minerals
- **Action on bones:** Calcitriol increases the activity of osteoblasts and hence mineralization of bones is increased. It remodels the activity of osteoclasts and osteoblasts. It prevents rickets and osteomalacia.

2. **Absorption of lipids (TAG): (Bergstrom theory) (Fig. 15).**

- Digestory products of lipids such as 2 monoacyl glycerol, long chain fatty acids, cholesterol and phospholipid are incorporated to form mixed micelle with the help of bile salts. Micelles are spherical particles with hydrophilic exterior and hydrophobic interior
- Micelles are aligned at the micro villous surface of jejunal mucosa and they diffuse passively into the mucosal cells
- Bile salts are reabsorbed from ileum and returned to liver for re-excretion— enterohepatic circulation
- Inside the mucosal cells-long chain fatty acids are re-esterified to form TAG.

Formation of Chylomicrons

- TAG, cholesterol ester and phospholipid molecules along with apo B 48 and apo A are incorporated into chylomicrons and transported through lacteals to enter into lymphatic circulation via thoracic duct
- Chylomicrons transported through lacteals into the thoracic duct and then into lymph circulation.

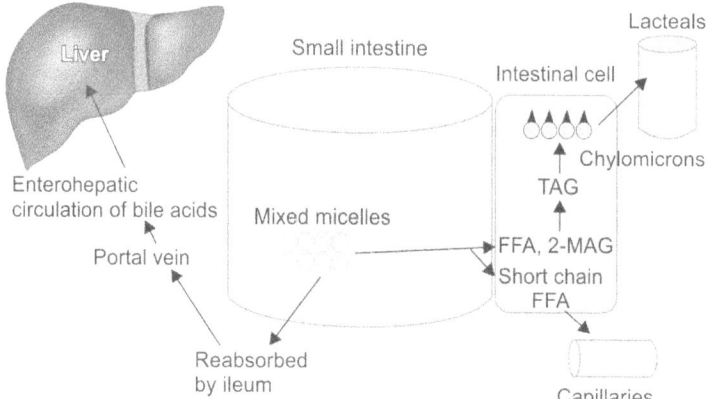

Fig. 15: Absorption of TAG.

3. Excretion of bilirubin and clinical importance of bilirubin estimations.

- End products of heme metabolism are bile pigments – bilirubin and biliverdin
- From Hb, globin chains are separated and hydrolysed and the amino acids are channelled into the amino acid pool
- The iron is re-utilized **(Fig. 16)**
- **About 6 g of Hb is broken down per day, from which about 250 mg of bilirubin is formed**
- Normal **plasma free bilirubin level is** -0.2 to 0.7 mg/dL
- Normal **plasma conjugated bilirubin level is** -0.1 to 0.4 mg/dL.

Transport of Bilirubin to Liver (Fig. 17)

- Bilirubin formed is insoluble and toxic and it is in unconjugated form. It is transported in plasma bound to albumin. 1 molecule of albumin can bind with 2 molecules of bilirubin
- **Uptake of bilirubin by liver parenchymal cells:** Done by carrier mediated active process. In liver cells bilirubin is bound to an intracellular protein called **ligandin.** This binding is inhibited by taking aspirin or penicillin and this will produce kernicterus in new born babies
- **Conjugation of bilirubin:** Unconjugated toxic bilirubin is conjugated with UDP

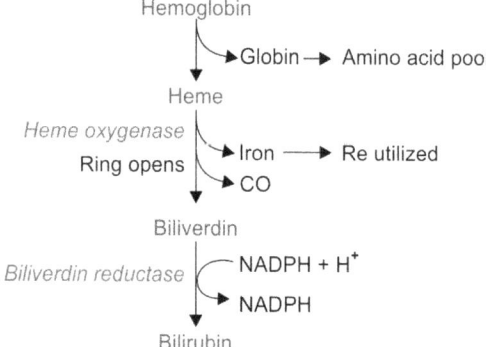

Fig. 16: Synthesis of bilirubin.

glucuronic acid by UDP glucuronyl transferase enzyme. Bilirubin monoglucuronide is formed first (20%) which is then converted to diglucuronate (80%). This conjugation process is interfered by drugs like primaquine, novobiocin and pregnenolone, etc.

- **Excretion of bilirubin to bile**: This is done by an active process against a concentration gradient. This is **the rate limiting step** for the entire process. This excretion is mediated by multispecific organic anion transporter
- **Fate of conjugated bilirubin in intestine**
- After the secretion of conjugated bilirubin into bile, it passes through hepatic and common bile duct into the intestinal lumen

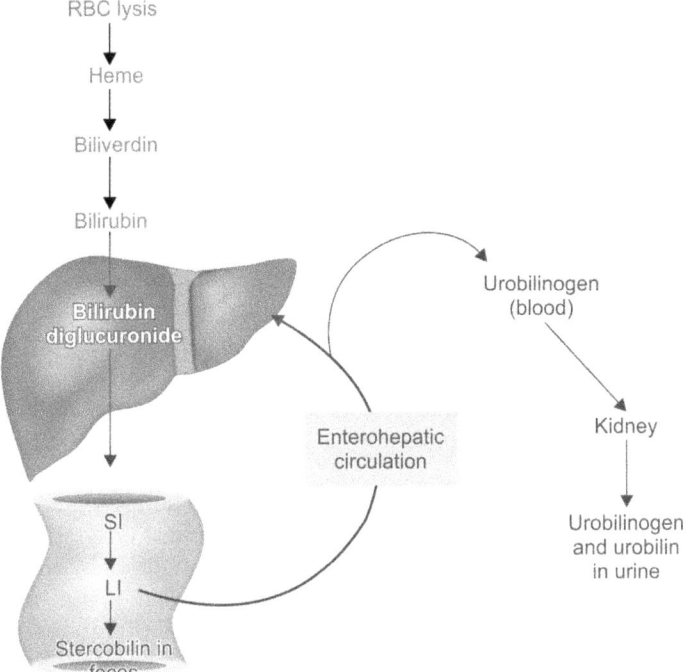

Fig. 17: Synthesis and excretion of bilirubin.

- In the intestine, the conjugated bilirubin is hydrolysed by the bacterial beta glucuronidase to get converted to unconjugated bilirubin
- Free bilirubin thus formed is reduced further into colorless tetrapyrrole urobilinogen, which is oxidized to an orange yellow pigment urobilin
- Rest of urobilinogen is reduced to stercobilinogen which is oxidized to a brown pigment called stercobilin, which is excreted in feces (250 to 300 mg/day)
- A part of urobilinogen (20%) enters into enterohepatic circulation to get re-excreted at the liver by portal circulation
- A small amount of urobilinogen is excreted through the urine (less than 4 mg/day)
- Finally both UBG and SBG are oxidized to urobilin and stercobilin by atmospheric O_2. Both these are present in urine as well as feces.

Bilirubin Estimation

- **Van den Bergh test:** Serum bilirubin is estimated by Van den Bergh test. Normal serum does not give positive Van den Bergh reaction.
  Principle: Diazotized sulfanilic acid reacts with bilirubin to form a purple color complex called as azobilirubin.

Reagents
- Sulfanilic acid in HCL
- Sodium nitrate
- **Types of Van den Bergh reaction and their significance.**
  - **Indirect van den Bergh test:** Unconjugated bilirubin in blood gives positive test. This test helps in diagnosing pre-hepatic and hepatic jaundice
  - **Direct van den Bergh test:** Conjugated bilirubin present in the blood give immediate positive test. This test helps in detection of post hepatic jaundice
  - **Biphasic test:** When both conjugated and unconjugated bilirubin present in higher amount in the sample, a purple color produced immediate and the color is intensified on adding alcohol. This is specific for hepatocellular jaundice.

4. Coupling of oxidative phosphorylation, uncouplers and their importance.

- Coupling of oxidation with phosphorylation is known as oxidative phosphorylation. Oxidative phosphorylation is explained by chemiosmotic theory by Peter Mitchell
- **Oxidative phosphorylation is comprised of the following processes**
  - Oxidation of reducing equivalents (NADH and $FADH_2$) **(Fig. 18)**
  - Electron transfer through 3 protein assemblies (complex I, III, and IV)
  - Transport of H^+ into intermembrane space
  - Transport of H^+ into the mitochondrial matrix
  - Synthesis of ATP by complex 5.
- The transport of protons from inside to outside of inner mitochondrial membrane is accompanied by generation of proton gradient across the membrane
- Protons (H^+ ions) accumulate outside the membrane to create an electrochemical potential difference and this force drives the synthesis of ATP by ATP synthase (V) complex
- There is also the creation of pH gradient on either side of membrane.

Complex V – ATP Synthase (Figs. 19 and 20)

- It is a proton assembly in the inner mitochondrial membrane
  It has 2 functional subunits – F_1 and F_0 and looks like a lollipop. F_0 is embedded in the membrane and water insoluble. Both F_0 and F_1 are connected by a protein stalk. Protons enter through F_0 subunit and it acts as a proton channel. F_1 unit projects into the matrix and catalyses ATP synthesis
- As per Boyer's hypothesis there will be a conformational change in the mitochondrial membrane proteins which leads to ATP synthesis. This is considered as rotary motor or energy driving model or binding change model
- ATP synthase enzyme has a central gamma unit surrounded by alternating α3 and β3 subunits. Due to the proton flux γ subunit rotates and that induces conformational changes in the β3 subunits which releases ATP. One β subunit has open (O) conformation, the second has loose (L) conformation and the third has tight (T) conformation
- Protons induce the rotation of γ subunit which in turn induces conformation changes in β subunits. ADP and Pi bind to β subunits in L conformation to form

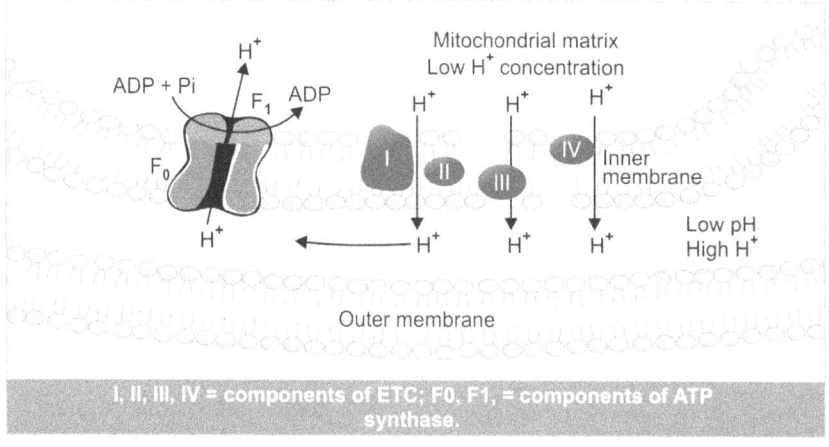

Fig. 18: Components of METC.

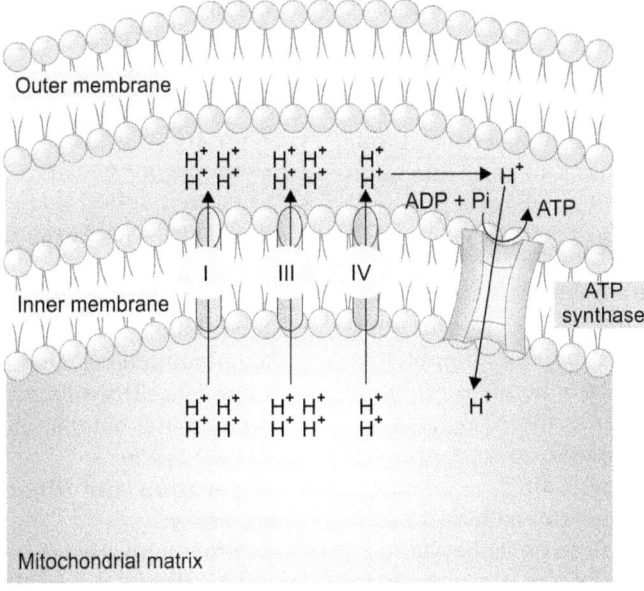

Fig. 19: Synthesis of ATP.

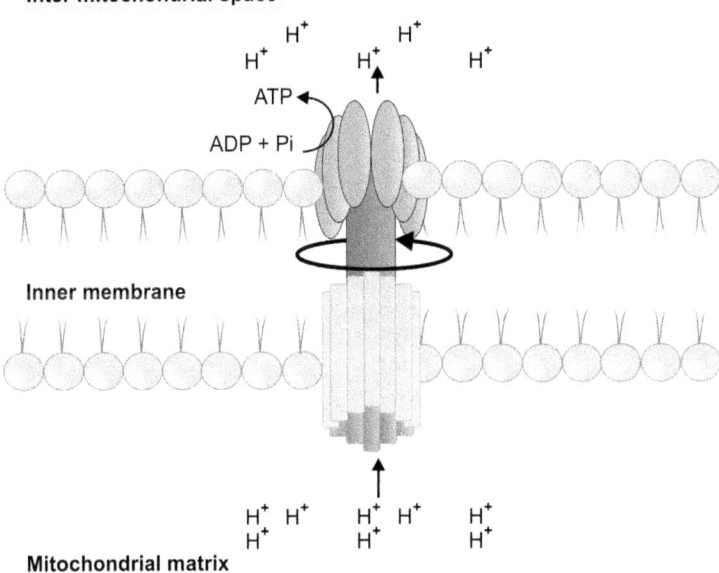

Fig. 20: ATP synthase enzyme.

ATP by changing site to L conformation and then T to O conformation and 3 ATP are generated for each revolution. So ATP synthase is considered as world's smallest molecular motor.

REGULATION OF ATP SYNTHESIS

- Availability of ADP—respiratory or acceptor control
- Source of NADH and FADH2 from TCA cycle.

Inhibitors of Oxidative Phosphorylation
- Atractyloside – inhibits translocase
- Oligomycin – inhibits flow of protons through Fo
- Ionophores, e.g. valinomycin – mobile ion carriers – allows K to permeate mitochondria; gramicidin – channel former.

Uncouplers of Oxidative Phosphorylation
- Uncouplers are amphipathic and increase the permeability of the lipoid inner mitochondrial membrane to protons, thus reducing the electrochemical potential and short-circuiting the ATP synthase. Therefore the oxidation can proceed without phosphorylation
- **Uncouplers** dissociate oxidation in the respiratory chain from phosphorylation
- These compounds are toxic in vivo, causing respiration to become uncontrolled, since the rate is no longer limited by the concentration of ADP or P_i. Example **2,4-dinitrophenol**
- **Atractyloside** inhibits oxidative phosphorylation by inhibiting the transporter of ADP into and ATP out of the mitochondrion
- The antibiotic **oligomycin** completely blocks oxidation and phosphorylation by blocking the flow of protons through ATP synthase
- **Thermogenin (or the uncoupling protein)** is a physiological uncoupler found in brown adipose tissue that functions to generate body heat, particularly for the newborn and during hibernation in animals.

Significance of Uncoupling
The cold habitat animals contain brown adipose tissue, which is rich in electron carriers and they are specialized to carry out an oxidation uncoupled form phosphorylation. This is essential to control body temperature.

---

5. Clinical importance of isoenzymes with suitable example.

- Multiple molecular forms of an enzyme catalyzing the same reaction are isoenzymes or isozymes, e.g. lactate dehydrogenase-5 isoenzymes (LDH 1, 2, 3, 4 and 5), creatine kinase-3 isoenzymes (CK-1, 2, 3) and alkaline phosphatase
- They are physically distinct forms of the same enzyme activity
- They are synthesised from various tissues and hence useful to study the disorders of those organs
- They are made up of different subunits. If the subunits are the same they are known as homomultimer. They are represented by same gene. If the subunits are different they are known as heteromultimer produced by different gene
- **Separation and identification of isoenzymes:**
  - **Electrophoresis:** Depends upon the mobility in electrical field
  - **Heat stability:** Some gets denatured by heat, e.g. bone isoenzyme of ALP
  - **Inhibitors:** Tartrate labile ACP
  - **Substrate specificity or K_m value:** Different for each isoenzyme, e.g. glucokinase and hexokinase
  - **Localization:** LDH-H4 form is present in heart; LDH-M4 – skeletal muscle.

Lactate Dehydrogenase
- Low density lipoprotein (LDL) catalyses the conversion of pyruvate to lactate and vice versa. LDL is concentrated in RBC cell; therefore minor hemolysis causes the false value. Normal values ranges from 100-200 U/L
- Elevation of LDH is seen in hemolytic anemia, hepatocellular damage, muscular dystrophy, cancer, etc.
- LDH is tetramer made up of two H (heart) bands and two M (muscle) bands. Both of these are same molecular weight and with minor amino acid variations
- There are 5 isoenzymes. They are LDH1, LDH2, LDH3, LDH4, and LDH5
- With two different polypeptide chains therefore 5 combinations of H and M are possible, namely H4, H3M, H2M2, M3H, M4. The tissue specificity and diagnostic importance of these 5 isoenzymes is as follows:

- H4 form found in heart, which is useful for diagnosing heart disease
- M4 form found in muscle, hence it is useful in diagnosing muscle diseases.
- Isoenzymes of LDH help in the diagnosis of heart and liver diseases
- Flipped pattern is observed in myocardial infarction (LDH-1 > LDH-2)
- Increased activity of LDH-5 is an indicator of liver diseases.

Creatine Kinase (CK)
- It catalysis the synthesis of creatine phosphate from creatine and ATP
- Normal blood ranges from 15-100 IU/L
- It is made up of 2 polypeptides namely M and B. Therefore 3 combinations of isoenzymes are possible. They are MM found in skeletal muscle, MB found in heart and BB found in brain
- CK subform is highly elevated in muscular dystrophies, acute cerebrovascular injuries. It is most reliable factor in diagnosing AMI
- Three isoenzymes - CK BB (1), CK MB (2), CK MM (3)
  1. CK BB (1) – present in brain
  2. CK MB (2) is the earliest reliable marker of myocardial infarction
  3. CK MM (3) is elevated in muscle diseases.

Alkaline Phosphatase (ALP)
- It is nonspecific enzyme which hydrolyses aliphatic, aromatic and heterocyclic compounds at pH 9-10 in the presence of Mn and Mg. Zinc is a constituent ion of ALP
- ALP produced by osteoblasts for the calcification process
- Normal serum levels are 40-125 u/L. Moderate increase seen in hepatic diseases, and very high levels are seen in extrahepatic obstruction or intrahepatic obstructions, and very high levels are seen in bone diseases
- ALP has nearly 6 types of iso-enzymes: Alpha-1 ALP, Alpha-2 heat labile ALP, Alpha-2 heat stable ALP, pre-beta ALP, Gamma- ALP, leucocyte ALP (LAP)
  - They are due to the difference in the carbohydrate content
- Alpha 1 ALP: It is about 10% total ALP, and is increased in obstructive jaundice
- Alpha 2 ALP: It is about 20% of total ALP – increased in hepatitis
- Alpha 2 heat stable ALP: It is about 1% of total ALP. It is heat stable above 65°C
- Pre beta ALP: It is about 50% of total ALP. It is elevated in bone diseases
- Gamma ALP: It is about 10%, it is increased in ulcerative colitis
- Leucocyte ALP (LAP) it is increased in lymphomas and decreased in chronic myeloid leukemia.

Acid Phosphatase (ACP)
- It acts at a pH between 4 and 6
- Normal value in serum is 2.5 to 12 U/L
- Secreted by prostate cells, RBCs, WBCs and platelets
- The value of ACP is increased in prostate cancer and it is an important tumor marker for prostate cancer
- It has got a tartrate labile isoenzyme which is helpful in follow up of prostate cancer. Its normal level is 1 U/L.

6. **Biochemical changes in von Gierke's disease and their relation to enzyme deficiency.**

- It is also called as glycogen storage disease type I and it is most common type
- Incidence: 1 in 100,000 births
- **Cause**: Glucose-6-phosphatase (G6P) enzyme is deficient which converts Glucose-6-phosphatase to glucose.
  - Glucose-6-phosphatase $\xrightarrow{\text{Glucose-6-phosphatase}}$ Glucose

Clinical Features
- As the glucose cannot be released from liver during overnight fasting it leads to **hypoglycemia**
- G6P may be diverted to glycogen synthesis. Therefore, the accumulation of large amount of glycogen in liver leads to **enlargement of liver and cirrhosis**. Due to this children my die in early age

- The excess G6P is then diverted to HMP shunt with increasing production of pentoses and nucleotides. Nucleotides are converted to uric acid, which is characterized as **hyperuricemia**
- Other symptoms include, hyperlipidemia, lactic acidosis and ketosis
- Early death in childhood.

Treatment

- Symptomatic treatment
- Gene therapy and genetic counseling.

7. Role of LDL receptors in metabolism of LDL and the disease caused by its defect.

LDL Metabolism (Fig. 21)

- LDL transports cholesterol from liver to peripheral tissues
- It has only ApoB100.

Production of LDL

- Most of the LDL is derived from VLDL but a small part is directly released from the liver
- LDL is taken by peripheral tissues and by hepatocytes by **receptor mediated** endocytosis. This is a regulated mechanism
- LDL is also removed by an unregulated independent mechanism by scavenger receptors by forming foam cells. This mechanism is active when blood cholesterol level is very high.

Structure of LDL Receptor (Fig. 22)

LDL receptor also called "apoB, E" receptor, since it is specific for ApoB100 and E. It looks like pits and occurs on the cell surface of all cells especially hepatocytes. These pits are coated with a protein called clathrin on the cytosolic side of the cell membrane. The glycoprotein receptor spans the membrane, the B-100 binding region being at the exposed amino terminal end.

Metabolic fate of LDL: LDL cholesterol after binding to LDL receptors is taken up by endocytosis. The apoprotein and cholesteryl ester are then hydrolysed in the lysosomes, and cholesterol is translocated into the cell. The receptors are recycled to the cell surface. This influx of cholesterol inhibits in a coordinated manner HMG-CoA synthase, HMG-CoA reductase, and, therefore, cholesterol synthesis. It stimulates

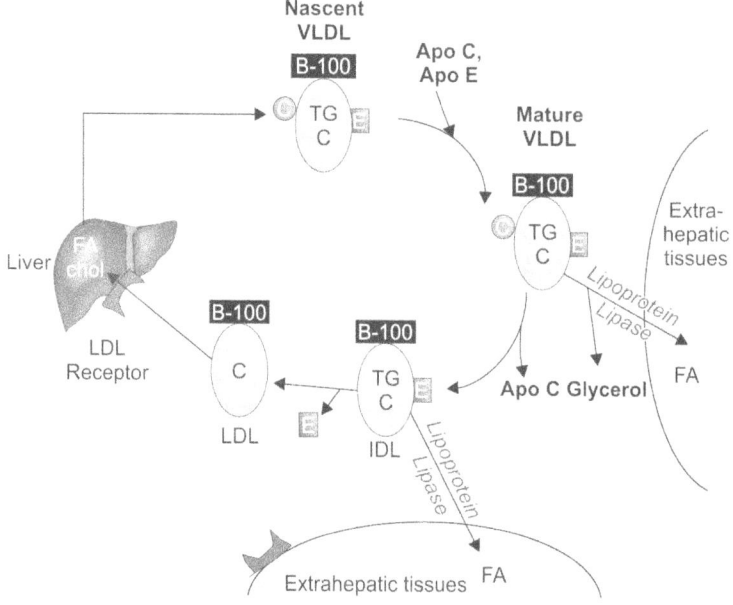

Fig. 21: LDL metabolism.

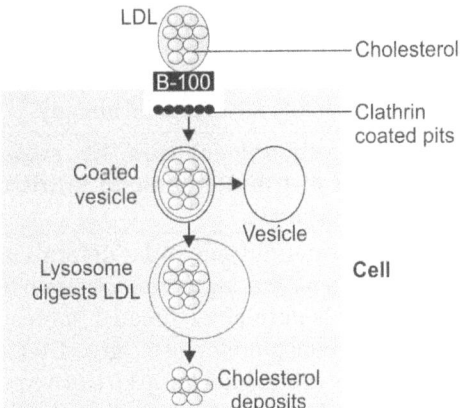

Fig. 22: LDL receptor.

ACAT activity; and down-regulates synthesis of the LDL receptor. Thus, the number of LDL receptors on the cell surface is regulated by the cholesterol requirement for membranes, steroid hormones, or bile acid synthesis.

Clinical Significance

- If LDL concentration is increased it will lead to higher incidence of atherosclerosis
- A fraction of cholesterol is taken by macrophages
- LDL infiltrates through arterial walls and the cholesterol gets deposited in the arterial walls and foam cells are formed by oxidation of LDL
- Atheromatous plaques are formed from the foam cells deposited on the walls causing increased thrombosis and coronary artery diseases
- Because of this complications, LDL cholesterol is known as **'bad cholesterol'**
- Insulin and thyroxine increase the binding of LDL to liver cells. This is the cause for hypercholesterolemia in diabetes and hypothyroidism.
- **Disorder:**

Familial hyper-cholesterolemia type IIa	Defective LDL receptors or mutation in ligand region of ApoB-100	Elevated LDL levels and hyper-cholesterolemia, resulting in atherosclerosis and coronary disease

8. Definition expression and significance of K_m value.

K_m Michaelis-Menten constant

- K_m is the substrate concentration at which v_i is half the maximal velocity ($V_{max}/2$) attainable at a particular concentration of enzyme. K_m thus has the dimensions of substrate concentration
- According to Michaelis theory, the formation of enzyme substrate complex is a reversible while the breakdown of complex to enzyme and product is irreversible

$$V_1 = \frac{V_{max}[S]}{K_m + [S]}$$

- The Michaelis-Menten equation illustrates in mathematical relationship between initial reaction velocity v_i and substrate concentration [S]
- $V_1 = V_{max}[S]/K_m + [S]$ where, V_1 = initial velocity, [S] = molar substrate concentration, K_m = Michaelis-Menten constant
- It denotes the affinity of enzyme for substrate. The lesser the value of K_m, the affinity of the enzyme for the substrate is more K_m value is substrate concentration at half maximal velocity - means 50% of enzyme molecules are bound with substrate molecules at that particular substrate concentration
- K_m is independent of enzyme concentration. If enzyme concentration is double, the V_{max} will be double, but ½ V_{max} will remain same. In other words irrespective of enzyme concentration, 50% molecules are bound to substrate at that particular substrate concentration
- K_m is the signature of enzymes and characteristic feature of a particular enzyme for a specific substrate
- K_m is a constant. K_m denotes the affinity of enzyme for substrate and it is inversely related to the dissociation constant.

9. Role of liver in integration of metabolism during postprandial state.

- Dietary nutrients are processed and distributed in liver as the venous drainage of gut and pancreas passes through hepatic portal vein before entering into general circulation
- After a meal, the liver is filled with absorbed nutrients like carbohydrates, lipids and amino acids. These nutrients are then metabolised in liver, stored or directed to other tissues. Insulin secreted from pancreas in excess also enters the liver.

Carbohydrate Metabolism

- Increased phosphorylation of glucose—by glucokinase to glucose 6 P
- Increased glycogenesis: Glucose 6 P is converted to glycogen by activation of glycogen synthase
- Increased activity of HMP pathway: Stimulated by NADPH
- Increased Glycolysis: Glucose is converted to pyruvate by increasing the activity of regulated enzymes – glucokinase, PFK-1, and pyruvate kinase. Pyruvate is converted to acetyl CoA which may be used as a substrate for fatty acid synthesis or it is oxidized to produce energy in TCA cycle
- Decreased production of glucose by decreasing gluconeogenesis and glycogenolysis.

Fat Metabolism

- **Increased fatty acid synthesis:** Denovo synthesis of fatty acids occur in liver in absorptive period from the increased production of acetyl CoA and NADPH
- **Increased triacylglycerol synthesis:** From fatty acyl CoA available from de novo synthesis from acetyl CoA and from the hydrolysis of TAG component of chylomicron remnant.

Amino Acid Metabolism

- **Increased amino acid degradation:** The excess amino acids are not stored but are released into blood and taken to other tissues to use in protein synthesis
- Increased protein synthesis to replace any proteins which are degraded already.

10. Caloric requirement and its recommended distribution among nutrients in an adult male.

- Energy expenditure can be determined directly by measuring heat output from the body but is normally estimated indirectly from the consumption of oxygen. There is an energy expenditure of 20 kJ/L of oxygen consumed regardless of whether the fuel being metabolized is carbohydrate, fat, or protein
- **Calorific value** of nutrients (Table 1) (energy density) is measured by using bomb calorimeter. More energy is produced from fat

Table 1: Calorific value of nutrients.

	Energy (KJ/g)	O_2 Consumed (L/g)	CO_2 produced (L/g)	RQ
Carbohydrate	16	0.8	0.8	1
Protein	17	0.9	0.8	0.8
Fat	37	2	1.4	0.7

- **Respiratory quotient (RQ):** It is the measurement of the ratio of the volume of carbon dioxide produced in L/g to volume of oxygen consumed in L/g. Respiratory quotient is an indication of the mixture of metabolic fuels being oxidized.
- **Energy requirement is calculated by the energy required for**
  - Maintenance for basal metabolic rate (BMR)
  - Specific dynamic action (SDA)
  - Extra energy expenditure for physical activity
- **Basal metabolic rate (BMR):** It is the energy needed for a person who is awake but is in a state of physical and mental rest. It is the minimum amount of energy required to perform vital functions such as circulation, respiration, working of heart, etc.

Normal value:
- **Men:** 34-37 k cal/m^2/hr

- **Women:** 30-35 k cal/m²/hr
  It is therefore possible to calculate an individual's energy requirement from body weight, age, gender, and level of physical activity.
- **Specific dynamic action:**
  - It is represented as thermogenic effect of food. The heat is produced after intake of food, which is due to energy expenditure for digestion and absorption of food form reserved energy (diet induced thermogenesis)
  - SDA can be considered as the activation of energy needed for various chemical reactions. This activation energy is varied to different food
    Example: For carbohydrate—5%, for proteins—30% and for fat—15%, etc.
- **Physical activity:**
  - Energy requirement of an individual depends upon—occupation, physical activity and lifestyle which can be divided into 3 groups—sedentary, moderate and heavy
  - Heavy workers need high BMR.

11. List various DNA repair mechanisms and give their biomedical importance.

- Synthesis of DNA is known as replication
- The process of replication occurs with high fidelity. Proofreading is done after replication to correct mistakes in arrangement of bases and base pairs
- Inspite of all these things alterations in base arrangements may occur due to various physical and chemical agents causing damage in DNA which can be corrected by the following mechanisms:
  - Mismatch repair
  - Nucleotide excision repair (NER)
  - Base excision repair
  - Double strand break.

Mismatch repair (Fig. 23)

- This may occur due to copying error
- During replication one to few bases may be unpaired in a DNA strand causing mismatch

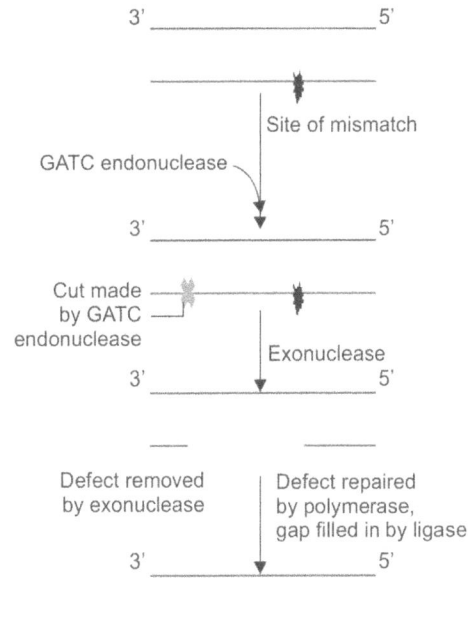

Fig. 23: Mismatch repair.

- Mut proteins identify the mismatched nucleotides based on the degree of methylation
- GATC sequences which are present 1/1000 nucleotides approximately are methylated on the adenine residue on the parent strand (not on the newly synthesized strand)
- GATC endonuclease cuts the strand bearing the mismatch and the mismatched nucleotide(s) is/are removed by an exonuclease
- The gap left is then filled in by DNA polymerase enzyme and the ends are joined to the 5'phosphate of the remaining original strand by DNA ligase enzyme.

Base excision repair (Fig. 24)

- **Depurination of DNA,** which happens spontaneously owing to the thermal lability of the purine N glycosidic bond, occurs at a rate of 5000–10,000/cell/d at 37 °C causing base alterations. Spontaneous deamination of cytosine to uracil may occur or by alkylating or deaminating compounds which will be repaired by this process

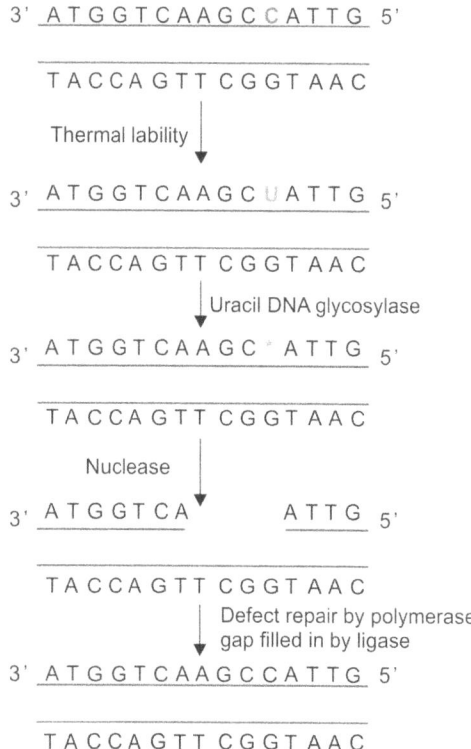

Fig. 24: Base excision repair.

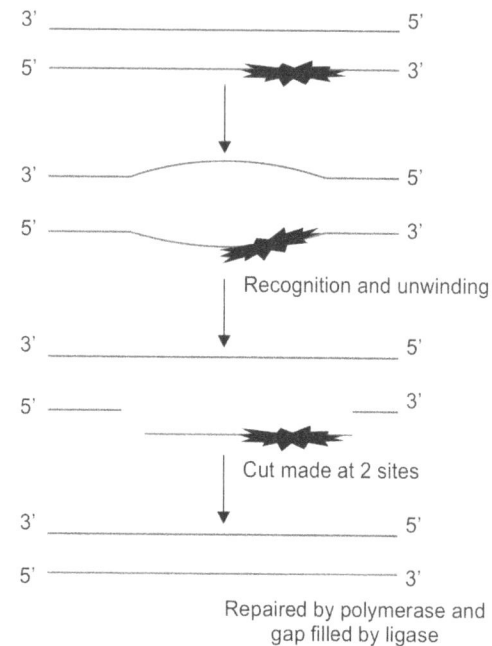

Fig. 25: Nucleotide excision repair.

- **Specific glycosylases** can recognize these abnormal bases and remove the base from the deoxyribose phosphate backbone of DNA. This will produce an apyrimidinic or apurinic site as per the base removed
- **Specific endonucleases** do the excision and a lyase enzyme removes it. The gap is then filled in by DNA polymerase and ligase enzymes.

Nucleotide excision repair (for thymine-thymine dimer) (Fig. 25)

- This mechanism is used to repair and replace regions of damaged DNA up to 30 bases in length due to damage by ultraviolet (UV) light causing joining of adjacent pyrimidines usually thymines producing dimers
- A special UV specific endonuclease (Uvr ABC excinuclease), recognizes the dimer and cleaves the damaged strand on either side of the dimer releasing a short oligonucleotide leaving a gap
- This gap is then filled in by normal cellular enzymes like DNA polymerase and ligase.

dsDNA repair (Fig. 26)

- Double-strand breaks can occur in DNA as a result of ionizing radiation or oxidative free radical generation. Some chemotherapeutic agents can destroy cells by causing double-strand breaks or preventing their repair
- DNA PK (protein kinase) has one binding site for the free ends of the DNA and another for dsDNA just inside these ends. It therefore allows for the approximation of these two separated ends
- The unwound, approximated DNA forms base pairs
- The extra nucleotide tails are removed by an exonuclease; and the gaps are filled and closed by DNA ligase.

BIOMEDICAL IMPORTANCE

Xeroderma pigmentosum (XP)

- It is an autosomal recessive condition in which there is defect in nucleotide excision repair mechanism

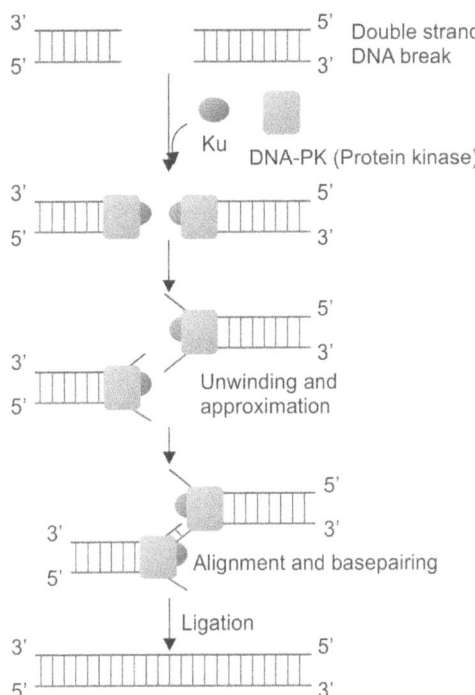

Fig. 26: dsDNA break repair.

- Pyrimidine dimers are formed in the skin cells which are exposed to UV light. The patient becomes highly sensitive to UV rays. Sunlight causes blisters in the skin
- Because of the defective repair system, the cells cannot repair the damaged DNA resulting in skin cancer. Death occurs in second decade due to skin cancer
- This is also caused by defects in the genes coding for any of the XP proteins required for the repair.

Ataxia telengiectasia:
- Autosomal recessive disease due to mutated ATM gene
- It is associated with DNA repair mechanisms
- Caused due to UV sensitivity
- Associated with cerebellar ataxia, telengiectasia in eyes, lymphoreticular neoplasms. It is present in 1:40000 persons.

Other diseases of defective DNA repair are Fanconi's anemia, Bloom's syndrome, Lynch syndrome, Cockayne syndrome and hereditary polyposis, colon cancer.

12. Enzyme defects and biochemical consequences of two inborn errors of phenylalanine metabolism—Phenylketonuria and Alkaptonuria.

PHENYLKETONURIA (PKU)

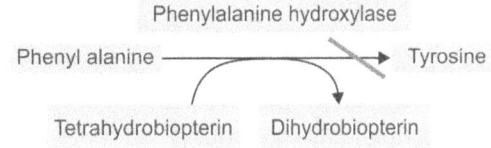

- It is an autosomal recessive disease with an incidence of 1:10,000 births
- It is due to deficiency of phenylalanine hydroxylase
- So phenylalanine is not converted into tyrosine and it accumulates hyperphenylalaninemia
- The excess of phenylalanine is converted to phenylpyruvate, phenyllactate, and phenylacetate and phenylacetylglutamine. Phenylpyruvate, phenyllactate, phenyl acetate are excreted in urine.

Clinical Manifestations

- The child is mentally retarded
- Convulsions, tremors, agitation, hyperactivity may be present
- The child often has hypopigmentation due to reduced availability of tyrosine for melanin production
- Phenyllactate in sweat causes mousy body odor.

Laboratory Diagnosis

- Blood level of phenylalanine is elevated – normal level is 1 mg/dL, which is elevated to >20 mg/dL
- This is confirmed by tandem mass spectroscopy
- Guthrie's test is confirmative
- Urine ferric chloride test is positive
- DNA probes-to diagnose the defects in phenylalanine hydroxylase and dihydrobiopterin reductase.

Treatment

- Early detection
- Low phenylalanine diet—tapioca based diet which has low phenylalanine is the treatment of choice
- Gene therapy is under trial.

ALKAPTONURIA

- It is an inborn error of metabolism in the metabolism of tyrosine/phenylalanine
- It is an autosomal recessive condition affecting 1:250,000 births
- It is due to the defect in homogentisate oxidase enzyme

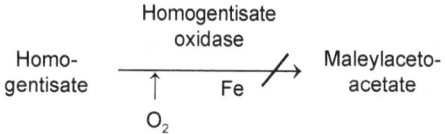

- Homogentisate gets accumulated and oxidised to benzoquinone acetate and forms alkaptone bodies
- Alkaptone bodies get deposited in intervertebral discs, cartilages of nose and pinna of ear developing ochronosis. Black pigments get deposited over joint cavities causing arthritis
- Urine turns black on standing. $FeCl_3$ test is positive. Benedict's test is strongly positive since homogentisate is a reducing agent
- Generally it is a harmless condition.

---

13. Name heavy metal poisons. Write biochemical consequences of any two.

Heavy metal poisons are lead, mercury, aluminium, arsenic, etc.

i. Lead poisoning

- It is a cumulative poison and is accumulated in tissues 90% lead is seen in bones, 9% in blood, and 1% in brain and kidneys
- There is no safe level. More than 25 µg/dL in adults and more than 10 µg/dL in children lead to toxicity
- It crosses the placenta and causes miscarriage, stillbirth and premature delivery
- Permanent neurological defects, cerebral palsy and optic atrophy may be seen
- In children mental retardation, learning disabilities, behavioral problems and seizures, etc.
- Anemia, abdominal colic and loss of appetite are common
- Discoloration and blue line among the gums are features of acute lead poisoning
- Lead inhibits heme synthesis by inhibiting the enzymes ALA dehydratase and ferrochelatase. Life span of RBC shortened. Anemia is predominent due to reduced heme synthesis and also lead inhibits iron absorption
- **Treatment:** Antidotes are used–calcium dodecyl edetate, penicillamine and BAL, dimercaprol and dimercaptosuccinic acid.

ii. Arsenic toxicity

- The oxides of arsenic are commonly used as fruit sprays, pesticides, rat poisons, etc.
- It acts on sulfhydryl enzymes and interferes with cell metabolism
- It may also cause intravascular hemolysis which leads to hemoglobinuria.
- There will be anaphylactic reactions
- Later complications are agranulocytosis, hepatitis, jaundice and encephalitis.

iii. Mercury poisoning

- Most common industrial poison
- It occurs due to inhalation of elementary mercury vapor from broken thermometer, sphygmomanometer
- In acute poisoning pulmonary edema and encephalopathy may result
- In chronic poisoning, there will be a classical triad of oral lesions, tremor and psychological changes may result—called erethism
- Organic mercury poisoning is called minamata disease which is characterized by dysarthria, ataxia and visual problems.

iv. Aluminium toxicity

- Common in paint workers and exposure from packing, building materials, cosmetics, antacids and aluminium cooking vessels
- A person can tolerate upto 1 mg/day of aluminium and usually 100 mg/day aluminium is excreted through urine

- Aluminium prevents absorption of calcium, phosphorus and iron. It also interferes heme synthesis
- Aluminium toxicity may lead to Alzheimer's disease and Parkinson's disease and also implicated in degeneration of dendrites.

14. Biochemical roles and nutritional importance of trace elements.

Trace elements are the minerals whose requirement is less than 100 mg/day. They are iron, iodine, copper, manganese, zinc, molybdenum, selenium and fluoride.

IRON

Sources: Leafy vegetables are a major source of iron followed by jaggery and liver. Pulses and cereals are a low source of iron. Milk is a very poor source of iron.

RDA: Adults—20 mg/day, pregnant women—40 mg/day, children—20-30 mg/day.

Metabolism: Only ferrous form is absorbed.
- HCl, vitamin C reduces iron to ferrous form, so increases its absorption. Phytic acid and oxalic acid form salts with iron so inhibits iron absorption
- Calcium and copper inhibits iron absorption
- Transport of iron is done by the transport protein-transferrin
- TIBC (total iron binding capacity) is provided by the transferrin. It increases in iron deficiency anemia. Soluble transferrin receptor levels also increased.

Storage

- Iron is stored as ferritin in mucosal cells, liver, spleen, bone marrow
- Apoferritin combines with iron to form ferritin. It is seen in intestinal mucosal cells, liver cells, bone marrow and spleen.

Functions of Iron

- Iron is the integral part of hemoglobin and myoglobin and is required for transport of oxygen
- Cytochromes and nonheme proteins of electron transport chain and oxidative phosphorylation need iron
- Peroxidase contains iron which is required for the phagocytosis of bacteria by neutrophils
- Iron is needed for the immune competence of body.

Deficiency

- Microcytic hypochromic anemia ensues
- In anemia body cells lack oxygen and the person becomes apathic
- Severe iron deficiency leads to heart failure
- Chronic deficiency leads to achlorhydria, impaired attention, irritability, lower memory, poor scholastic performance.

ZINC

- Total zinc content of body is 2 g, out of which 60% is in skeletal muscle and 30% in bones
- Rich dietary sources are grains, beans, nuts, cheese, meat and shellfish
- Copper, cadmium, calcium will interfere with the absorption of zinc
- In liver, zinc is stored in combination with a specific protein, metallothionein
- Zinc is excreted through pancreatic juice and lesser extent through sweat
- More than 300 enzymes are zinc dependent
  - Example: Carboxypeptidase- cleaves C-terminal ends of dietary proteins
  - Carbonic anhydrase—$H^+ + HCO_3^- \rightarrow H_2CO_3 \rightarrow H_2O + CO_2$
  - Alkaline phosphatase- needed for bone formation.

Functions of Zinc

- It is a component of RNA polymerase. It is also needed for protein synthesis
- Superoxide dismutase contains Zn, which is an antioxidant enzyme and so zinc is also an antioxidant
- Zinc stabilizes insulin. Insulin when stored in beta cells of pancreas contains zinc, which stabilizes the hormone

- Gusten is a salivary protein which contains zinc. It is needed for taste sensation.

RDA: For adults is 10 mg/day; children: 10 mg/day.

SELENIUM

- Selenium intake is dependent on the nature of soil in which food crops growing.
- Requirement is 50-100 µg/day
- In mammals glutathione peroxidase is the important selenium containing enzyme. RBC contains large quantity of glutathione peroxidase
- 5-deiodinase enzyme which is involved in the synthesis of thyroid hormone—in the conversion of thyroxin to T3-depends on selenium. Selenium deficiency leads to hypothyroidism
- Selenium concentration in testis is the highest in adult tissue. It is necessary for development of spermatozoa
- Selenium acts as nonspecific intracellular antioxidant
- Selenocysteine is considered as 21st amino acid which is genetically coded with UGA as codon.

Functions of Selenium

- Antioxidant function—the requirement of vitamin E reduces with increase in selenium intake. Both spare the action of one another
- Glutathione peroxidase-antioxidant enzyme which protects RBC from free radicals
- 5-deiodinase (thyroid metabolism)
- It is necessary for spermatogenesis
- Selenium is a constituent of selenocysteine, an amino acid.

IODINE

- **RDA:** 150-200 µg/day
- Iodine deficiency is common in India and iodized salt can prevent this.

Functions

- Only biological role of iodine is it helps in the formation of thyroxine and triiodothyronine
- About 80% of body iodine is stored in thyroglobulin as iodothyroglobulin in thyroid glands
- Radioactive iodine is useful in thyroid scanning I^{131}.

FLUORIDE

- Fluoride prevents dental caries. Residual food in the teeth undergoes bacterial fermentation and leads to acid production which causes dental caries. Fluoride when supplied in drinking water or tooth paste at about 1 ppm, coats the teeth and exchanges acid and also kills the bacteria, preventing dental caries
- But when fluoride in water exceeds more than 2 ppm it will cause chronic intestinal upset, gastroenteritis, loss of appetite and loss of weight. Level more than 5 ppm will cause mottling of enamel, stratification and discoloration of teeth
- A level more than 20 ppm is toxic leading to fluorosis, which causes osteoporosis, osteosclerosis and brittle bones. Genu valgum is the characteristic feature. Fluorosis leads to blood concentration of fluoride of 50 µg/dL.

COPPER

- Copper is needed for absorption of iron and incorporation of iron into Hb
- Necessary for the action of tyrosinase enzyme
- It is a co-factor for hydroxylation reactions done by vitamin C.

---

15. (a) List the different mechanisms involved in hormone action and (b) write about the mechanism of action of hormones using cAMP as second messenger.

(a) Different mechanisms involved in hormone action

- Hormones are substances released from endocrine glands which are ductless glands present in the body
- From the glands they are transported to their target organs through blood circulation.
- Based on the mechanism of action the hormones are classified into 2 types:

1. Hormones with intracellular receptors (Type I)
2. Hormones with cell surface receptors (Type II).

1. **Hormones with intracellular receptors (Type I)**
   Examples: Glucocorticoids, mineralocorticoids, sex hormones, calcitriol, thyroxine

2. **Hormones with cell surface receptors (Type II)**
   - Type IIA - Hormones acting through cyclicAMP as second messenger, e.g. ACTH, TSH, glucagon, calcitonin, catecholamines
   - TYPE IIB - Hormones acting through cyclic GMP as second messenger, e.g. nitric oxide (NO), atrial natriuretic factor (ANF)
   - Type IIC - Hormones acting through calcium or phosphatidylinositol (PIP2), e.g. TRH, CCK, vasopressin, oxytocin
   - Type IID - Hormones mediated through tyrosine kinase, e.g. somatomedin, insulin, EGF, IGF
   - TYPE IIE - Hormones with intracellular messenger which may be a kinase or utilize. Phosphatase cascade, e.g. IL, GH, PRL, TNF, erythropoietin.

(b) **Mechanism of action of hormones using cAMP as second messenger (Fig. 27)**
- CyclicAMP - Adenosine 3'5' monophosphate
- It is a cyclic nucleotide of adenine
- It is synthesised from ATP by the action of adenylate cyclase which is an enzyme of integral membrane
- Its activity is regulated by many peptide hormones which may stimulate or inhibit the production of cAMP from ATP, e.g. glucagon
- cAMP is degraded by phosphodiesterase enzyme which hydrolyses cyclicAMP to AMP
- cAMP acts as a second messenger for hormones like calcitonin, epinephrine, glucagon, etc.
- It is produced in the cell in response to activation of adenylate cyclase in response to active G protein

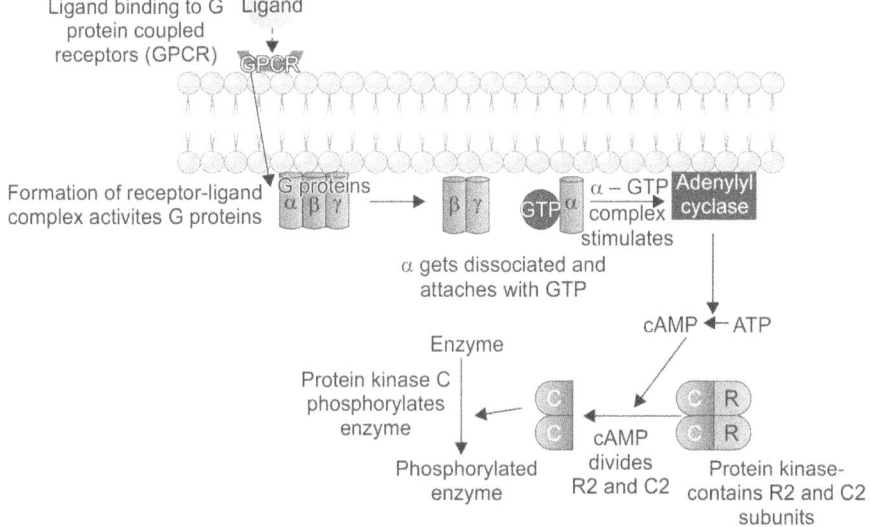

Fig. 27: Mechanism of second messenger action of cAMP.

- In eukaryotic cells, cAMP binds to a protein kinase called cAMP dependent protein kinase A (PKA) that is a heterotetrameric molecule consisting of two regulatory subunits (R) and two catalytic subunits (C)
- cAMP binds to the regulatory subunits and dissociates the tetramer unto regulatory and catalytic subunits
- The active C subunit catalyzes the transfer of the phosphate of ATP to a serine or threonine or tyrosine residues in a variety of proteins
- The effects of cAMP in eukaryotic cells are mediated by protein phosphorylation-dephosphorylation, principally on serine and threonine/tyrosine residues
- The end result is the formation of phosphorylated protein. This causes a change in its function, e.g. epinephrine stimulates cAMP production leading to phosphorylation of phosphorylase kinase which is the active form, leading to glycogenolysis
- Glycogen phosphorylase and hormone sensitive lipase are controlled by cyclic AMP.

16. List various thyroid function test and give the importance of free thyroid hormones in assessing thyroid function test.

- Thyroid gland synthesise the thyroid hormones—thyroxine (T3 and T4) and calcitonin
- Thyroid function tests are useful in assessing the functioning of thyroid gland and to diagnose the hyper and hypothyroidism

In Vitro TFT

ASSAY OF HORMONES
- **Serum Total T3 and T4 by immunoassay**
  - **RIA/ ELISA**
    - Normal T3 = 70-200 ng/dL; T4 = 5-12.5 µg/dL
  - In hyperthyroidism, thyroid hormone levels-both T3 and T4 levels are increased but TSH levels decreased
  - In hypothyroidism T3 and T4 are reduced in serum but TSH level is increased.
- **Free T3 and T4 (fT3 and fT4)**
  - More reliable test
  - Normal value of free T4 = 10 to 27 pmol/L; T3 = 3 to 9 pmol/L
  - Values increased in hyperthyroidism and thyrotoxicosis and decreased in hypothyroidism.
- **Thyroid binding proteins-Thyroid binding globulin (TBG)**
  - Normal level of TBG = 12 to 28 µg/ml
  - TBG - increased in hypothyroidism, pregnancy and in estrogen therapy
  - Level decreased in hyperthyroidism, nephrotic syndrome.
- **Resin uptake test (T_3RU or T_3U)**
  - Indirect estimate of binding capacity of plasma TBG
  - Radioactive iodine labelled- $^{125}I\text{-}T_3$ is added to the patient's serum which will occupy the free binding sites on TBG. Excess unattached $^{125}I\text{-}T_3$ is removed and the amount taken up by the resin is estimated
  - Normal value of T_3U is 25 to 35%
  - Values increased in hyperthyroidism and decreased in hypothyroidism.
- **Plasma TSH (RIA method)**
  - Normal value = 2 to 6 µU/ml
  - In primary hyperthyroidism TSH level is elevated due to lack of feedback but in secondary hyperthyroidism, TSH and T3 and T4 levels are low.
- **Thyroid antibodies:** To detect auto-immune disorders of thyroid gland caused due to the antibodies against thyroid tissues.

In Vivo Tests
- **Thyroid iodine uptake test:** Using ^{131}I. Normal value - 1 to 13% absorbed after 2

hours and 15 to 45 and absorbed after 24 hours
- **TRH stimulation test:** An abnormal response is observed in hyperthyroidism and hypopituitrism
- **TSH stimulation test:** IV administration of TSH will increase radioactive iodine thyroid uptake and blood thyroid hormone level
- **Thyroid scanning:** Ultrasonogram.

Importance of Free Thyroid Hormones: (Free T3 and T4)

- Free T3 and T4 are active molecules
- This can be measured by ELISA, CLIA or FIA accurately
- Free T4 constitutes only 0.03% of total T4 and free T3 forms 0.3% of free T3
- Values of free hormones are not affected by the amount of carrier proteins in the blood and so variations in binding proteins will not affect the results in hyper and hypothyroidism.

17. Alternations in biochemical investigations in cirrhosis liver.

- Cirrhosis of liver is characterized by parenchymal damage of liver, fibrosis and regeneration of liver cells
- Liver has a major role in metabolism and storage of most of the biomolecules and so the clinical abnormalities will not be manifested till the damage of liver is well advanced
- Common causes for cirrhosis are alcoholic abuse, chronic hepatitis, toxic drugs, hemochromatosis, Wilson's disease, etc.

BIOCHEMICAL ALTERATIONS

1. **Plasma proteins** (all except immunoglobulin are synthesised in liver):
   - Low total protein and albumin
   - Increased prothrombin time
   - Hyperglobulinemia
   - Reduction of clotting factors which need vitamin K for activation - bleeding tendency is more
   - Serum electrophoresis-albumin band is thin and less prominent and increased globulin band.
2. **Bilirubin:** Increase of both conjugated and unconjugated bilirubin - hepatic jaundice and van den Bergh may be biphasic.
3. **Enzymes:**
   - Transaminases - Variable depending of the severity. Values of AST higher in alcoholic diseases
   - Alkaline phosphatase (ALP) - Higher if there is cholestasis
   - Gamma-glutamyl transferase (GGT) increased in alcoholics- marker enzyme in alcoholics
   - 5-nucleotidase-elevated if there is obstruction to biliary passage.
4. **Others:**
   - Electrolytes - hyponatremia - increased secretion of ADH due to reduced plasma volume
   - Lactic acidosis-due to reduced plasma volume because of edema and ascites.

18. Metabolically important products formed from methionine.

Metabolic products formed from methionine:
- S-adenosyl methionine - active methionine involved in transmethylation reactions
- Creatinine and creatine
- Epinephrine - through transmethylation
- Choline
- Melatonin
- Amino acid cysteine during catabolism of methionine and cystine from cysteine.

Active form of methionine (S-Adenosyl Methionine)

- S-adenosyl methionine (SAM) is obtained by accepting adenosyl group from ATP by methionine by methionine adenosyl transferase

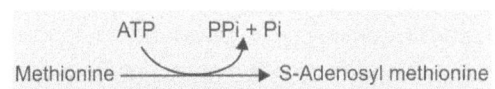

- The function of SAM is transmethylation reactions

- **Transmethylation reaction** is acceptance of a methyl group from a donor like SAM by a compound resulting in another compound.

The transmethylation reactions are

Methyl acceptor	Methylated product
Guanidoacetic acid	**Creatine**
Serine	**Choline**
Epinephrine	Metanephrine
Norepinephrine	**Epinephrine**
Transfer RNA	Methylated tRNA

Creatine and creatinine production (Fig. 28)

- Creatine and creatinine are the non-protein nitrogenous substances present in normal urine. They are synthesized by 3 amino acids—Arginine, glycine and methionine. The synthesis occurs in kidney, liver and muscles
- **Step 1: At the Mitochondria of kidney.** Glycine combines with arginine and aminidino group is transferred from arginine to glycine to form guanidoacetic acid and ornithine by an amido transferase
- **Step 2: At liver**—Guanidoacetic acid receives a methyl group from S-adenosyl methionine (SAM) to form creatine
- **Step 3: In the muscles**—Creatine kinase (CK) in muscles converts creatine to creatine phosphate which acts as a high energy molecule involved in resynthesis of ATP from ADP during muscle contraction. Lohmann's reaction is the storage form of energy in muscles
- **Step 4:** Creatine loses water to form creatinine which is excreted by the kidneys by a non-enzymatic spontaneous reaction.

Clinical Application

- Normal serum level of creatinine is 0.7 to 1.4 mg/dL; serum creatine is 0.2 to 0.4 mg/dL
- Serum creatinine is a marker of renal failure. Creatinine clearance test is used to measure GFR
- Creatine kinase has many isoenzymes and is elevated in muscular dystrophies and myocardial infarction. It is the first enzyme to be elevated in myocardial infarction.

Epinephrine: Catecholamines

- Tyrosine is first hydroxylated to DOPA by tyrosine hydroxylase. It requires tetrahydro—Biopterin and NADPH
- DOPA is decarboxylated to form dopamine by DOPA decarboxylase, a PLP dependent enzyme. Dopamine is a catecholamine which is a neurotransmitter. In Parkinsonism dopamine level is reduced. L-DOPA is used as a drug in Parkinsonism
- Dopamine is hydroxylated to norepinephrine by dopamine hydroxylase
- Norepinephrine is methylated to epinephrine by methyl transferase which needs SAM which is the methyl donor
- **Epinephrine is methylated to metanephrine** and oxidized to Vanillylmandelic acid (VMA) and excreted in urine. Level of VMA is elevated in pheochromocytoma and in neuroblastoma.

Choline

- Ethanolamine produced by the decarboxylation of serine
- Then ethanolamine is methylated three times by SAM to form trimethyl ethanolamine which is choline
- Choline is an important one carbon donor
- Choline is acetylated to form acetyl choline which is a neurotransmitter.

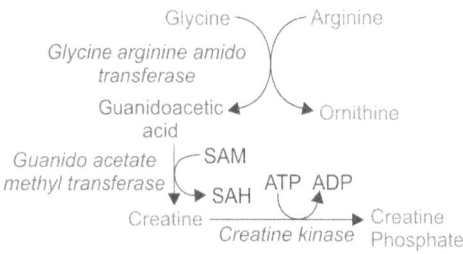

Fig. 28: Synthesis of creatine.

Melatonin

- It is the acetylated and methylated product of serotonin secreted by pineal gland
- Serotonin is 5 hydroxytryptomine
- Meatonin is involved in diurnal variations, sleep wake cycles and biological rhythms
- It is also a neurotransmitter.

Cysteine and Cystine

- During methionine catabolism, methionine is converted to SAM
- SAM donates methyl group to methyl acceptors by methyl transferases to form S-adenosyl homocysteine (SAH)
- SAH loses adenosine using adenosine homocysteinase to form homocysteine.
- Homocysteine combines with serine to form cystathionine using cystathionine synthase
- Cystathionine is hydrolyzed **to cysteine** and homoserine by cystathioninase
- Cysteine is needed for the formation of glutathione along with glutamic acid and glycine
- It also forms taurine - a conjugating agent
- 2 molecules of cysteine combine to form cystine.

19. Clinical application of DNA recombinant technology.

When a gene of one species is transferred to another gene of different species, it is called recombinant DNA technology or genetic engineering. Usually there will be combination of human DNA and bacterial DNA. The DNA thus formed is called as recombinant DNA or chimeric DNA or hybrid DNA.

Applications

- Large scale production of therapeutic human proteins can be obtained, e.g. human recombinant insulin for diabetic patients
- Vaccines with genetic material of bacteria and viruses can be produced
- Genetic probes can be produced to
  - Identify genetic diseases during antenatal period
  - Diagnosis of virus and bacteria in blood using their DNA
  - To pinpoint location of a gene in chromosome
  - To identify mutations in genes
  - To detect activation of oncogenes.
- **Gene therapy:** Normal genes could be inserted into the patient's cells where it is defective, e.g. Adenosine deaminase deficiency.

20. Biochemical application of tumor markers.

Definition: They are also known as tumor index substances.

- They are the biological substances synthesised and released by cancer cells
- They are found in an increased level in blood and other body fluids and tissues
- Tumor markers are substances whose presence or elevation in body is used to identify or confirm the presence or to monitor the prognosis of the cancer.

Uses of Tumor Markers

- Detection and diagnosis of cancer
- To assess the prognosis – whether curable or not
- To monitor the treatment effectivity and follow up
- Localize the tumor by using radiolabelled antibodies.

Types of Tumor Markers

- Oncofetal antigens
- Carbohydrate markers
- Enzymes
- Hormones
- Serum proteins
- Catabolic product.

Oncofetal Antigens

- Proteins produced in fetal life which may be decreased or absent in blood after birth
- They reappear in cancer patients because of reactivation of the genes of the protein by transformation
- **Example** - Alpha fetoprotein
  - Hepatoma, germ cell tumors
  - Carcinoembryogenic antigen
  - Colorectal and GI tumors.

Carbohydrate Markers

- They are either antigens on the tumor cell surface or secreted by tumor cells
- High molecular weight glycoproteins - abbreviated as CA - carbohydrate antigen
- **Example** CA 12—increased in ovarian cancer.

Enzymes

- Enzymes are present in high concentration inside the cells and released into circulation due to tumor necrosis
- This also leads to tumor metastasis

Example

Alkaline phosphatase	Bone secondaries, liver secondaries
Prostatic acid phosphatase	Prostate cancer
Prostate specific antigen	Prostate cancer
Neuron specific enolase	Nervous system tumors.

Hormones

- Endocrine tissues which produce hormones in normal conditions will produce the hormones in excess during certain neoplastic conditions
- Non-endocrine tissues which are situated away from the endocrine sites will produce the hormone in excess - ectopic syndrome

Example

Human beta HCG	Choriocarcinoma
Calcitonin	Medullary Ca of thyroid
Big ACTH	Lung oat cell cancer
Vasoactive intestinal polypeptide (VIP)	APUDomas
Vanllylmandelic acid (VMA)	Pheochromocytoma, neuroblastoma.

Serum Proteins

Example

Immunoglobulins (Ig)	Multiple myeloma, macrogobulinemia
Bence Jones proteins in urine	Multiple Myeloma.

Catabolic Product

Hydroxy proline—bone metastasis.

MBBS Examination 2004

ANSWER ALL QUESTIONS

I. Essay questions (10 Marks each)

1. Describe TCA cycle and its inhibitors and energetics. Add a note on the amphibolic role of TCA cycle. How is TCA cycle regulated?
2. Discuss cholesterol synthesis and its regulation. Mention the various substances obtained from cholesterol.
3. Discuss the metabolism of glycine. Add a note on metabolic disorders associated with glycine metabolism.
4. What is the normal serum calcium level? Discuss the distribution of calcium in the body. Describe the sources, daily requirement, absorption and excretion of calcium. Explain how serum calcium level is maintained?

II. Short notes (5 Marks each)

1. Phospholipids.
2. Biotin.
3. Isoenzymes.
4. Protein-energy malnutrition.
5. Obstructive jaundice (posthepatic jaundice).
6. Uncouplers of oxidative phosphorylation.
7. Absorption of carbohydrates from the intestines.
8. Structure of hemoglobin.
9. Bile salts—synthesis and biological role.
10. Vitamin E.
11. Alkaptonuria.
12. Transfer RNA.
13. Metabolism of zinc.
14. Detoxication by conjugation.
15. Salvage pathway of purine synthesis.
16. Metabolic acidosis.
17. Tumor markers.
18. Clearance tests.
19. Lac operon.
20. Cytochrome P450.

I. ESSAY QUESTIONS

1. Describe TCA cycle and its inhibitors and energetics. Add a note on the amphibolic role of TCA cycle. How is TCA cycle regulated?

The TCA cycle is a series of reactions in mitochondria that oxidize acetyl residues and reduce coenzymes which on re-oxidation are linked to the formation of ATP.

- **Other name:** *Citric acid cycle or Krebs cycle or Tricarboxylic acid cycle*
- **Intracellular location:** Mitochondria.

STEPS OF TCA CYCLE (FIGS. 1 AND 2)

Preparatory phase: Acetyl-CoA enters into the TCA cycle in the mitochondria and joins with 4C oxaloacetate which is considered as a catalyst.

Sources of Acetyl-CoA

- Glycolysis (aerobic) ends in pyruvate. Then pyruvate ⟶ acetyl-CoA
- Beta oxidation of fatty acid ⟶ acetyl-CoA
- Ketogenic amino acids ⟶ acetyl-CoA

Step 1: Formation of Citric Acid

- Oxaloacetate condenses with acetyl-CoA to form citrate.
- It is catalyzed by citrate synthase
- It is an irreversible step.

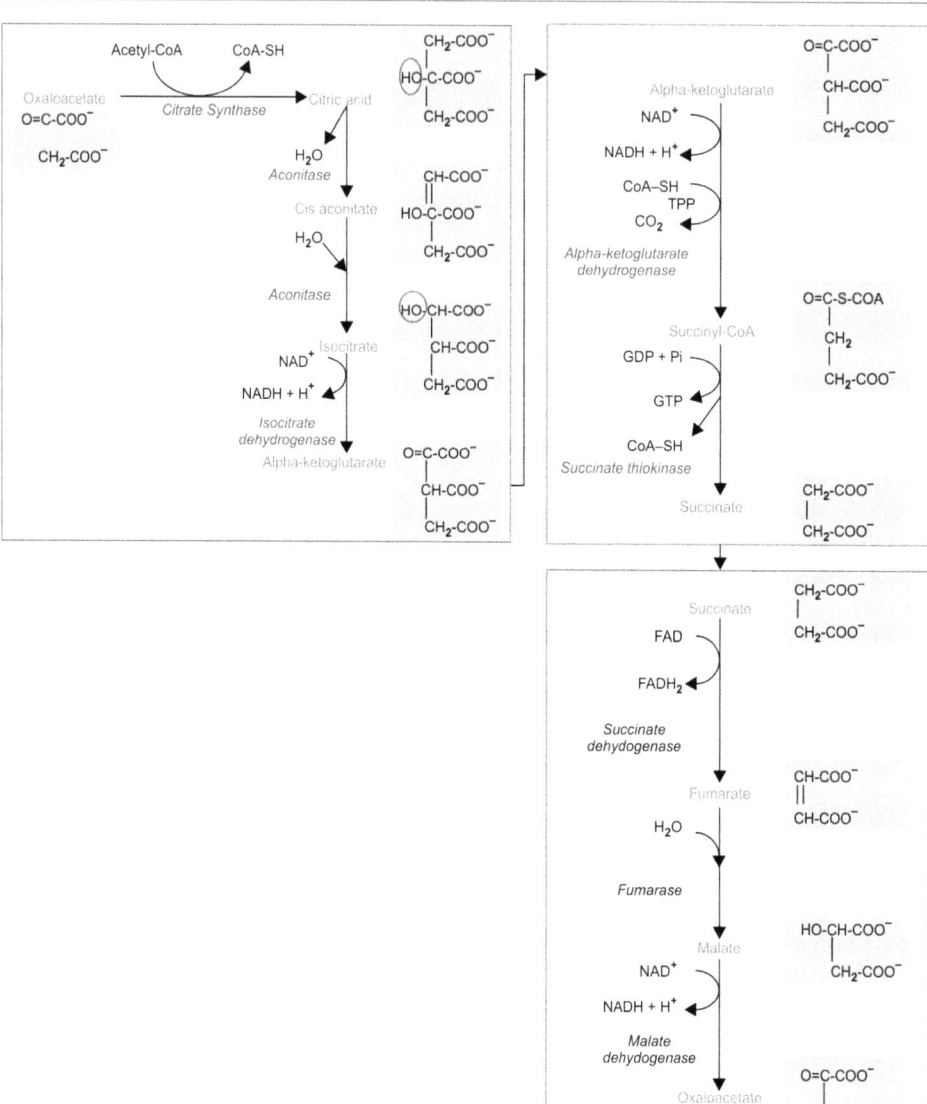

Fig. 1: Steps of TCA cycle.

Step 2: Formation of Isocitrate

- Citrate is isomerized to isocitrate by aconitase
- Here the intermediate is cis-aconitate
- It is a reversible step.

Step 3: Formation of α-KG

- Isocitrate is dehydrogenated to form oxalosuccinate
- It is unstable and undergoes spontaneous decarboxylation to form α-ketoglutarate. It is catalyzed by isocitrate dehydrogenase. NADH generated enters into ETC to generate ATP (2-5).

Step 4: Formation of Succinyl-CoA

- α-KG is oxidatively decarboxylated to form succinyl CoA by α-ketoglutarate dehydrogenase

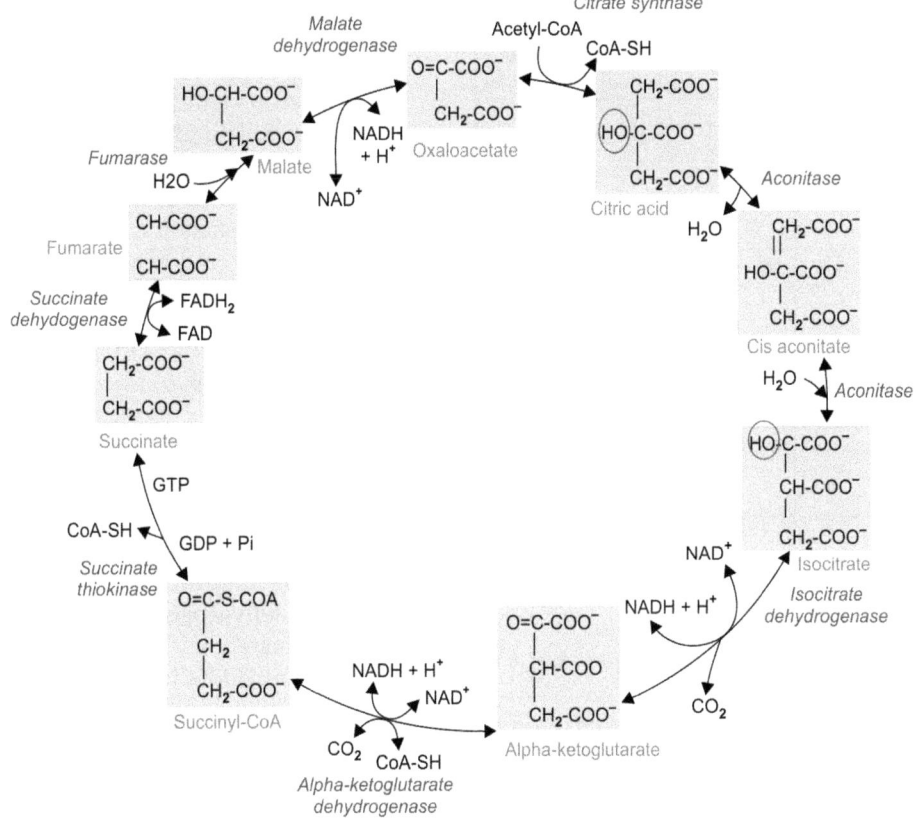

Fig. 2: TCA cycle.

- It is a multienzyme complex with 3 sub-units. It is an irreversible step. NADH enters into ETC. Five co-enzymes are needed—NAD, FAD, TPP, CoA and Lipoate.

Step 5: Generation of Succinate (Substrate Level Phosphorylation)

- This reaction is an example for substrate level phosphorylation
- Succinyl COA ⟶ Succinate
- It is catalyzed by succinate thiokinase.

Step 6: Formation of Fumarate

Succinate is dehydrogenated to fumarate by succinate dehydrogenase.

Oxidative phosphorylation-through FAD to produce 1.5 ATP.

Step 7: Formation of Malate

Fumarate to malate conversion is done by fumarase.

Step 8: Regeneration of Oxaloacetate

Finally malate is oxidized to oxaloacetate by malate dehydrogenase.

Malate ⟶ oxaloacetate ⟶ acetyl-CoA

- Oxaloacetate acts as a catalyst which again joins with another molecule of acetyl-CoA to continue another cycle.

Significance

- Complete oxidation of acetyl-CoA
- ATP generation
- Final common oxidative pathway
- Anaplerotic role.

Energetics

Step No.	Reactions	Co-enzyme	ATP (old calculation)	ATP (new calculation)
3	Isocitrate to α-KG	NADH	3	2.5
4	α-KG to succinyl-CoA	NADH	3	2.5
5	Succinyl-CoA to succinate	GTP	1	1
6	Succinate to fumarate	FADH2	2	1.5
8	Malate to oxaloacetate	NADH	3	2.5
Total ATP			12	10

Regulation

- Citrate synthase: Inhibited by ATP (allosteric inhibitor)
- Isocitrate dehydrogenase: Activated by ADP; inhibited by ATP and NADH
- α-KG dehydrogenase: Inhibited by succinyl CoA and NADH
- Availability of ADP: Cellular need of ATP and availability of ADP inside the cells regulate TCA cycle.

Amphibolic Pathway (AMPHI = both)

- The citric acid cycle is both anabolic and catabolic and so called as amphibolic
- It is not only a pathway for oxidation of two-carbon units—it is also a major pathway for interconversion of metabolites arising from **transamination** and **deamination** of amino acids
- It also provides the substrates for **amino acid synthesis** by transamination, as well as for **gluconeogenesis** and **fatty acid synthesis**
- Anabolic or synthetic reactions of TCA cycle:
  - Oxaloacetate and α-ketoglutarate serve as precursor for aspartate and glutamate respectively. These 2 amino acids are utilized for the synthesis of other amino acids by transamination and also for the synthesis of purines and pyrimidines
  - Succinyl CoA is utilized for the synthesis of heme and porphyria
  - Citrate from mitochondria is transported to cytosol by tricarboxylic acid transporter where it is cleaved to form oxaloacetate and acetyl-CoA by ATP citrate lyase. Acetyl-CoA is utilized for fatty acid synthesis.

Inhibitors of TCA Cycle

- **Aconitase:**
  - Inhibited by fluroacetate
  - It is a noncompetitive inhibition.
- **α-KG dehydrogenase:**
  - Inhibited by arsenite
  - It is a noncompetitive inhibition.
- **Succinate dehydrogenase:**
  - By malonate
  - It is a competitive inhibitor.

2. **Discuss cholesterol synthesis and its regulation. Mention the various substances obtained from cholesterol (Figs. 3 and 4).**

Major sites of cholesterol synthesis: Liver, adrenal cortex, testes, ovaries and intestines.

Enzymes of this synthesis are present in cytosol and endoplasmic reticulum of all nucleated cells.

First 2 steps are similar to the 2 steps of ketogenesis.

Step 1: Condensation of acetyl CoA: Cytosol

Two molecules of acetyl CoA condense to form acetoacetyl-CoA by the enzyme acetoacetyl-CoA synthase.

Step 2: Production of HMG CoA: Cytosol

Third molecule of acetyl-CoA joins with acetoacetyl-CoA to form hydroxymethylgutaryl-CoA (HMG-CoA) by the enzyme HMG-CoA synthase.

Step 3: Rate limiting step

HMG-CoA is reduced by a NADPH dependent enzyme—HMG-CoA. Reductase to form mevalonate (6C).

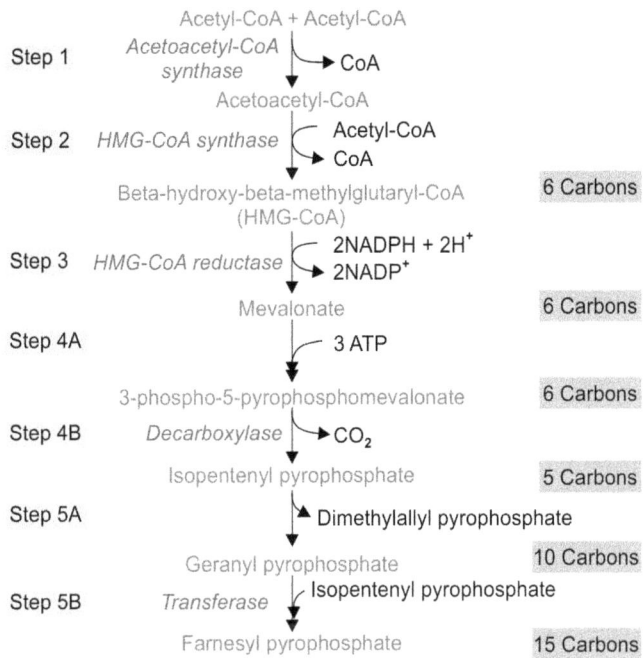

Fig. 3: Synthesis of cholesterol (Steps 1 to 5B).

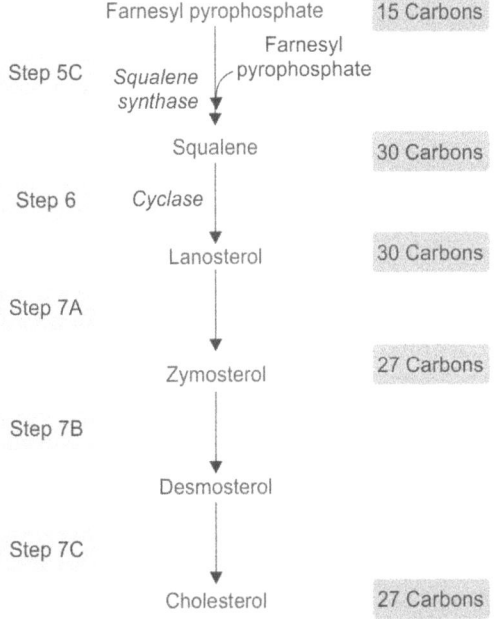

Fig. 4: Synthesis of cholesterol (Steps 5C to 7C).

Step 4A and B: Production of 5C units

4A: Mevalonate is phosphorylated to phosphomevalonate, pyrophosphomevalonate and 3P 5-pyrophosphomevalonate by kinase enzymes in 3 steps.

4B: Decarboxylation of 3P 5-pyrophosphomevalonate to form 5C compound—isopentenyl-PP (5C).

Step 5: Condensation of 5C units (5A, 5B and 5C)

Six numbers of 5C units are condensed to form gPP, farnesyl PP and then to squalene in a stepwise process to form 30 C squalene.

Step 6: Cyclization

Squalene undergoes oxidation by epoxidase with molecular oxygen and NADPH to form squalene epoxide which on cyclization is converted to lanosterol (30 C) – the first sterol formed.

Step 7:

- **7A:** Removal of 3 additional methyl group on C4 and 14 to form Zymosterol (27 C)
- **7B:** Migration of double bond from 8-9 position to 5-6 position to form desmosterol—which is present in fetal

brain but not in adult brain. It reappears in certain brain tumors like glioma
- **7C: Double bonds** in the side chain between C 24-25 is reduced by NADPH to form the 27 carboned cholesterol with cyclopentanoperhydrophenanthrene ring and side chain.

Regulation of Cholesterol Synthesis
- **Rate limiting enzyme:** HMG-CoA reductase is regulated at the transcription level of its gene as per the availability of cholesterol
- **Hormonal regulation:** Insulin and thyroxin increase the activity of HMG-CoA reductase whereas cortisol and glucagon decrease its activity
- **Drugs:** Statin group of drugs like lovastatin, compactin competitively inhibit HMG-CoA reductase enzyme
- **Bile acids:** Inhibit HMG-CoA reductase activity.

Products formed from Cholesterol
- **Bile acids and bile salts**
  - **Primary bile acids:** Cholic acid and chenodeoxycholic acids
  - **Secondary bile acids:** Lithocholic acid and deoxycholic acid and their conjugated Na and potassium salts.
- **Steroid and sex hormones**
  - Steroid hormones—glucocorticoids and mineralocorticoids
  - Sex hormones from pregnenolone-progesterone, androgens—testosterone and pestrogens
- Vitamin D and calcitriol.

---

3. **Discuss the metabolism of glycine. Add a note on metabolic disorders associated with glycine metabolism.**

Glycine is the simplest, nonessential and glucogenic amino acid.

Synthesis of Glycine

Glycine is derived from serine, threonine and from CO_2 and NH_3 by glycine synthase.

Serine: Beta carbon of serine is carried by tetra hydrofolate to channel into the one carbon pool and the alpha carbon serine forms glycine.

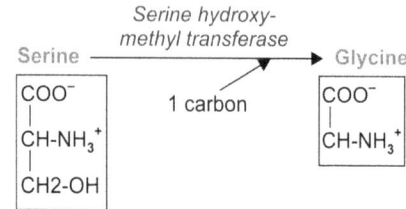

- **Threonine:** Threonine aldolase enzyme cleaves it into glycine and aldehyde
- **Glycine synthase:** This multienzyme complex reacts with CO_2, NH_3 and one carbon unit to form glycine. NAD, lipoamide, PLP and THFA are the co-enzymes of this step. Reversal of this reaction leads to glycine cleavage system.

Catabolism and Utilization of Glycine
- **Glycine cleavage system:** This is the reversal of the multienzyme complex—glycine synthase reaction mentioned above by means of oxidative deamination

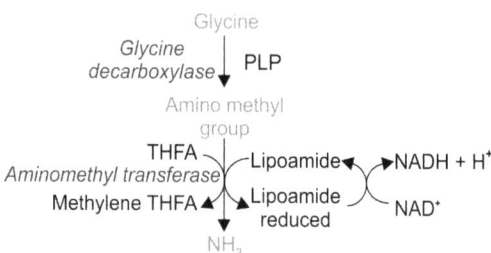

- **Glucogenic pathway:** Glycine is first converted to serine which is then acted be serine dehydratase to form pyruvate which enters into gluconeogenic pathway by reversal of glycolysis.

Compounds formed from Glycine (Fig. 5A)
- Creatine, creatine phosphate and creatinine (glycine + arginine + S adenosylmethionine)
- Heme (glycine + succinyl-CoA)
- Purine bases and nucleotides—C4, C5 and N7
- Glutathione (gamma glutamyl cysteinyl glycine)
- Conjugation for xenobiotics
- Constituent of proteins like collagen (glycine + proline + hydroxyproline)

- Methylene tetrahydrofolate by glycine cleavage system
- Glucose—it is glucogenic.

Products Derived from Glycine (Fig. 5B)
- **Creatine production from glycine:**
  - Creatine and creatinine are the non-protein nitrogenous substances present in normal urine. They are synthesised by 3 amino acids—arginine, glycine and methionine. The synthesis occurs in kidney, liver and muscles
  - Normal serum level of creatinine is 0.7 -1.4 mg/dL; serum creatine is 0.2–0.4 mg/dL
  - Serum creatinine is a marker of renal failure. Creatinine clearance test is used to measure GFR.

- **Production of heme (Fig. 6):** Succinyl-CoA combines with glycine catalyzed by the enzyme ALA synthase in the presence of the coenzyme pyridoxal phosphate in the mitochondria to form alpha-amino-beta-ketoadipic acid which is converted by the same enzyme to delta amino levulinic acid. It is the rate limiting step in heme synthesis.

Metabolic disorders of Glycine Metabolism
- **Nonketotic hyperglycinemia**
  - This is due to defect in glycine cleavage system
  - Glycine level is increased in blood, urine and CSF

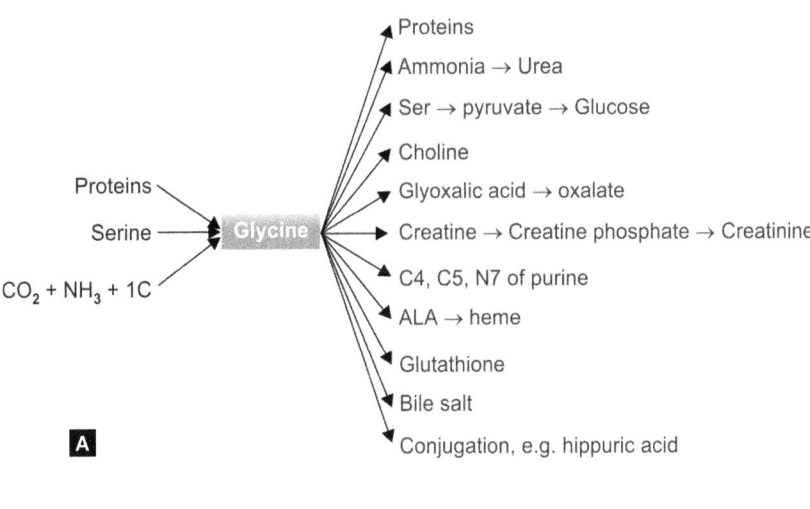

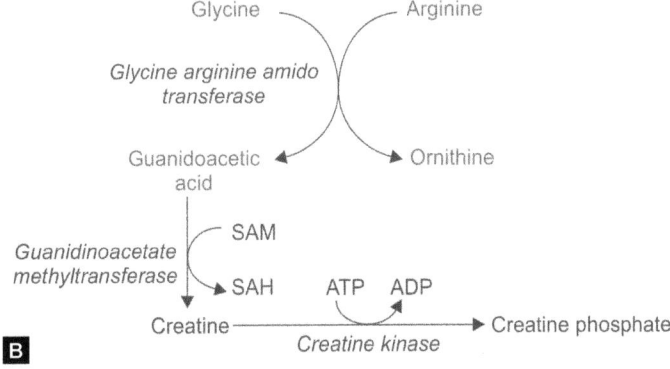

Figs. 5A and B: A. Fate of glycine; B. Synthesis of creatine from glycine.

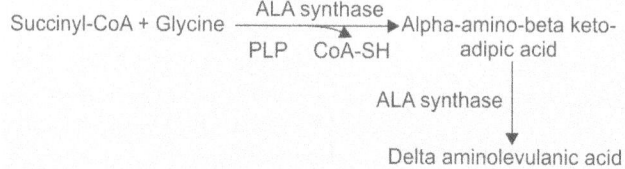

Fig. 6: Role of glycine in heme synthesis.

- Severe mental retardation and seizures are present.
- **Glycinuria:**
  - Rare disorder
  - Blood glycine level normal but urine contains increased amount of glycine (normal 0.5 to 1 g/day)
  - Glycinuria is due to defective renal reabsorption of glycine
  - Formation of oxalate renal stones but urinary oxalate level is normal.
- **Primary hyperoxaluria—Type I and II**
  - **Type I hyperoxaluria:**
    - It is an autosomal recessive trait
    - Due to protein targeting defect
    - The enzyme alanine glyoxylate aminotransaminases which is normally present in hepatic peroxisomes is located in mitochondria and so the enzyme becomes inactive.
    - This leads to excessive production of oxalate which gets deposited in the kidney causes nephrolithiasis, renal colic and hematuria
    - External oxalosis is seen in heart, blood vessels and bones.
  - **Type II primary oxaluria:**
    - It is a milder condition presented with urolithiasis only
    - It also results from deficient activity of cytoplasmic glyoxylate oxidase.

Management

- Increase the excretion of oxalates by increasing the water intake
- Restrict the dietary intake of oxalates—leafy vegetables, seasame seeds, tea, cocoa, beetroot, spinach, increased intake of vitamin C.

4. What is the normal serum calcium level? Discuss the distribution of calcium in the body. Describe the sources, daily requirement, absorption and excretion of calcium. Explain how serum calcium level is maintained?

Calcium: Calcium is one of the major minerals needed for the body.

Normal Blood level of Calcium

Total calcium level is 9–11 mg/dL

Distribution of Calcium

Three forms of calcium in blood:
1. Ionized calcium (active form) – 5 mg/dL.
2. Protein bound Ca – 4 mg/dL
3. Protein complexed with phosphate, HCO_3^-, Citrate – 1 mg/dL.

Sources: Good source—milk; medium sources—egg, fish, vegetables.

Cereals: Rice, wheat contain small amounts of calcium but they are the good source of calcium in India.

Daily Requirement

- Adult — 500 mg
- Children — 1200 mg
- Pregnancy and lactation — 1500 mg
- Above 50 years — 1500 mg + Vitamin D (20 mg)

Absorption of Calcium

- Absorption of calcium takes place from the first and second part of duodenum
- Calcium is absorbed against concentration gradient and requires energy

- Absorption requires a carrier protein, helped by calcium dependent ATPase.

Factors Promoting Calcium Absorption
- Vitamin D induces the synthesis of the binding protein—calbindin in the intestinal epithelial cells, and facilitates calcium absorption
- Parathyroid hormone enhances calcium absorption through the increased synthesis of calcitriol
- Acidity favors calcium absorption
- Amino acids lysine and arginine facilitate calcium absorption
- Lactose promotes calcium uptake by intestinal cells.

Factors Inhibiting Calcium Absorption
- Phytates and oxalates form insoluble salts and interfere with calcium absorption
- High dietary phosphate results in the formation of insoluble calcium phosphate and prevents calcium uptake
- Malabsorption syndromes—impaired fat absorption leads to formation of insoluble calcium soaps with fatty acids
- Alkaline condition is unfavorable for calcium absorption
- High content of dietary fiber interferes with calcium absorption.

Excretion of Calcium
- Calcium is excreted partly through the kidneys and intestines. Renal threshold for serum calcium is 10 mg/dL. Beyond this level calcium gets excreted in urine
- Excretion of calcium into feces is a continuous process and it is increased in vitamin D deficiency.

Factors Regulating Calcium Level
- Hormones:
    - Vitamin D—calcitriol
    - Parathyroid hormone (PTH)
    - Calcitonin—thyroid
- Phosphorus
- Serum proteins
- Alkalosis and acidosis
- Renal threshold
- Children.

HORMONAL REGULATION

Vitamin D (Calcitriol-1, 25-dihydroxycholecalciferol)

The active vitamin D (Calcitriol) acts as a steroid hormone. It is synthesised in kidney.
- **Effect on intestine:** Calcitriol binds to specific cytoplasmic receptors which interacts with DNA and induces the synthesis of mRNA for specific proteins Calbindin which is a calcium binding protein which helps in the absorption of calcium and phosphorus from the intestines
- **Effects on bone:** Calcitriol stimulates the activity of osteoblasts which help in mineralization of bones. They secrete alkaline phosphatase enzyme which in turn increases the ionic concentration of phosphate and calcium
- **Effects on kidney:** Calcitriol increases the reabsorption of calcium and phosphorous from the renal tubules thereby conserving both minerals.

Parathyroid Hormone (PTH)
- Parathyroid hormone (PTH) is secreted by four parathyroid glands present at the posterior aspect of thyroid gland
- Decreased serum calcium level leads to release of PTH from parathyroids. PTH activates the enzyme adenylcyclase in target cells and increases intracellular calcium concentration
- **PTH and bones:** PTH causes demineralization of bones. It activates pyrophosphatase in osteoclasts leading to bone resorption and decalcification. Calcium is released into the bloodstream and increases blood calcium level. This leads to loss of bone matrix
- **PTH and kidneys**: PTH causes decreased renal excretion of calcium and increased excretion of phosphates and increased reabsorption of calcium leading to increased blood calcium level
- **PTH and intestines**: PTH stimulates increased production of calcitriol which

acts on intestine to absorb more calcium leading to increased calcium level in blood.

Calcitonin

- Secreted by parafollicular cells of thyroid gland
- It is a polypeptide of 32-34 amino acids and its secretion is stimulated by serum calcium, gastrin, glucagon and biological amines
- It decreases serum calcium level by inhibiting resorption of bone and decreases the activity of osteoclasts and increases the activity of osteoblasts
- Calcitonin and PTH are antagonistic to each other but both together promote growth and remodeling of bone
- In kidney—calcitonin increases excretion of phosphates in urine like PTH.

OTHER FACTORS

Phosphorus

- There is a reciprocal relationship of calcium with phosphorus
- Ionic product of Ca × P is kept as a constant
- Normally—(Ca) 10 mg/dL × (P) 4 mg/dL = 40; ionic product is 40
- In renal insufficiency—↓ excretion of P - ↑ level of P in blood—↓ level of calcium -tetany.

Serum Proteins

- Total calcium level is decreased in hypoalbuminemia—for reduction of each 1 g/dL of albumin there will be reduction of 0.8 mg/dL of calcium
- Ionized calcium level will be normal and so no deficiency manifestations will be present.

Alkalosis and Acidosis

- Alkalosis favors binding of more calcium with proteins by lowering of ionized calcium but the total calcium level is normal. Calcium deficiency is manifested
- Acidosis favors ionization of calcium.

Renal Threshold for Calcium

Renal threshold for calcium is 10 mg/dL and calcium gets excreted at this level.

Children

In children the normal calcium level will be near the upper limit and the ionic product of calcium × P = 50 (adult –40).

II. SHORT NOTES

1. Phospholipids.

Definition: They are compound lipids which contain esters of fatty acids with alcohol - glycerol or sphingosine – amino alcohol, nitrogenous base and phosphate group.

Classification of Phospholipids

Glycerophospholipids

They are made up of esters of fatty acid with glycerol, phosphate, and nitrogenous group as functional group. Alcohol is glycerol.

Glycerophospholipids are further classified as:

- **Those containing nitrogen group:** They are lecithin, cephalin, phosphatidylserine
  - **Lecithin** (phosphatidylcholine)—the functional group is choline. It is the most abundant group of phospholipid present in cell membrane. It is the storage form of choline in the body
    - **Dipalmitoyl lecithin**—it has two palmitic acids, it serves as surface active agent and major constituent of lung surfactant preventing adherence of inner surface of lungs in newborn children. Its absence in premature infants causes respiratory distress syndrome
    - **Lysolecithin**—formed by the removal of fatty acid either at C1 or C2 of lecithin.
  - **Cephalin**—phosphatidylethanolamine – found in biomembranes. They are amphipathic
  - **Phosphatidylserine**—functional group is serine.

- **Nonnitrogenous glycerophospholipids**
  - **Phosphatidylinositol**—functional group is inositol. Phosphatidylinositol bisphosphate (PIP2) acts as second messenger in hormonal action
  - **Phosphatidic acid**—is the simplest phospholipid and it is made up of glycerol + 2 fatty acids attached to C1 and 2, and the third OH is esterified to phosphoric acid
  - **Cardiolipin**—diphosphatidylglycerol - it is made up of two phosphatidic acids linked to central glycerol. It is a major lipid of mitochondrial membrane having antigenic property.

Sphingophospholipids

They are made up of esters of fatty acids with sphingosine as the alcohol (FA + Sphingosine = Ceramide)

Example: Sphingomyelin - it is a constituent of myelin sheath of axon.

Functions of Phospholipids

- They are amphipathic in nature
- They are structural components of cell membrane and regulate membrane permeability
- They are structural components of lipoproteins and help in the transport of lipids
- They help in fat absorption in the form of micelle
- They prevent fatty liver by acting as lipotropic factors
- They are helpful in insulating the nerve impulse, e.g. sphingomyelin
- Arachidonic acid liberated from phospholipids serves as a source of synthesis of prostaglandins
- Dipalmitoyl lecithin acts as a lung surfactant to prevent respiratory distress syndrome
- Cephalin participates in blood clotting
- Phosphatidyl inositol is the source of second messengers- inositol trisphosphate and diacylglycerol which are involved in hormonal action.

2. Biotin.

Other name: egg white injury factor

Source

Normal bacterial flora of gut will provide adequate quantities of biotin.

Other sources are liver, yeast, soyabean, eggyolk.

RDA: 200-300 mg

Biochemical Functions

- Biotin acts as co-enzymes for carboxylation reactions.
- CO_2 fixation reactions:
  - Acetyl-CoA carboxylase
  - Acetyl-CoA + CO_2 + ATP $\longrightarrow$ Malonyl CoA + ADP + Pi
  - Propionyl CoA carboxylase
  - Propionyl CoA + CO_2 + ATP $\longrightarrow$ Methylmalonyl CoA + ADP + Pi
  - Pyruvate CoA Carboxylase
  - Pyruvate + CO_2 + ATP $\longrightarrow$ oxaloacetate + ADP + Pi

Deficiency Symptoms

- Dermatitis
- Muscle pain
- Anorexia
- Glossitis.

Treatment

Injection of biotin 100-300 mg.

3. Isoenzymes.

Refer 2003 Short Note 5.

4. Protein-energy malnutrition.

Disorders of malnutrition commonly manifested as protein-energy malnutrition (PEM). There are two major types of malnutritional diseases:

Marasmus: This is due to severe deficiency of both dietary energy and proteins. Primary calorie insufficiency and secondary protein deficiency. Marasmus means to waste.

Kwashiorkor: This is due to isolated deficiency of proteins with Sufficient calorie intake.

Kwashiorkor means sickness the older child gets, when the next child is born.

The differences between these two malnutrition conditions are tabulated.

	Marasmus	Kwashiorkor
Age of onset	Below one year	1-5 years
Deficiency of	Calorie and proteins	Proteins alone
Cause	Early weaning and repeated infection	Starchy diet after weaning. Precipitated by acute infection
Growth retardation of child	Marked	Severe
Attitude	Irritable and fretful	Lethargic and apathetic
Appearance	Shrunken skin and bones, dehydrated	Looks plump due to edema of face and lower limbs
Appetite	Normal	Anorexia
Skin	Dry and atrophic	Crazy pavement dermatitis due to peeling and cracking of skin
Hair	No change	Sparse, soft and thin
Other features	Watery diarrhea, weakness and other nutritional deficiencies	Angular stomatitis, cheilosis, watery diarrhea, muscle wasting
Serum albumin	2-3 g/dL	< 2 g/dL
Serum cortisol	Increased	Decreased

5. Obstructive jaundice (Postheptic jaundice).

This is due to cholestasis or obstruction in the passage of conjugated bilirubin from liver cells to the intestine. The obstruction may be intrahepatic or extrahepatic.

Common Causes of Obstructive Jaundice

- Intrahepatic cholestasis—due to chronic active hepatitis, biliary cirrhosis, lymphomas, obstructive stage of viral hepatitis
- Extrahepatic cholestasis—due to stones in gallbladder or biliary tract, stricture of biliary canaliculi, carcinoma of head of pancreas or enlarged lymph glands pressing on the bile duct.

Biochemical Findings in Obstructive Jaundice

- Increased total bilirubin in serum (normal—0.2-1 mg/dL)
- Conjugated bilirubin is increased in blood and urine (normal 0.2-0.4 mg/dL)
- Increased level of serum alkaline phosphatase enzyme (normal 40-125 IU/L)
- Absence of urobilinogen in urine
- Absence of stercobilinogen in feces—clay colored stools
- Presence of bile salts and bilirubin in urine —dark colored urine.

6. Uncouplers of oxidative phosphorylation.

Refer 2003 Short Notes 4.

- In METC, oxidation and phosphorylation proceed simultaneously. The compounds which uncouple the ETC from oxidative phosphorylation are called uncouplers
- Uncouplers are amphipathic and increase the permeability of the lipid inner mitochondrial membrane to protons, thus reducing the electrochemical potential and short-circuiting the ATP synthase
- Therefore the oxidation can proceed without phosphorylation
- ATP synthesis will not occur and the energy is dissipated as heat
- **Uncouplers** dissociate oxidation in the respiratory chain from phosphorylation.
- These compounds are toxic in vivo, causing respiration to become uncontrolled, since the rate is no longer limited by the concentration of ADP or P_i
- Example: 2,4-dinitrophenol, di-nitrocresol, pentachlorophenol, trifluorocarbonyl cyanide phenylhydrazone (FCCP), chlorocarbonyl cyanide phenylhydrazone (CCCP) and aspirin in high doses
- **Physiological uncouplers:**
  - **Thermogenin (or the uncoupling protein)** is a physiological uncoupler found in brown adipose tissue that functions to generate body heat, particularly for the newborn and during hibernation in animals

- Thyroxin
- Long chain free fatty acid.

7. Absorption of carbohydrates from the intestines.

The digested products of carbohydrates – the monosaccharides mainly glucose/galactose are absorbed from the lumen of duodenum and upper jejunum. Hexoses are absorbed more rapidly and galactose is absorbed more efficiently.

Absorption occurs by 2 mechanisms:
1. Active transport against concentration gradient – requires energy
2. Facilitated transport with concentration gradient.

a. **Active transport against concentration gradient (from low glucose concentration to higher concentration) SGLUT-1 and 2:**
   - This requires energy, specific transport proteins and sodium ions
   - It is a co-transport or symport mechanism
   - Absorption of glucose is carried through sodium dependent glucose transporter-1 (SGLUT-1) which is specific to intestine and SGLUT-2 which is specific to kidney
   - Energy is provided by the hydrolysis of ATP linked to sodium pump. By this Na^+ is expelled from the cell in exchange of K^+. So energy is needed indirectly
   - This principle is applied in common treatment for diarrhea by **oral rehydration fluid** which **contains glucose and sodium**. Presence of glucose in fluid allows uptake of sodium to replenish body NaCl
   - Active transport is inhibited by the cardiac glycoside—ouabain which inhibits sodium pump and phlorizin which inhibits reabsorption of glucose in kidney tubules.

b. **Facilitated bidirectional transport with concentration gradient (GLUT):**
   - Glucose is transported by this mechanism by various glucose transporters— Types 1, 2, 3, 4, 5, and 7
   - GLUT1 is the most common transporter in brain, kidney, colon, placenta, retina and RBCs
   - Type 2 (GLUT2) (**Fig. 7**) is an uniport and the delivery is by ping pong mechanism by the inversion of the transporter into the inner side of membrane–found in liver, beta cells of pancreas–glucose sensors, low affinity for glucose but high K_m for glucose
   - Type 3 (GLUT3)—high affinity for glucose present in neurons, brain, kidney
   - Type 4 (GLUT4) (**Fig. 8**)—major transporter in skeletal muscle. Heart muscle and adipose tissues. It is the only transporter **under the control of insulin**
   - In type II diabetes mellitus there is reduction in membrane GLUT4 to produce insulin resistance in muscle cells and adipocytes

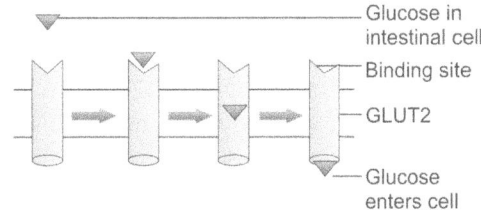

Fig. 7: GLUT2.

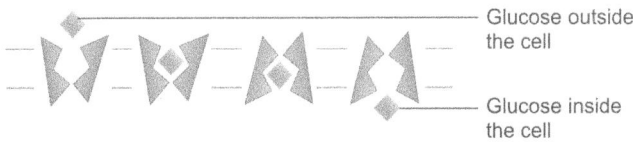

Fig. 8: GLUT4.

- GLUT5 – in intestines, testes, sperms and kidney – specific for fructose and mannose.

8. Structure of hemoglobin.

- The adult hemoglobin is represented as HbA
- It is made up of 2 alpha chains and 2 beta chains and each polypeptide contains a non-protein part/prosthetic group called heme.

Other Forms

- Fetal Hb (HbF)—made up of 2 alpha and 2 gamma chains
- HbA2 (adult Hb)—made up of 2 alpha and 2 delta chains
- Normal adult blood contains 97% HbA, 2% HbA2 and 1% HbF
- Molecular weight 67KD
- Each alpha chain has 141 amino acids and each beta and gamma and delta chains have 146 amino acids
- There are 36 histidine residues in Hb, these are important in buffering action
- The 58th histidine residue in alpha chain is called distal histidine
- The 87th histidine residue is called proximal histidine
- The alpha and beta/delta polypeptide chains are connected by relatively weak noncovalent bonds like vander walls forces, hydrogen bonds and electrostatic forces.

Assembling of heme with globin and its functions

- There are total four heme molecules in one Hb
- Heme is a cyclic molecule made up of 4 pyrrole rings and ferrous iron with its center
- Ferrous iron has 6 valences. Ferrous iron is oxidized to ferric form
- This ferrous iron linked to pyrrole nitrogen by 4 co-ordinate valancy bonds and fifth one is attached to imidazole nitrogen of the proximal histidine of polypeptide chain. The 6th valence is bound to O_2 and it oxidized to ferric form of Hb.

9. Bile salts—synthesis and biological role.

- Bile salts are derivatives of cholesterol
- Cholesterol is catabolized to bile acids and salts, vitamin D and sex and steroid hormones.

Bile Acids and Bile Salts

- **Primary bile acid:** Cholic acid and chenodeoxycholic acids-synthesised in liver
- **Secondary bile acids:** Lithocholic acid and deoxycholic acid. They are derived from primary bile acids in intestines by deconjugation and 7α dehydroxylations
- **Bile salts are** the conjugated Na and potassium salts of bile acids.

Synthesis of Bile Acids/Bile Salts

Bile acids are synthesised in the liver form cholesterol. They contain 24 carbon atoms.

Steps

- Cholesterol is hydroxylated at 7th position by **7 α-hydroxylase** enzyme which is **the rate limiting enzyme** which needs NADPH and vitamin C and converted into 7 α-hydroxycholesterol
- This in turn is acted by 12 α-hydroxylase with the addition of CoASH in the presence of NADPH to form Cholyl-CoA and chenodeoxycholyl-CoA with the removal of 3C propionate. This forms 24 carbon cholic acid or chenodeoxycholic acid—primary bile acids with the removal of CoASH
- The so formed 24C bile acids conjugated with glycine/taurine to produce glycocholicacid or taurocholicacid and glycochenodeoxycholic acid/taurochenodeoxycholic acid
- These primary bile acids are converted to secondary bile acids by intestinal bacteria by deconjugation and 7α dehydroxylation to form deoxycoholic acid and lithocholic acid respectively
- **Bile salts:** They are the sodium or potassium salts of primary and secondary bile acids.

Biological Role of Bile Salts

- They facilitate the lipid digestion
- They act as detergent in the formation of lipid micelle
- They emulsify the lipids into droplets to form mixed micelles and thereby increase the surface area of the particles and lower the surface tension
- Micelle formation helps in absorption of lipids.

10. Vitamin E.

It is a fat soluble vitamin.

Other names: Alpha Tocopherol (tokos-childbirth; pheros- to bear; ol-alcholol) or anti-infertility vitamin, anti-sterility vitamin, antioxidant vitamin.

- α-tocopherol is the active form of **vitamin E**
- **Normal level in blood: 0.5-1 mg/dL.**
- **RDA:**
  - Males – 10 mg/day
  - Females – 8 mg/day.
- **Sources:** Vegetable oils (wheat germ oil, sunflower oil, safflower oil, cotton seed oil)
- **RDA:** I mg = 1.5 IU
  - RDA of this vitamin is linearly with the consumption of PUFA
  - Men = 10 mg/15 IU, Women = 8 mg/12 IU.
- **Structure:** It is made up of 6-hydroxychromane ring and 3-isoprenoid units.

This vitamin is of 3 types:
1. Alpha-tocopherol – 5, 7, 8 – tri-methyltocol
2. Beta-tocopherol – 5, 8 – di-methyltocol
3. Gama-tocopherol – 7, 8 – di-methyltocol.

Absorption

- Since it is a fat soluble vitamin, it needs bile salts for absorption
- It is transported as chylomicron. It is stored in adipose tissue.

Biochemical Role

It is natural antioxidant. This vitamin is found at cell membranes, fat deposits and it self oxidized to quinone form by oxidants (free radicals-O_2^-, H_2O_2, OH^-, etc. and spares the others form oxidation such as unsaturated fatty acids, other vitamins, and other essential biomolecules.

Other Functions

- **Antioxidant**—most powerful natural-chain breaking antioxidant
- It protects RBC from hemolysis and also keeps the integrity of all cells
- It prevents peroxidation of PUFA
- It protects the germinal epithelium of gonads and prevents sterility
- It is involved in storage of creatine in muscle
- It is involved in amino acid absorption
- It protects the other vitamins from oxidation
- It boosts immune response
- It reduces premature aging
- It reduces the risk of atherosclerosis by reducing oxidation of LDL
- **Inter-relationship with selenium:** Both selenium and vitamin E act synergistically to minimize lipid peroxidation. Selenium spares the requirement of vitamin E and vice versa.

Deficiency

- Increased fragility of RBC
- Muscular dystrophy
- Weakness of muscles and creatinuria.

11. Alkaptonuria.

Alkaptonuria

- It is an inborn error of metabolism in the metabolism of tyrosine/phenylalanine
- It is an autosomal recessive condition affecting 1:250,000 births
- It is due to the defect in homogentisate oxidase enzyme

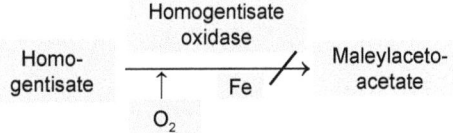

- Homogentisate gets accumulated and oxidized to benzoquinone acetate and forms alkaptone bodies
- Alkaptone bodies get deposited in intervertebral discs, cartilages of nose and pinna of ear developing ochronosis. Black pigments get deposited over joint cavities causing arthritis
- Urine turns black on standing. $FeCl_3$ test is positive. Benedict's test is strongly positive since homogentisate is a reducing agent
- Generally it is a harmless condition.

12. Transfer RNA (Fig. 9).

Transfer RNA or soluble RNA is a type of RNA
- It shows extensive internal base pairing
- It has clover leaf-like structure
- It contains unusual bases. They are dihydrouracil (DHU), pseudouridine (Ψ) and hypoxanthine. Many bases are methylated
- It acts as an adapter molecule in carrying a specific amino acid for a particular codon in mRNA and helps in protein synthesis – translation
- It has an acceptor arm, anticodon arm, DHU arm and pseudouridine arm
  - **Acceptor arm is at 3′ end:** It carries the amino acids. It has seven base pairs. The end sequence is CCA-3′. The 3′ end hydroxyl group is bonded with carboxyl end of amino acids
  - **Anticodon arm of tRNA:** It is present at the opposite side of acceptor arm. It recognizes the triplet nucleotide codon present in mRNA
  - **DHU arm of tRNA:** It contains dihydrouridine. DHU arm serves as the recognition site for enzymes
  - **Pseudouridine arm of tRNA:** It contains pseudouridine and it is involved in binding tRNA to ribosomes.

Function of tRNA

- tRNA has got a major role in translation (protein synthesis)
- The tRNA molecules carry the specific amino acid at the CCA-3′ end of the acceptor arm. There are about 20 tRNA molecules available, one specific for each amino acid
- The three nucleotide base sequences at the anticodon arm of the tRNA recognize the corresponding complimentary codons in the mRNA to form base pairs to continue the protein synthesis.

13. Metabolism of zinc.

- Total zinc content of body is 2 g, out of which 60% is in skeletal muscle and 30% in bones
- In liver, zinc is stored in combination with a specific protein, metallothionein
- More than 300 enzymes are zinc dependent
  - Example: Carboxypeptidase—cleaves C-terminal ends of dietary proteins
  - Carbonic anhydrase—$H^+ + HCO_3^- \rightarrow H_2CO_3 \rightarrow H_2O + O_2$
  - Alkaline phosphatase—needed for bone formation
  - Lactate dehydrogenase—pyruvate to lactate
  - Glutamate dehydrogenase—deamination process.

Functions of Zinc

- It is a component of RNA polymerase. It is also needed for protein synthesis
- Superoxide dismutase contains zn, which is an antioxidant enzyme and so zinc is also an antioxidant

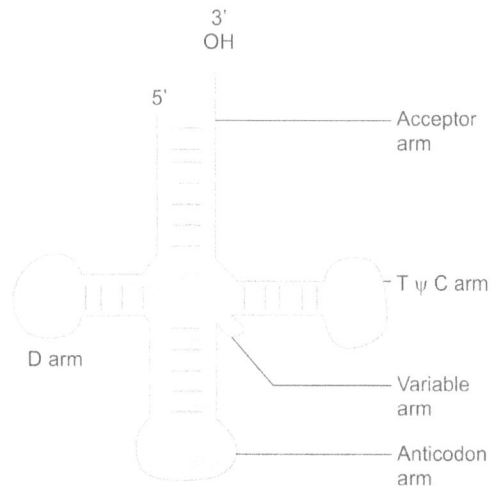

Fig. 9: Transfer RNA.

- Zinc stabilizes insulin. Insulin when stored in beta cells of pancreas contains zinc, which stabilizes the hormone
- Gusten is a salivary protein which contains zinc. It is needed for taste sensation.

14. Detoxication by conjugation.

- It is the second phases of detoxification of xenobiotics which is also known as biotransformation
- Here the toxic foreign substances are made to less harmful, water soluble substances and get excreted from the body.

Detoxification by Conjugation

- A xenobiotic which undergoes phase 1 reaction has become a new metabolite which contains chemical groups like hydroxyl (OH), amino (NH_2) and carboxyl (COOH) groups
- Phase 2 reactions are **conjugation reactions** - addition of **conjugating agents** like: glucuronic acid, glutathione, glutamine, glycine, cysteine, acetylation – CH_3 – acetyl-CoA, methylation – CH_3, S-adenosylmethionine (SAM) and sulfation – SO^{4-} PAPS
- **Conjugation by glucuronic acid:** The most common phase II reaction
  - Active glucuronide – UDP glucuronide by UDP-glucuronyltransferase in ER. It is induced by barbiturates
  UDP–glucuronyl transferase
  - UDP glucuronic acid + R-OH ⟶ UDP + R - Glucuronide
  - Unconjugated bilirubin is conjugated with glucuronic acid to form bilirubin diglucuronide in liver and excreted through bile.
- **Conjugation by glutathione (GSH):** Glutathione is a tripeptide containing glycine, cysteine and glutamic acid. It conjugates aliphatic halides, aromatic nitro compounds, halogenated compounds and epoxides formed in Phase I reactions and detoxify them. In the body it is done by the enzyme glutathione S-transferase.
  Glutathione S-transferase
  Xenobiotics + G-SH ⟶ X-S-G

- **Conjugation with glutamine:** In phenylalanine metabolism, phenyl acetic acid is conjugated with glutamine to form phenylacetylglutamine which is excreted in urine
- **Conjugation with glycine:** Aromatic carboxylic acids are conjugated with glycine
  - Example: Benzoic acid is conjugated with glycine to form hippuric acid
  - **Bile acids:** Cholic acid is conjugated with glycine to form glycocholic acid and deoxycholic acid is conjugated to deoxyglycocholic acid.
- **Conjugation with cysteine:** Cysteine is first acetylated to form acetyl cysteine which gets conjugated with toxic substances like chlorobenzene, bromobenzene, naphthalene and other compounds to nontoxic mercapturic acid. Example: Bromobenzene + Cysteine + Acetic acid Bromophenyl mercapturic acid.
- **Conjugation with acetic acid: (Acetylation):** Acetic acid is conjugated to compounds with amino group by the enzyme acetyl transferase
  - Some drugs like sulfanilamide, INH (isoniazide) and PABA are acetylated before excretion.
- **Conjugation by methylation:**
  - S-adenosyl methionine is the active methyl donor
  - The reaction is catalysed by the enzyme methyl transferase
  - Example:
    - Nicotinic acid and thyroxine – N–methylated
    - Estrogens – O-methylated
    - Epinephrine and norepinephrine – are methylated at phenolic hydroxyl group.
- **Conjugation by sulfation (with active sulphate):**
  - Phosphoadenosine phosphosulphate (PAPS) is the active sulphate formed by the addition of ATP with sulphates
  - Sulphotransferase enzyme transfers sulfate group from PAPS to the OH of

phenol, cresol, steroids or to NH_2 of aliphatic amines to form etheral sulphate.

15. Salvage pathway of purine synthesis.

- Routinely purine nucleotides are synthesised by De Novo synthetic pathway
- Purine salvage pathway recycles the purines and make it available for nucleic acid synthesis.

Purine Salvage Pathway

- PRPP is the starting material and it is also a substrate for de novo synthesis of purines. So these 2 pathways are interlinked
- There are 2 enzymes involved in salvage pathways:
  1. Adenine phosphoribosyltransferase (APRTase)
  2. Hypozanthine guanine phosphoribosyltranferase(HGPRTase).
- Adenine is converted to AMP using PRPP by adenine phosphoribosyltransferase
- Guanine is converted to GMP and hypoxanthine is converted to IMP using PRPP by hypoxanthine guanine phosphoribosyl transferase
- The salvage pathway is important for RBC and brain since De novo synthesis of purine nucleotides are not operative in these areas
- A defect in HGPRTase will lead to Lesch-Nyhan syndrome.

Adenine + PRPP $\xrightarrow{APRTase}$ AMP + PPi

Guanine + PRPP $\xrightarrow{HGPRTase}$ GMP + PPi

Hypoxanthine + PRPP $\xrightarrow{HGPRTase}$ IMP + PPi

Lesch-Nyhan Syndrome

- It is an X-linked inborn error of purine metabolism, incidence 1:10,000
- It is due to the complete deficiency of HGPRTase which is an enzyme of salvage pathway
- So the salvage pathway is stopped and PRPP accumulates which will go for increased purine synthesis and catabolism of purines to uric acid
- Hyperuricemia leads to nephrolithiasis and gout in later life
- It is also characterized by self-mutilation and mental retardation.

16. Metabolic acidosis.

- Acidosis is reduction of pH less than 7.38. It is classified into metabolic and respiratory acidosis
- Metabolic acidosis is primarily due to base deficit. The bicarbonate deficit may occur due to excess acid production or depletion of bicarbonate
- **Anion gap**: It is difference between measured cations and measured anions. Usually it shows the unmeasured anions. **The normal value is 12 mmol/L**
- Anion gap is calculated as the difference between $(Na^+ + K^+)$ and $(HCO_3^- + Cl^-)$
- Decreased anion gap is seen in hypoalbuminemia, multiple myeloma.

Metabolic acidosis is classified into

- **High anion gap metabolic acidosis (HAGMA)** accumulation of acid anions
  - Due to accumulation of acid anions - value between 15 and 20
  - **Causes**:
    - Renal failure H^+ excretion is less.
    - Diabetic ketoacidosis—ketoacid production is more acetoacetate and beta hydroxybutyrate
    - Lactic acidosis—hypoxia, circulatory failure, many drugs, and bacterial metabolism increase lactic acid. Methanol, ethanol also cause lactic acidosis.
- **Normal anion gap metabolic acidosis (NAGMA)**
  - Loss of both anions and cations, the anion gap is normal, but acidosis may prevail
  - **Causes:**
    - Diarrhea—loss of bicarbonate and cations—Na or K or both from intestinal secretions
    - Hyperchloremic metabolic acidosis in renal tubular acidosis, acetazolamide therapy and ureteric transplantation into large gut.

- **Metabolic acidosis is compensated by**
  - Respiratory compensation hyperventilation so that pCO_2 comes down. There will be Kussmaul respiration, low pH, bicarbonate will be low. pCO_2 starts decreasing due to respiratory compensation
  - Renal compensation—increased excretion of acid and conservation of base occurs. This sets within 2 to 4 days
  - Associated hyperkalemia is seen commonly due to distribution of K^+ and H^+.

Clinical Features

- Hyperventilation
- Kussmaul respiration
- Depressed myocardial contractility.

Treatment

- To stop production of acid by giving IV fluids and insulin
- Oxygen to be given to patients with lactic acidosis
- Potassium level to be monitored
- Required bicarbonate should be given by intravenous route.

17. Tumor markers.

Definition: They are also known as tumor index substances.

- They are the biological substances synthesised and released by cancer cells.
- They are found in an increased level in blood and other body fluids and tissues
- Tumor markers are substances whose presence or elevation in body is used to identify or confirm the presence or to monitor the prognosis of the cancer.

Uses of Tumor Markers

- Detection and diagnosis of cancer
- To assess the prognosis—whether curable or not
- To monitor the treatment effectivity and follow-up
- Localize the tumor by using radiolabelled antibodies.

Types of Tumor Markers

- Oncofetal antigens
- Carbohydrate markers
- Enzymes
- Hormones
- Serum proteins
- Catabolic product.

Oncofetal Antigens

- Proteins produced in fetal life which may be decreased or absent in blood after birth
- They reappear in cancer patients because of reactivation of the genes of the protein by transformation
- **Examples:**
  - Alpha fetoprotein
  - Hepatoma, germ cell tumors
  - Carcinoembryogenic antigen
  - Colorectal and GI tumors.

Carbohydrate Markers

- They are either antigens on the tumor cell surface or secreted by tumor cells
- High molecular weight glycoproteins - abbreviated as carbohydrate antigen (CA)
- **Example:** CA 12—increased in ovarian cancer.

Enzymes

- Enzymes are present in high concentration inside the cells and released into circulation due to tumor necrosis
- This also leads to tumor metastasis
- **Examples:**
  - Alkaline phosphatase
  - Bone secondaries, liver secondaries
  - Prostatic acid phosphatase
  - Prostate cancer
  - Prostate specific antigen
  - Prostate cancer
  - Neuron specific enolase
  - Nervous system tumors.

Hormones

- Endocrine tissues which produce hormones in normal conditions will produce the hormones in excess during certain neoplastic conditions

- Nonendocrine tissues which are situated away from the endocrine sites will produce the hormone in excess—ectopic syndrome
- **Examples:**
  - Human Beta hCG
  - Choriocarcinoma
  - Calcitonin
  - Medullary Ca of thyroid
  - Big ACTH
  - Lung oat cell cancer
  - Vasoactive intestinal polypeptide (VIP)
  - APUDomas
  - Vanillylmandelic acid (VMA)
  - Phaeochromocytoma, neuroblastoma.

Serum Proteins
- **Examples:**
  - Immunoglobulins (Ig)
  - Multiple myeloma, macrogobulinemia
  - Bence-Jones proteins in urine
  - Multiple myeloma.

Catabolic Product
Hydroxyproline—bone metastasis.

18. Clearance tests.

- Measurement of clearance is a test for glomerular filtration rate (GFR)
- It provides most useful general index for the assessment of the severity of the renal damage
- A decrease in renal function is assumed due to the loss of functional nephrons, rather than decrease in the function of individual nephrons
- Normal GFR for young adults is 120—130 mL/min/1.73 m^2
- **Clearance tests**: Done to assess the glomerular filtration and renal blood flow
- Renal clearance of a substance is the volume of plasma from which the substance is completely cleared by the kidney in 1 minute
- **Clearance** = mg of substance excreted per min/mg of substance per ml of plasma
  - $C = U \times V/P$
  - C = Clearance of the substance
  - U = Concentration of the substance in urine
  - P = Concentration of the substance in plasma
  - V = Volume of urine passed per minute.
- Clearance is expressed as milliliter of plasma per unit time
- **Clearance tests:** These tests are done by using either endogenous markers such as urea or creatinine or exogenous markers like Inulin, ^{51}Cr-labelled EDTA, ^{99}Tec-labelled EDTA, etc.
- Out of all creatinine clearance test is the best
- **Creatinine clearance test**: It is based on the rate of excretion of metabolically produced creatinine which is excreted through urine
  - Creatinine is freely filtered by the glomeruli but not reabsorbed by the tubules. A small amount of creatinine is secreted by the tubules
  - 24 hours urine is collected and blood is also collected for estimation of creatinine. Urinary volume is measured (V) and the concentration of creatinine in urine (U) and plasma (P) are estimated and by using the formula $C = U \times V/P$ the creatinine clearance is calculated
  - Normal range for creatinine clearance is 90–120 mL/min
  - Reduced creatinine clearance indicates chronic renal damage and reduced blood flow to glomeruli
  - Urea clearance is the ml of blood which is cleared of urea per minute. Patient is asked to empty the bladder and 200 ml of water is given to drink. After one hour the volume of voided urine is measured, blood urea and urine urea are estimated.
  - Urea clearance = UV/P (where U = mg of urea/ml of urine, P = mg of urea/ml of plasma, v = volume of urine excreted)
  - Normal value is about 75 mL/min
  - Values below that shows a deteriorating renal function (progression to renal failure).

19. Lac operon (Fig. 10).

- Operon is a unit of gene expression mainly in prokaryotes. It was introduced by Jacob and Monod
- In prokaryotes the genes involved in a metabolic pathway are called as operons
- **Lac operon** (Lactose operon): This explains the gene expression in lactose metabolism in *E. coli*
- It includes:
  - Regulatory gene (lac I—for inhibition)
  - Operator gene (O)
  - Three structural genes—Z, Y, A
  - Promoter site (P) next to operator gene and
  - Control elements.
- In the bacterial cell the structural genes – (Z, Y, A)
  - **Z gene** encodes for the enzyme beta-galactosidase which hydrolyses lactose to galactose and glucose
  - **Y gene** is responsible for the production of galactose permeases which transports galactose and lactose into the cell
  - **A gene** codes for the thiogalactoside transacetylase.
- The transcription of these genes start from common promoter (p), located close to Z gene
- The RNA polymerase binds to the promoter and transcribes the three structural genes as single mRNA
- Regulation of lac operon is explained by the concept of induction, repression, derepression, positive regulator under 3 mechanisms.

20. Cytochrome P450 (Fig. 11).

- During Phase I reactions of detoxification, reactions are involved with oxidation by hydroxylase enzymes present in endoplasmic reticulum. There are 150 isoforms. They are monooxygenases – cytochrome P450. They are mixed function oxidases containing hemre. NADPH is its coenzyme
  $RH + O_2 + NADPH \rightarrow ROH + H_2O + NADP^+$
- They are inducible enzymes. Phenobarbital - ↑ their activity. It is involved in metabolism of drugs and aromatic hydrocarbon
- Mitochondrial P450 enzymes present in mitochondria and microsomal P450 system is involved in steroid synthesis in adrenal cortex
- Cytochromes P450 are an important superfamily of heme-containing monooxygenases
- These enzymes are present in the endoplasmic reticulum of liver and intestine – (microsomal) and in the mitochondria in other tissues (mitochondrial)
- In the cytochromes of electron transport chain, NADH and NADPH are involved in donation of reducing equivalents to cytochrome P450 through two types of reactions—Class I and Class II systems
  1. Class I system has FAD containing reductase enzyme and P450 heme protein.
  2. Class II system has cytochrome reductase which passes electrons from $FADH_2$ to FMN
- Finally electrons from cytochrome P-450 are accepted by oxygen leading to

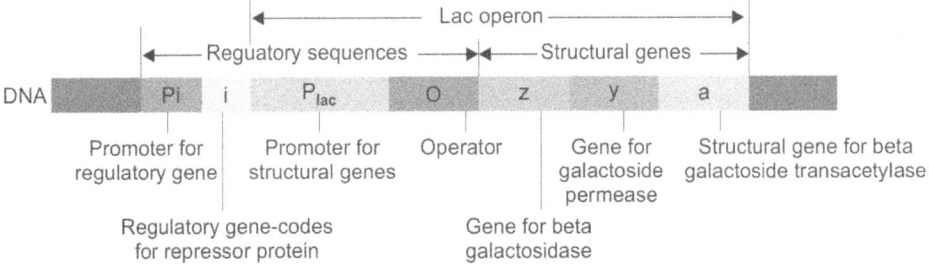

Fig. 10: Lac operon.

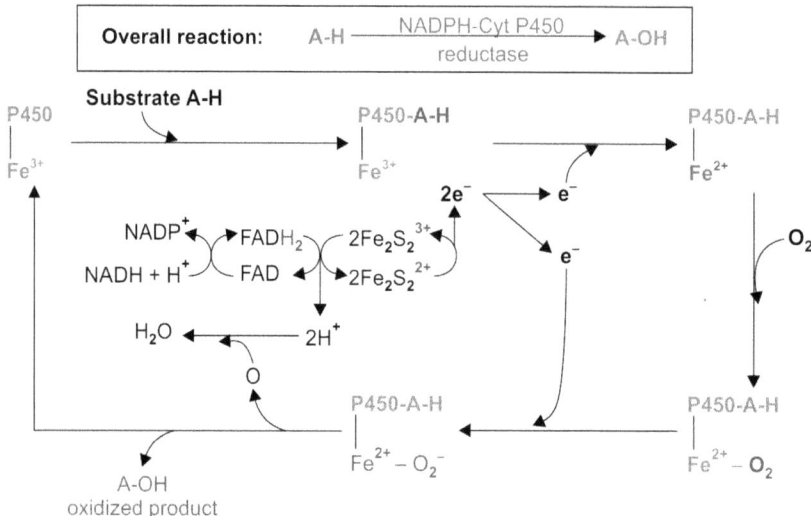

Fig. 11: Mechanism of detoxification by vytochrome P450.

hydroxylation. These series of reactions are known as hydroxylase cycle
- In liver endoplasmic reticulum, another heme containing protein called cytochrome b_5 acts along with cytochrome P450 and is involved in drug metabolism and detoxification
- Example for hydroxylation of drugs—aminopyrine, aniline, morphine, benzpyrene and benzphetamine
- Many drugs induce the synthesis of cytochrome P450 enzyme, e.g. phenobarbitone
- The steps of detoxification of compounds is given in the **Figure 11**.

MBBS Examination 2005

ANSWER ALL QUESTIONS

I. Essay questions (10 Marks each)

1. What is enzyme inhibition? Describe different kinds of enzyme inhibitions with example.
2. Describe in detail the synthesis and utilization of ketone bodies. Name any three conditions of increased production of ketone bodies and mention laboratory evaluation of ketoacidosis.
3. Describe the metabolism of phenylalanine in the body and discuss the inborn errors of metabolism.
4. What is the normal pH of blood? Explain the various mechanisms by which the normal pH of the blood is maintained.
5. What are the sources, properties, functions, deficiency manifestation and RDA for ascorbic acid?
6. What is the normal fasting and post prandial blood glucose level? Explain how normal blood glucose level is maintained. Add a note on the disruption of hormonal regulation of blood glucose.
7. Why ammonia is toxic to the body? What are the ways by which ammonia is disposed in the body? Add a note on hyperammonemia conditions.
8. What is the normal serum calcium level? Explain how serum calcium is maintained. Name the hypocalemia conditions.

II. Short notes (5 Marks each)

1. Lipoproteins and their functions.
2. Significance of HMP shunt pathway.
3. Synthesis and conjugation of bilirubin.
4. Sources of acetyl-CoA and fate of acetyl-CoA.
5. Functions and deficiency of vitamin A.
6. Isoenzymes and their diagnostic importance.
7. Galactosemia.
8. Cyclic AMP.
9. Recommended daily dietary allowance.
10. Essential fatty acids.
11. Role of vitamin D in calcium metabolism.
12. Iron.
13. Prostaglandins.
14. Ketone bodies.
15. Degeneracy of code.
16. Detoxification.
17. Gout.
18. Antioxidants.
19. Genetic code.
20. Proto-oncogenes and oncogenes.
21. Allosteric enzymes and its feedback regulation.
22. Phospholipids and their clinical importance.
23. Kwashiorkor.
24. Inhibitors of electron transport chain.
25. Diagnostic value of isoenzymes.
26. Basal metabolic rate (BMR).
27. Fatty acid synthesis.
28. Heme degradation (bilirubin synthesis).
29. Eicosanoids.
30. LDL metabolism.
31. Synthetic nucleotides and their importance.
32. Liver function tests.
33. Anion gap and its diagnostic importance.

34. Tumor markers.
35. Salvage pathways.
36. Mechanism of action of thyroid hormones.
37. Detoxification by hydroxylation.
38. Blotting techniques.
39. Glutathione—role in amino acid transport.
40. Essential amino acids.

I. ESSAY QUESTIONS

1. **What is enzyme inhibition? Describe different kinds of enzyme inhibitions with example.**

- Enzyme inhibition is one of the factors influencing enzyme activity
- Enzyme inhibitors are organic or inorganic substances which can bind reversibly or irreversibly with the enzymes and alter the catalytic activity of the enzyme, e.g. drugs, toxins, etc.

Reversible Inhibition

In this type, the inhibitors bind noncovalently with the enzymes and the inhibition will be reversed when the inhibitors are removed.

This type is further divided into:
- **Competitive inhibitors (substrate analogue inhibitors):**
  - Usually they are structural analogue of the substance
  - They bind and compete to the substrate binding site of the enzyme forming an enzyme inhibitory (EI) complex
  - K_m value is increased but no change in V_{max}
  - Example: Competitive inhibition of succinate dehydrogenase by malonate which resembles succinate (TCA cycle)
  - Many drugs act as competitive inhibitors, e.g. sulphonamide is an analogue of PABA and inhibits pteroid synthetase in the folic acid synthesis
  - Allopurinol inhibits xanthine oxidase.
- **Noncompetitive reversible inhibitors:**
  - These inhibitors are structurally different from the substrate. So they bind on the enzyme molecule other than the substrate binding site. There is no competition between inhibitor and substrate
  - V_{max} is reduced, K_m is not altered
  - The enzyme reaction is slowed but not stopped
  - Example: Heavy metal poisoning inhibiting enzyme.
- **Uncompetitive inhibitors:** Rare
  - They can bind only to enzyme substrate (ES) complex but not to free enzyme
  - They decrease both V_{max} and K_m.

Irreversible Inhibitors

- They bind with enzyme tightly by covalent bonds and form stable complex
- It is irreversible
- Example: Iodoacetate—irreversible inhibitor of glyceraldehyde 3P dehydrogenase (glycolysis)
- **Suicide inhibition**: Here the original inhibition is converted to a more potent form by the same enzyme and inhibits the reaction
- Example: Aspirin inhibits cyclo-oxygenase of prostaglandin synthesis.

Allosteric Inhibition

- Allosteric enzyme has one catalytic site where the substrate binds and there is an allosteric site where the positive or negative modifier binds
- Greek: Allo = Other, e.g. Phosphofructokinase
- The inhibitor is not a substrate analog
- K_m is increased but V_{max} is reduced, e.g. aspartate transcarbamoylase
- If the regulatory molecule enhance the activity of the enzyme it is known as positive modulator and if it inhibits the enzyme activity it is known as negative modulator

- Allosteric regulators are divided into two classes based on the influence of allosteric effector on K_m and V_{max}.

2. **Describe in detail the synthesis and utilization of ketone bodies. Name any three conditions of increased production of ketone bodies and mention laboratory evaluation of ketoacidosis (Fig. 1).**

- The ketone bodies (KB) are three in number, namely—**acetoacetate, β-hydroxybutyrate and acetone**. Acetoacetate is primary ketone bodies and the other 2 are secondary ketone bodies
- Acetyl-CoA formed from fatty acids can enter and get oxidized in TCA cycle only when carbohydrates are available. During starvation and in uncontrolled diabetes mellitus, the acetyl-CoA takes the alternate fate of formation of ketone bodies
- Level of KB in blood is **less than 1 mg/dL**
- **Site of formation:** Liver-mitochondrial matrix of liver cells
- **Site of utilization of KB:** Extrahepatic tissues
- **Uses:** During starvation, it is the major fuel for brain, heart and muscles. Brain gets 75% of energy from KB during starvation
- **Precursor:** Acetyl-CoA.

Synthesis of Ketone Bodies (Ketogenesis) (Fig. 1)

Reactions

- **Condensation:** Two molecules of acetyl-CoA condense to form acetoacetyl-CoA, this reaction is catabolized by thiolase
- **Production of HMG-CoA:** Acetoacetyl-CoA condenses with another molecule of acetyl-CoA to produce β-hydroxy-β-methylglutaryl-CoA (HMG-CoA) by the enzyme HMG-CoA synthase. This is the key regulatory enzyme of ketogenesis
- **Lyase reaction:** HMG-CoA is cleaved to acetoacetate and acetyl-CoA by the action of HMG-CoA lyase present only in liver
- **Reduction and spontaneous decarboxylation:** Acetoacetate is reduced by dehydrogenase to β-hydroxybutyrate in the presence of NADH or it undergoes spontaneous decarboxylation to form acetone.

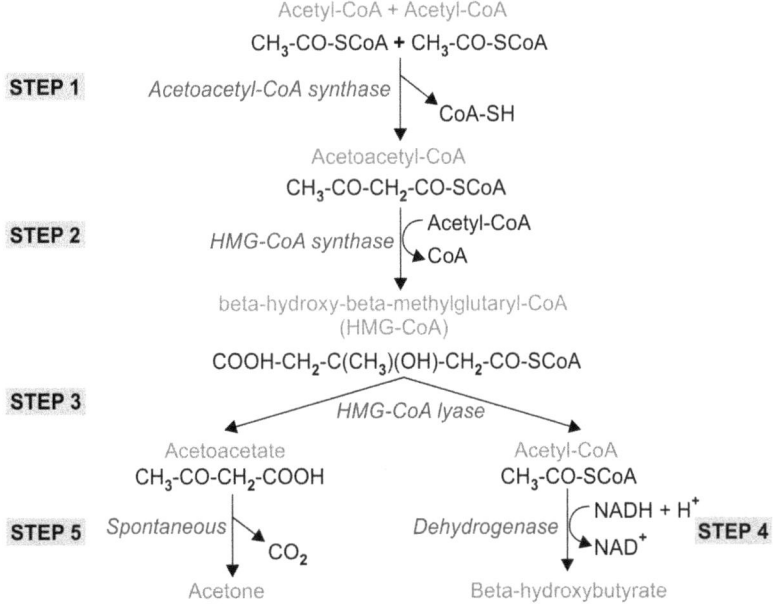

Fig. 1: Synthesis of ketone bodies.

Utilization of ketone bodies: Ketone body utilization takes place in extrahepatic tissues for energy production. Tissues like heart, renal cortex, prefer ketone bodies than glucose for energy production.

Ketolysis Reactions

Acetoacetate is activated to acetoacetyl-CoA by thiophorase enzyme
1. Acetoacetate + succinyl-CoA → acetoacetyl-CoA + succinate
2. Then acetoacetyl-CoA enters into beta-oxidation pathway to produce energy.

Conditions which lead to elevated ketone bodies (Ketosis)

- Diabetic ketoacidosis
- Prolonged fasting
- Muscle wasting diseases.

When the blood level of ketone bodies is more than 1 mg/dL that will lead to ketonemia, ketonuria—excretion of KB in urine and smell of acetone in breath.

Features of Ketosis

- Metabolic acidosis
- Kussmaul's respiration—acidotic breathing due to compensatory hyperventilation
- Breath—smells of acetone
- Osmotic diuresis
- Dehydration
- Sodium loss
- Coma.

Laboratory Evaluation of Ketoacidosis

Ketone bodies appear in urine under pathological conditions, such as uncontrolled diabetes mellitus, persistent vomiting, von Gierke disease. The major ketone bodies are three—acetoacetic acid, beta-hydroxybutyric acid and acetone.

Ketone bodies in urine are analyzed by Rothera's test, rapid tests, such as ketostix strips and acetest tablets.

Rothera's Test

Principle: Freshly prepared sodium nitroprusside reacts with ketone bodies and form a purple colored ferropentacyanide complex. This test is specific for acetoacetate and beta-hydroxybutyrate.

Procedure: 5 mL of urine is saturated with solid ammonium sulphate. 3 drops of sodium nitroprusside is added and then strong ammonia is poured along the sides of the tube to get a purple ring.

3. Describe the metabolism of phenylalanine in the body and discuss the inborn errors of metabolism (Figs. 2 and 3).

METABOLISM OF PHENYLALANINE

Phenylalanine is an essential aromatic amino acid. It is partly glucogenic and partly ketogenic.

Major Catabolic Pathway of Phenylalanine

Conversion of Phenylalanine to Tyrosine by Hydroxylation (Fig. 2)

Phenylalanine hydroxylase enzyme hydroxylates. Phenylalanine to tyrosine in the presence of the cofactor tetrahydrobiopterin, and coenzymes—NADPH and NADH. It is an irreversible reaction. Further tyrosine is catabolized by various steps to form fumarate (glucogenic pathway) and acetoacetate (ketogenic pathway).

Tyrosine is an aromatic amino acid. It is synthesized from phenylalanine. It is both glucogenic and ketogenic.

Catabolism of Tyrosine (Fig. 3)

Step 1: Transamination: Tyrosine is transaminated by tyrosine transaminase using PLP and alpha-ketoglutarate to form p-hydroxyphenylpyruvate and glutamic acid. This step is induced by glucocorticoids.

Step 2: Synthesis of homogentisic acid: (Dihydroxyphenyl acetate) p-hydroxyphenylpyruvate is converted to homogentisate by hydroxylase enzyme. It is a copper containing enzyme. Ascorbic acid is required for this reaction.

Step 3: Formation of maleylacetoacetate: By the cleavage of aromatic ring homogentisate is converted to maleylacetoacetate by a dioxygenase called homogentisate oxidase which contains an iron atom at its active site

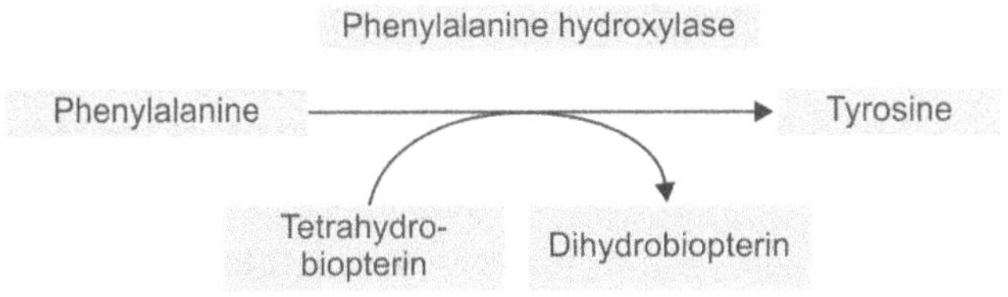

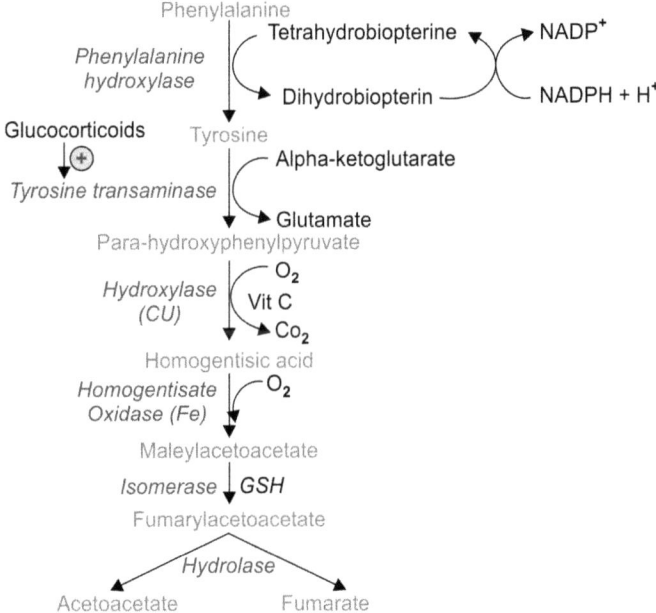

Fig. 2: Phenylalanine hydroxylation.

Fig. 3: Catabolism of tyrosine.

Step 4: Isomerization of maleyl- to fumaryl-acetoacetate: Maleylacetoacetate is converted to its isomer fumarylacetoacetate by isomerase using glutathione (GSH) as its cofactor.

Step 5: Hydrolysis of fumarylacetoacetate: Fumarylacetoacetate is cleaved into fumarate (glucogenic) and acetoacetate (ketogenic) by a hydrolase enzyme.

Alternate Pathway of Phenylalanine Catabolism (Fig. 4)

- Phenylalanine is transaminated by a specific transaminase to form phenylpyruvate which is dehydrogenated to form phenylacetate in the presence of NAD
- Phenylpyruvate is reduced by LDH to synthesise phenyllactate

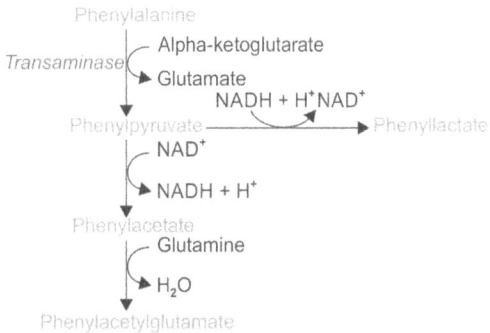

Fig. 4: Alternate pathway of phenylalanine catabolism.

- Phenylacetate is conjugated with glutamine to form phenylglutamine which is excreted in urine

- All these products are excreted through urine.

Other Products formed from Tyrosine
- Thyroxine
- Catecholamines
- Melanin pigments.

Inherited disorder associated with Phenylalanine metabolism-Phenylketonuria (PKU)
- It is an autosomal recessive disease with an incidence of 1:10,000 births
- It is due to deficiency of phenylalanine hydroxylase
- So phenylalanine is not converted into tyrosine and it accumulates hyperphenylalaninemia
- The excess of phenylalanine is converted to phenylpyruvate, phenyllactate, and phenylacetate and phenylacetyl glutamine. Phenylpyruvate, phenyllactate, phenylacetate are excreted in urine.

Clinical Manifestations
- The child is mentally retarded
- Convulsions, tremors, agitation, hyperactivity may be present
- The child often has hypopigmentation due to reduced availability of tyrosine for melanin production
- Phenyllactate in sweat causes mousy body odor.

Laboratory Diagnosis
- Blood level of phenylalanine is elevated—normal level is 1 mg/dL which is elevated to >20 mg/dL.
- This is confirmed by Tandem mass spectrometry
- Guthrie's test is confirmative
- Urine ferric chloride test is positive
- DNA probes—to diagnose the defects in phenylalanine hydroxylase and dihydrobiopterin reductase.

Treatment
- Early detection
- Low phenylalanine diet—Tapioca based diet which has low phenylalanine is the treatment of choice.

4. **What is the normal pH of blood? Explain the various mechanisms by which the normal pH of the blood is maintained.**

Refer 2003 Essay Questions 4.
- Normal blood pH is between 7.38-7.42 (7.4)
- pH is the negative logarithm of hydrogen ion concentration
- As per Henderson-Hasselbalch equation, $pH = pKa + \log x [Base]/[Acid]$
- If the concentration of base and acid are equal, $pH = pKa$.

Mechanisms Maintaining pH
- Buffers of body fluids—first line of defence
- Respiratory mechanism—second line of defence
- Renal mechanism—third line of defence.

Role of Buffers in Body Fluids

Buffers resist changes in pH when small quantities of an acid or an alkali are added. Various buffers in blood are:
- **Bicarbonate buffer system**
- **Phosphate buffer system**
- **Protein buffer system**

a. **Bicarbonate buffer system: (Bicarbonate- Carbonic acid system)** ($NaHCO_3/H_2CO_3$)
   - It is the most important buffer in plasma and is formed by ($NaHCO_3/H_2CO_3$)
   - It accounts for 40% in whole body and 65% in plasma
   - The base HCO_3^- is the **metabolic component** and it is regulated by kidney and carbonic acid (H_2CO_3) is called **respiratory component** since it is regulated by the lungs
   - The **normal bicarbonate level** in plasma is 24 mmol/L.
     - The normal PCO_2 of arterial blood is 40 mm of Hg
     - The **normal carbonic acid concentration** in blood is 1.2 mmol/L.
   - Carbonic acid has a pKa of 6.1 so it is a poor buffer. But the high blood concentration and the ratio of base to salt is high (20:1) which makes it an effective buffer

- Under physiological conditions with pH 7.4 the ratio of bicarbonate to carbonic acid is **20:1**
- When **strong acid such as HCl (H^+)** is added to the bicarbonate buffer then
- $H^+ + HCO_3^- \rightarrow H_2CO_3 \rightarrow H_2O + CO_2$
- CO_2 stimulates respiratory center and it is excreted by lungs—respiratory compensation
- When **strong alkali like NaOH** is added to the bicarbonate buffer then
- $NaOH + H_2CO_3 \rightarrow NaHCO_3 + H_2O$
- Level of H_2CO_3 decreases because it reacts with NaOH
- $H_2O + CO_2 \rightarrow H_2CO_3 \rightarrow H^+ + HCO_3^-$
- The rise in bicarbonate is compensated by increased excretion through kidney (renal compensation).

b. **Phosphate buffer system**—it is an intracellular buffer with low concentration in plasma
   - It is made of $NaHPO_4/NaH_2PO_4$. It has a pKa of 6.8. It is an effective buffer system because its pKa value 6.7 is nearer to physiological pH.
   - **The ratio of $HPO_4 : H_2PO_4 = 4:1$**
   - In acidosis—$Na_2HPO_4 + H^+ \rightarrow NaH_2PO_4$ → excreted by the kidneys
   - In alkalosis—$NaH_2PO_4 + NaOH \rightarrow Na_2HPO_4 + H^+ + H_2O$.

c. **Protein buffer system**
   - **Extracellular (Na protein/H protein)**
     - Buffering capacity of proteins depend on the pKa value of ionisable side chains
     - The most effective buffer is imidazole group of **Histidine** molecules with a pKa value of 6.1
     - Albumin contains 16 histidine residues and so albumin accounts for the nonbicarbonate buffer system.
     - In acidosis $H^+ + Pr \rightarrow HPr$
     - In alkalosis $HPr \rightarrow H^+ + Pr$.

- **Intracellular – Hb buffer system (KHb/HHb) (Fig. 5)**
  - Hb is the major blood buffer in RBCs and it acts along with bicarbonate system
  - It has 38 histidine residues

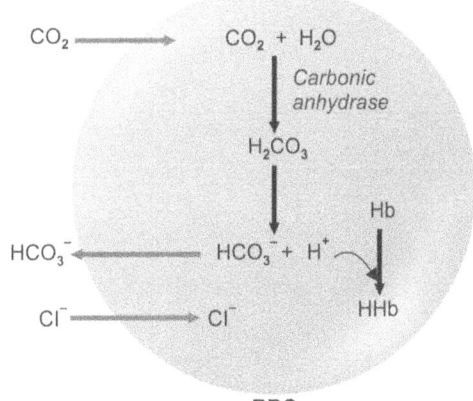

Fig. 5: Hb buffer system.

- **In the tissue level:** The oxyHb releases O_2 to the tissues which is facilitated by low pO_2, low pH and high pCO_2 and CO_2 produced is returned to the lungs, carried by Hb where CO_2 is eliminated in expired air
- **In the RBC:** CO_2 is converted to carbonic acid by carbonic anhydrase resulting in decrease in pH and Hb becomes deoxyHb
- DeoxyHb neutralises carbonic acid to increase the pH and there will be increase in bicarbonate and decrease in pCO_2
- To maintain electroneutrality chloride ions enter into RBC for each bicarbonate leaves. This is called **Chloride shift**
- **In the lungs:** OxyHb releases H^+ which is buffered by bicarbonate to form carbonic acid which is converted by carbonic anhydrase to CO_2 and water which get eliminated by ventilation.

Role of Respiratory System in Acid-Base balance (Second line of Defence)
- When there is fall in pH (acidosis) the respiratory rate is stimulated resulting in hyperventilation. This would eliminate more CO_2 thereby lowering H_2CO_3
- In the lungs, H^+ combines with HCO_3^- to form H_2CO_3 which becomes H_2O and CO_2. This CO_2 is released into the lungs. So lungs reduce the acid load of H_2CO_3 by excretion of CO_2 **(Fig. 6)**

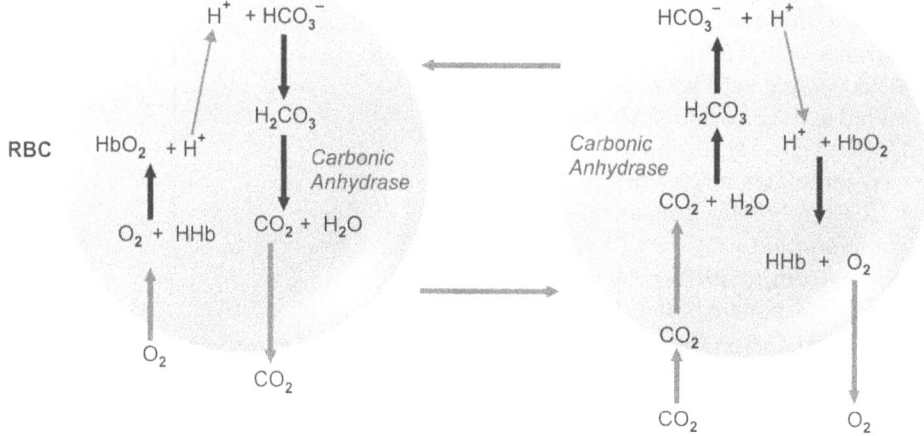

Fig. 6: Reactions in lungs.   **Fig. 7:** Reaction in tissues.

- In tissues, pCO_2 is high and pH is low to the formation of acids by the cells like lactate and production of CO_2 by cells. CO_2 diffuses into RBC. It combines with water to form carbonic acid by carbonic anhydrase. And dissociates into H^+ and HCO_3^-. So RBC traps H^+ from the tissues. Some of the HCO_3^- diffuses out of the cell in exchange for chloride **(Fig. 7)**
- In metabolic acidosis lungs hyperventilate to excrete more acid. In metabolic alkalosis the reverse happens.

Renal Regulation of Acid-base Balance (Third line of defence)

- Kidneys regulate pH of extracellular fluid
- Normal urine has pH around 6. This pH is lower than that of ECF (7.4). This is called **acidification of urine**
- The steps of this mechanism are:
  - Excretion of H^+
  - Reabsorption of bicarbonate
  - Excretion of titratable acid
  - Excretion of ammonia.
- **Excretion of H^+ (Fig. 8)** (generation of bicarbonate)—in proximal convoluted tubular cells, CO_2 combines with water to form carbonic acid using carbonic anhydrase.

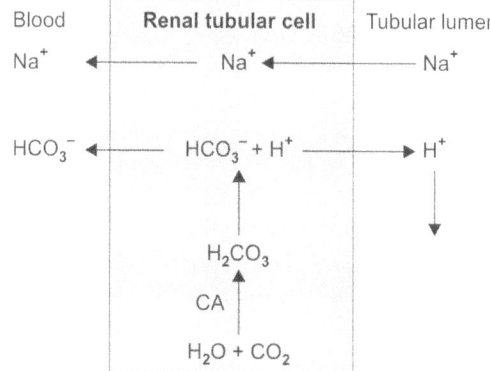

Fig. 8: Excretion of H^+.

  - Then it ionizes to H^+ and HCO_3^-. This H^+ is then secreted into the tubular lumen in exchange for Na^+
  - There is net excretion of hydrogen ions and net generation of bicarbonate. This increases the alkali reserve.
- **Reabsorption of bicarbonate (Fig. 9)**
  - Sodium bicarbonate in the lumen becomes sodium and bicarbonate
  - Sodium is taken up by PCT cells in exchange of hydrogen ions. H^+ combines with HCO_3^- in the tubular lumen to form carbonic acid which forms CO_2 and water and both are diffused into the cell and converted back to carbonic acid

- In the cell again it dissociates to H^+ and HCO_3^-. HCO_3^- is taken into blood with sodium
- There is no net excretion of H^+ or generation of new bicarbonate. The net effect is the reabsorption of filtered bicarbonate mediated by sodium - hydrogen exchanger
- By this base reaction is conserved.
- **Excretion of H^+ as titratable acid (Fig. 10)**
  - In the distal convoluted tubules, hydrogen ions are secreted into the tubular fluid in exchange of sodium
  - This sodium is obtained from Na_2HPO_4—disodium hydrogen phosphate which is a base
  - Na_2HPO_4 combines with H^+ to form the acid NaH_2PO_4 which is the major form of titratable acid in urine
  - Titratable acidity of urine refers to number of milliliters of N/10-NaOH required to titrate 1 liter of urine to pH 7.4. This is a measure of net acid excretion by kidney
  - As the tubular fluid moves down the renal tubules, more H^+ ions are added causing more acidification of urine with fall in pH of urine upto pH 4.5
  - The acid and basic phosphate pair is considered as urinary buffer.
- **Excretion of NH_4^+ (Fig. 11):** Occurs mostly at DCT. This helps to excrete H^+ and reabsorb HCO_3^-
  - This is another mechanism to buffer H^+ ion into the tubular fluid
  - H^+ ions combine with NH_3 to form ammonium ions (NH_4)
  - The enzyme glutaminase deamidates glutamine in DCT becomes glutamate and ammonia
  - This ammonia is secreted into the lumen which combines with hydrogen ions to become ammonium ions and get excreted in urine.

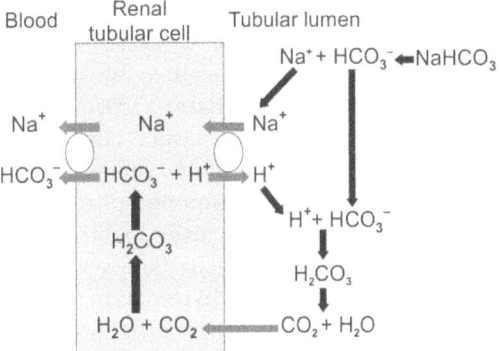

Fig. 9: Reabsorption of bicarbonate.

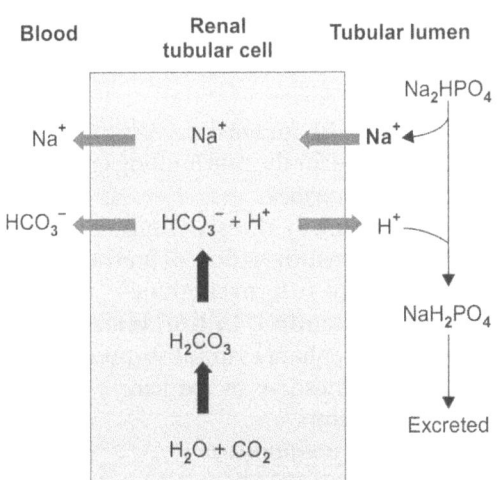

Fig. 10: Excretion of titratable acid as phosphate.

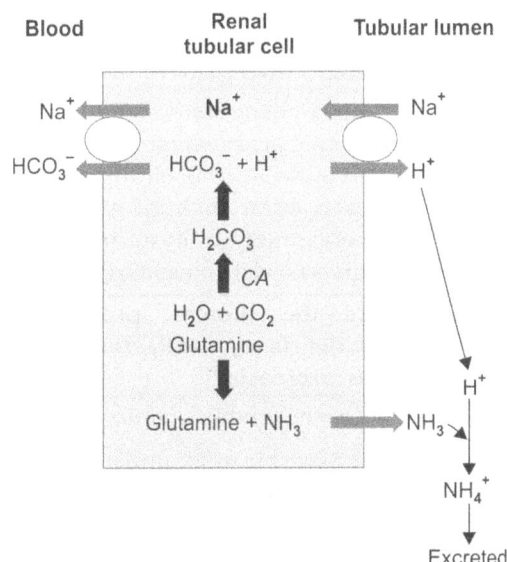

Fig. 11: Excretion of titratable acid as ammonium acids.

Disorders of Acid–Base Balance

- **Acidosis:** Accumulation of acids and loss of bases causing fall of pH. They are of 2 types which are as follows:
  1. **Metabolic acidosis:**
     - Primary change is decrease in plasma bicarbonate concentration which is compensated by $\downarrow pCO_2$ by hyperventilation
     - This occurs in diabetic ketoacidosis, lactic acidosis, renal failure, renal tubular acidosis, etc.
  2. **Respiratory acidosis:**
     - Primary excess of carbonic acid with $\uparrow pCO_2$. This is compensated by increase in bicarbonate
     - This occurs in chronic obstructive airways diseases, asthma, emphysema, paralysis of respiratory muscles, respiratory depressant toxic drugs, etc.
- **Alkalosis:** Loss of acid or accumulation of bases causing increased pH. They are 2 types which are as follows
  1. **Metabolic alkalosis:**
     - Primary change is excess of bicarbonate which is compensated by $\uparrow pCO_2$ by hypoventilation
     - This is seen in vomiting, hypokalemia, Cushing's syndrome, diuretic therapy.
  2. **Respiratory alkalosis:**
     - Primary change is deficit of pCO_2 (carbonic acid) which is compensated by decrease in bicarbonate
     - This is seen in high altitude, hyperventilation, hysteria, septicemia, salicylate poisoning, etc.

---

5. What are the sources, properties, functions, deficiency manifestation and RDA for ascorbic acid?

Vitamin C is a water-soluble vitamin.

Other name: Ascorbic acid, antiscorbutic vitamin.

Sources: Vegetables and Fruits

Rich sources: Gooseberry (amla), citrus fruits, guava, green vegetables, tomatoes, potatoes.

RDA

- 75 mg/day (equal to 50 mL orange juice)
- Pregnancy and lactation and aged persons: 100 mg/day

Structure

It is similar to hexose sugar. L-ascorbic acid and L-dehydroascorbic acid are the two forms of this vitamin, both are interconvertible.

Biochemical Functions of Vitamin C

- **Reversible oxidation and reduction:** Vitamin C can change between ascorbic acid and dehydroascorbic acid
- **Vitamin C is the coenzyme for hydroxylase**
  - **Hydroxylation of proline and lysine:** Post-translational hydroxylation of proline and lysine residues are necessary for the formation of cross-links in collagen to give strength to the fibers
  - **Tyrosine metabolism: a) Dopamine hydroxylase** is a copper containing enzyme involved in the synthesis of the catecholamines—norepinephrine and epinephrine from tyrosine in the adrenal medulla and central nervous system
    b) Vitamin C helps in oxidation of para-hydroxyphenylpyruvate to homogentisic acid
  - **Hydroxylation of Tryptophan** to 5 hydroxytryptophan (serotonin) by hydroxylase enzyme needs vitamin C
  - **Steroid synthesis:** Vitamin C is needed for the hydroxylation reactions in adrenal cortex
  - **Bile acid formation:** Vitamin C is required for the rate limiting enzyme—7α hydroxylase
  - **Carnitine synthesis:** Vitamin C helps in the hydroxylation of gamma-butyrobetaine to form carnitine
- **Role of vitamin C in iron metabolism:** Vitamin C enhances the absorption of iron from the intestines by reducing ferric iron to ferrous iron
- **Folic acid metabolism**

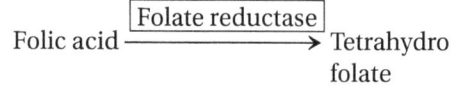

Folic acid $\xrightarrow{\text{Folate reductase}}$ Tetrahydrofolate

- **Hb metabolism**

  MetHb $\xrightarrow{\text{Vitamin C}}$ Hb

- **Antioxidant property:** It prevents cancer formation—especially bladder cancer caused by aniline dye.
- **Immune functions:** Vitamin C stimulates phagocytic action of leukocytes and produces antibodies.
- **Prevention of cataract:** Vitamin C reduces the risk of cataract formation.

Vitamin C Deficiency

- **Scurvy:** Skin changes, fragility of blood capillaries, gum decay, tooth loss, and bone fracture, many of which can be attributed to deficient collagen synthesis
- **Infantile scurvy:** Other name: Barlow's disease
  In infants between 6 to 12 months, diet should be supplemented with vitamin C
- **Hemorrhagic tendency:** Collagen is abnormal and intercellular cement substance is brittle. So capillaries are fragile leading to the tendency to bleed even under minor pressure. It results in **ecchymoses and petechiae**
- **Internal hemorrhage:** Hemorrhage may occur in the **conjunctiva and retina**. Bleeding may be seen as epitaxis, hematuria or melena
- **Oral cavity:** Painful swollen gums. Loosening of teeth due to separation of dentine
- **Bones**: Bones become weak due to failure of osteoblasts. Bleeding into joint cavities
- **Anemia:**
  - Microcytic, hypochromic anemia
  - Poikilocytosis and anisocytosis are seen
  - Anemia may be due to loss of blood by bleeding, decreased iron absorption.

---

6. **What is the normal fasting and postprandial blood glucose level? Explain how normal blood glucose level is maintained. Add a note on the disruption of hormonal regulation of blood glucose.**

Refer 2003 Essay Question 2
- Normal fasting blood glucose—70–110 mg/dL
- Normal postprandial blood glucose—120–140 mg/dL.

BLOOD GLUCOSE HOMEOSTASIS

Blood glucose is maintained at the normal range for optimal utilization of glucose by the body. In our body, certain tissues like brain, retina and testes are solely dependent on glucose for their energy at certain concentration.

Sources of Blood Glucose

- **Dietary sources:** Plant starch—which is degraded to glucose in the intestine and absorbed into blood
- **Gluconeogenesis:** Glucose is formed from noncarbohydrates sources like pyruvate, lactate, glycerol and glucogenic amino acids
- **Glycogenolysis:** The stored glycogen present in liver and muscle is broken down to glucose.

Utilization of Glucose

- **Glycolysis and TCA cycle:** Glucose is used as main energy source by all cells to produce ATP
- **Glycogenesis:** Excess glucose is converted to glycogen and stored in liver and muscle
- Glucose is utilized for synthesis of nonessential amino acids and fat
- Glucose is utilized for synthesis of amino sugars.

Excretion of Glucose

The kidney is the major organ which regulates the glucose excretion. In normal healthy persons there is no excretion of glucose in urine.

Glucose is excreted through urine if blood glucose is more than 180 mg/dL. This is called as **renal threshold level**.

The maximum reabsorption of glucose by renal tubules is 350 mg/minute (tubular maximum).

Blood Glucose Regulation during Fed State

Following a meal, glucose level is increased in circulation. This high concentration of glucose is regulated via two processes:

1. **Action of glucokinase:** Glucokinase found only in liver and is having high Km and low affinity to glucose. During postprandial conditions glucose level is high and so glucose binds with this enzyme. Hence, immediately after meals the glucose is acted upon by glucokinase in liver and utilized for energy production through glycolysis
2. **Action of insulin:** High concentration of glucose in blood in the fed stage stimulates the production of insulin from pancreas. Uptake of glucose by most of extrahepatic tissues except brain is dependent on insulin.

Blood Glucose Regulation during Fasting

After meals, after about 2.5 hours the blood glucose level is regulated to the normal range. After another 3 hours, the glucose is supplied through glycogenolysis, and there after by gluconeogenesis.

REGULATION OF GLUCOSE BY HORMONES

The various hormones play significant role in regulation of blood glucose concentrations. They are as follows:

Hypoglycemic Hormone

Insulin: It is 51 amino acid peptide hormone produced from β-cells of islets of Langerhans of pancreas. Insulin is a hypoglycemic hormone. It lowers the blood glucose by means of following mechanisms:
- Insulin stimulates glycolysis, glycogenesis, HMP shunt, fat synthesis
- Insulin suppresses gluconeogenesis, glycogenolysis.

Hyperglycemic Hormones

- **Glucagon:**
  - It is produced form α-cells of islets of Langerhans of pancreas
  - Its functions are agonist to the insulin actions anti-insulin action
  - It stimulates gluconeogenesis, glycogenolysis.
- **Epinephrine or Adrenaline—from adrenal medullary gland**
- **Thyroxine—from thyroid gland**
- **Glucocorticoids—from adrenal cortex**
  - These hormones are hyperglycemic in nature
  - They stimulate gluconeogenesis, and glycogenolysis
  - Glucocorticoids stimulates protein metabolism.
- **Growth hormone:**
  - It inhibits the glucose utilization by cells
  - It stimulates protein synthesis
  - Disruption of hormonal regulation of blood glucose is mainly the deficiency of insulin
  - The metabolic disorder associated with insulin deficiency is diabetes mellitus.

Two Types of Diabetes Mellitus

1. Type I DM—Insulin dependent DM (IDDM)
2. Type II—Non-insulin-dependent (NIDDM)

Type I: It is due to decreased insulin production. Onset is below 30 years. It is common during adolescence. These patients are more prone to ketosis.

Type II: It is due to insulin resistance. It is seen in 95% of patients with diabetes mellitus. Seen in individuals above 40 years. They are less prone for ketosis 60% cases are obese.

Diagnosis of DM

- Blood glucose level—by OGTT
  - Fasting—more than 126 mg/dL
  - Two hours after glucose—more than 200 mg/dL
- Other laboratory tests to be done:
  - Fasting and postprandial blood glucose estimation—once in 3 months for monitoring
  - Complete lipid profile—total cholesterol, TAG, HDL and LDL cholesterol once in 6 months
  - Kidney function tests—blood urea and serum creatinine—twice a year

- Microalbuminuria and frank albuminuria—once in a year
- Microalbuminuria—presence of 50 to 300 mg/day albumin in urine—predictor of renal damage; Albumin >300 mg/day—overt diabetic nephropathy.
• Glycated Hb—best index of long-term control of DM–HbA1C levels reveals mean glucose level over the previous 10-12 weeks
• Fructosamines
• Advanced glycation end products.

7. **Why ammonia is toxic to the body? What are the ways by which ammonia is disposed in the body? Add a note on hyperammonemia conditions.**

FORMATION OF AMMONIA

- Ammonia is produced in human body mostly by the catabolism of amino acids and by other nitrogenous substances like amino sugars, purines, pyrimidines and biological amines
- **Ammonia is toxic to the body and so it should be eliminated or detoxified. Very minute amount of ammonia may produce toxicity in CNS**
- Production of ammonia from amino acids are done by the following steps:
  - Transamination
  - Transdeamination—(oxidative deamination)
  - Nonoxidative deamination.
- **Transamination (Fig. 12):** Transamination is the exchange of the alpha amino group between one alpha amino acid and another alpha ketoacid forming a new alpha amino acid (II) and a new ketoacid (II). This is catalyzed by a group of enzymes known as transferases or aminotransferases with pyridoxal phosphate (PLP) as its coenzyme. It is a reversible reaction.
- **Reaction sequence:** Amino acid 1 + keto acid 1 → Amino acid 2 + Keto acid 2
  For example, Alanine + Alpha-ketoglutarate → Glutamate + Pyruvate (alanine amino transferase, PLP)
  (1AA)   (1KA)   (II AA)   (II KA)

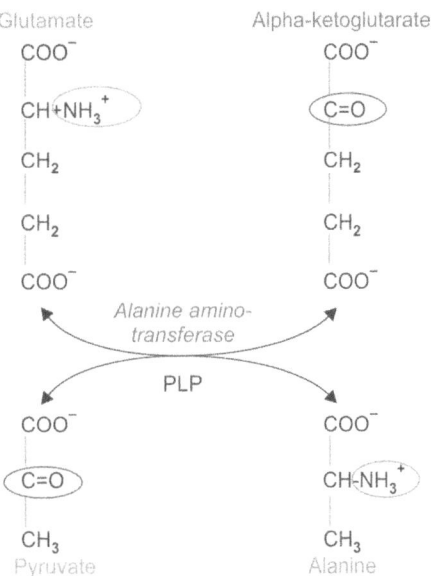

Fig. 12: Transamination.

acts as an acceptor of amino group forming a Schiff's base. In the above example, first the amino group from alanine (amino acid 1) is removed to form pyruvate (keto acid 2). Then this amino group is taken up by alpha ketoglutarate (keto acid 1) to form glutamate (amino acid 2)
- **Exception:** Transamination will not occur in lysine, threonine, proline and hydroxyproline.

Transdeamination (Fig. 13)

- Oxidative deamination of glutamate:
  - Transamination followed by deamination is known as transdeamination
  - Transamination takes place in the cytoplasm of all the cells of body. After transamination, the amino group is transported to liver as glutamic acid
  - In the liver, mitochondria, glutamate dehydrogenase enzyme deaminates glutamate to form ammonia and alpha-ketoglutarate with the help of NAD.
- **Other pathways of deamination:**
  - This is done by L and D amino acid oxidases and monoamine oxidase.
  - **L-amino acid oxidase**—acts on all amino acids except hydroxyl group con-

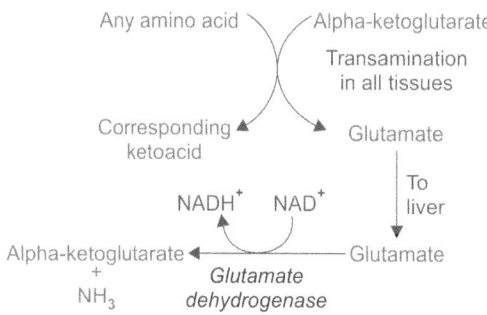

Fig. 13: Transdeamination.

taining amino acids and acidic amino acids with FMN as coenzyme to form ketoacid and peroxides which is acted by catalase enzymes in peroxisomes
- **D-amino acid oxidase:** This oxidises glycine and all D amino acids (bacterial metabolism) using FAD as coenzyme to liberate ammonia and ketoacids
- **Monoamine oxidases:** Oxidation of monoamines—mainly in tyrosine metabolism.

Nonoxidative Deamination

- Done by—
  a. Dehydratase—acts on hydroxy amino acids,
     For example, serine → pyruvate + ammonia
     Threonine → α-ketobutyric acid + ammonia
  b. Desulfhydratase—deamination + trans - sulfuration
     For example, cysteine → H_2S + pyruvate + ammonia (through imino acid)
     Histidase—histidine → urocanate + NH_3
- GIT – NH_3 formed by bacterial putrefaction.

TRANSPORT OF AMMONIA

- Ammonia is toxic to brain, so it has to be eliminated or detoxified quickly
- So it combines with glutamate to form glutamine especially in brain cells
- This glutamine is taken into liver and by glutaminase; it is converted back to ammonia
- Glutamic acid acts as a link between amino groups of amino acids and ammonia
- Concentration of glutamic acid is 10 times more than other amino acids in blood
- Major form of transport of ammonia is glutamine from brain and intestines to liver
- Alanine is the transport form of ammonia from muscles.

FINAL DISPOSAL OF AMMONIA/FORMATION OF UREA

- First line of defence against ammonia is done by trapping of NH_3 by glutamic acid to form glutamine especially in brain cells
- Second line of defence is by the formation of urea which is the end product of protein metabolism in the liver.

Steps of Urea Formation (Fig. 14)

- The urea cycle is the first metabolic pathway to be elucidated in 1932. This cycle is also called as Krebs-Henseleit urea cycle or ornithine cycle
- **Site:** In liver. First two steps of urea cycle are taken place in liver mitochondria and other steps are taken place in cytosol
- The two nitrogen atoms of urea derived from two different sources, one from ammonia and other directly from aspartic acid (α amino group).

Step 1: Formation of Carbamoyl Phosphate

- One molecule of ammonia condenses with CO_2 in the presence of two molecules

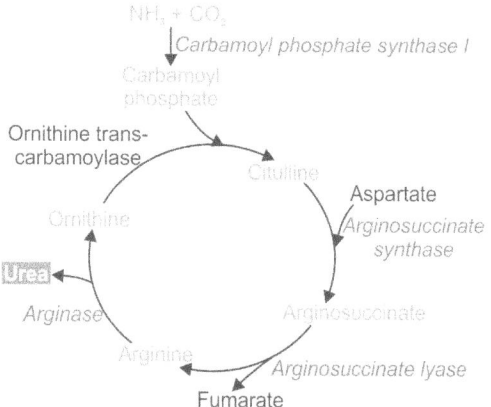

Fig. 14: Steps of urea formation.

of ATP to form carbamoyl phosphate by the enzyme carbamoyl phosphate synthetase-I. (CPS-1). This occurs in liver mitochondria
- This is the rate limiting step. It is an irreversible step and regulated allosterically by (NAG) (N acetylglutamate).

Step 2: Formation of Citrulline (Mitochondria)
- The carbamoyl group is transferred to the NH_2 group of ornithine by ornithine transcarbamoylase (OTC)
- Citrulline enters into the cytoplasm to continue further reactions

Step 3: Formation of Argininosuccinate
- One molecule of aspartic acid adds to citrulline forming a carbon to nitrogen bond which provides second nitrogen of urea by argininosuccinate synthetase
- Two high energy phosphate bonds are utilized.

Step 4: Formation of Arginine
- Argininosuccinate is cleaved by argininosuccinate lyase (argininosuccinase) to arginine and fumarate. Fumarate inhibits this step
- Fumarate enters into TCA cycle to be converted to malate which is then converted to oxaloacetate
- Oxaloacetate is transaminated to aspartate. This is a link between TCA cycle and urea cycle.

STEP 5: Formation of Urea
- Hydrolysis of arginine gives rise to urea and ornithine by the enzyme arginase
- Ornithine returns to the mitochondria to react with another molecule of carbamoyl phosphate to proceed the next cycle.

HYPERAMMONEMIA

Urea Cycle Disorders—due to Defect in the Enzymes of Urea Cycle

- **Hyperammonemia type I**
  - Enzyme deficient is carbamoyl phosphate synthetase I. Incidence is 1 in 100,000
  - It is an autosomal recessive disease
  - Very high level of ammonia in blood, mental retardation.
- **Hyperammonemia type II**
  - Enzyme deficient is ornithine transcarbamylase
  - X-linked
  - Ammonia, glutamine increased in blood. Orotic aciduria due to channeling of carbamoyl phosphate to pyrimidine synthesis.
- **Citrullinemia**
  - Enzyme deficient is argininosuccinate synthetase
  - It is autosomal recessive disorder
  - High blood levels of ammonia and citrulline. Citrullinuria—1–2 g/day.
- **Argininosuccinic aciduria**
  - Enzyme deficient is argininosuccinate lyase. Incidence 3/200,000
  - Argininosuccinate in blood and urine
  - Friable brittle tufted hair (trichorrhexis nodosa).
- **Hyperargininemia**
  - Enzyme deficient is arginase. Incidence 1 in 100,000
  - Arginine increased in blood and CSF
  - Instead of arginine, cysteine and lysine are lost in urine.
- **Hyperornithinemia**
  - Due to defective ornithine transport protein due to defect in *ORNT1* gene
  - Autosomal recessive condition
  - Hyperornithinemia, hyperammonemia and homocitrullinuria are seen (HHH syndrome).

8. **What is the normal serum calcium level? Explain how serum calcium is maintained. Name the hypocalemia conditions.**

NORMAL BLOOD LEVEL OF CALCIUM

- Total calcium level—9-11 mg/dL
- Three forms of calcium in blood
- Ionized calcium (active form)—5 mg/dL
- Protein-bound Ca—4 mg/dL
- Protein complexed with phosphate, HCO_3^- citrate—1 mg/dL.

Factors Regulating Calcium Level

- Hormones:
  - Vitamin D—calcitriol
  - Parathyroid hormone (PTH)
  - Calcitonin—thyroid
- Phosphorus
- Serum proteins
- Alkalosis and acidosis
- Renal threshold for calcium
- Product of calcium and phosphorus.

Hormonal Regulation

Vitamin D: (Calcitriol—1,25-dihydroxycholecalciferol)

The active vitamin D (calcitriol) acts as a steroid hormone. It is synthesized in kidney.

- **Effect on intestine:** Calcitriol binds to specific cytoplasmic receptors which interacts with DNA and induces the synthesis of mRNA for specific proteins: Calbindin which is a calcium binding protein which helps in the absorption of calcium and phosphorus from the intestines.
- **Effects on bone:** Calcitriol stimulates the activity of osteoblasts which help in mineralization of bones. They secrete alkaline phosphatase enzyme which in turn increases the ionic concentration of phosphate and calcium
- **Effects on kidney:** Calcitriol increases the reabsorption of calcium and phosphorous from the renal tubules thereby conserving both minerals.

Parathyroid Hormone

- Parathyroid hormone is secreted by four parathyroid glands present at the posterior aspect of thyroid gland
- Decreased serum calcium level leads to release of PTH from parathyroids. PTH activates the enzyme adenylyl cyclase in target cells and increases intracellular calcium concentration
- **PTH and bones**—PTH causes demineralization of bones. It activates pyrophosphatase in osteoclasts leading to bone resorption and decalcification. Calcium is released into the bloodstream and increases blood calcium level. This leads to loss of bone matrix
- **PTH and kidneys**—PTH causes decreased renal excretion of calcium and increased excretion of phosphates and increased reabsorption of calcium leading to increased blood calcium level
- **PTH and intestines**—PTH stimulates increased production of calcitriol which acts on intestine to absorb more calcium leading to increased calcium level in blood.

Calcitonin

- Secreted by parafollicular cells of thyroid gland
- It is a polypeptide of 32–34 amino acids and its secretion is stimulated by serum calcium, gastrin, glucagon and biological amines
- It decreases serum calcium level by inhibiting resorption of bone and decreases the activity of osteoclasts and increases the activity of osteoblasts
- Calcitonin and PTH are antagonistic to each other but both together promote growth and remodeling of bone
- In kidney—calcitonin increases excretion of phosphates in urine like PTH.

Phosphorus

- There is a reciprocal relationship of calcium with phosphorus
- Ionic product of Ca x P is kept as a constant
- Normally—(Ca) 10 mg/dL x (P) 4 mg/dL = 40; ionic product is 40
- In renal insufficiency—↓ excretion of P → ↓ level of P in blood → level of calcium → tetany.

Serum Proteins

- Total calcium level is decreased in hypoalbuminemia—for reduction of each 1 g/dL of albumin there will be reduction of 0.8 mg/dL of calcium
- Ionized calcium level will be normal and so no deficiency manifestations will be present.

Alkalosis and Acidosis

- Alkalosis favors binding of more calcium with proteins by lowering of ionized calcium but the total calcium level is normal. Calcium deficiency is manifested
- Acidosis favors ionization of calcium.

Renal Threshold for Calcium

Renal threshold for calcium is 10 mg/dL and calcium gets excreted at this level.

Ionic Product of Calcium and Phosphorus

In children the normal calcium level will be near the upper limit and the ionic product of calcium and phosphorus = 50 (adult -40).

Hypocalcemia Conditions

- Deficiency of vitamin D
- Hypoparathyroidism
- Carcinoma of thyroid—medullary
- Malabsorption of calcium in intestines
- Hyperphosphatemia—renal failure
- Hypoalbuminemia.

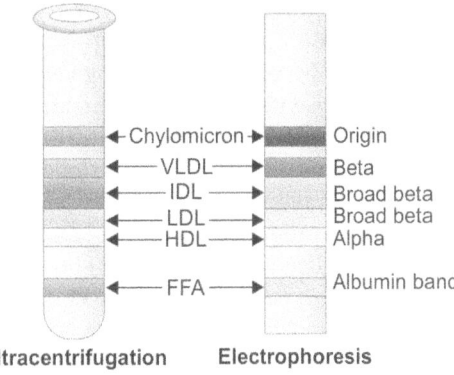

Fig. 15: Separation of lipoproteins.

II. SHORT NOTES

1. Lipoproteins and their functions.

Lipoproteins are conjugated proteins. These are spherical bodies made up of lipid and proteins. The outer layer has polar heads—phospholipid, apoproteins and free cholesterol and inner core contains nonpolar lipids such as TAG, tails of PL, cholesteryl esters.

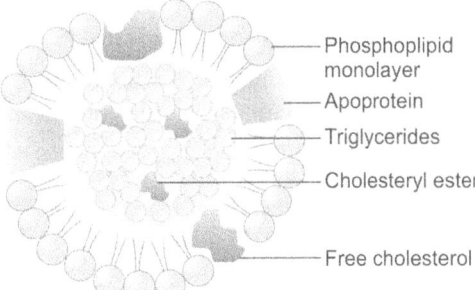

Fig. 16: Structure of chylomicron.

General Structure of Lipoproteins

They are classified according to their density into 4 major types **(Fig. 15)**:
1. Chylomicron
2. Very low density lipoproteins (VLDL)/pre-beta lipoproteins
3. Low density lipoproteins (LDL)/beta lipoproteins
4. High density lipoproteins (HDL)—alpha lipoprotein.

1. **Chylomicron (Fig. 16):**
   - Rich in TAG
   - The TAG of CM are derived from dietary lipids—exogenous
   - These are very larger molecules having lower density than VLDL
   - They contain high concentrations of lipid and lower concentrations of proteins
   - It is synthesized in intestine and it contains apo B-48, apo A. Apo C and E are added from HDL

   Function: They transport dietary TAG from intestines to adipose tissues.

2. **Very low density lipoproteins (VLDL)/prebeta lipoproteins**
   - These are synthesized in liver from TAG which is endogenous—synthesized in liver
   - It has the apoproteins B-100 and CII and E derived from HDL

   Function: VLDL are involved in transport of TAG from liver to peripheral tissues.

3. **Low density lipoproteins (LDL)/beta-lipoproteins**
   - These molecules are rich in cholesterol and contain apo B-100
   - They are derived from VLDL and their half life is 2 days

   Function: LDL is directly linked to CVD risk as it is involved in transport of cholesterol from liver to peripheral tissues. Hence, it is called as bad cholesterol.

4. High density lipoproteins (HDL)/alpha-lipoprotein

- These are very small having very high density with lower concentrations of lipid and higher concentrations of proteins
- They have the apoproteins A-I, A-II, Apo C and Apo E
- HDL is involved in reverse cholesterol transport catabolized by LCAT

Function: Cholesterol present in the peripheral tissues is transported to liver for further catabolism. Hence, it is called as "good cholesterol".

2. Significance of HMP shunt pathway.

Biochemical Significance (Oxidative Phase)

- Biosynthesis of pentoses ribose-5 phosphate for the synthesis of nucleotides and nucleic acids
- Provides way for interconversion of pentoses and hexoses (both phases)
- Generation of NADPH reducing equivalents for:
  - Reductive synthesis of fatty acids, bile acids, cholesterol
  - NADPH is needed for the integrity of RBC membrane
  - Antioxidant—free radical scavenger
  - Helps to prevent metHb
  - Detoxifies drugs by liver microsomes P450 enzymes.

Clinical Significance

- Glucose-6-phosphate dehydrogenase deficiency
  - X-linked recessive trait
  - Cells having the deficient enzyme have lower rate of NADPH production and deficiency of reduced glutathione leading to hemolysis
  - This deficiency is manifested only when exposed to certain drugs, such as primaquine (antimalarial)
  - Fava beans consumption and sulfa drugs also precipitate hemolysis
  - Methemoglobinemia will be seen in circulation in glucose-6-phosphate deficiency. There is no cyanosis

- Transketolase activity of RBC is used to measure the deficiency level of thiamine
- Genetic defect in transketolase enzyme will lead to Wernicke-Korsakoff syndrome (encephalopathy) seen in alcoholics.

3. Synthesis and conjugation of bilirubin.

Catabolism of hemoglobin (Hb) (Synthesis of Bilirubin) (Fig. 17)

- Occurrence: **Endothelial cells of liver, bone marrow, spleen**
- End product of heme metabolism is bile pigments—bilirubin and biliverdin
- From Hb, globin chains are separated and hydrolyzed and amino acids are channeled into the amino acid pool
- The iron is re-utilized
- About 6 g of Hb is broken down per day, from which about 250 mg of bilirubin is formed
- **Normal plasma—free bilirubin level is:** 0.2–0.7 mg/dL
- **Normal plasma—conjugated bilirubin level is:** 0.1–0.4 mg/dL.

Steps

- This occurs at the microsomal fraction of cells by the microsomal enzyme system—heme oxygenase in the presence of NADPH, cytochrome C and O_2.
- Ferric iron (Fe^{3+}) and CO are released with the production of linear tetrapyrrole green pigment biliverdin. Iron is taken up by the

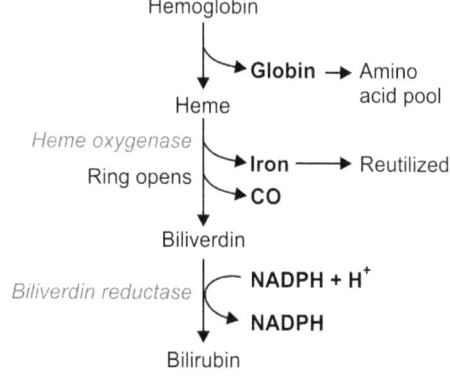

Fig. 17: Synthesis of bilirubin.

protein transferrin. Biliverdin is reduced to red yellow pigment called bilirubin by NADPH dependent reductase. Bilirubin is conjugated and water soluble

- **Transport of bilirubin to liver:** Bilirubin thus formed is insoluble and toxic and it is in unconjugated form. It is transported in plasma bound to albumin. 1 molecule of albumin can bind with 2 molecules of bilirubin
- **Uptake of bilirubin by liver parenchymal cells:** Done by carrier mediated active process. In liver cells bilirubin is bound to an intracellular protein called **ligandin.** This binding is inhibited by taking aspirin or penicillin and this will produce kernicterus in newborn babies
- **Conjugation of bilirubin (Fig. 18):** Unconjugated toxic bilirubin is conjugated with UDP glucuronic acid by UDP glucuronyl transferase enzyme. Bilirubin monoglucuronide is formed first (20%) which is then converted to diglucuronide (80%).

This conjugation process is interfered by drugs like primaquine, novobiocin and pregnenolone, etc.

- **Excretion of bilirubin to bile:** This is done by an active process against a concentration gradient. This is **the rate limiting step** for the entire process. This excretion is mediated by multispecific organic anion transporter
- **Fate of conjugated bilirubin in intestine (Fig. 19):**

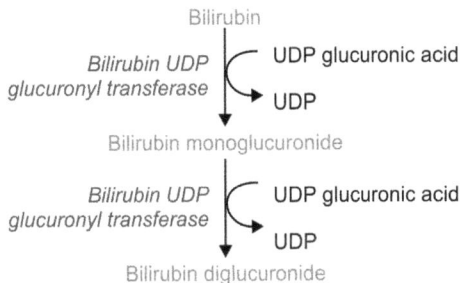

Fig. 18: Conjugation of bilirubin.

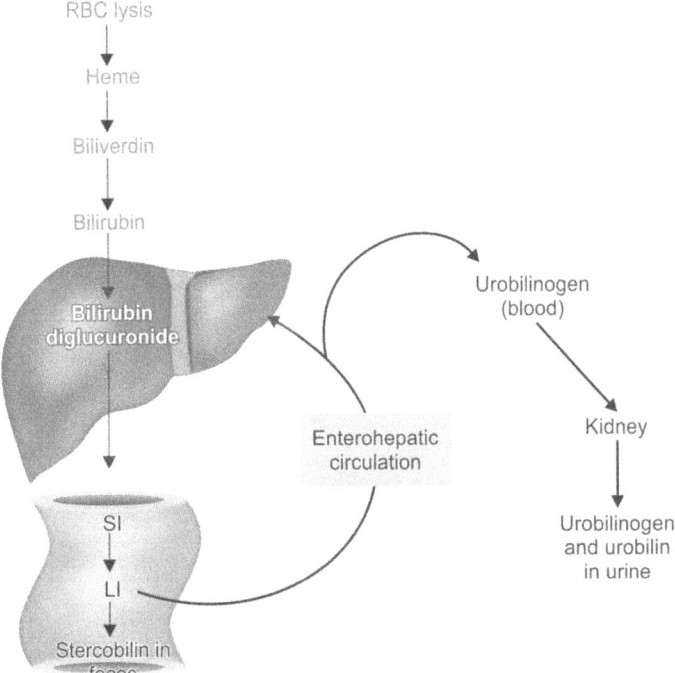

Fig. 19: Fate of conjugated bilirubin in intestine.

- After the secretion of conjugated bilirubin into bile, it passes through hepatic and common bile duct into the intestinal lumen
- In the intestine, the conjugated bilirubin is hydrolyzed by the bacterial beta-glucuronidase to get converted to unconjugated bilirubin
- Free bilirubin thus formed is reduced further into colorless tetrapyrrole urobilinogen which is oxidized to an orange yellow pigment urobilin
- Rest of urobilinogen is reduced to stercobilinogen which is oxidized to a brown pigment called stercobilin which is excreted in feces (250–300 mg/day)
- A part of urobilinogen (20%) enters into enterohepatic circulation to get re-excreted at the liver by portal circulation. A small amount of urobilinogen is excreted through the urine.

4. **Sources of acetyl-CoA and fate of acetyl-CoA (Fig. 20).**

Sources of Acetyl-CoA
- Pyruvate derived from aerobic glycolysis is oxidatively decarboxylated to acetyl-CoA by pyruvate dehydrogenase in mitochondria
- Beta-oxidation of even chain fatty acids like palmitic acid (16 C) and stearic acid (18 C) will produce acetyl-CoA occurs in mitochondria
- Carbon skeleton of ketogenic amino acids like phenylalanine, tyrosine, leucine are catabolized to produce acetyl-CoA.

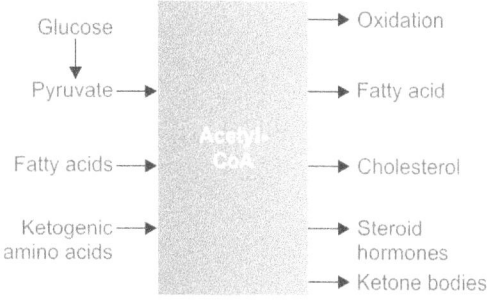

Fig. 20: Sources and fate of acetyl-CoA.

Fate of Acetyl-CoA
- **Tricarboxylic acid cycle (TCA Cycle):** Two carboned acetyl-CoA enter into the citric acid cycle in the mitochondria and condenses with 4C oxaloacetate and completely oxidized to produce energy in the forms of ATP, CO_2 and water. It is the final common oxidative pathway of all foodstuffs
- **Synthesis of fatty acids:** Acetyl-CoA enters into the cytoplasm through the inner membrane of mitochondria as citrate by ATP citrate lyase to synthesize fatty acids (de novo synthesis) with the help of NADPH—reductive synthesis
- **Ketone body synthesis:** During starvation and other conditions like uncontrolled diabetes mellitus three molecules of acetyl-CoA condense to form ketone bodies—acetone, acetoacetate, beta-hydroxy-butyrate-occurs in cytoplasm
- **Cholesterol synthesis:** Three molecules of acetyl-CoA are condensed to form cholesterol by reductive synthesis with the help of NADPH. In adrenal cortex and in reproductive organs like testes, ovaries cholesterol is converted to steroid and sex hormones, respectively
- **AcetylCholine formation:** Acetyl-CoA combines with choline to form acetylcholine which is a neurotransmitter in brain and in nerve synapses
- **Detoxication:** Acetyl-CoA acts as a detoxifying agent to detoxify sulphonamide drugs by acetylation
- **Acetylation** of amino sugars for **glycoprotein synthesis**
- **Acetylation** of neuramnic acid to synthesise gangliosides
- **N-acetylglutamate (NAG):** It acts as an activator of the rate limiting enzyme of urea cycle—carbamoyl phosphate synthetase I.

5. **Functions and deficiency of vitamin A.**

Function in Vision

In the retina, retinaldehyde functions as the prosthetic group of the light-sensitive opsin proteins forming rhodopsin (in rods) and iodopsin (in cones).

Wald's visual cycle (Fig. 21)

- Rhodopsin plays the pivotal role in vision. It is the membrane protein found in the photoreceptor cells of the retina
- Rhodopsin is made up of the protein opsin and 11-cis-retinal
- When light falls on the retina, 11-cis-retinal isomerizes to all-trans-retinal
- A single photon can excite the rod cell. The photon produces immediate conformational changes
- The unstable intermediates produced are Rhodopsin → bathorhodopsin → lumirhodopsin → metarhodopsin → and finally opsin + all-trans-retinal
- The all-trans-retinal is then released from the protein and transported out of the retinal epithelium by an ABC protein. The all-trans-retinal is isomerized to 11-cis retinal in the retina itself in the dark by the enzyme **retinal isomerase.** This reaction takes place in the retinal pigment epithelium
- The 11-cis–retinal combines with opsin to generate **rhodopsin.** Alternatively the all–trans-retinal is transported to liver and then reduced to all–trans-retinol by alcohol dehydrogenase (ADH)
- The all-trans-retinol is isomerized to 11-cis-retinol and then oxidized to 11-cis–retinal in liver. This is then transported to retina. This completes the Wald's visual cycle
- Visual pigments are G protein coupled receptors **(Fig. 22).** 11-cis-retinal keeps it in an inactive form which gets activated by photoexcitation. Cyclic GMP is also generated at the same time and it acts as a gate for cation specific channels
- G protein of retina is transducin
- Nerve impulse thus generated is transmitted to visual centers in brain.

Dark Adaptation

Bright light depletes rhodopsin stores in rods. When a person enters into a dim area from bright light there is difficulty in seeing which will be improved within few minutes by the resynthesis of rhodopsin. This is called dark adaptation time. This time is increased in vitamin A deficiency.

Functions of Rods and Cones

Rhodopsin in rods is responsible for dim light and iodopsin in cones is responsible for color vision. Both proteins contain 11-cis-retinal.

- **Retinol:**
  - Acts like steroid hormone and regulates expression of genes

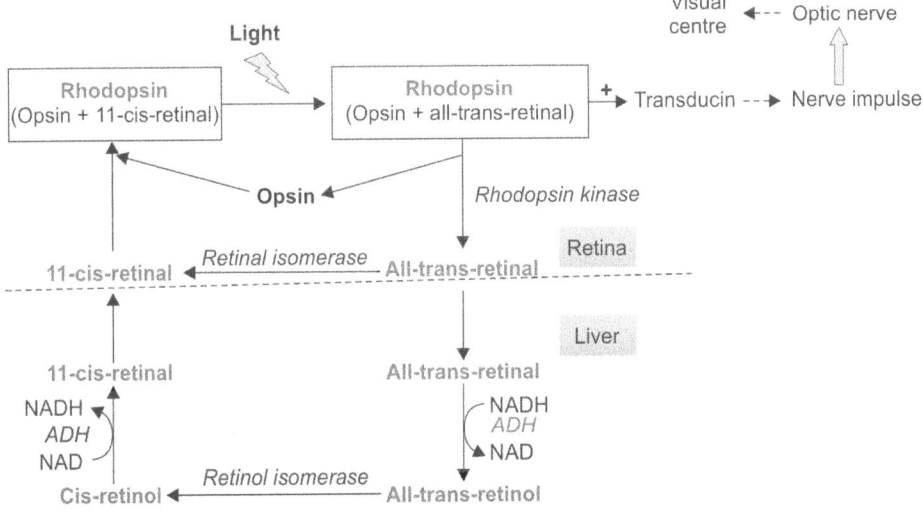

Fig. 21: Wald's visual cycle.

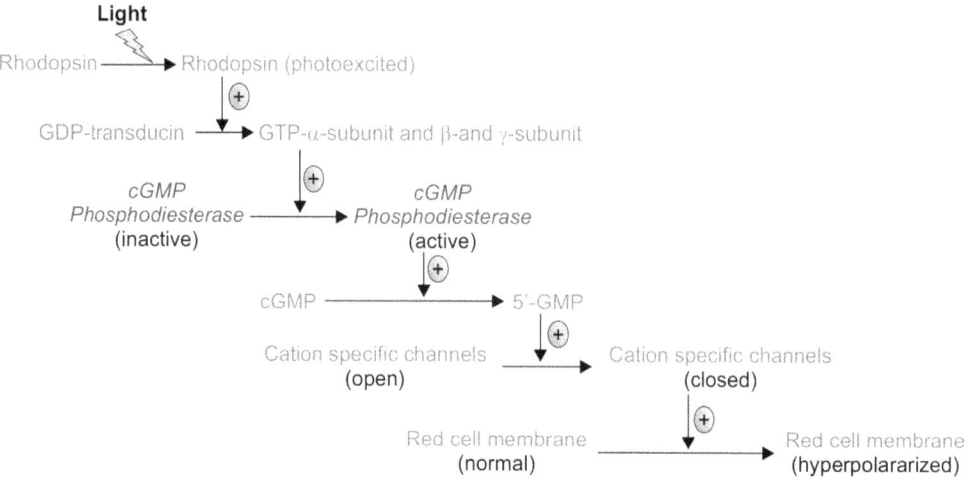

Fig. 22: Cyclic GMP mediated rhodopsin cycle.

- It is needed for reproductive system functions.
- **Retinoic acid:**
  - Regulates gene expression and cellular differentiation during growth and development
  - **Metabolic effect of retinoic acid:** It controls gluconeogenesis in liver and regulates the synthesis of glycoproteins and GAGs as carrier of oligosaccharides. It also controls cholesterol synthesis
  - They act as steroids.
- **Carotenoids:** Precursor form act as antioxidants.

Deficiency

Ocular Manifestations

- **Night blindness or nyctalopia:** Earliest symptoms of vitamin A deficiency. Impaired dark adaptation
- More prolonged deficiency leads to **Xerophthalmia**—dryness of conjunctiva which may spread to cornea
- **Bitot's spots:** Grayish white triangular plaques are seen adherent to conjunctive due to increased thickness
- **Keratomalacia:** Softening of cornea and keratinization which may lead to total blindness due to corneal opacity.

Skin and Mucous Membrane Lesions

- **Hyperkeratosis or phrynoderma:** Due to hyperkeratinization of epithelium. Rough skin. Epithelium gets keratinized and become atrophied in respiratory, gastrointestinal and genitourinary tracts and got atrophied
- Keratinization of urinary tract leads to formation of urinary calculi
- Acne formation.

Immunity

- Vitamin A also has an important role in differentiation of immune system cells, and mild deficiency leads to increased susceptibility to infectious diseases
- Furthermore, the synthesis of retinol-binding protein in response to infection is reduced (it is a negative **acute phase protein**).

6. **Isoenzymes and their diagnostic importance.**

Refer 2003 Short Note 5.

- Multiple molecular forms of an enzyme catalyzing the same reaction are isoenzymes or isozymes, e.g. lactate dehydrogenase—5 isoenzymes (LDH-1, 2, 3, 4 and 5), creatine kinase—3 isoenzymes (CK-1, 2, 3) and alkaline phosphatase

- They are physically distinct forms of the same enzyme activity
- They are synthesized from various tissues and hence useful to study the disorders of those organs
- They are made up of different subunits. If the subunits are the same they are known as homomultimer. They are represented by same gene. If the subunits are different they are known as heteromultimer produced by different gene.

Separation and Identification of Isoenzymes

- Electrophoresis—depends upon the mobility in electrical field
- Heat stability—some gets denatured by heat, e.g. bone isoenzyme of ALP
- Inhibitors—tartrate labile ACP
- Substrate specificity or K_m value—different for each isoenzyme, e.g. glucokinase and hexokinase
- Localization—LDH-H4 form is present in heart; LDH-M4 in skeletal muscle.

Lactate Dehydrogenase

- LDL catalyzes the conversion of pyruvate to lactate and vice versa. LDL is concentrated in RBC cell; therefore minor hemolysis causes the false value. Normal values ranges from 100-200 U/L
- Elevation of LDH is seen in hemolytic anemia, hepatocellular damage, muscular dystrophy, cancer, etc.
- LDH is tetramer made up of two H (heart) bands and two M (muscle) bands. Both of these are same molecular weight and with minor amino acid variations
- There are 5 isoenzymes. They are LDH-1, LDH-2, LDH-3, LDH-4, and LDH-5
- With two different polypeptide chains therefore 5 combinations of H and M are possible namely H4, H3M, H2M2, M3H, M4. The tissue specificity and diagnostic importance of these 5 isoenzymes is as follows:
  - H4 form found in heart which is useful for diagnosing heart diseases
  - M4 form found in muscle hence it is useful in diagnosing muscle diseases
  - Isoenzymes of LDH help in the diagnosis of heart and liver diseases
  - Flipped pattern is observed in myocardial infarction (LDH-1 > LDH-2)
  - Increased activity of LDH-5 is an indicator of liver diseases.

Creatine Kinase

- It catalysis the synthesis of creatine phosphate from creatine and ATP
- Normal blood ranges from 15-100 IU/L
- It is made up of 2 polypeptides namely M and B. Therefore 3 combinations of isoenzymes are possible. They are MM found in skeletal muscle, MB found in heart and BB found in brain
- CK subform is highly elevated in muscular dystrophies, acute cerebrovascular injuries. It is most reliable factor in diagnosing AMI
- Three isoenzymes—CK BB(1), CK MB(2), CK MM(3):
  1. CK BB(1)—present in brain
  2. CK MB(2)—is the earliest reliable marker of myocardial infarction
  3. CK MM(3)—is elevated in muscle diseases.

Alkaline Phosphatase

- It is nonspecific enzyme which hydrolyses aliphatic, aromatic and heterocyclic compounds at pH 9-10 in the presence of Mn and Mg. Zinc is a constituent ion of ALP
- ALP produced by osteoblasts for the calcification process
- Normal serum levels are 40-125 U/L. Moderate increase seen in hepatic diseases, and very high levels are seen in extrahepatic obstruction or intrahepatic obstructions, and very high levels are seen in bone diseases
- ALP has nearly 6 types of isoenzymes are—Alpha-1 ALP, Alpha-2 heat labile ALP, Alpha-2 heat stable ALP, pre-beta ALP, gamma-ALP, leucocyte ALP(LAP)
- They are due to the difference in the carbohydrate content

- Alpha-1 ALP—it is about 10% total ALP, and is increased in obstructive jaundice
- Alpha-2 ALP labile—it is about 20% of total ALP, increased in hepatitis
- Alpha-2 heat stable ALP—it is about 1% of total ALP. It is heat stable above 65°C
- Pre-beta ALP—it is about 50% of total ALP. It is elevated in bone diseases
- Gamma-ALP—it is about 10%, it is increased in ulcerative colitis
- Leucocyte-ALP(LAP)—it is increased in lymphomas and decreased in chronic-myeloid leukemia

Acid Phosphatase
- It acts at a pH between 4 and 6
- Normal value in serum is 2.5 to 12 U/L
- Secreted by prostate cells, RBCs, WBCs and platelets
- The value of ACP is increased in prostate cancer and it is an important tumor marker for prostate cancer
- It has got a tartrate labile isoenzyme which is helpful in follow-up of prostate cancer. Its normal level is 1U/L.

7. Galactosemia.

- It is an inborn error of metabolism in galactose metabolism **(Fig. 23)**
- **Incidence:** 1 in 35,000 births
- **Defect**: Deficiency of galactose-1 phosphate uridyltransferase enzyme. Inherited defects of galactokinase, uridyl-transferase, or 4-epimerase can also cause galactosemia.
- **Features:**
  - Hypoglycemia—due to accumulation of galactose-1-phosphate which inhibits galactokinase and glycogen phosphorylase
  - Unconjugated bilirubin is increased—due to reduced conjugation of bilirubin
  - Enlargement of liver (jaundice)
  - Severe mental retardation
  - Congenital cataract—due to enzyme deficiency. Galactose is reduced to dulcitol which gets accumulated in lens causing cataract due to its osmotic effect
  - Amino aciduria—due to renal tubular damage due to deposition of galactose-1-phosphate in renal tubules
  - Galactosemia—due to accumulation of galactose in blood and galactosuria.
- **Diagnosis:** Presence of galactose in urine (galactosuria), congenital cataract, amniocentesis—for prenatal diagnosis
- **Treatment:** Lactose free diet. Mental retardation cannot be corrected.

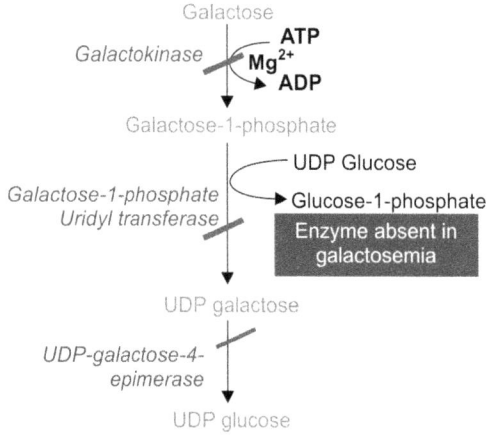

Fig. 23: Galactosemia.

8. Cyclic AMP.

- Cyclic AMP—adenosine 3'5' monophosphate
- It is a cyclic nucleotide of adenine
- It is synthesized from ATP by the action of adenylate cyclase which is an enzyme of integral membrane.
- Its activity is regulated by many peptide hormones which may stimulate or inhibit the production of cAMP from ATP, e.g. glucagon
- cAMP is degraded by phosphodiesterase enzyme which hydrolyses cyclic AMP to AMP
- cAMP acts as a second messenger for hormones like calcitonin, epinephrine, glucagon, etc **(Fig. 24)**.
- It is produced in the cell in response to activation of adenylate cyclase in response to active G protein
- In eukaryotic cells, cAMP binds to a protein kinase called cAMP dependent protein kinase A (PKA) that is a heterotetrameric

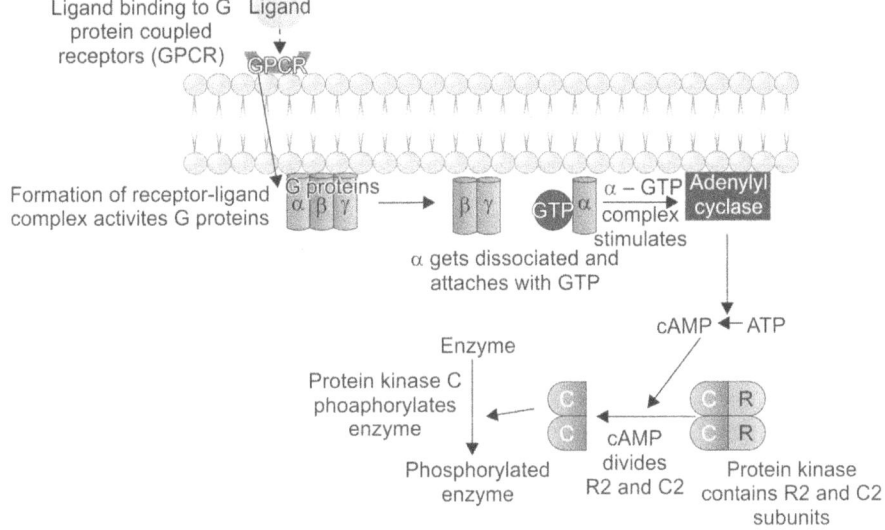

Fig. 24: Mechanism of second messenger action of cAMP.

molecule consisting of two regulatory subunits (R) and two catalytic subunits (C)
- cAMP binds to the regulatory subunits and dissociates the tetramer unto regulatory and catalytic subunits
- The active C subunit catalyzes the transfer of the phosphate of ATP to a serine or threonine or tyrosine residues in a variety of proteins
- The effects of cAMP in eukaryotic cells are mediated by protein phosphorylation—dephosphorylation principally on serine and threonine/tyrosine residues
- The end result is the formation of phosphorylated protein. This causes a change in its function, e.g. epinephrine stimulates cAMP production leading to phosphorylation of phosphorylase kinase which is the active form leading to glycogenolysis
- Glycogen phosphorylase and hormone sensitive lipase are controlled by cyclic AMP **(Fig. 24)**.

9. **Recommended daily dietary allowance.**
- Recommend daily dietary allowance (RDA)—it represents the quantities of the nutrients to be provided in the diet daily to maintain good health and physical efficiency of the body
- RDA for an adult of 70 kg weight is as follows: Carbohydrates—400 g/day, fats —70 g/day, proteins—56 g/day, ascorbic acid—60 mg/day
- The daily need for essential nutrients has been published by the food and nutrition board of the National Research Council as recommended dietary allowances.

FACTORS AFFECTING DAILY ALLOWANCE

- **Sex**: RDA is higher in men than women (around 20%) except that of iron for menstruating women. Extra requirement is needed for pregnant and lactating women
- **Age**: Requirement is higher in growing age, e.g. for a growing child protein requirement is about 2 g/kg body weight and for an adult protein requirement is 1 g/kg body weight
- **Diseases**: Certain common diseases are associated with excess intake of nutrients. Obesity, diabetes, CVD, cancer due to high fat intake, cerebrovascular disease due to high salt intake
- The allowances are to provide for individual variations among most normal

persons depending upon the environment conditions.

10. Essential fatty acids.

Essential fatty acids (EFA) cannot be synthesized by the body but have to be supplemented in diet. They are polyunsaturated fatty acids. They are:
- Linoleic acid (18 C)-ω6
- Linolenic acid (18 C)-ω63
- Arachidonic acid (20 C)-ω6—can be formed, if the dietary supply of linolenic acid is sufficient. So it cannot be strictly categorized under essential fatty acid.

All the essential fatty acids are unsaturated fatty acids which mean their aliphatic chain, contain one or more double bonds.

Significance of PUFA (EFA)
- Used for esterification and excretion of cholesterol
- They form the components of biological membranes and increase the fluidity of membranes of cells
- Eicosanoids (prostaglandin, prostacycline and thromboxanes) are derived from arachidonic acid
- They are antiatherogenic.

Deficiency of EFA

Causes acanthocytosis, acrodermatitis, hyperkeratosis and hypercholesterolemia. Deficiency of unsaturated fatty acid leads to improper synthesis of skin this is called as phrynoderma or toad skin, it is characterized by horny eruptions on the posterior and lateral parts of limbs, back and on the buttocks, hair loss, poor wound healing.

Sources

They are present in vegetable oils and fish oils.
- Linoleic acid (all-cis-9-12-octadecadienoic acid)—present in corn, peanut, cotton seed, soybean and other plant oils
- Linolenic acid (all-cis-6,9,12-octadecatrienoic acid)—present in oils of evening-primrose, borage
- Arachidonic acid (all-cis-5, 8,11,14-eicosatetraenoic acid)—found in animal fats.

- **Arachidonic acid is semiessential because it can be produced form linoleic acid.**

11. Role of vitamin D in calcium metabolism.
Refer 2005, Essay Question 8

12. Iron.

Iron is a trace element needed for human beings.

SOURCES

Leafy vegetables are a major source of iron followed by jaggery, liver. Pulses and cereals are a low source of iron. Milk is a very poor source of iron.

RDA: Adults—20 mg/day, pregnant women—40 mg/day, children—20-30 mg/day.

ABSORPTION

- Only ferrous form is absorbed
- HCl, vitamin C reduces iron to ferrous form, so increases its absorption. Phytic acid and oxalic acid form salts with iron so inhibits iron absorption
- Calcium and copper inhibits iron absorption
- Duodenum and jejunum are the sites of absorption
- When iron stores in the body are depleted, absorption is enhanced. When iron stores are adequate, absorption is decreased. This is called mucosal block theory
- Ferrous iron in the intestinal lumen binds to mucosal cell protein called divalent metal transporter-1 (DMT-1). This iron is transported into the mucosal cell. The unabsorbed iron is excreted
- Inside the mucosal cell, iron is incorporated into apoferritin to form ferritin. Whenever there is iron deficiency this ferritin supplies the iron. In iron deficiency erythropoietin is produced in kidney which enhances iron absorption.

TRANSPORT OF IRON

- Transport of iron is done by the transport protein transferrin

- Ceruloplasmin, the ferro-oxidase enzyme—oxidises ferrous iron to ferric state
- Iron is taken up by the peripheral cells through transferrin receptors
- Total iron binding capacity (TIBC) is provided by the transferrin. It increases in iron deficiency anemia **(Fig. 25)**.

Storage
Iron is stored as ferritin in mucosal cells, liver, spleen, bone marrow.

Functions of Iron
- Iron is the integral part of hemoglobin and myoglobin and is required for transport of oxygen
- Cytochromes and nonheme proteins of electron transport chain and oxidative phosphorylation need iron
- Peroxidase contains iron which is required for the phagocytosis of bacteria by neutrophils
- Iron is needed for the immune competence of body.

Deficiency of Iron

Causes
- Indian diet contains less iron
- Hookworm infestation
- Repeated pregnancies
- Chronic blood loss in piles, peptic ulcer and uterine bleeding
- Nephrosis, subtotal gastrectomy and lead poisoning are the other causes of iron deficiency.

Clinical Features
- Microcytic hypochromic anemia ensues
- In anemia body cells lack oxygen and the person becomes apathic
- Severe iron deficiency leads to heart failure
- Chronic deficiency leads to achlorhydria, impaired attention, irritability, lower memory, poor scholastic performance.

Toxic Manifestations
Acute intoxication—diarrhea, nausea, abdominal pain.

Hemosiderosis: It occurs in patients receiving repeated blood transfusions. Hemosiderin pigments deposit in spleen and liver.
- Hemosiderin is an iron storage protein which can hold about 35% of iron by weight
- It accumulates in the body (spleen and liver as golden brown granules) when the supply of iron is in excess, e.g. repeated blood transfusions
- Hemosiderosis is commonly observed among Bantu tribe in South Africa. This is attributed to a high intake of iron from their staple diet corn which is low in phosphate content and their habit of cooking foods in iron pots.

Hemochromatosis
- It is a disease in which iron is directly deposited in the tissues (liver, spleen, pancreas and skin)
- The manifestations are bronzed pigmentation of the skin, cirrhosis of liver and pancreatic fibrosis.
- The triad of cirrhosis, hemochromatosis, and diabetes are referred to as bronze diabetes
- **Iron vessels:** Cooking in iron utensils causes iron overload
- Bantu siderosis, hemochromatosis are other causes of iron overload.

13. Prostaglandins.

Eicosanoids are 20 carbon containing fatty acids (FA). They are derived from 20 carbon FA namely prostanoic acid. They are also called as group of local hormones.

Precursor for Eicosanoids
The precursor molecule for eicosanoids is arachidonic acid.

Types of Eicosanoids
They are 4 types of eicosanoids:
1. Prostaglandins (PGs)
2. Prostacyclins (PGI)
3. Thromboxanes (TXs)
4. Leukotrienes (LTs).

Classification of Prostaglandins
According to the attachment of different substituent groups to the ring prostaglandins

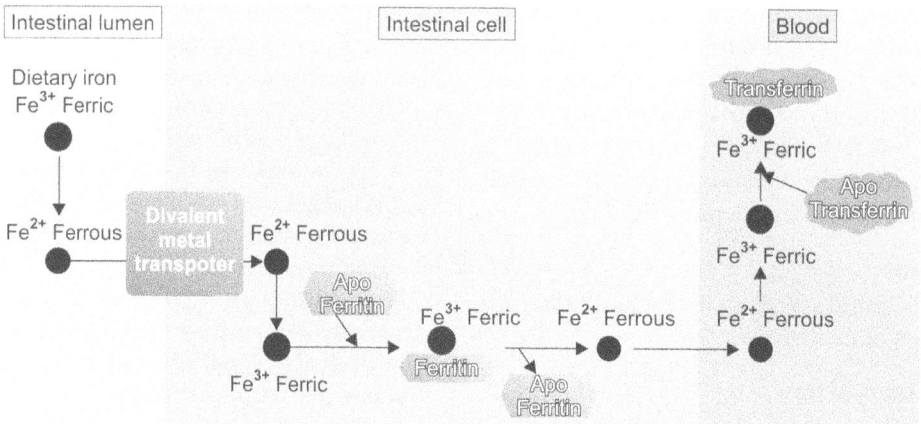

Fig. 25: Absorption and transport of iron.

are classified as A, B, D, E, F, G and H. Prostacyclins (PGI).

Synthesis of Prostaglandins

All the tissues are able to synthesise eicosanoids from PUFA.
- Series-1 double bond—from linoleic acid
- Series-2 double bonds—from arachidonic acid
- Series-3 double bonds—from eicosa pentaenoic acid.

Synthesis of Prostaglandins (PGs) (Fig. 26)

- **Cyclo-oxygenase pathway**—in this pathway all the prostaglandins, prostacyclines and thromboxanes are produced except LTs
- Phospholipids in the membranes are acted by phospholipases to release arachidonic acid
- Arachidonic acid is acted by cyclo-oxygenase enzyme to produce PGG_2, H_2 which are converted to PGD_2, E_2, F_2
- **It is also diverted to synthesize PGI_2 by prostacycline synthase and TXA_2 by thromboxane synthase.**

Functions of Prostaglandins and Related Compounds

On CVS
- PGI_2—is a powerful vasodilator, hence used in treatment of hypertension. PGI_2 inhibits vasodilatation and inhibits platelet aggregation to promote thrombus formation
- TXA_2 produced by platelets are vasoconstrictors and cause platelet aggregation. PGI and TX are having opposite actions.

On Ovary and Uterus

PGF_2—induces termination of pregnancy and induction of labor by stimulating uterine muscles. So it is used in medical termination of pregnancy and to arrest postpartum bleeding.

On Respiratory Tract
- PGE is a potent bronchodilator whereas PGF is bronchoconstrictor
- PGE 1 and 2 are used in treatment of asthma.

On Immunity and Inflammation
- PGE_2 and D_2—induce inflammation by increasing the permeability of capillaries.
- On gastrointestinal tract **(GIT)** PGE—it inhibit gastric secretion so it is used for treating gastric ulcers
- **Metabolic effects** PGE_2 stimulates glycogenesis, induces calcium mobilization form bones and inhibits lipolysis.

14. Ketone bodies.

Refer 2005 Essay Question 2.
- Acetyl-CoA formed from fatty acids can enter and get oxidized in TCA cycle only when carbohydrates are available. During

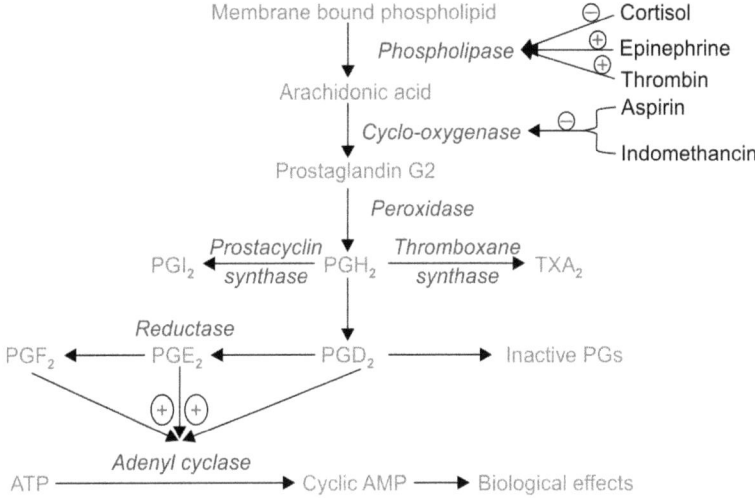

Fig. 26: Synthesis of prostaglandins.

starvation and in uncontrolled diabetes mellitus, the acetyl CoA takes the alternate fate of formation of ketone bodies (KB)
- Level of KB in blood is **less than 1 mg/dL**
- **Site of formation:** Liver
- **Site of utilization of KB:** Extrahepatic tissues
- **Uses:** During starvation, it is the major fuel for brain, heart and muscles. Brain gets 75% of energy from KB during starvation
- The ketone bodies are mainly three— namely-**acetoacetate, β-hyroxybutyrate and acetone**. The later one is volatile in nature. Ketone bodies are water-soluble and on oxidation produce high range of energy.

Synthesis of Ketone bodies (Ketogenesis): Ketogenesis takes place during high production of FA from liver.
Site: Mitochondrial matrix of liver cells
Precursor: Acetyl-CoA.

KETOGENESIS (FIG. 27)

Reactions

- **Condensation:** Two molecules of acetyl-CoA condense to form acetoacetyl-CoA, this reaction is catabolized by thiolase
- **Production of HMG-CoA:** Acetoacetyl-CoA condenses with another molecule of acetyl-CoA to produce β-hydroxy-β-methylglutaryl-CoA (HMG-CoA) by the enzyme HMG-CoA synthase. This is the key regulatory enzyme of ketogenesis
- **Lyase reaction:** HMG-CoA is cleaved to acetoacetate and acetyl-CoA by the action of HMG-CoA lyase present only in liver
- **Reduction and spontaneous decarboxylation:** Acetoacetate is reduced by dehydrogenase to beta–hydroxybutyrate in the presence of NADH **or** it undergoes spontaneous decarboxylation to form acetone.

Utilization of Ketone bodies: Ketone body utilization takes place in extrahepatic tissues for energy production. Tissues like heart, renal cortex, prefer KA than glucose for energy production.

15. Degeneracy of code.

- It is one of the salient features of genetic code
- 61 codons code for 20 amino acids so most of the amino acids have more than 1 codons, e.g. serine has 6 codons and glycine has 4 codons this is called degeneracy of code
- The codons that degenerate the same amino acid are called synonyms which mostly differ in the 3' end or third base of codon.

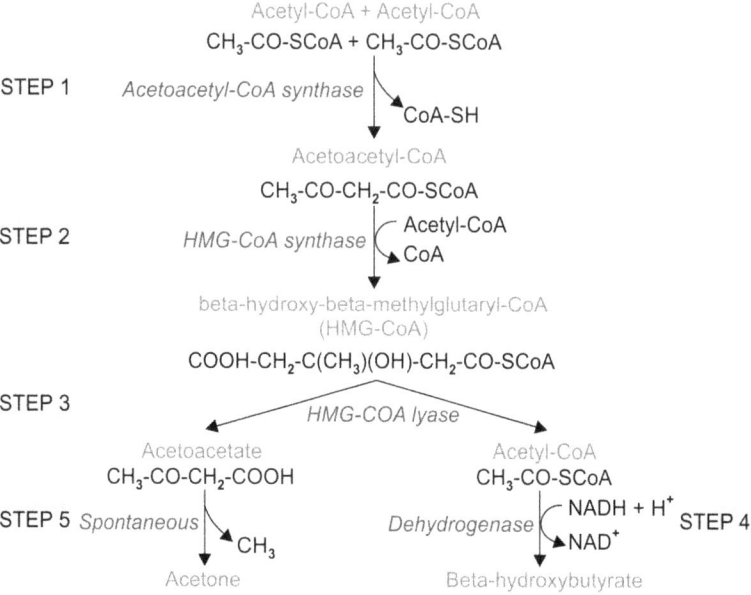

Fig. 27: Ketogenesis.

16. Detoxification.

Xenobiotics are strange or foreign compounds which may be accidentally ingested or taken as drugs or compounds produced in the body by bacterial metabolism.

VARIOUS XENOBIOTICS

- Compounds accidentally ingested like preservatives, food additives and adulterants
- Drugs taken for therapeutic purposes
- Endogenous compounds which has to be eliminated by body like bilirubin, steroids
- Compounds produced by bacterial metabolism, e.g. amines produced by decarboxylation of amino acids like histamine from histidine; cadaverine from lysine; putrescine from ornithine; tyramine from tyrosine and tryptamine from tryptophan.

Detoxification is the process by which these xenobiotics are detoxified in the body. It is also known as biotransformation.

PHASES OF DETOXIFICATION (FIG. 28)

There are 3 phases of detoxification—phase I, II and III

1. Phase I—Hydroxylation—oxidation, reduction, hydrolysis—products are excreted via Phase II
2. Phase II—conjugation—by conjugating agents
3. Phase III—combination of all these reactions.

Phase 1 Reactions

- It is the alteration of foreign molecule by adding a functional group by hydroxylation, oxidation, reduction and hydrolysis. The main function of phase 1 is to convert it into nontoxic metabolite
- By the end of this phase the toxicity may be decreased.

Hydroxylation

It is the chief reaction involved with oxidation by hydroxylase enzymes present in endoplasmic reticulum. There are 150 isoforms. They are—cytochrome P450 monooxygenases. They are mixed function oxidases. NADPH is its coenzyme

$$RH + O_2 + NADPH \rightarrow ROH + H_2O + NADP^+$$

- They are inducible enzymes. Phenobarbital -↑ their activity. It is involved

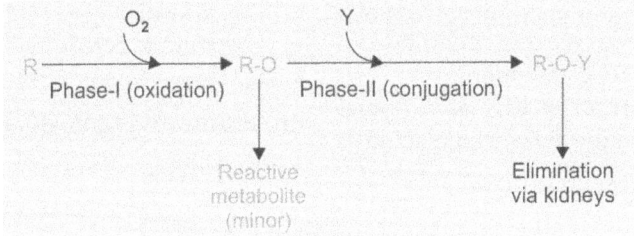

Fig. 28: Phases of detoxification.

in metabolism of drugs and aromatic hydrocarbon
- Mitochondrial P450 enzymes present in mitochondria
- Microsomal P450 system is involved in steroid synthesis in adrenal cortex.

Oxidation
By oxidation alcohols and aldehydes are converted to their corresponding acids.
For example: Ethyl alcohol ⟶ acetaldehyde ⟶ acetic acid
Benzaldehyde ⟶ benzoic acid

Reduction
Done by cytochrome P450 reductases in liver.
- Nitro compounds are reduced to amine, e.g. picric acid → picramic acid
- Aldehydes/ketones are reduced to alcohols.

Hydrolysis
Esters, amines, hydrazines, amides and glycosidic bonds are biotransformed by hydrolysis by hydrolases like esterases, etc.
For example, aspirin ⟶ salicylic acid + acetic acid.

Phase 2 Reactions: (Conjugation)
Refer 2004 Short Note 14.

Phase 3 Reactions: May or May Not Occur
- The product of phase II is further conjugated with glutathione
- In certain cases the xenobiotics may be converted to harmful carcinogens.

17. Gout.
- Uric acid is the catabolic end product of purine nucleotides. When uric acid level is increased in blood it tends to get deposited as crystals in synovial fluid of joints leading to inflammation and acute arthritis. This disease is called gout.

TYPE OF GOUT
Two types of gout—primary and secondary gout.

Primary Gout
About 10% is idiopathic. Others are due to inherited disorders due to defective enzymes.

Causes of Primary Gout
- Super active 5-phosphoribosyl amido transferase enzyme which is not sensitive to feedback regulation leads to increased uric acid production
- Abnormal PRPP synthetase—not subjected to allosteric regulation which leads to increased uric acid production
- Salvage pathway enzyme deficiencies—this causes increased availability of PRPP and decreased purines. So no feedback inhibition
- Glucose-6-phosphatase (G6P) deficiency-von Gierke's Disease—in this condition, G6P cannot be converted to glucose and so glucose enters HMP pathway to produce more Ribose 5P. This will lead to high production of PRPP which leads to more purines and more uric acid by catabolism of purines.

Secondary Gout
- Increased production of uric acid—due to increased turnover of cells as in

malignancy lymphomas, leukemia, polycythemia, psoriasis, after treatment of cancer, trauma and starvation
- Reduced excretion of uric acid—renal failure, thiazide diuretics, lactic acidosis and ketoacidosis.

Clinical Features
- Uric acid gets deposited in the cooler areas of body like distal joints to form tophi
- Hyperuricemia leads to increased excretion of uric acid through kidneys, so uric acid crystals get deposited in the urinary tract leading to renal calculi.

Treatment
Combination of nutritional and drug therapy.
- **Dietary purine**—intake should be reduced, alcohol should be restricted
- **Uricosuric drugs**—which increases the excretion of uric acid like probenecid should be used
- **Allopurinol**—competitive inhibitor of Xanthine. Oxidase can be used to reduce urate production and calculi
- **Colchicine**—an anti-inflammatory drug can be used to reduce inflammation in joints.

18. Antioxidants.

Antioxidants are compounds which prevent lipid peroxidation or rancidity by free radicals or control the oxidation process.

Types
I. **As per the nature**
   - **Naturally occurring antioxidants**—For example vitamin E and C, selenium, β-carotene
   - **Chemicals**: Butylated hydroxyanisole (BHA), butylated hydroxytoluene (BHT).
II. **As per their action:** Two types: a) Preventive and b) Chain breaking antioxidants.

Preventive Antioxidants
- They will inhibit the initial production of free radicals. They are catalase, glutathione peroxidase and EDTA

- Catalase: $2H_2O_2 \longrightarrow O_2 + H_2O$
- Glutathione peroxidase: $2H_2O_2 \longrightarrow 2H_2O$
- EDTA.

Chain Breaking Antioxidants
- They inhibit the propagative phase:

$$O_2 + O_2 + 2H^+ \longrightarrow H_2O_2 + O_2$$

- They include—superoxide dismutase, uric acid and vitamin E
- Vitamin E would intercept the peroxyl free radical and inactivate it before PUFA can be attacked

$$T\text{-}OH + ROO' \longrightarrow TO' + ROOH$$

- The phenolic hydrogen of alpha tocopherol reacts with the peroxyl radical converting it to a hydroperoxide product
- The tocoperoxyl radical thus formed is stable and will not propagate the cycle any further
- This oxidative form of vitamin E is converted to vitamin E by ascorbic acid. Ascorbic acid becomes dehydroascorbate by reacting with vitamin E radical. Two molecules of dehydroascorbate combine together to form ascorbate
- Other antioxidants are ceruloplasmin, caffeine and β-carotene
- Some antioxidants used in therapy are vitamin C, vitamin E, dimethylthiourea, dimethylsulfoxide, allopurinol.

19. Genetic code.

- It is a triplet codon in mRNA
- The letters A, G, U, and C correspond to the nucleotides found in DNA
- Within the protein coding genes these nucleotides are organized into three-letter code words called codons, and the collection of these codons makes up the genetic code
- There are four different bases that can generate 64 codons.

Salient Features
- **Triplet codons:** Each codon is consecutive sequence of three bases on the mRNA, e.g. UUU codes for phenylalanine

- **Nonoverlapping:** The codes are read one after another in a continuous manner, e.g. AUG,CAU,GAU,GCA, etc.
- **Nonpunctuated:** There is no punctuation in between codons and they are comma less
- **Degenerate:** 61 codon codes for 20 amino acids so most of the amino acids have more than 1 codons, e.g. serine has 6 codons and glycine has 4 codons this is called degeneracy of code. The codons that degenerate the same amino acid are called synonyms which mostly differ in the 3' end or third base of codon
- **Unambigous:** Codons are unambiguous that means one codon stands only for one amino acid
- **Universal:** The codons are same for same amino acids in all species. Exception is AUA codes for methionine in mitochondria and it codes for isoleucine in cytoplasm
- **Wobbling hypothesis:** Put forth by Crick. Reduced stringency between the third base of the codon and the complementary nucleotide in the anticodon is wobbling, e.g. GGU, GGC, and GGA code for glycine all the three pair with the anticodon CCI (I-Inosinic acid). A single tRNA can recognize more than one codon
- **Terminator codon:** There are three codon which do not code for any amino acids. They are nonsense codons or terminator codonsor punctuate codons. These three codons are UGA, UAG, UAA collectively known as amber, ochre and opal codons. In special cases, UGA stands for selenocysteine
- **Initiator codon:** AUG acts as initiator codon. For few proteins GUG may be the initiator codon.

20. Proto-oncogenes and oncogenes.

- Oncogenes are genes capable of causing cancer. They have the potential to cause cancer
- Oncogenes were originally discovered in tumor causing viruses—viral oncogenes – e.g. rous sarcoma virus—which causes sarcoma in avians. A strain of virus deficient in particular gene cannot cause this disease and named as *sarcoma* gene (Src)
- These are similar to certain genes present in normal avian cells called as proto-oncogenes
- Viral genes are denoted as V-src and cellular genes as C-src
- Oncogenes are the sequence of DNA which has been altered or mutated from the proto-oncogenes
- Oncogenes encode for certain proteins known as oncoproteins
- Products of many oncogenes are polypeptide growth factors, e.g. sis gene produces platelet derived growth factors (PDGF) needed for wound healing
- Some of the products act as receptors for growth factors, e.g. erb-B—produces receptors for—epidermal growth factor (EGF).

Activation of Oncogenes

Viruses, chemical carcinogens, chromosome translocations, gamma rays, spontaneous mutations may activate the oncogenes which lead to malignancy.

Examples for Oncogenes causing Cancer

- Erb-B1—lung cancer
- Erb-B2—gastric tumors.

Proto-oncogenes

- Proto-oncogenes are normal regulatory genes of cells
- Their products are mostly:
  - Growth factors for the cells, e.g. *sis* gene for PDGF needed for wound healing B-receptors for growth factors. e.g. erb-B-receptor for EGF
  - Those involved in intracellular growth signaling pathways, e.g. src products.
- C-oncogenes are under the control of these regulatory genes and expressed whenever needed
- When proto-oncogenes are mutated, they become oncogenes, which cannot be controlled and increased growth signaling leads to cancer, e.g. Ras, src, etc.

Antioncogenes or Oncosuppressor Gene

- These are the genes which protect a person from getting cancer
- When the gene is deleted or mutated, cancer results
- Antioncogenes are written in capital letters, whereas oncogenes are written in small letters, e.g. retinoblastoma – RB (antioncogene).

21. Allosteric enzymes and its feedback regulation.

- Allosteric enzymes have two individual sites—one for binding of substrate and the other for modifier/regulator
- Enzymes which have one catalytic site where the substrate binds and another separate site where the modifier binds are known as allosteric enzymes [Greek: Allo S = other], e.g. phosphofructokinase.
- The binding of regulatory molecule can either enhance the activity of the enzyme (**allosteric activation**) or inhibit the activity of the enzyme (**allosteric inhibition**)
- The inhibitor is not a substrate analog.
- K_m is increased but V_{max} is reduced, e.g. aspartate transcarbamoylase
- If the regulatory molecule enhance the activity of the enzyme it is known as positive modulator and if it inhibits the enzyme activity it is known as negative modulator
- Negative feedback regulation—inhibition of enzyme activity by product is called as negative feedback regulation. It is necessary to control metabolic pathways for efficient cellular functions
- Positive feedback regulation—it is quite opposite to negative feedback regulation
- Allosteric regulators are divided into two classes based on the influence of allosteric effector on K_m and V_{max}
- K-class of allosteric enzymes—effector changes K_m but not V_{max}, e.g. phosphofructokinase
- V-class of allosteric enzymes—effector alters the V_{max}, but not K_m, e.g. acetyl-CoA carboxylase.

For example, allosteric enzymes and their modifiers.

S. No.	Allosteric enzyme	Allosteric activator	Allosteric inhibitor
1	ALA synthase		Heme
2	Aspartate transcarbamoylase	ATP	CTP
3	HMG-CoA reductase		Cholesterol
4	PFK	AMP, F-2,6-P	ATP, citrate
5	Acetyl-CoA carboxylase	Citrate	Acyl-CoA
6	Citrate synthase		ATP

22. Phospholipids and their clinical importance.

Refer 2004 Short Note 1.

23. Kwashiorkor.

This is due to the malnutrition of proteins with adequate energy intake. Kwashiorkor means sickness the older child gets when the next child is born. This is the most common nutritional disorder in many parts of the world. It is entirely preventable if children are given a well-balanced diet with adequate amount of protein and essential amino acids.

The salient features of kwashiorkor is tabulated below:

Features	Kwashiorkor
Age of onset	1-5 years
Growth retardation of child	Severe
Attitude	Lethargic and apathetic
Appearance	Edema on face and limbs
Appetite	Anorexia
Skin	Crazy pavement dermatitis
Hair	Sparse, soft and thin
Other	Angular stomatitis, cheilosis, watery diarrhea, muscle wasting, fatty liver
Serum albumin	<2 g (hypoalbuminemia)

24. Inhibitors of electron transport chain (Fig. 29).

Site Specific Inhibitors

- **Complex I—CoQ specific inhibitors.**
  - Barbiturates—amobarbital
  - Antibiotic—piercidin
  - Rotenone, insecticide, fish poison
  - Alkylguanidines—hypotensive drugs.
- **Complex II to coenzyme Q:** Carboxin.
- **Complex III to cytochrome c inhibitors:**
  - Antimycin
  - British anti-lewisite (BAL)
  - Naphthoquinone.
- **Complex IV—cytochrome oxidase inhibitors:**
  - CO - Carbon monoxide
  - CN - Cyanide
  - H2S - Hydrogen sulphide
  - Azide.
- **Site between succinate dehydrogenase and CoQ:**
  - Carboxin—inhibits transfer of ions from FADH2
  - Malonate—competitively inhibits succinate dehydrogenase.

Inhibitors of Oxidative Phosphorylation

- Atractyloside—inhibits translocase
- Oligomycin—inhibits flow of protons through Fo
- Ionophores—For example valinomycin—mobile ion carriers—allows K to permeate mitochondria; Gramicidin—channel former.

Uncouplers of Oxidative Phosphorylation

- 2,4-dinitrophenol (2,4 DNP)
- 2,4-dinitrocresol (2,4 DNC)
- Chlorocarbonylcyanidephenyl hydrazone (CCCP).

Physiological Uncouplers

- Thyroxine
- Thermogenin in brown adipose tissue.

25. Diagnostic value of isoenzymes.

Refer 2003, Short Note 5.

26. Basal metabolic Rate (BMR)

Definition: The energy required by an awake individual during physical, emotional and digestive rest. It is the minimum amount of energy required to perform vital functions such as circulation, respiration, working of heart, etc.

Normal value:

- Men—34-37 kcal/m^2/hr (24 kcal/kg body weight/day)
- Women—30-35 kcal/m^2/hr.

Resting metabolic rate: 3% higher than BMR. It is the energy required to maintain life or vital functions of the body.

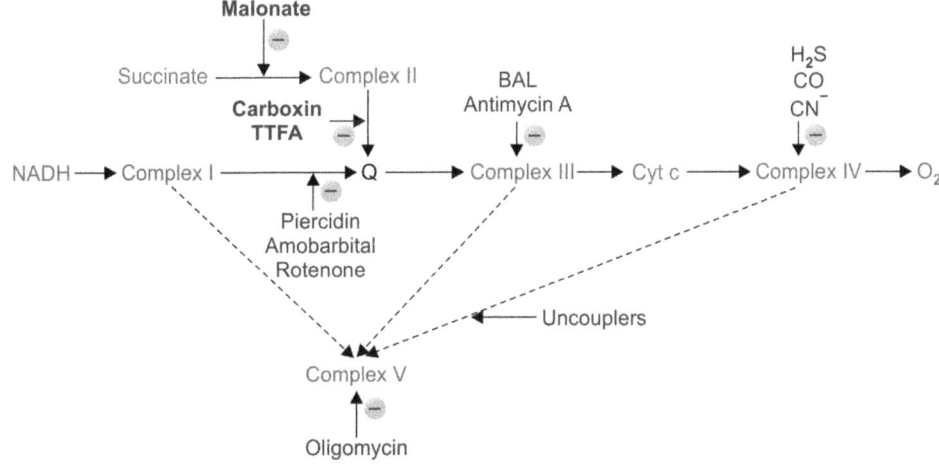

Fig. 29: Inhibitors of Electron transport chain.

Measurement of BMR: (direct method—by the heat evolved; indirect method—by volume of O_2 consumed and CO_2 evolved).

Factors Affecting BMR

- **Age:** In old age, BMR is lowered
- **Sex:** Males have a higher value
- **Temperature:** BMR increases in cold climate
- **Exercise:** It increases during exercise
- **Fever:** 12% increase during fever
- **Thyroid hormones:** BMR is raised in hyperthyroidism.

27. Fatty acid synthesis.

De novo synthesis of fatty acid—Lynen's spiral.

Site of Synthesis

- Cytosol (extra mitochondrial fractions) of liver, adipose tissue, kidney, brain and mammary glands
- Major fatty acid is synthesized by palmitic acid (16 C).

Importance

- The excess consumption of carbohydrates and proteins are converted to fatty acids
- Fatty acids are building blocks of fats in the form of triacylglycerol.

Precursor Molecule for Fatty Acid Synthesis

Acetyl-CoA is the starting molecule in fatty acid synthesis. Sequential addition of 2 carbon acetyl-CoA molecules results in the formation of long fatty acid chain.

Reactions (Fig. 30): All the reactions in the fatty acid synthesis are taken place in multi-functional enzyme called fatty acid synthase complex. It is a dimer; each monomer consists of 7 enzymes and 1 acyl carrier protein.

The total reactions are divided into 3 phases:

1. Production of acetyl-CoA, NADPH
2. Conversion of acetyl-CoA into malonyl-CoA
3. Synthesis of fatty acid chain.

Preparatory Phase: Production of acetyl-CoA molecules

The acetyl-CoA molecules are synthesized from—aerobic glycolysis, pyruvate oxidation, oxidation of even chain fatty acids and by the metabolism of certain amino acids in the mitochondria which is then transferred to the cytosol through citrate.

NADPH is mainly produced from HMP shunt.

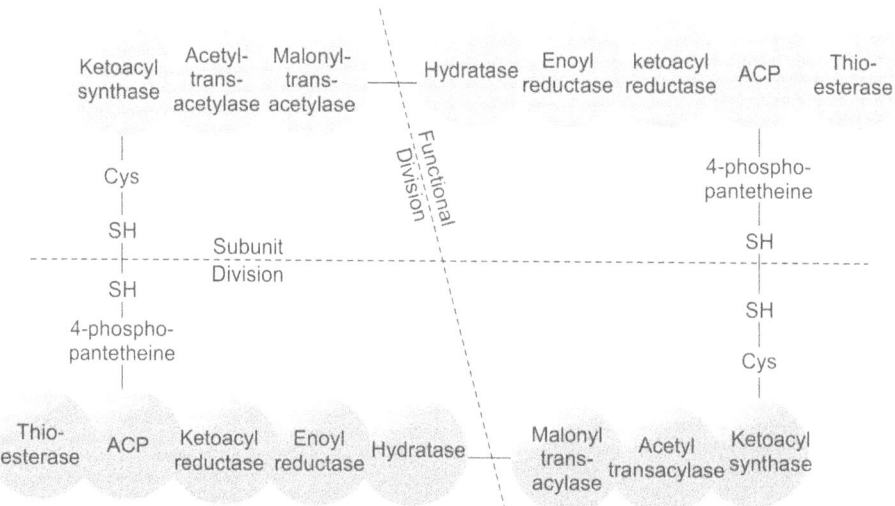

Fig. 30: Fatty acid synthase complex.

Step 1: Conversion of acetyl-CoA to Malonyl-CoA by Carboxylation (Fig. 31)

In the presence of acetyl-CoA carboxylase, acetyl-CoA is converted into malonyl-CoA. This is the rate limiting step. Biotin is the co-enzyme

$$\text{Acetyl-CoA} + CO_2 \xrightarrow{\text{Acetyl-CoA carboxylase}} \text{Malyonyl-CoA}$$

Step 2: Formation of Fatty Acid Chain

- **Step 2A:** Acetyl transacylase enzyme transfers acetyl group to SH group of condensing enzyme which is otherwise known as ketoacyl synthase. Now the enzyme is called as acetyl S-Condensing enzyme.
- **Step 2B:** Then Malonyl-CoA is bound to SH group of ACP component in the presence of malonyl transacylase. Now the enzyme is called as acyl-malonyl enzyme.

Step-3: Condensation

- The acetyl and malonyl units are then condensed to form β-ketoacyl-ACP or acetoacetyl-ACP by the condensing enzyme. During this process decarboxylation occurs and one carbon is lost.

Step 4: Reduction

β-ketoacyl (acetoacetyl)—ACP is reduced to β-hydroxyacyl-ACP in the presence of β-ketoacyl-ACP reductase, and NADPH.

Step 5: Dehydration

B-hydorxyacyl-ACP is then dehydrated to form 2 enoyl ACP by dehydratase enzyme.

Step 6: Second Reduction

- 2 enoyl ACP is again reduced to acyl-ACP (Butyryl-ACP) by enoyl reductase enzyme
- The carbon chain from the ACP is shifted to SH group of ketoacyl synthase
- Completion of 1 cycle occurs with the formation of 4 carbon fatty acid chain.

Cycling Reactions

In next preceding cycle additions of 2 carbon malonyl-CoA to growing chain takes place. Sequence of reactions—condensation, reduction, dehydration and reduction are repeated for 7 times to get 16 carbon palmitic acid with total 8 cyclic reactions.

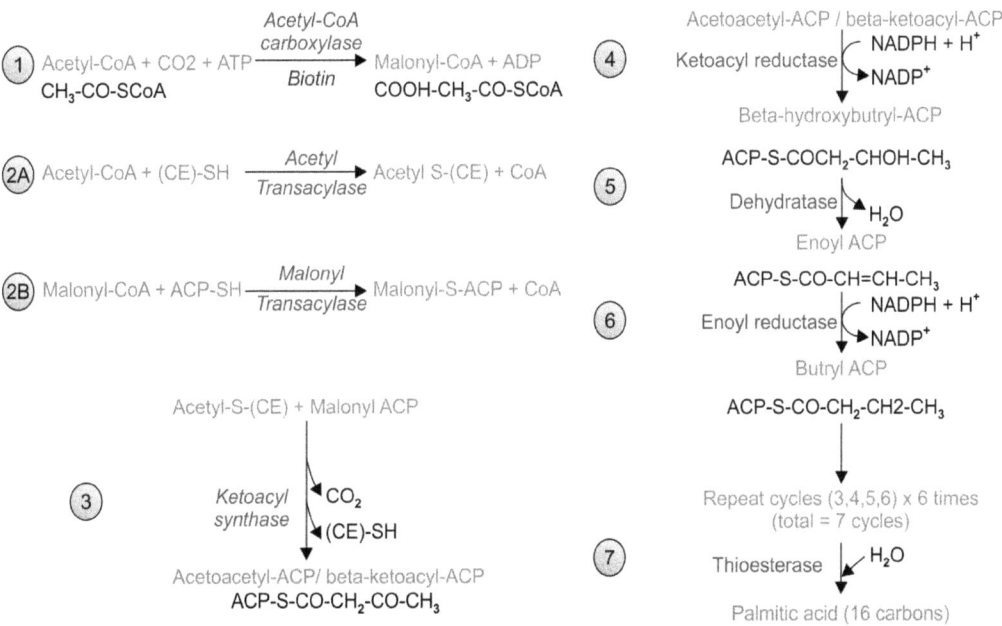

Fig. 31: Fatty acid synthesis.

Step 7: Release of Palmitic Acid

Thioesterase or decyclase enzyme releases palmitic acid from the multienzyme complex.

Regulation of Fatty Acid Synthesis

- Availability of substrates—high carbohydrate level and citrate increase lipogenesis
- Key enzyme—acetyl-CoA carboxylase is activated by citrate and by covalent modification by dephosphorylation
- The hormones like insulin stimulates the synthesis—whereas glucagon, epinephrine, norepinephrine inhibit the synthesis by inactivating acetyl-CoA carboxylase.

28. Heme degradation (Bilirubin synthesis).

Refer 2005 Short Note 3.

29. Eicosanoids.

Refer 2005 Short Note 13.

Leukotriens

Lipoxygenase Pathway (Fig. 32)

- In this pathway arachidonic acid is converted to various LTs which are synthesized in WBC, lung, heart, spleens.
- LT B4—is produced in neutrophils and it is a potent chemotactic agent.
- The slow reacting substances of anaphylaxis (SRS-A) contains LTC4, D4 and E4. They are very active than histamine and cause violent allergic reactions. They cause contraction of smooth muscles, bronchoconstriction, vasoconstriction, clumping of RBCs, and increase capillary permeability. SRS is the mediator of asthma.

30. LDL metabolism.

LDL Metabolism (Fig. 33)

- LDL transports cholesterol from liver to peripheral tissues
- It has only apo B100.

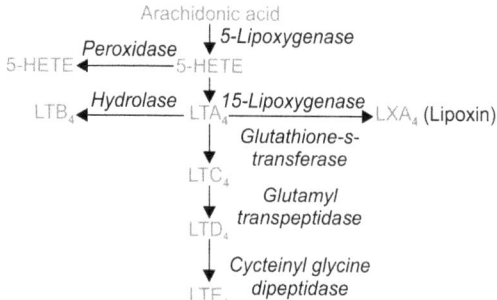

Fig. 32: Lipoxygenase pathway.

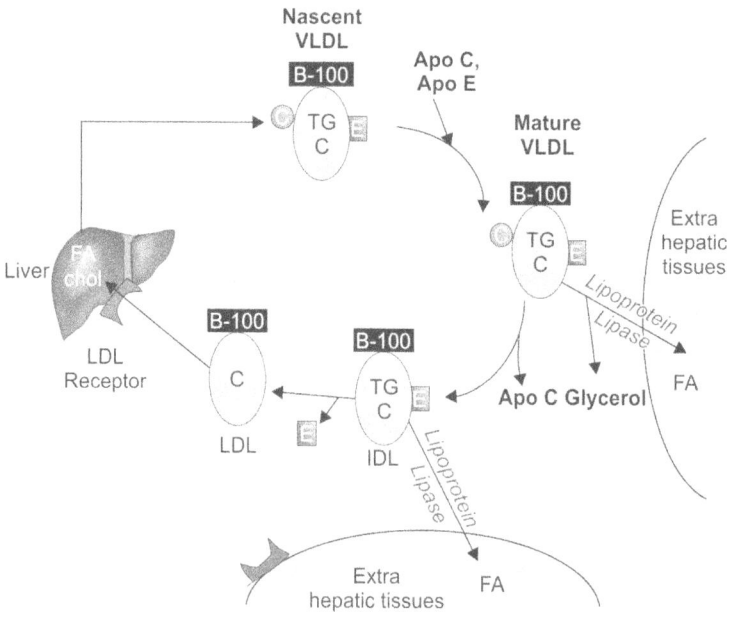

Fig. 33: LDL metabolism.

Production of LDL

- Most of the LDL is derived from VLDL but a small part is directly released from the liver
- LDL is taken by peripheral tissues and by hepatocytes by **receptor mediated** endocytosis—this is a regulated mechanism
- LDL is also removed by an unregulated independent mechanism by scavenger receptors by forming foam cells. This mechanism is active when blood cholesterol level is very high.

Structure of LDL Receptor (Fig. 34)

LDL receptor also called "apo B, E" receptor, since it is specific for apo B100 and E. It looks like pits and occurs on the cell surface of all cells especially hepatocytes. These pits are coated with a protein called clathrin on the cytosolic side of the cell membrane. The glycoprotein receptor spans the membrane, the B100 binding region being at the exposed amino terminal end.

Metabolic fate of LDL: LDL cholesterol after binding to LDL receptors is taken up by endocytosis. The apoprotein and cholesteryl ester are then hydrolyzed in the lysosomes, and cholesterol is translocated into the cell. The receptors are recycled to the cell surface. This influx of cholesterol inhibits in a coordinated manner HMG-CoA synthase, HMG-CoA reductase, and, therefore, cholesterol synthesis. It stimulates ACAT activity; and down-regulates synthesis of the LDL receptor. Thus, the number of LDL receptors on the cell surface is regulated by the cholesterol requirement for membranes, steroid hormones, or bile acid synthesis.

Clinical Significance

- If LDL concentration is increased it will lead to higher incidence of atherosclerosis
- A fraction of cholesterol is taken by macrophages
- LDL infiltrates through arterial walls and cholesterol gets deposited in the arterial walls and foam cells are formed by oxidation of LDL
- Atheromatous plaques are formed from the foam cells deposited on the walls causing increased thrombosis and coronary artery diseases
- Because of this complications, LDL cholesterol is known as **'bad cholesterol'**
- Insulin and thyroxine increase the binding of LDL to liver cells. This is the cause for hypercholesterolemia in diabetes and hypothyroidism.

Disorder

| Familial hyper-cholesterolemia type IIa | Defective LDL receptors or mutation in ligand region of Apo B100 | Elevated LDL levels and hypercholesterolemia, resulting in atherosclerosis and coronary disease |

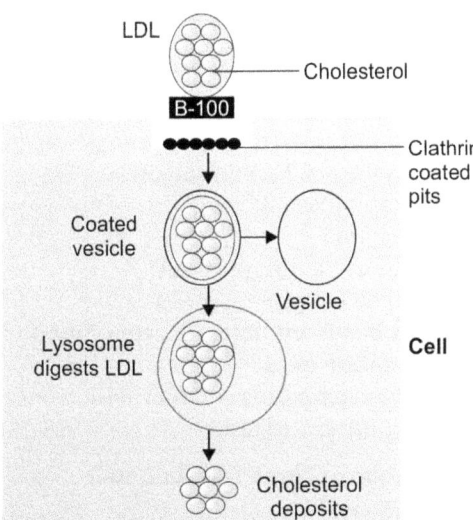

Fig. 34: LDL receptor.

31. Synthetic nucleotides and their importance.

- These are structurally similar nucleotides but functionally opposite—mild variation in structural configuration either in heterocyclic ring or in sugar moiety
- They inhibit enzymes of nucleic acid synthesis
- Disruption of base pairing

Hence they are used for the treatment for: a) cancer; b) for gout—allopurinol; c) drugs for immunosuppresants to be given in organ transplant cases, e.g. azathioprine.

Synthetic Analogues of Purines

- **6 mercaptopurine** (purenethol)—used for treating acute leukemia, immunosuppresant. It acts by inhibiting protein synthesis
  Side effects—bone marrow depression, nausea, vomiting
- **6 thioguanine**—inhibits enzymes of purine nucleotide pathway
- **Acyclovir** (acycloguanine)—used to treat herpes zoster by inhibiting DNA polymerase of herpes virus
- **Allopurinol**—for the treatment of gout, uric acid calculus, leukemia.
- **Azathioprine**—(imidazole derivative of 6 mercaptopurine)
  - It inhibits synthesis of DNA, RNA
  - It is an immunosuppresant.

Synthetic Analogues of Pyrimidines

- **5' flurouracil**—(thymidine analogue)
  - ↓ DNA—thymineless death, ↓ thymidilate synthesis and prevents protein synthesis
  - **Treatment:** Adenocarcinoma—breast, cancer stomach, colon
  - **Toxicity:** Myelosuppresant.
- **5'flurocytosine** 5-FC—thymidine analogue—antifungal
  - **Treatment**—cryptococosis, candidiasis
  - **Side effects** - hepatotoxicity, rashes
- **5' iodo 2' deoxyuridine (IudR)**
  - Antiviral - ↓ viral DNA synthesis— Inhibits DNA viral replication—pox and herpes
  - Local application—effective for herpes simplex keratitis.
- **6-AzaCytidine** (mylosar)/5-azacytidine
- ↓ Pyrimidine synthesis → ↓ orotic decarboxylase. More side effects
- **Cytarabine (ara-c)** - Arabinosyl-cytosine S-phase antimetabolite
  - Blocks DNA synthesis alone, interferes chain elongation
  - **Treatment of cancer**—acute myeloblastic leukemia; viral infection
  - **Side effects**—bone depression, oral ulcers, GI disorders, conjunctivitis.
- **AZT:** Taken up by lymphocytes and converted to AZT triphosphate—inhibits HIV
  - **Reverse transcriptase:** It competes with dTPP, synthesis of DNA from viral RNA
  - **Side effects:** Bone marrow depression, anemia.

32. Liver function tests.

The tests used to diagnose liver disease are called liver function tests. They are:

- **Tests based on hepatic excretory function:**
  - Serum bilirubin
  - Urine bile pigments - bilirubin, bile salts, urobilinogen.
  - Fecal urobilinogen
  - Dye excretion test - bromsulphophthalein (BSP) test.
- **Markers of liver injury—estimation of liver enzymes:**
  - Serum alanine aminotransferase (ALT)
  - Serum aspartate aminotransferase (AST)
  - Serum alkaline phosphatase (ALP)
  - Serum gamma-glutamyl transferase (GGT).
- **Tests based on synthetic function: (Synthesis of plasma proteins):** Estimation of:
  - Total plasma proteins
  - Serum albumin, globulin, A/G ratio
  - Prothrombin time (PT).
- **Special tests: Estimation of:**
  - Ceruloplasmin
  - Ferritin
  - Alpha-1 antitrypsin (AAT)
  - Alpha fetoprotein (AFP).
- **Tests based on detoxification function:** Estimation of:
  - Blood ammonia and bilirubin
  - Hippuric acid test.

Explanation of Three Tests in Detail

- **Synthetic function: Total plasma proteins, serum albumin, globulins**

- Almost all plasma proteins with exception of immunoglobulins are synthesized by liver. Normal total serum proteins level is 6 to 8 g/dL
- Albumin is quantitatively the most important protein synthesized by the liver, and reflects the extent of functioning liver cell mass. Normal albumin level is 2.5 to 3.5 g/dL
- In hepatocellular diseases hypoalbuminemia occurs
- Normal serum globulin level is 2 to 3.5 g/dL. In chronic inflammatory disorders such as hepatitis and in cirrhosis of liver hyperglobulinemia will be present
- A/G Ratio: Since albumin has a half life of 20 days, in all chronic diseases of liver, the albumin level is decreased. A reversal of A/G ratio is seen in cirrhosis of liver. Normal A/G ratio is 1.2:1 to 2.5:1
- Estimation of total proteins is done by Biuret method and serum albumin is estimated by Bromocresol green method. Globulin is calculated by subtracting albumin values from total protein
- It is also estimated by doing electrophoresis of proteins and calculated by densitometry.
- **Prothrombin Time (Synthetic function)**
  - Since prothrombin is synthesized by the liver, it is a useful indicator of liver function
  - The half life of prothrombin is 6 hours only. Therefore PT indicates the recent function of liver
  - PT is prolonged only when more than 80% of liver function is lost
  - In vitamin K deficiency PT is prolonged. To differentiate liver dysfunction from that of vitamin K deficiency, vitamin K is given to the patient and PT is measured. Elevated PT even after administration of vitamin K indicates liver dysfunction.
- **van den Bergh test: (Hepatic excretory function) – Estimation of Bilirubin**
  - The serum bilirubin estimation is based on van den Bergh reaction in which diazotised sulfanilic acid reacts with bilirubin to form a purple colored complex, azobilirubin. Normal serum does not give a positive van den Bergh test
  - When bilirubin is conjugated, the purple color is produced immediately on mixing with the reagent, the response is said to be van den Bergh direct positive
  - When the bilirubin is unconjugated, the color appears only after addition of alcohol, so it is said to be van den Bergh indirect positive
  - When both conjugated and unconjugated bilirubin are present, it produces an immediate color, which intensifies on adding alcohol. It is then said to be biphasic
  - In hemolytic jaundice—unconjugated bilirubin is elevated so indirect positive
  - In obstructive jaundice—conjugated bilirubin is elevated so direct positive
  - In hepatic jaundice—both conjugated and unconjugated bilirubin are elevate—so biphasic.

33. Anion gap and its diagnostic importance.

- The sum of cations and anions in ECF is always the same to maintain the electrical neutrality
- Sodium and potassium together form 95% of cations
- Chloride and bicarbonate form 86% of the anions. So these electrolytes are commonly measured
- Hence there is always a difference between the measured anions and cations
- **The unmeasured anions constitute the anion gap.** This is due to the presence of protein anions, sulfate, phosphate and organic acids
- **The normal value is 12 mmol/L.** It is increased in some forms of metabolic acidosis
- It is calculated as difference between $(Na^+ + K^+)$ and $(HCO_3^- + Cl^-)$.

High Anion Gap Metabolic Acidosis (HAGMA)

- In metabolic acidosis, accumulation of acid anions will make the anion gap between 15 and 20
- This anion gap is increased when there is a decrease in cations as in hypokalemia, hypocalcemia. When the cations are increased anion gap is altered as in hypoalbuminemia
- HAGMA is seen in a) renal failure—he excretion of H⁺ and generation of bicarbonate both are deficient, b) diabetic ketoacidosis, (c) lactic acidosis—lactic acid is increased in tissue hypoxia, circulatory failure. (Normal lactic acid is less than 2 mmol/L).

Normal Anion Gap Metabolic Acidosis (NAGMA)

- When there is a loss of both anion and cation, the anion gap is normal but acidosis may prevail
- Causes of NAGMA:
  - Diarrhea—loss of intestinal secretion leads to acidosis. The bicarbonates, sodium and potassium are lost
  - Hyperchloremic acidosis—occurs in renal tubular acidosis, acetazolamide therapy and in ureteric transplantation.

Decreased anion gap—it is seen in hypoalbuminemia, multiple myeloma, and in hypercalcemia.

34. Tumor markers.

Refer 2004 Short Note 17.

35. Salvage pathways.

- **Purine salvage**
  Refer 2004 Short Note 15
- **Pyrimidine salvage pathway (Fig. 35)**
  - Uridine cytidine kinase enzyme converts uridine and cytidine to UMP and CMP in the presence of ATP
  - Deoxythymidine is converted to TMP by thymidine kinase with the help of ATP
  - Deoxycytidine is converted to dCMP by deoxycytidine kinase with the help of ATP.

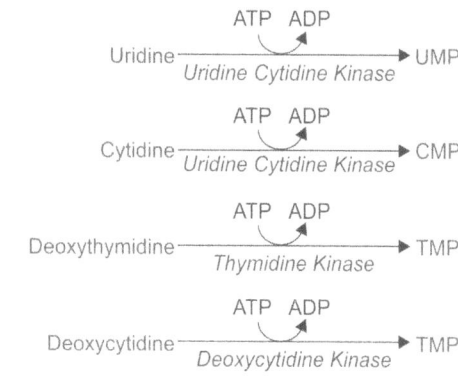

Fig. 35: Pyrimidine salvage pathway.

36. Mechanism of action of thyroid hormones.

- Thyroid hormones are:
  - Triiodothyronine – T3
  - Tetraiodothyronine – T4 – Thyroxine
- Thyroid hormones are synthesized from the amino acid tyrosine
- Protein bound iodine (PBI); Normal total PBI—10 µg/dL
- It is the transport form of thyroid hormones in plasma
- It is biologically inactive
- Normal values of thyroid hormones in blood
- Free triiodothyronine – Free T3—80 to 220 ng/dL
- Free tetraiodothyronine – Free T4—0.8 to 2.4 ng/dL
- Total thyroxine (T4) – 5 to 12 µg/dL.

Mechanism

- Thyroid hormone attaches to specific nuclear receptors to form hormone receptor complex which then binds with DNA to form thyroid responsive element (TRE)
- T3 binding results in increase of transcription.

Metabolic Effects

- **T3** is more active than T4
- **Metabolic rate:** BMR is increased by increasing the cellular metabolism

- **Thermogenesis:** Major effect mediated through uncoupling of oxidative phosphorylation
- **Synthesis of RNA and protein:** T4 increase the synthesis of RNA and protein; T3 causes protein catabolism and negative nitrogen balance
- **Hyperthyroidism:** Loss of body weight
- **Glucose metabolism:** Increased gluconeogenesis.
- **Fatty acid metabolism:** Increased cholesterol degradation and so level of cholesterol decreased which is an indicator of hyperthyroidism.

37. Detoxification by hydroxylation.

Phase one reaction of detoxication
- It is the alteration of foreign molecule by adding a functional group by hydroxylation, oxidation, reduction and hydrolysis. The main function of phase 1 is to convert it into a nontoxic metabolite
- By the end of this phase the toxicity may be decreased.
- **Hydroxylation:** It is the chief reaction involved with oxidation by hydroxylase enzymes present in endoplasmic reticulum. There are 150 isoforms. They are cytochrome P450 Mono-oxygenases. They are mixed function oxidases. NADPH is its coenzyme

$RH + O_2 + NADPH * ROH + H_2O + NADP^+$

- They are inducible enzymes. Phenobarbital ↑ their activity. It is Involved in metabolism of drugs and aromatic hydrocarbon
- Mitochondrial P450 enzymes present in mitochondria
- Microsomal P450 system is involved in steroid synthesis in adrenal cortex.

38. Blotting techniques (Fig. 36).

Blotting is a technique for transferring DNA, RNA and proteins on to a carrier so they can be separated, and often follows the use of a gel electrophoresis. The southern blot is used for transferring DNA, the northern blot for RNA and the western blot for protein.

- **Northern blot (Fig. 37)**
  - Northen blot technique is used for detection of specific RNA sequences. It was developed by James Alwine and George stark at Stanford University
  - RNA is isolated from several biological samples, e.g. tissues → then electrophoresed and blotted on to a membrane. This is then probed with radioactive cDNA. There will be RNA-DNA hybridization. This is used to detect gene expression in a tissue.
- **Western blot (Fig. 38)**
  - The proteins are isolated from the tissue and electrophoresis is done
  - The separated proteins are then transferred on to a nitrocellulose membrane

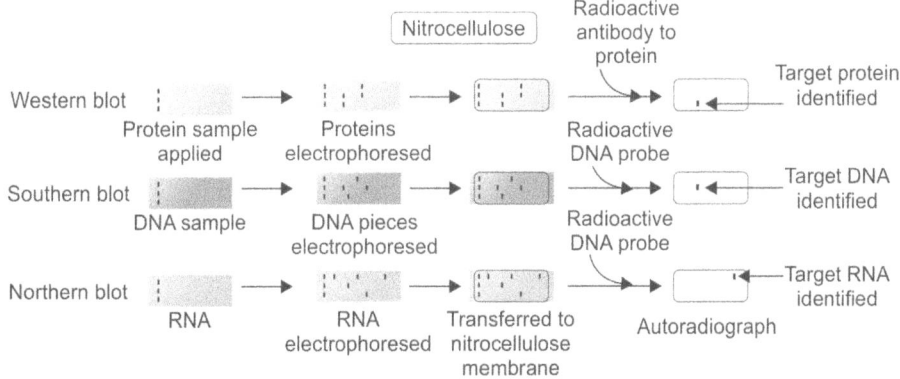

Fig. 36: Blotting technique.

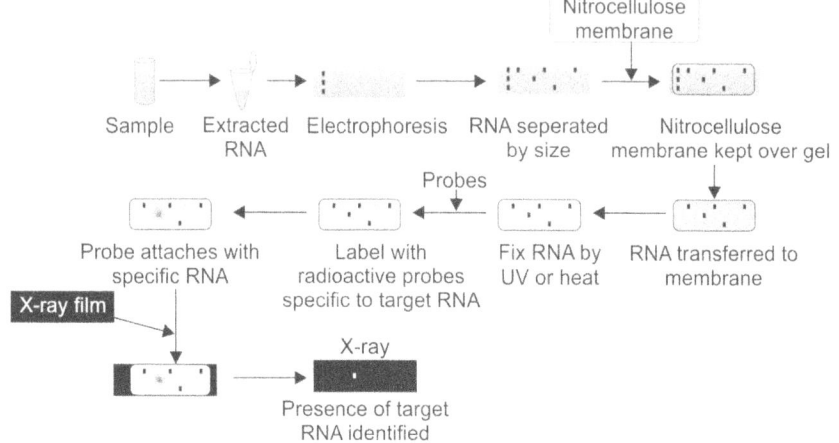

Fig. 37: Northern blot.

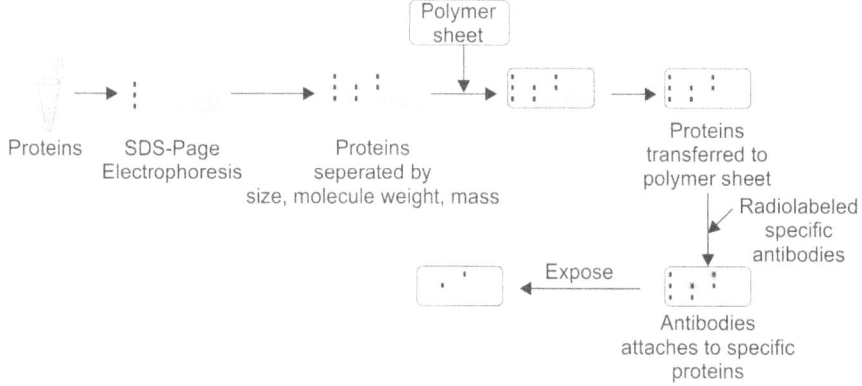

Fig. 38: Western blot.

- After fixation, it is probed with radioactive antibody and autoradiographed
- Alternately the specific antibody is poured over, washed and a second antibody carrying horse radish peroxidase is added. Hydrogen peroxide and a chromogen are layered. This technique is useful to identify the specific protein.
- **Southern blot (Fig. 39)**
  - This technique was found out by EM Southern (Aug, 2005)
  - This technique is based on DNA hybridization technique
  - Used to detect specific DNA segment.
- Steps:
  - DNA is extracted from the tissues.
  - It is fragmented using restriction endonucleases
  - The cut fragments are electrophoresed in agarose gel
  - It is then treated with NaOH to convert DNA to single stranded DNA
  - The gel is then blotted over a nitrocellulose membrane
  - An exact replica of the pattern in the gel is reproduced in the membrane. The DNA gets attached to the membrane

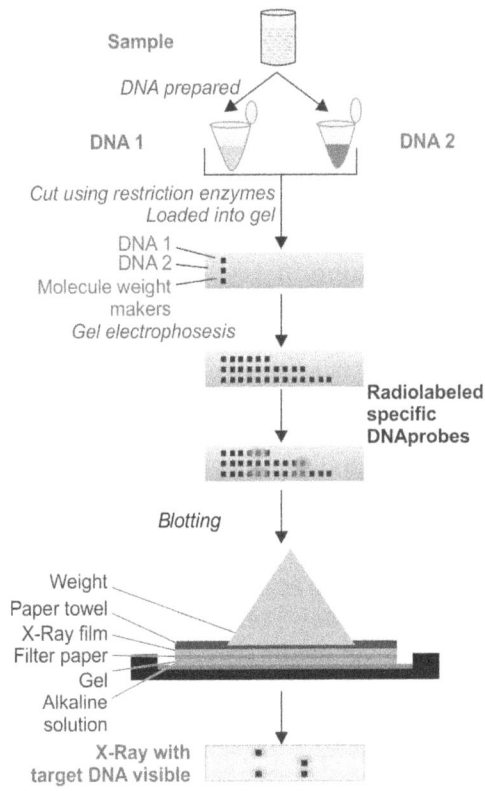

Fig. 39: Southern blot.

- The DNA is fixed to the membrane at 80 C
- A radioactive DNA probe which is complementary to the desired DNA fragment is applied
- This probe gets attached to the desired DNA (DNA hybridization)
- The membrane is washed and a radiographic film is exposed on the membrane
- The X-ray is developed to identify the DNA.

39. Glutathione role in amino acid transport.

Role in absorption of amino acids in intestines, kidney tubules and in brain—Meister cycle **(Fig. 40)**. Role of glutathione in amino acid transport.

- Glutathione is involved in Meister cycle which is needed for absorption and transport of neutral amino acids in intestines, kidney tubules and brain
- Glutathione reacts with the amino acid to be transported to form gamma-glutamyl amino acid by the enzyme gamma-glutamyl tranferase (GGT)

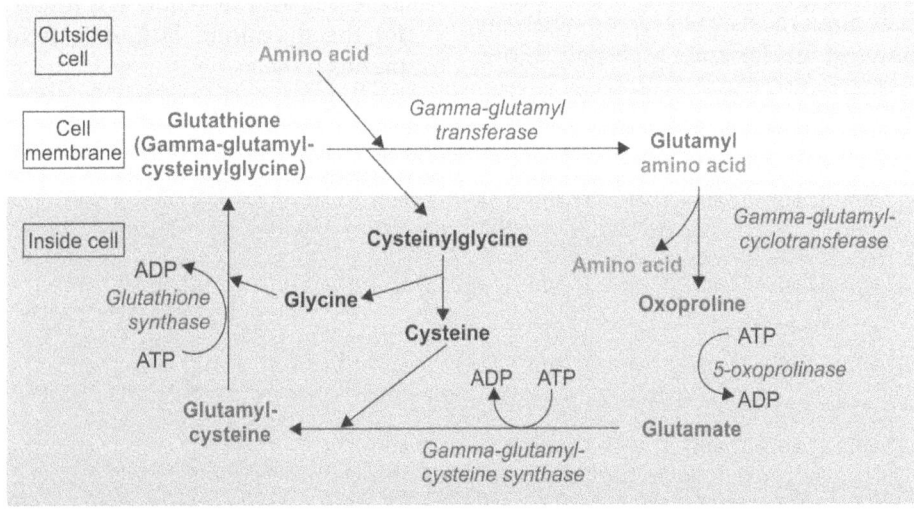

Fig. 40: Meister cycle.

- Gamma-glutamyl amino acid is then acted by gamma-glutamyl cycle transferase to release the free amino acid and oxoproline. 5-oxoprolinase enzyme converts oxoproline to glutamate. 5-oxoprolinase enzyme deficiency will cause oxoprolinuria
- Free amino acid is thus transported across the membrane and glutathione is reformed by combining with cysteine and glycine.

40. Essential amino acids.

Essential amino acids are indispensable amino acids which cannot be synthesized in the body but have to be supplemented by diet. They are:
- Arginine, histidine, isoleucine, leucine. threonine, lysine, methionine, phenylalanine, tryptophan and valine
- **Phenylalanine-tyrosine** is derived from phenylalanine, from which catecholamines—dopamine, norepinephrine and adrenaline, melanin pigment and thyroid hormones are produced
- **Tryptophan**: Necessary for the synthesis of neurotransmitter serotonin. It helps to relieve migraine and depression. It is also a precursor of niacin and its coenzymes—NAD, NADP
- **Valine, isoleucine and leucine**: Branched chain amino acids. They serve as alternate source of fuel for brain especially during starvation. Leucine is the major ketogenic amino acid
- **Lysine:** Component of muscle protein, collagen and is needed in the synthesis of enzymes and hormones. It is also a precursor for carnitine which is essential for transport of long chain fatty acids through mitochondrial membrane
- **Methionine:** It is a sulfur containing amino acid involved in transmethylation reactions. Homocystine is an intermediate in the metabolism of methionine
- **Threonine:** Hydroxyl group containing amino acid. Glycine is produced from threonine and it helps in phosphorylation reactions.

Semiessential Amino Acids

- Arginine and histidine are **semiessential amino acids** which can be synthesized in adults but not by growing children. Both are basic amino acids.
- **Arginine** is the precursor of polyamines, nitric oxide, creatine and creatinine. It is an intermediate in urea cycle.
- **Histidine** gives rise to histamine by decarboxylation. Histamine causes hypotension. It also produces smooth muscle contraction, enhances vascular permeability and increased acid secretion. It is responsible for the maximum buffering action of plasma proteins.

MBBS Examination 2006

ANSWER ALL QUESTIONS

I. Essay questions (10 Marks each)

1. Describe the process of glycogen synthesis and glycogenolysis.
2. What is normal serum cholesterol level? Describe the process of synthesis of cholesterol.
3. Describe the metabolism of tryptophan and add a note on inborn errors associated with it.
4. Describe the De novo synthesis of purine nucleotides.
5. Write detail about β-oxidation of fatty acids (FA) oxidation of FA under following headings:
   a. Definition   b. Site
   c. Steps and   d. Energetics
6. Discuss citric acid cycle under following headings:
   a. Location
   b. Reaction and
   c. Energetics
7. Write an essay on chemistry, functions, deficiency manifestations and hypervitaminosis state of vitamin A.
8. Describe the sources, requirement, absorption, transport, storage forms, functions, deficiency and toxic manifestations of Iron.
9. Discuss urea cycle under the following headings—(a) Site (b) Sources of amino group (c) Steps and (d) Regulation.
10. Discuss about nucleic acids under following headings—types, functions, components, chargaff's rule of DNA composition, different forms of DNA double helix and differences between DNA and RNA.

II. Short notes (5 Marks each)

1. Mutarotation.
2. Factors regulating the enzyme action.
3. Anaplerotic reactions of TCA cycle.
4. What are ketone bodies? Describe the formation of ketone bodies.
5. Chemiosmotic theory/oxidative phosphorylation.
6. Justify the statement that vitamin D is a hormone.
7. Thiamine.
8. Vitamin B12 (extrinsic factor of castle).
9. Acute intermittent porphyria (AIP).
10. Physiological jaundice (neonatal jaundice).
11. Isoelectric pH.
12. Thin layer chromatography.
13. Functions of plasma proteins.
14. Zinc.
15. Metabolic acidosis.
16. Gamma-aminobutyric acid (GABA).
17. Methylmalonic aciduria.
18. Structure of tRNA.
19. LAC operon.
20. Insulin.
21. Define and classify polysaccharides with examples.
22. Define and classify enzymes with examples.
23. Protein-energy malnutrition.
24. Acute intermittent porphyria.
25. Role of cytochromes in ETC.
26. Comparison between prokaryotic and eukaryotic cells.
27. Post-translational modifications with two examples.

28. Alpha-helical structure of a peptide/ secondary structure of proteins.
29. Buffer system in the body.
30. Principles of electrophoresis and its clinical applications.
31. Applications of genetic engineering.
32. G proteins.

I. ESSAY QUESTIONS

1. Describe the process of glycogen synthesis and glycogenolysis.

Glycogen Metabolism (Fig. 1)

Glycogen is the storage form of glucose mainly in liver and in skeletal muscles.

Glycogen is a homopolysaccharide made up of glucose units linked by $\alpha 1,4$ and $\alpha 1,6$ glycosidic linkages.

Glycogenesis: (Synthesis of Glycogen) (Fig. 1)

It is the synthesis of glycogen. It needs 2 ATP.

Glycogenolysis: It is the degradation of glycogen to glucose but not the reversal of each.

Glycogenesis - Steps

1. Glucose is phosphorylated to glucose-6 phosphate (G6P) by hexokinase in muscle and glucokinase in liver
2. Glucose-6-phosphate is converted to glucose-1-phosphate by phosphoglucomutase enzyme
3. Synthesis of UDP glucose—glucose-1-phosphate reacts with UTP to form UDP-glucose by the enzyme UDP-glucose pyrophosphorylase
4. Glycogen primer—to initiate glycogen synthesis, a pre-existing glycogen may act as a primer. There is a specific protein-glycogenin which accepts glucose from UDP-glucose
5. Glycogen synthesis—by glycogen synthase enzyme: Glycogen synthase helps in the formation of 1, 4 glycosidic linkages by transferring the glucose from UDP-glucose to the nonreducing end of glycogen
6. Formation of branches—branching enzyme (glucosyl alpha 4, 6 transferase).

This enzyme transfers a small fragment of 5 to 8 glucose residues from the non-reducing end of glycogen to another glucose residue where it is linked by alpha-1-6 linkage. This leads to the formation of another new nonreducing end. Further elongation of glycogen occurs with branches to form a fully formed glycogen.

Glycogenolysis (Fig. 1)

It is the degradation of glycogen to glucose-6-phosphate in muscle and glucose in liver. It is not the reverse of glycogenesis but it is a separate pathway.

- **Action of glycogen phosphorylase: Rate-limiting enzyme**
  - **Glycogen phosphorylase** catalyzes the phosphorylytic cleavage by inorganic phosphate (phosphorylysis) of the $1 \rightarrow 4$ linkages of glycogen to yield glucose-1-phosphate
  - The terminal glucosyl residues from the outermost chains of the glycogen molecule are removed sequentially until approximately four glucose residues remain on either side of a $1 \rightarrow 6$ branch.
- **Action of glucan transferase: Debranching enzyme**
  - Another enzyme **glucan transferase** transfers a trisaccharide unit from one branch to the other, exposing the $1 \rightarrow 6$ branch point
  - **Hydrolysis** of the $1 \rightarrow 6$ linkages requires the **debranching enzyme.**
  The combined action of phosphorylase and these other enzymes leads to the complete breakdown of glycogen).
- **Phosphoglucomutase—reversible action**
  - The reaction catalyzed by phosphoglucomutase is reversible, so that glucose-6-phosphate can be formed from glucose-1-phosphate.
- **Glucose phosphatase**
  - Present only in **liver** and **kidney**, but not in muscle
  - A specific enzyme, **glucose-6-phosphatase,** that hydrolyzes glucose-6-phosphate yielding glucose that is

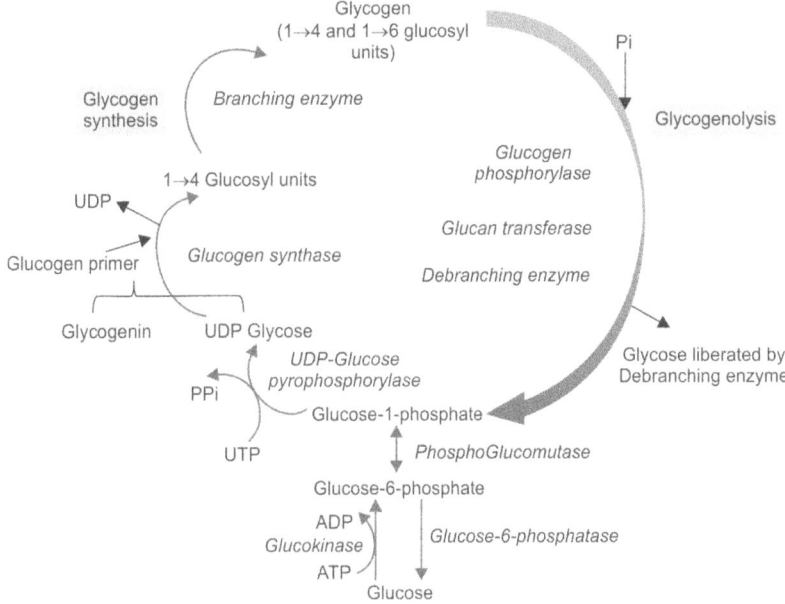

Fig. 1: Glycogen metabolism.

exported leading to an increase in the blood glucose concentration. **It is absent in muscle.**

Glycogenolysis

Regulation of Glycogen Metabolism
- **Allosteric regulation** of activation and deactivation of glycogen synthase and phosphorylase by phosphorylation or dephosphorylation.
- **Hormonal regulation:**
  - Glycogenesis—activated by insulin
  - Glycogenolysis—activated by glucagon, epinephrine
  - These regulations are mediated by cAMP in a cascade pathway.
- **Glycogen phosphorylase: Regulatory enzyme.**
  It exists in 2 forms.
  1. Glycogen phosphorylase a-active or phosphorylated form
  2. Glycogen phosphorylase b - inactive or dephosphorylated form
     - This activation and deactivation occur by stimulation by epinephrine (muscle) and glucagon (liver) via activation of adenylate cyclase by cascade pathway
     - **Allosteric regulation of phosphorylase:** It is allostearically inhibited by glucose-6-phosphate and ATP.

2. **What is normal serum cholesterol level? Describe the process of synthesis of cholesterol.**

Refer 2004 Essay Question 2.
Normal blood cholesterol levels—150–200 mg/dL.

3. **Describe the metabolism of tryptophan and add a note on inborn errors associated with it?**

- The aromatic amino acids are phenylalanine, tyrosine, tryptophan
- Tryptophan is an essential amino acid containing indole group
- It is both glucogenic and ketogenic amino acid.

Metabolism of Tryptophan
- **Major pathway (Kynurenine-Anthralinate pathway)—97% (Fig. 2)**

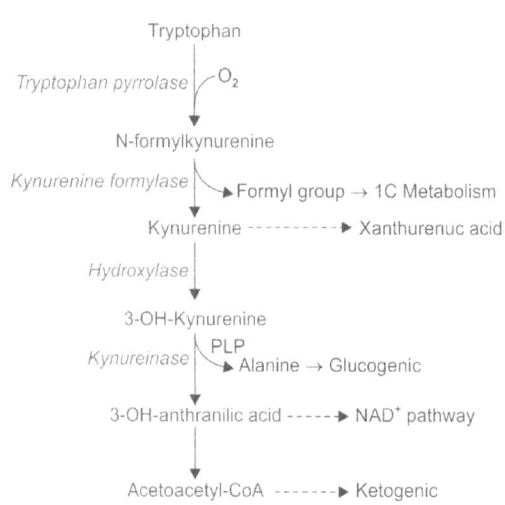

Fig. 2: Kynurenine-anthralinate pathway.

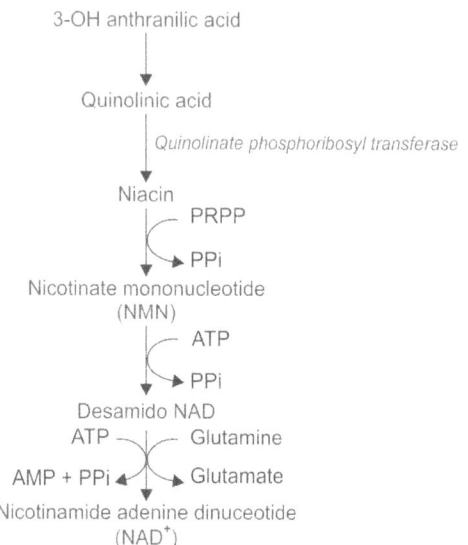

Fig. 3: Niacin pathway.

- Tryptophan is oxidized by **tryptophan pyrrolase**—a dioxygenase enzyme to form N-formylkynurenine. This enzyme is a heme containing enzyme induced by glucocorticoids
- Formylkynurenine is converted to kynurenine by the enzyme **kynurenine formylase**
- Kynurenine is then hydroxylated to 3-hydroxy kynurenine by a **hydroxylase enzyme**
- 3-hydroxykynurenine is converted to 3-hydroxyanthranlinate and alanine by a PLP dependent enzyme **kynureinase**. Alanine enters into glucogenic pathway after converted to pyruvate
- In **B6 deficiency** hydroxykynurenine is converted to xanthurenic acid which gets excreted in urine
- 3-hydroxyanthranilate undergoes either decarboxylation to form niacin or it is catabolized to ketoadipic acid and decarboxylated to Acetoacetyl-CoA which enter to the ketogenic pathway.

Niacin Pathway—3% (Fig. 3)

- 3-hydroxyanthranlinate undergoes decarboxylation to form nicotinic acid by the action of the rate limiting enzyme quinoline phosphoribosyl transferase (QPRTase) NAD and NADP are formed
- 60 mg of tryptophan will give rise to 1mg of niacin.

Serotonin Pathway—1% (Fig. 4)

This pathway occurs in brain, mast cells, platelets and gastrointestinal tract.

- **Step-1 (hydroxylation of tryptophan):** Tryptophan is hydroxylated to 5-hydroxytryptophan by tryptophan hydroxylase which needs a cofactor tetrahydrobiopterin and NADPH
- **Step-2 (decarboxylation):** 5-hydroxytryptophan is decarboxylated to serotonin which is 5-hydroxytryptamine (5-HT). Decarboxylase enzyme requires pyridoxal phosphate as coenzyme
- **Degradation of serotonin:** Serotonin **undergoes** acetylation by acetyl-CoA and methylation by S-adenosylmethionine to form **Melatonin** (N-acetyl-5-methoxyserotonin)
- **Serotonin**—It is also oxidized by mono amine oxidase to form 5-hydroxyindoleacetic acid (5-HIA) which is excreted in urine.

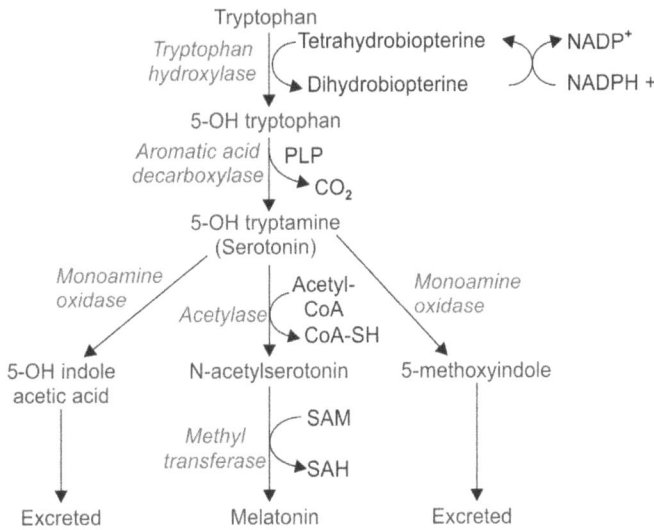

Fig. 4: Serotonin pathway.

Melatonin

- It is the acetylated and methylated product of serotonin secreted by Pineal gland
- It is involved in diurnal variations, sleep wake cycles and biological rhythm
- It is also a neurotransmitter.

Functions of Serotonin

- Serotonin is synthesized by neurons and by the argentaffin cells of gastrointestinal tract
- It is a neurotransmitter in the brain and an antidepressant
- It is a vasoconstrictor and induces smooth muscle contraction
- Serotonin level is low in cases of depressive psychosis and it is involved in inducing sleep, appetite, mood and temperature regulation
- It decreases the sensitivity to pain.

Products formed from Tryptophan

- Serotonin
- Melatonin
- Vitamin Niacin and its coenzymes – NAD, NADP
- Alanine
- Formyl group (one carbon unit)
- 5-HIAA
- Indican

Disorders Associated with Tryptophan Metabolism

Malignant Carcinoid syndrome (Carcinoid tumors)

- Serotonin is synthesized by the argentaffin cells of gastrointestinal tract and it is necessary for GI motility
- Carcinoid tumors are malignant tumors of argentaffinomas in small intestines and appendix
- There will be increased secretion of serotonin from these tumors (> 40 mg/dL)
- Oat cell carcinoma of lung also produce increased serotonin secretion
- Flushing, diarrhea, sweating and hypertension will be present as symptoms
- Pellagra may be associated with this condition due to niacin deficiency
- Estimation of urinary 5-HIAA is diagnostic of malignant carcinoid tumor. Normal level of urinary-5-HIAA is < 5 mg/day and in carcinoid tumor the level is increased more than that.

Hartnup disease—autosomal recessive disorder.

- It is named after the family of Hartnup in whom the disorder was described first
- It is due to defective amino acid transport during absorption of amino acids from the intestines and also during reabsorption of amino acids from renal tubules
- This leads to the deficiency of tryptophan and nicotinic acid and NAD
- Neurological and pellagra like symptoms are present
- Aminoaciduria will be present due to failure of amino acid transport in renal tubules
- Increased excretion of indole compounds will be detected by Obermeyer test

Treatment: Supplementation of niacin and high protein diet.

4. Describe the De novo synthesis of purine nucleotides.

Site of synthesis: Liver, erythrocytes, polymorphs—not in brain.

Sources of Purine Ring

- N1—aspartate; N3, N9—glutamine
- C4, C5 and N7—glycine
- C2—formyltetrahydrofolic acid
- C8—methenyl-tetrahydrofolic acid
- C6—respiratory CO_2

Steps of purine nucleotides synthesis: De novo synthesis (Fig. 5)

- **Synthesis of PRPP:** Ribose 5-phosphate becomes phosphoribosyl pyrophosphate (PRPP) by the enzyme PRPP synthetase using ATP
- **Formation of N_9:** The rate-limiting enzyme PRPP amidotransferase catalyses addition of ammonia group from glutamine to PRPP forming 5-phosphoribosyl amine liberating glutamate
- **Addition of C_4, C_5 and N_7:** Next a whole molecule of glycine (C4,5 and N7) is inserted forming glycinamide ribosyl 5- phosphate by the enzyme **PR-glycinamide synthase**
- **Addition of C_8:** Formyl transferase enzyme inserts a formyl group from N5, N10-methenyl-THF to form **formylglycinamide R5P**
- **Formation of N_3:** By the action of the enzyme **formylglycinamidine synthase** one molecule of ammonia is added from one more molecule of glutamine to form **formylglycinamidine R5P**

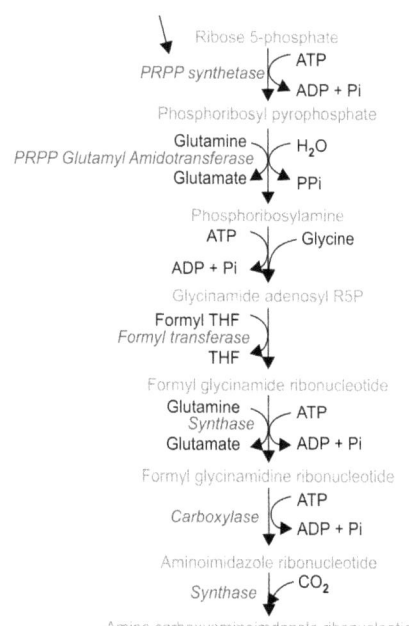
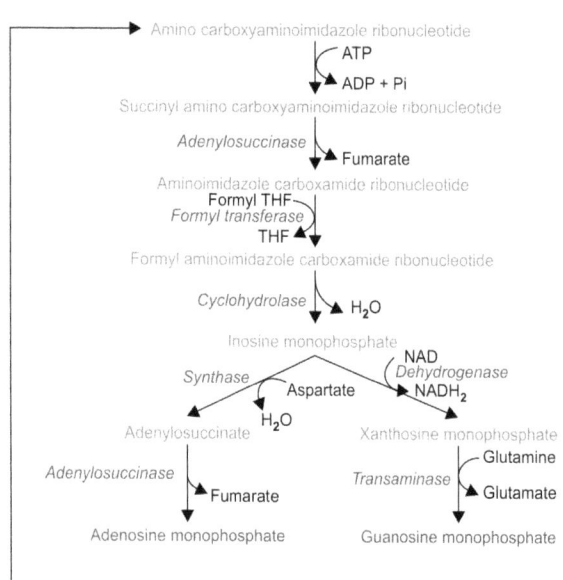

Fig. 5: Synthesis of purine nucleotides.

- **Ring closure:** By the enzyme **aminoimidazole synthase,** one molecule of water is removed and ring is closed to form **aminoimidazole R5P**
- **Addition of C_6: Carboxylase** enzyme adds CO_2 to form **aminoimidazole carboxylate R5P**
- **Addition of N_1:** By the enzyme succinycarboxamide R5P synthase aspartate is added with the removal of water to form **aminoimidazole succinyl carboxamide R5P**
- **Removal of Fumarate: Adenylosuccinase enzyme** removes fumarate to form **aminoimidazole carboxamide R5P** (AICAR)
- **Addition of C_2:** One formyl group obtained from N10-formyl-THF is added to form formimino imidazole carboxamide R5P by the enzyme **formyl transferase**
- **Complete closure of purine ring:** By the enzyme **cyclohydrolase** the ring is closed to form the **first purine nucleotide** — the parent nucleotide—inosine monophosphate (IMP)
- **Conversion of IMP to AMP and GMP:**
  - **Inosine 5'-monophosphate (IMP)** undergoes dehydrogenation by **dehydrogenase** using NAD and becomes xanthosine monophosphate (XMP). XMP take ammonia from Glutamine to form **guanosine monophosphate (GMP)**
  - It takes succinate from aspartate by the **adenylosuccinate synthase** enzyme to form **adenylosuccinate** which liberates fumarate to form **adenosine monophosphate (AMP).**

Regulation of Purine Synthesis

- The rate-limiting step of purine synthesis is amidotransferase (step 1). It is inhibited by AMP and GMP
- The availability of PRPP—depends on availability of Ribose 5-P (HMP pathway)
- The activity of PRPP synthetase is regulated by:
  - Negative modifiers like purines and pyrimidine (↑Pi) (↓ - ATP, GTP)
  - Feedback inhibition by products—ADP and AMP, GMP and GDP.
- PRPP glutamyl amidotransferase—key enzyme inhibited by purine nucleotides.

5. **Write detail about β-oxidation of fatty acid (FA) under following headings**
   a. Definition   b. Site
   c. Steps and   d. Energetics

Beta-oxidation of palmitic acid (16 C fatty acid) and its regulation is discussed below:

Definition: Palmitic acid is 16 carboned saturated long-chain fatty acid
Beta-oxidation is the process of oxidation and splitting of 2 carbon units which are sequentially removed at the beta carbon of fatty acids

- **Site of occurrence:** All tissues predominantly in liver and skeletal muscle
- **Intracellular location:** Mitochondria.
- **Substrate:** Palmitic acid
- **Product:** Acetyl-CoA, NADH, $FADH_2$.

Steps

- Preparative steps—activation of fatty acids (palmitic acid) and transport of fatty acids across mitochondrial membranes into mitochondrial matrix
- Beta-oxidation of fatty acids.

Preparative Step 1: Activation of Palmitic Acids (Fig. 6)

Palmitic acids are activated by ATP to form their acyl-CoA derivatives by the enzyme thiokinase or fatty acyl-CoA synthetase.

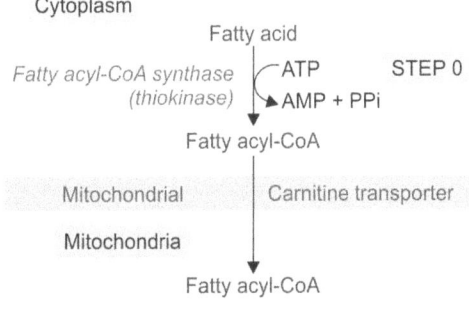

Fig. 6: Activation of fatty acid (palmitic acid).

Two high-energy bonds are utilized in this step. This step occurs at cytoplasm.

Fatty acid + ATP + CoA Acyl-CoA + PPi + AMP

Preparative Step 2: Role of Carnitine as a Carrier (Fig. 7)

- Palmitic acyl-CoA cannot pass through inner mitochondrial membrane. Hence activated fatty acids are transported to the mitochondria by carnitine shuttle
- Carnitine is synthesized from lysine and methionine in liver and kidney and it is beta-hydroxy-gamma-trimethyl ammonium butyrate
- Carnitine carries fatty acyl groups across the inner mitochondrial membrane. Transfer of acyl group to carnitine occurs by the enzyme carnitine acyltransferase (CAT-1) at the cytosolic side of inner mitochondrial membrane to form acylcarnitine
- Translocase enzyme carries acylcarnitine across the membrane to the matrix of mitochondria where carnitine acyltransferase II (CAT-II) transfers acyl group to coenzyme. Free carnitine will return back to cytosol by translocase.

Beta-Oxidation Steps

Four steps are involved in Beta-oxidation. They are (Fig. 8):
1. FAD dependent dehydrogenation
2. Hydration
3. NAD dependent dehyrogenation
4. Thiolytic cleavage.

FAD dependent dehydrogenation: By FAD linked fatty acyl-CoA dehydrogenase: Fatty acyl-CoA is dehydrogenated to α,β unsaturated fatty acyl-CoA (trans-enoyl-CoA) by FAD dependent dehydrogenase. FAD is converted to $FADH_2$ to produce 1.5 ATPs at electron transport chain.

Hydration: Enoyl-CoA hydratase enzyme helps in adding one molecule of water to α, β unsaturated fatty acyl-CoA to form β-hydroxy fatty acyl-CoA.

NAD dependent dehydrogenation: β-hydroxy fatty acyl-CoA is oxidized to form β-keto fatty acyl-CoA with NAD as coenzyme to generate 2.5 ATP.

Thiolytic cleavage: β-keto fatty acyl-CoA undergoes thiolytic cleavage to split one molecule of acetyl-CoA. A fatty acid with 2 carbon atom less (14 C) is produced.

Further cycles of step 1,2,3 and 4 of β-oxidation are repeated till the fatty acid

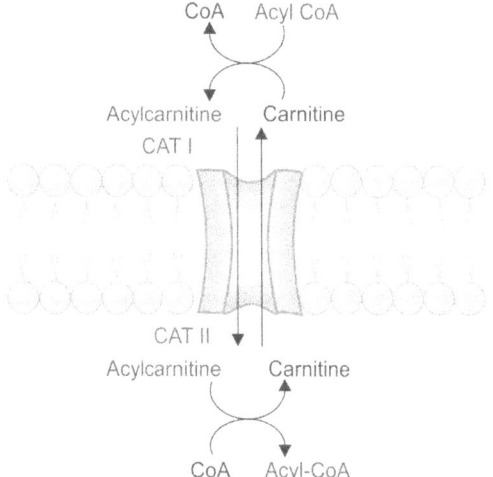

Fig. 7: Carnitine shuttle.

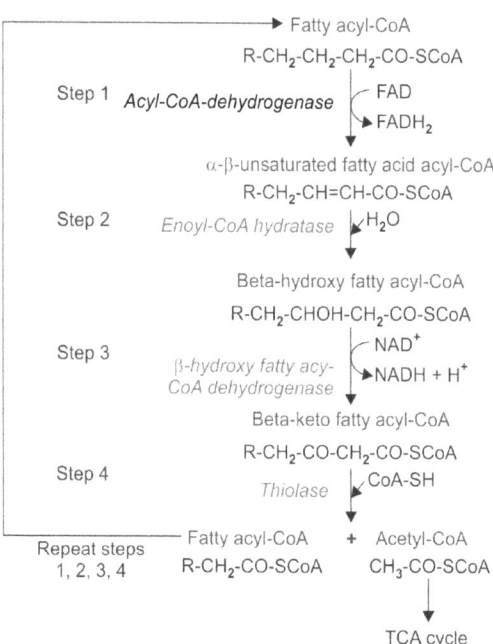

Fig. 8: Beta-oxidation of fatty acid.

Box 1: Summary of beta-oxidation.

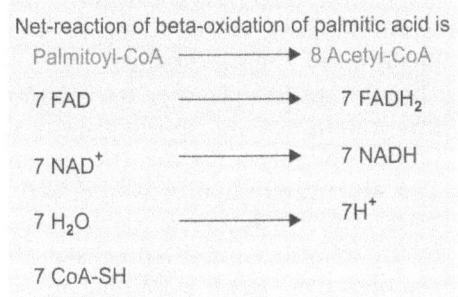

is completely converted to acetyl-CoA. Summary of beta oxidation is given in Box 1.

Energetics of Beta-Oxidation of Palmitic Acid

From palmitoyl CoA to acetyl-CoA: ATP
Acyl—CoA dehydrogenase 7 FADH2 7 × 1.5 10.5
Beta-OH dehydrogenase 7 NADH 7 × 2.5 17.5
From 8 acetyl-CoA 8 × 10 80
Total energy yield   108
ATP used for activation of FA   2
Hence net gain of ATP = 108 − 2 = 106

Regulation of Beta-Oxidation
- Availability of free fatty acid
- Hormones—glucagon increases FFA level and insulin decreases
- CAT-1 enzyme is the regulator of fatty acid enter into the mitochondria. This enzyme is inhibited by malonyl-CoA.

6. **Discuss citric acid cycle under following headings:**
   a. **Location**
   b. **Reaction and**
   c. **Energetics.**

Refer 2004 Essay Question 1.

7. **Write an essay on chemistry, functions, deficiency manifestations and hypervitaminosis state of vitamin A.**

Vitamin A is a fat-soluble vitamin.

Common names: Antixerophthalmic vitamin.

Chemical name: Retinol (vitamin A—alcohol), retinal (vitamin A—aldehyde), retinoic acid (vitamin A—acid)

Sources
Animal (Preformed Vitamin A)
Milk, butter, cheese, liver, egg yolk, fish liver oil (cods and shark liver).

Plant: Vegetable Sources
- Provitamin form beta-carotene
- Carrot, papaya, mango, spinach and green leafy vegetables.

Chemistry
Beta-Carotene
- The precursor form in plants has two β-ionone rings
- One molecule of beta-carotene can give rise to two molecules of vitamin A.
- Vitamin A consists of β-ionone ring and one isoprenoid side chain
- Retinoids—natural and synthetic form of vitamin A
- Various forms of vitamin A: Retinol (alchol), retinal (aldehyde) and retinoic acid (acid).
- **Retinol** (alcohol) containting beta-ionone ring. Side chain has two isoprenoid units with four double bonds and one OH group.
- **Retinal**—obtained by oxidation of retinol. Retinal may be reduced to retinol by reductase enzyme.
  Retinol ⟷ retinal ⟶ retinoic acid
- Vitamin A1 - all-trans retinal
- Vitamin A2 - 11-cis retinal (fish oil)
- **Retinoic acid**—produced by oxidation of retinal.

Absorption
- Plant source—β-carotene is cleaved by dioxygenase to from two molecules of retinal
- Retinal is reduced to retinol by NADH/NADPH dependent reductase present in intestinal mucosa
- Animal retinly esters of diet—are hydrolysed by pancreatic or intestinal hydrolase present in the brush border of the intestine to produce retinol. it occurs at the intestine. It needs bile salts.

Transport
- Inside the mucosal cells, retinol is re-esterified with fatty acids, incorporated

into chylomicrons and transported to liver. In the liver, it is stored as retinol palmitate
- Transport from liver to target organ is done by plasma retinol binding protein (RBC). One molecule of RBP binds with one molecule of retinol
- Zn plays important role in transport.

Uptake by Tissues
- By specific receptors found on retina, skin, gonads and other target tissues
- Then the vitamin is bound to cellular retinol binding protein (CRBP) and carried to the nucleus and bound to hormone response elements of DNA **(Fig. 9)**.

Biochemical Role of Vitamin A

Function in Vision
- In the retina, retinaldehyde functions as the prosthetic group of the light-sensitive opsin proteins forming **rhodopsin** (in rods) and **iodopsin** (in cones).

Wald's Visual Cycle (Figs. 10 and 11)
- Rhodopsin plays the pivotal role in vision. It is the membrane protein found in the photoreceptor cells of the retina
- Rhodopsin is made up of the protein opsin and 11-cis retinal
- When light falls on the retina, 11-cis retinal isomerizes to all-trans retinal
- A single photon can excite the rod cell. The photon produces immediate conformational changes
- The unstable intermediates produced are—rhodopsin → bathorhodopsin → lumirhodopsin → metarhodopsin → and finally opsin + all-trans retinal
- The all-trans retinal is then released from the protein and transported out of the retinal epithelium by an ABC protein. The all-trans retinal is isomerized to 11-cis retinal in the retina itself in the dark by the enzyme **retinal isomerase.** This reaction takes place in the retinal pigment epithelium
- The 11-cis retinal combines with opsin to generate **rhodopsin.** Alternatively the all-trans retinal is transported to the liver and then reduced to all-trans retinol by alcohol dehydrogenase (ADH)
- The all-trans retinol is isomerised to 11cis-retinol and then oxidised to 11 cis –retinal in liver. This is then transported to retina. This completes the Wald's visual cycle
- Visual pigments are G-protein coupled receptors. 11-cis retinal keeps it in an inactive form which gets activated by photoexcitation. Cyclic GMP is also generated at the same time and it acts as a gate for cation specific channels
- G-protein of retina is transducin
- Nerve impulse thus generated is transmitted to visual centers in brain.

Dark Adaptation
Bright light depletes rhodopsin stores in rods. When a person enters into a dim area from

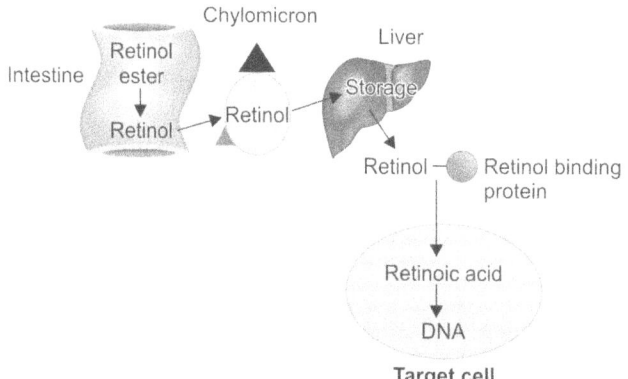

Fig. 9: Metabolism of vitamin A.

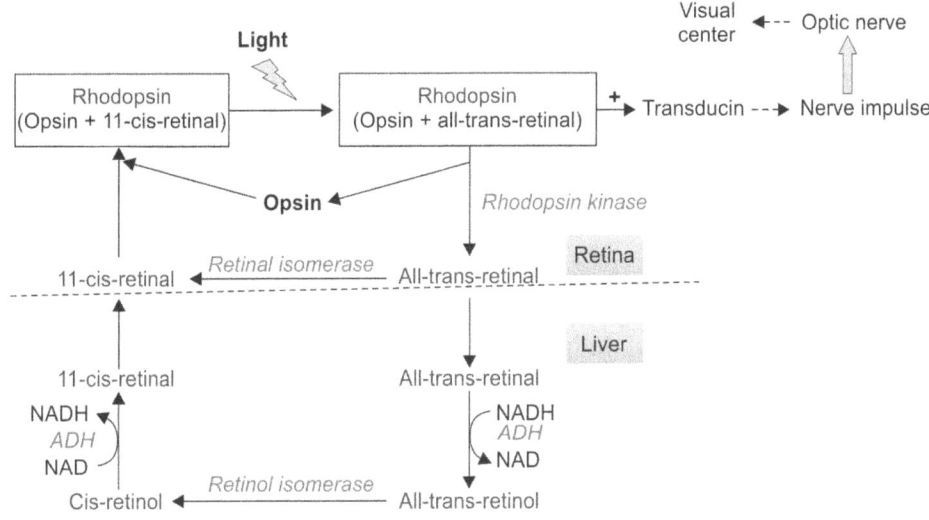

Fig. 10: Wald's visual cycle.

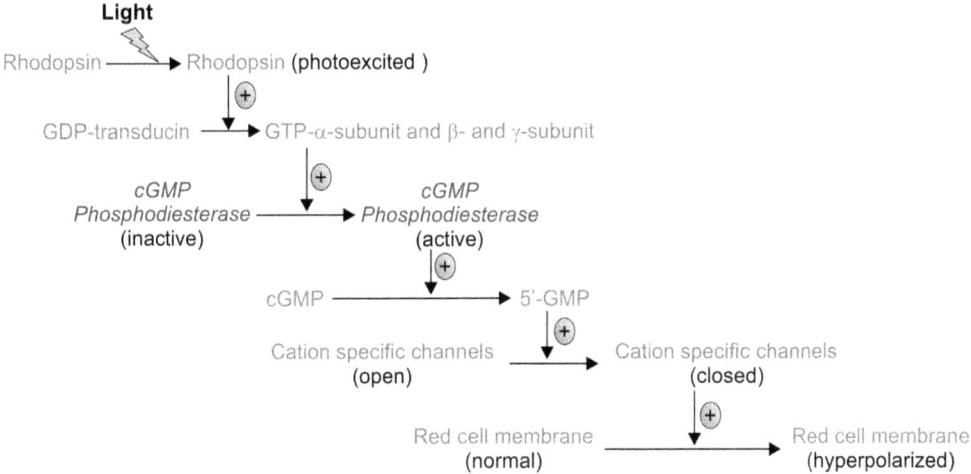

Fig. 11: Role of cGMP in visual cycle.

bright light there is difficulty in seeing which will be improved within few minutes by the resynthesis of rhodopsin. This is called dark adaptation time. This time is increased in vitamin A deficiency.

Functions of Rods and Cones

Rhodopsin in rods is responsible for dim light and iodopsin in cones is responsible for color vision. Both proteins contain 11-cis retinal.

Biochemical Functions of Retinol

- Acts like steroid hormone and regulates expression of genes
- It is needed for reproductory system functions.

Retinoic Acid

- Regulates gene expression and cellular differentiation during growth and development
- **Metabolic effect of retinoic acid:** It controls gluconeogenesis in liver and regulates the synthesis of glycoproteins and GAGs as carrier of oligosaccharides. It also controls cholesterol synthesis
- They act as steroids

- **Carotenoids:** Precursor form—act as antioxidants.

Recommend Daily Allowance (RDA)
- Adults: 750–1,000 µg/day
- Pregnancy: 1,000 µg/day
- Children: 400–600 µg/day.

Deficiency

Ocular Manifestations
- **Night blindness or nyctalopia**: Earliest symptoms of vitamin A deficiency. Impaired dark adaptation
- More prolonged deficiency leads to **xerophthalmia**—dryness of conjunctiva which may spread to cornea
- **Bitot's spots:** Grayish-white triangular plaques are seen adherent to conjunctiva due to increased thickness
- **Keratomalacia:** Softening of cornea and keratinization which may lead to total blindness due to corneal opacity.

Skin and Mucous Membrane Lesions
- **Hyperkeratosis** or phrynoderma—due to hyperkeratinization of epithelium. Rough skin. Epithelium gets keratinized and become atrophied in respiratory, gastrointestinal and genitourinary tracts and got atrophied
- Keratinization of urinary tract leads to formation of urinary calculi
- Acne formation.

Immunity
- Vitamin A also has an important role in differentiation of immune system cells, and mild deficiency leads to increased susceptibility to infectious diseases.

Furthermore, the synthesis of retinol-binding protein in response to infection is reduced (it is a negative **acute phase protein**).

Hypervitaminosis

Excessive intake of vitamin A leads to accumulation of vitamin A which causes tissue damage. Symptoms of toxicity affect the central nervous system (headache, nausea, ataxia, and anorexia, all associated with increased cerebrospinal fluid pressure), the liver is enlarged—hepatomegaly, hyperlipidemia and the skin lesions like excessive dryness, desquamation and alopecia.

---

8. Describe the sources, requirement, absorption, transport, storage forms, functions, deficiency and toxic manifestations of Iron.

Iron is a trace element needed for human beings.

Sources: Leafy vegetables are a major source of iron followed by jaggery, liver. Pulses and cereals are a low source of iron. Milk is a very poor source of iron.

Requirement
Adults: 20 mg/day, pregnant women: 40 mg/day, children: 20–30 mg/day.

Absorption (Fig. 12)
- Only ferrous form is absorbed
- HCl, vitamin C reduces iron to ferrous form, so increases its absorption. Phytic acid and oxalic acid form salts with iron so inhibits iron absorption
- Calcium and copper inhibits iron absorption
- Duodenum and jejunum are the sites of absorption
- When iron stores in the body are depleted, absorption is enhanced. When iron stores are adequate, absorption is decreased. This is called mucosal block theory
- Ferrous iron in the intestinal lumen binds to mucosal cell protein called divalent metal transporter (DMT1). This iron is transported into the mucosal cell. The unabsorbed iron is excreted
- Inside the mucosal cell, iron is incorporated into apoferritin to form ferritin. Whenever there is iron deficiency this ferritin supplies the iron. In iron deficiency erythropoietin is produced in kidney which enhances iron absorption.

Transport of Iron (Fig. 12)
- Transport of iron is done by the transport protein-transferrin

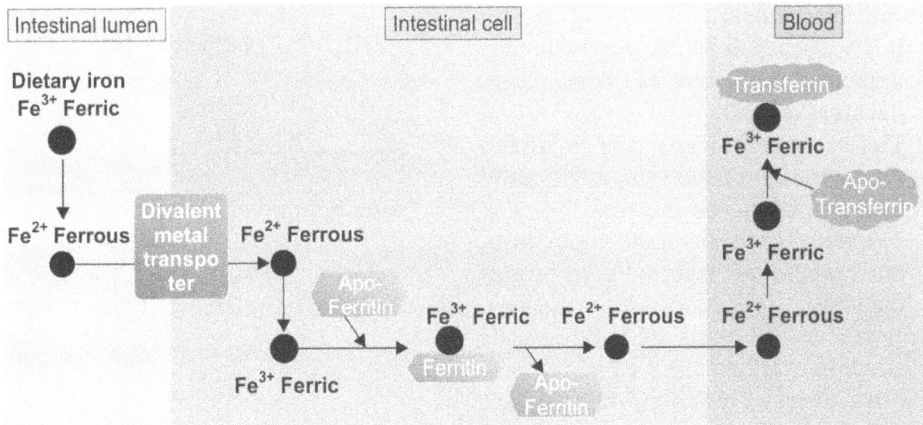

Fig. 12: Absorption and transport of iron.

- Ceruloplasmin, the ferro-oxidase enzyme oxidises ferrous iron to ferric state
- Iron is taken up by the peripheral cells through transferrin receptors
- Total iron binding capacity (TIBC) is provided by the transferrin. It increases in iron deficiency anemia.

Storage

Iron is stored as ferritin in mucosal cells, liver, spleen, bone marrow.

Functions of iron

- Iron is the integral part of hemoglobin and myoglobin and is required for transport of oxygen
- Cytochromes and nonheme proteins of electron transport chain and oxidative phosphorylation need iron
- Peroxidase contains iron which is required for the phagocytosis of bacteria by neutrophils
- Iron is needed for the immune competence of body.

Deficiency of Iron

Causes

- Indian diet contains less iron
- Hookworm infestation
- Repeated pregnancies
- Chronic blood loss as in piles, peptic ulcer and uterine bleeding
- Nephrosis, subtotal gastrectomy and lead poisoning are other causes of iron deficiency.

Clinical Features

- Microcytic hypochromic anemia ensues.
- In anemia body cells lack oxygen and the person becomes apathic
- Severe iron deficiency leads to heart failure
- Chronic deficiency leads to achlorhydria, impaired attention, irritability, lower memory, poor scholastic performance.

Toxic Manifestations

- Acute intoxication—diarrhea, nausea, abdominal pain
- **Hemosiderosis**—it occurs in patients receiving repeated blood transfusions. Hemosiderin pigments deposit in spleen and liver.
  - Hemosiderin is an iron storage protein which can hold about 35% of iron by weight
  - It accumulates in the body (spleen and liver as golden brown granules) when the supply of iron is in excess, e.g. repeated blood transfusions
  - Hemosiderosis is commonly observed among Bantu tribe in South Africa. This is attributed to a high intake of iron from their staple diet corn which is low in phosphate content and their habit of cooking foods in iron pots.

- **Hemochromatosis**
  - It is a disease in which iron is directly deposited in the tissues (liver, spleen, pancreas and skin)
  - The manifestations are bronzed pigmentation of the skin, cirrhosis of liver and pancreatic fibrosis
  - The triad of cirrhosis, hemochromatosis, and diabetes are referred to as bronze diabetes.
- Iron vessels—cooking in iron utensils causes iron overload
- Bantu siderosis, hemochromatosis are other causes of iron overload.

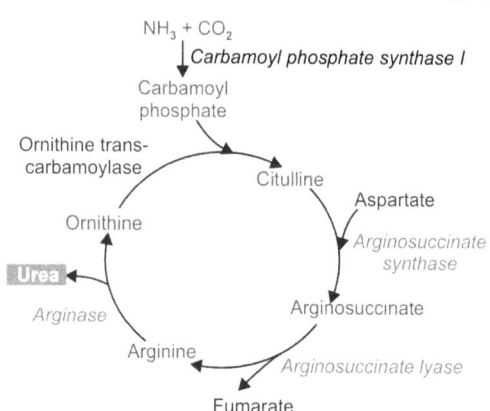

Fig. 13: Urea cycle.

9. Discuss urea cycle under the following headings—(a) Site (b) Sources of amino group (c) Steps and (d) Regulation.

- Urea is the end product of protein catabolism. It is synthesized in the liver mitochondria and cytoplasm. The two nitrogen atoms of urea derived from two different sources, one from ammonia and the other directly from aspartic acid (amino group)
- This cycle is also called as Krebs-Henselit urea cycle or ornithine cycle
- First line of defense against ammonia is done by trapping of NH_3 by glutamic acid to form glutamine in the brain cells
- Second line of defense is by the formation of urea which is the end product of protein metabolism in liver.

Steps of Urea Formation

The urea cycle is the first metabolic pathway to be elucidated in 1932. This cycle is also called as Krebs-Henselit urea cycle or ornithine cycle **(Fig. 13)**.

Site

In **Liver**. First two steps of urea cycle are taken place in liver mitochondria and other steps are taken place in cytosol.

Sources of Amino Group

The two nitrogen atoms of urea derived from two different sources, one from ammonia and other directly from aspartic acid (α-amino group).

STEP 1: Formation of Carbamoyl Phosphate

- One molecule of ammonia condenses with CO_2 in the presence of two molecules of ATP to form carbamoyl phosphate by the enzyme carbamoyl phosphate synthetase 1 (CPS 1). This occurs in liver mitochondria
- This is the **rate-limiting step**. It is an irreversible step and regulated allostearically by N-acetylglutamate (NAG)

STEP 2: Formation of Citrulline: Mitochondria

- The carbamoyl group is transferred to the NH_2 group of ornithine by ornithine transcarbamoylase (OTC)
- Citrulline enters into the cytoplasm to continue further reactions.

STEP 3: Formation of Argininosuccinate

- One molecule of aspartic acid adds to citrulline forming a carbon to nitrogen bond which provides second nitrogen of urea by argininosuccinate synthetase
- Two high-energy phosphate bonds are utilized.

STEP 4: Formation of Arginine

- Argininosuccinate is cleaved by argininosuccinate lyase (argininosuccinase) to arginine and fumarate. Fumarate inhibits this step

- Fumarate enters into TCA cycle to be converted to malate which is then converted to oxaloacetate
- Oxaloacetate is transaminated to aspartate. This is a link between TCA cycle and urea cycle.

STEP 5: Formation of Urea
- Hydrolysis of arginine gives rise to urea and ornithine by the enzyme arginase
- Ornithine returns to the mitochondria to react with another molecule of carbamoyl phosphate to proceed the next cycle.

Urea level in Blood

Normal blood urea level is 20–40 mg/dL Urinary excretion of urea is 15–30 g/day.

Urea level may be increased due to high protein intake and inborn errors of urea cycle. Increased blood urea level leads to uremia. Causes for elevation in urea level are as follows:
- Prerenal:
  - Increased protein breakdown—after surgery, fever
  - Diabetic coma, thyrotoxicosis
  - Dehydration—vomiting, diarrhea
  - Intestinal obstruction.
- Renal: Acute glomerular nephritis, nephrosis, pyelonephritis, hypertension, polycystic kidney
- Postrenal: Obstruction—stones, stricture, enlarged prostate, tumor—growth in bladder.

Regulation of Urea Cycle
- The enzyme levels change with protein content in diet. During starvation, the urea cycle enzymes activity increases due to increased catabolism
- N-acetylglutamate (pasteur effect)—it is the positive activator of CPS1. It is produced from acetyl-CoA and glutamate
- Compartmentalization—the first two enzymes are located in mitochondria. Fumarate inhibits its own formation because argininosuccinate lyase is in cytosol, while fumarase is in mitochondria.

10. Discuss about nucleic acids under following headings—types, functions, components, Chargaff's rule of DNA composition, different forms of DNA double helix and differences between DNA and RNA.

Types of Nucleic Acids
- Nucleic acids are classified into deoxyribonucleic acid (DNA) and ribonucleic acid (RNA)
- DNA is further classified into B-DNA, A-DNA, and Z-DNA
- RNA can be classified into messenger RNA (mRNA), ribosomal RNA (rRNA), Transfer RNA (tRNA), small nuclear RNA (snRNA).

Functions of Nucleic Acids

DNA
- DNA is the genetic material in the cell. It is the chemical basis of hereditary and it is organized into genes which are the fundamental units of genetic information
- The genes in DNA encode proteins which are necessary for cellular function
- It is involved in the synthesis of RNA —by transcription. Proteins are then synthesized by translation
- It provides template for replication of the information into daughter DNA.

RNA
- Messenger RNA (mRNA)—it is synthesized from DNA by transcription. It contains the codons for protein synthesis which serve as a template for protein synthesis. It is attached to ribosome on which protein synthesis occurs
- Transfer RNA (tRNA)—acts as an adapter molecule in carrying a specific amino acid for a particular codon in mRNA and helps in protein synthesis—translation
- Ribosomal RNA (rRNA)—is component of ribosomes. Ribosomes are made up of many polypeptides and rRNA
- Small nuclear RNA (snRNA)—these are small nuclear RNAs. They are involved

in the process of removal of introns and splicing of exons of mRNA precursors
- **Ribozymes**—some RNA are capable of enzymatic functions like peptidyl transferases.

Components

- **DNA**—it contains four deoxyribonucleotides as backbone—deoxyadenylate, deoxyguanylate, deoxycytidylate and thymidylate units which are held by 3'5'-phosphodiester bonds
- **RNA**—it is a polymer of purine and pyrimidine ribonucleotides of adenine, guanine, cytosine and uracil linked by 3'5'- phosphodiester bonds.

Structure of DNA: (Watson–Crick Model) (Fig. 14)

- **Right handed double helix**: DNA consists of two helical polynucleotide chains twisted around in right handed double helix. Purine and pyrimidine bases are inside the helix. Phosphate and deoxyribose units are on the outside. The planes of bases are perpendicular to the helical axis. Sugars are kept at right angles to the bases.
- **Base pairing rule – Chargaff's rule**:
  - In DNA, the two strands are complementary to each other
  - The number of adenine molecules are equal to thymine molecules (A=T) and number of cytosine molecules are equal to guanine molecules (C=G)
  - Adenine pairs with thymine by two hydrogen bonds (A=T); guanine pairs with cytosine by 3-hydrogen bonds (G≡C). This is called Chargaff's rule.
- **Hydrogen bonding**—adenine pairs with thymine by two hydrogen bonds (A=T); guanine pairs with cytosine by three hydrogen bonds (G≡C). GC bond is stronger than AT bond
- **Antiparallel**—the two strands of DNA run antiparallel to each other. One strand runs in 5' to 3' direction, while the opposite strand runs in 3' to 5' direction
- **Structure of helix**:
  - Diameter or width of the helix is 20 Å (1.9–2.0 nm)
  - It has a pitch of 3.4 nm per turn
  - Within a single turn 10 base pairs are seen
  - Adjacent pairs are separated by 0.34 nm
  - It has a major groove (1.2 nm) and a minor groove (0.6 nm) which wind along the molecule parallel to the phosphodiester backbone
  - Proteins interact with the bases in these grooves.

Different forms of DNA Double Helix

DNA exists in six structural forms. They are: A-DNA, B-DNA, C-DNA, D-DNA, E-DNA and Z-DNA. Out of these A, B, and Z forms are important.

- **B-DNA**—it has the classic Watson–Crick model. It is the most common form. The DNA is a right handed helix. It has two polydeoxyribonucleotide strands twisted around each other. The two strands are

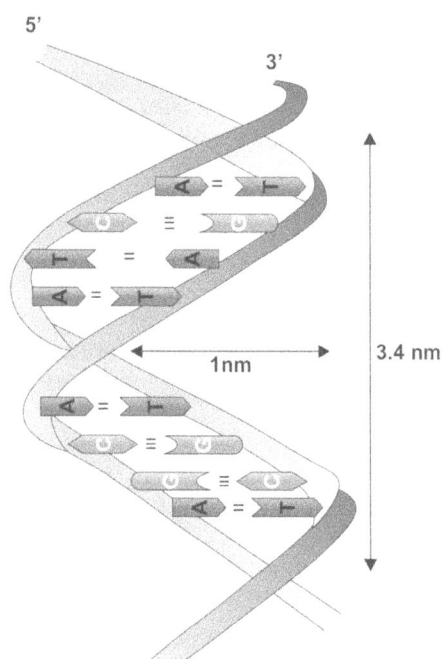

Fig. 14: Structure of DNA.

antiparallel. One strand runs from 5' to 3' direction and other on 3' to 5' direction. The width of double helix is 2 nm. Each turn of helix is 3.4 nm with 10 pairs of nucleotides. The sugar forms as backbone in which base is attached. The bases in two strands form hydrogen bonds and they are arranged according to Chargaff's rule

- **A-DNA**—is right handed helix having 11 base pairs per turn
- **Z-DNA**—is a left handed helix containing 12 base pairs per turn. The polynucleotide strands of DNA move in a zigzag fashion.

S. No.	Property	A-DNA	B-DNA	Z-DNA
1.	Shape	Broadest	Medium	Narrow
2.	Type of helix	Right handed	Right handed	Left handed
3.	Base pairs per turn	11	10	12
4	Helix diameter	25.5Å	23.7Å	18.4Å
5.	Pitch per turn of helix	25.3Å	35.4Å	45.6Å
6.	Major groove	Narrow	Wide	Flat
7.	Minor groove	Very broad	Narrow	Very narrow

Differences between DNA and RNA

S. No.	Characteristics	DNA	RNA
1.	Monomeric units	A,G,C, and thymidylate	A,G,C, and uridylate
2.	Sugar	Deoxyribose	Ribose
3.	Nature of strand/s	Double stranded helix	Single stranded
4.	Base pairs	A=T; G≡C	A= U; G≡C
5.	Types	A-DNA; B-DNA; Z-DNA	mRNA, tRNA, rRNA, snRNA
6.	Function	Carry genetic information. Synthesis of RNA —transcription	Involved in the synthesis of proteins — translation

II. SHORT NOTES

1. Mutarotation.

Definition: Mutarotation is defined as the change in the specific optical rotation representing the interconversion of α and β form of the D-glucose to an equilibrium mixture with respect to time

- Cyclic sugars show mutarotation as α and β anomeric forms interconvert.
- The specific opticalrotation of a freshly prepared glucose (α-anomer) solution in water is +112°

$$\alpha\text{-D-glucose} \rightleftarrows \text{Equilibrium mixture of } \alpha \text{ and } \beta\text{-D-glucose}$$
$$+112° \quad\quad +52.7°$$
$$\rightleftarrows \beta\text{-D-glucose}$$
$$+18.7°$$

- The specific optic rotation of α- and β-D-glucose are +112° and + 18.7°, respectively
- Freshly prepared α-D-glucose solution dissolved in water gradually changes its optic rotation from +112° to +52.7° with respect to time to form an equilibrium mixture containing 1/3 of α-anomers and 2/3 of β-anomers
- Similarly α and α forms of both pyranose and furanose forms of fructose interconvert through open chain form and at equilibrium, fructose has a specific rotation of –92°.

2. Factors regulating the enzyme action.

Regulation of enzyme activity occurs at different stages and in different ways in an enzyme catalyzed reaction.

There are regulatory enzymes in each metabolic pathway to regulate overall sequences and also to increase or decrease the catalytic activities. They act by following ways:

- Allosteric or noncovalent regulation
- Covalent regulation
- Activation of latent enzyme
- Induction and repression of enzyme synthesis
- Enzyme degradation
- Isoenzymes.

Regulation of Enzyme by Allosteric Regulation (noncovalent regulation)

- Allosteric enzymes act at other sites than the active site of enzymes or catalytic

site. The allosteric sites are for binding regulatory metabolites which are called effectors or modulators
- If the effectors inhibit the enzyme activity, they are called as negative effectors
- Allosteric enzymes do not obey the Michaelis-Menton behavior
- When the substrate itself serves as an effector, the effect is called as homotropic
- If the effector is different from the substrate, the effect is said to be heterotropic.

Feedback Allosteric Inhibition
- The process of inhibiting the first step of a metabolic pathway by the final product is called feedback inhibition or end product inhibition.

$$A \xrightarrow{E1} B \xrightarrow{E2} C \xrightarrow{E3} D \xrightarrow{E4} Product$$

- For example, aspartate transcarbamoylase is an allosteric enzyme in pyrimidine synthesis. The product CTP inhibits this enzyme by feedback inhibition
- The rate-limiting enzyme of heme synthesis—ALA synthase is inhibited by heme which is the final product by the mechanism.

Covalent Regulation
- Reversible regulation by addition of phosphate group (phosphorylation) or removal of phosphate group by dephosphorylation, e.g. glycogen phosphorylase—phosphorylation increased the activity.

Activation of Latent Enzymes
- Inactive precursor form of enzymes is called proenzymes or zymogens. They get activated by proteolytic cleavage of one or more peptide bonds, e.g.
  Chymotrypsinogen ⟶ Chymotrypsin
  Pepsinogen ⟶ Pepsin

Induction and Repression of Enzyme Synthesis
- Most of the enzymes are present in very small concentration and they have short half lives.

Two Types
a. **Constitutive enzymes**—housekeeping enzymes which cannot be controlled and their levels are always constant
b. **Adaptive enzymes**—their concentration increases or decreases as per the body needs.

Induction—means increased synthesis of enzyme, while repression indicates the decreased synthesis. This occurs at the gene level through the mediation of hormones and other substances. Glycogen synthase is induced by the hormone insulin pyruvate carboxylase is repressed by glucose.

Enzyme Degradation
- Half life of each enzyme defect in each enzyme ranges from minutes to hours or days
  - Amylase—3-5 hours
  - LDH-4—5-6 days.
- Usually the key enzymes get degraded rapidly. If they are not needed they get disappear and get resynthesized quickly when is needed.

Isoenzymes
- Multiple forms of the same enzymes also help to regulate the enzyme activity. They are tissue specific, e.g. isoenzymes of LDL and CPK which differ in their km value, V_{max} or both.

3. **Anaplerotic reactions of TCA cycle (Fig. 15).**

TCA cycle is considered as major metabolic cycle in living organism. The cycle will cease to work if the essential metabolites formed from intermediates of this cycle are deficient. So replenishment of deficient intermediates is needed to operate the cycle. This filling up reactions or influx reactions are termed as anaplerotic reactions.

Anaplerotic reactions are filling up reactions or influx reactions or replenishing reactions which supply 4-carbon units to the TCA cycle. By this, the intermediates of TCA cycle can serve as a source of precursors of biosynthetic pathways such as:

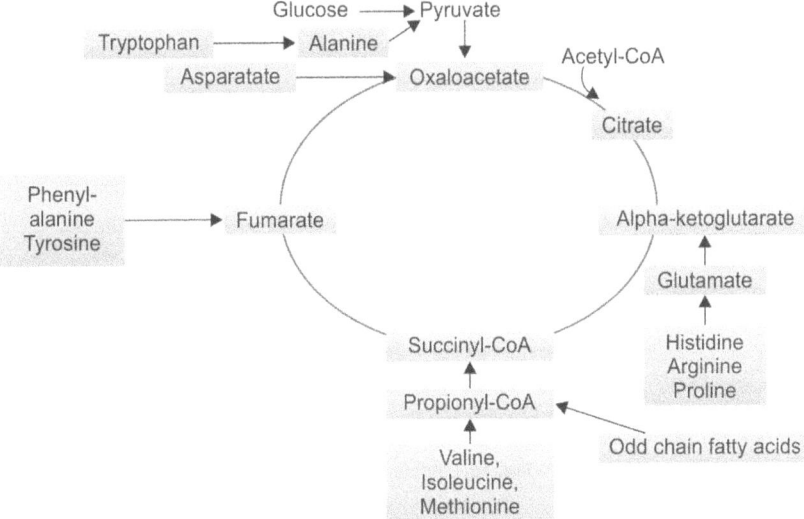

Fig. 15: Influx of intermediates (anaplerotic reactions of TCA cycle).

- Succinyl-CoA for heme synthesis
- Amino acids can be derived from the intermediates, e.g. glutamic acid from alpha-ketoglutarate, aspartate from oxaloacetate.

To make all these intermediates available continuously, anaplerotic reactions will fill up the supply. The anaplerotic reactions are:

- Conversion of pyruvate and CO_2 to oxaloacetate by pyruvate carboxylase which require biotin, ATP and Mg^{++}
- Transamination of aspartate to form oxaloacetate and transamination of glutamate to form α-ketoglutarate by transaminase enzymes with PLP as the coenzyme
- A cytoplasmic enzyme—NADP-dependent malic enzyme converts pyruvate to malate which can enter into mitochondria as an intermediate of TCA cycle
- Aromatic amino acids, such as phenylalanine and tyrosine are degraded to form fumarate
- Deamination of glutamate by glutamate dehydrogenase irreversibly to produce a ketoglutarate
- Succinyl-CoA can be synthesized from carbon skeletons of amino acids— valine, isoleucine and methionine and also from odd chain fatty acid propionyl-CoA **(Fig. 15)**.

4. What are ketone bodies? Describe the formation of ketone bodies.

Refer 2005 Essay Question 2.

5. Chemiosmotic theory/oxidative phosphorylation.

- Coupling of oxidation with phosphorylation is known as oxidative phosphorylation. Oxidative phosphorylation is explained by chemiosmotic theory given by Peter Mitchell
- **Oxidative phosphorylation is comprised of the following processes are here:**
  - Oxidation of reducing equivalents (NADH and $FADH_2$)
  - Electron transfer through 3 protein assemblies (Complex I, III, and IV) **(Figs. 16 and 17)**
  - Transport of H^+ into intermembrane space
  - Transport of H^+ into the mitochondrial matrix
  - Synthesis of ATP by complex 5.

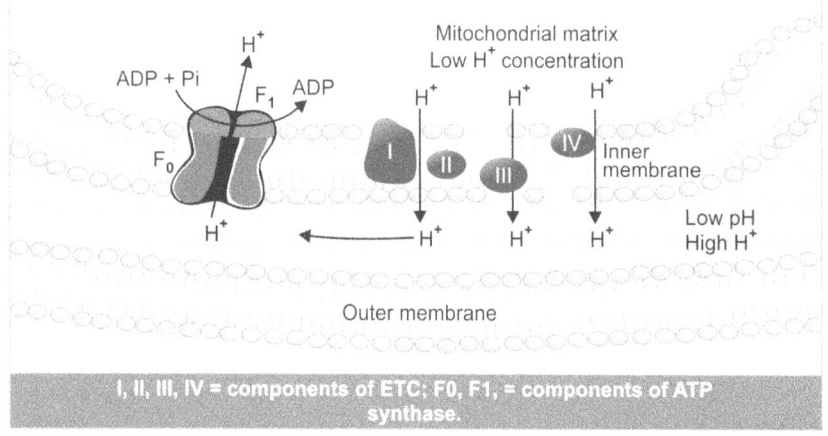

Fig. 16: Components of METC.

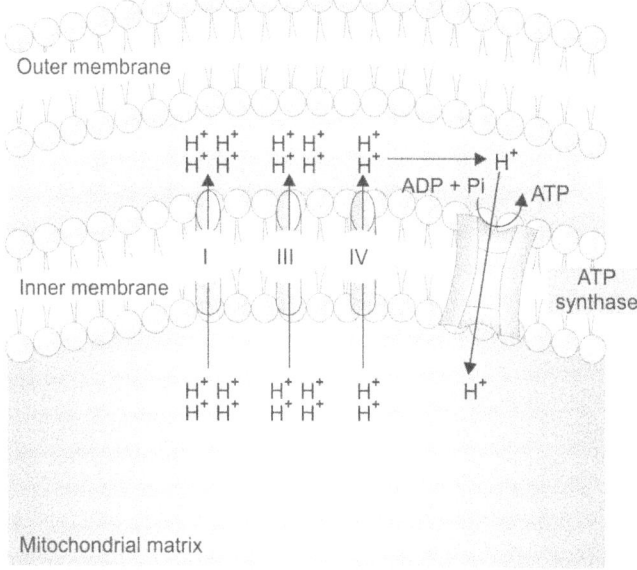

Fig. 17: Complex I, III, IV of METC.

- The transport of protons from inside to outside of inner mitochondrial membrane is accompanied by generation of proton gradient across the membrane
- Protons (H⁺ ions) accumulate outside the membrane to create an electrochemical potential difference and this force drives the synthesis of ATP by ATP synthase (V) complex
- There is also the creation of pH gradient on either side of membrane.

COMPLEX V—ATP SYNTHASE (FIG. 18)

- It is a proton assembly in the inner mitochondrial membrane. It has 2 functional subunits—F_1 and F_0 and looks like a lollipop. F_0 is embedded in the membrane and water insoluble. Both F_0 and F_1 are connected by a protein stalk. Protons enter through F_0 subunit and it acts as a proton channel. F_1 unit projects into the matrix and catalyses ATP synthesis

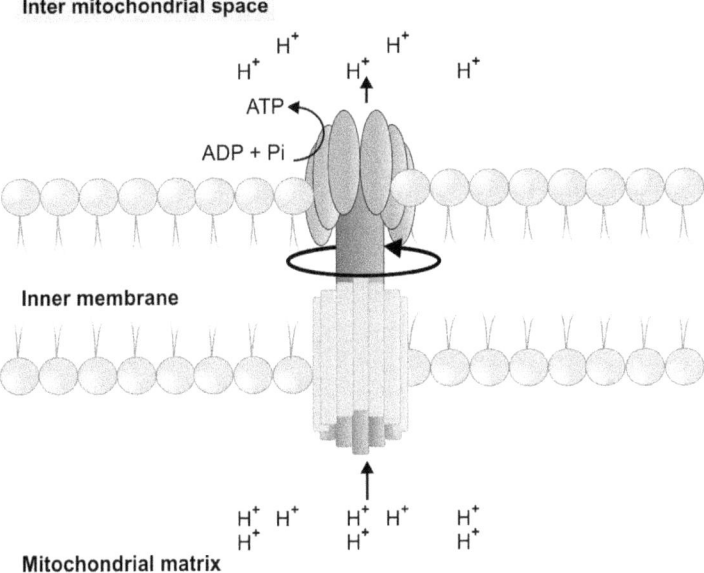

Fig. 18: ATP synthase.

- As per Boyer's hypothesis there will be a conformational change in the mitochondrial membrane proteins which leads to ATP synthesis. This is considered as rotary motor or energy driving model or binding-change model
- ATP synthase enzyme has a central gamma unit surrounded by alternating α3 and β3 subunits. Due to the proton flux γ subunit rotates and that induces conformational changes in the β3 subunits which releases ATP. One b subunit has open (O) conformation, the second has loose (L) conformation and the third has tight (T) conformation
- Protons induce the rotation of γ subunit which in turn induces conformation changes in β subunits. ADP and Pi bind to β subunits in L conformation to form ATP by changing site to L conformation and then T to O conformation and 3 ATP are generated for each revolution. So ATP synthase is considered as world's smallest molecular motor.

REGULATION OF ATP SYNTHESIS

- Availability of ADP—respiratory or acceptor control
- Source of NADH and FADH2 from TCA cycle.

INHIBITORS OF OXIDATIVE PHOSPHORYLATION

- Atractyloside—inhibits translocase
- Oligomycin—inhibits flow of protons through F_o
- Ionophores—e.g. valinomycin—mobile ion carriers allows K to permeate mitochondria; Gramicidin channel former.

Uncouplers of oxidative phosphorylation: 2,4-dinitrophenol (2,4-DNP), 2,4-dinitrocresol (2,4-DNC), chlorocarbonylcyanidephenyl hydrazone (CCCP).

6. **Justify the statement that vitamin D is a hormone.**

The active form of vitamin D is calcitriol (1, 25-dihydroxycholecalciferol)

Synthesis of active vitamin D

- 7-dehydrocholesterol found on the **skin** is activated by ultraviolet radiation from sunlight to form cholecalciferol
- Cholecalciferol is transported to **liver** where hydroxylation occurs at 25th position to form 25-hydroxylcholecalciferol

- Then it is carried in plasma bound to vitamin D binding protein and taken to **kidney**
- **In kidney** next hydroxylation occurs at 1st position to form 1, 25-dihydroxy-cholecalciferol or calcitriol which is the active form of vitamin D
- Active form of vitamin D (calcitriol) is considered **as calcitropic hormone**, while cholecalciferol is the prohormone
- The following characteristic features will demonstrate that the vitamin D is a hormone:
  - Cholecalciferol (prohormone) is synthesized in **skin** from 7-dehydrocholesterol by the action of UV light
  - The biologically active form (calcitriol) is synthesized in **kidney**
  - Calcitriol acts on specific **target organs such as bone, intestine and kidney.**
- Calcitriol exactly **acts as steroid hormones**—for instance, it induces the synthesis of calcium binding protein (calbindin/calmodulin) from intestinal cells at mRNA level **(Fig. 19)**
  - **Actinomycin D** inhibits the action of calcitriol. This supports the view that calcitriol exerts its effect on DNA leading to the synthesis of RNA
  - Calcitriol synthesis **is self-regulated by feedback mechanism**

Because of the above said reasons, vitamin D is considered as a hormone.

7. Thiamine.

Sources

- Plant sources like cereals (outer layer), pulses, oil seeds, nut and yeast
- Animal sources like organ meats, pork, milk, etc.

RDA

1–1.5 mg/day

Chemistry

Thiamine consists of a pyrimidine ring attached to a thiazole ring connected by methylene bridge.

Active form of Thiamine

- The coenzyme form of vitamin is thiamine pyrophosphate (TPP)
- It is synthesized by phosphorylation of thiamine by kinase
  Thiamine + ATP $\longrightarrow$ TPP + AMP.

Biochemical Functions

The thiamine pyrophosphate acts as co-decarboxylase, and involved in oxidative decarboxylation reactions, and transketolase reactions.

Oxidative Decarboxylation

- Conversion of pyruvate to acetyl-CoA by pyruvate dehydrogenase complex:

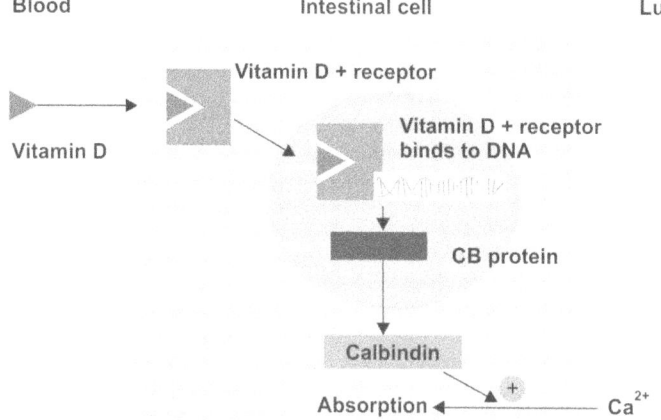

Fig. 19: Absorption of calcium.

$$\text{Pyruvate} \xrightarrow[\text{TPP, NAD} \quad CO_2, \text{NADH} + H^+]{\text{PDH Complex}} \text{Acetyl-CoA}$$

- TCA cycle: Alpha-ketoglutarate dehydrogenase:

$$\alpha\text{-ketoglutarate} \xrightarrow[\text{TPP, NAD} \quad CO_2, \text{NADH} + H^+]{\alpha\text{-KG Dehydrogenase}} \text{Succinyl-CoA}$$

- Branched-chain amino acid metabolism— alpha-keto acid dehydrogenase:

$$\alpha\text{-keto amino acid} \xrightarrow[\text{TPP, NAD} \quad CO_2, \text{NADH} + H]{\alpha\text{-keto acid dehydrogenase}} \text{Respective thioesters}$$

Transketolase Reaction – HMP Pathway

Involved in HMP pathway for the synthesis of pentoses and NADPH

Deficiency: Beriberi

The deficiency of thiamine leads to disease called beriberi, its features are depending on its type which are as follows:

Wet beriberi: Affects cardiovascular system.

It is related to edema of face, trunk, and serous cavities. Breathlessness, palpitation, swollen calf muscles, elevated systolic pressure, fast and bouncing pulse. Heart is weak.

Dry beriberi: Affects central nervous system (CNS)
- It is mostly related to degeneration of nervous system (peripheral neuritis)
- Muscles are weak and unable to walk
- There will be peripheral neuritis and sensory disturbances leading to complete paralysis.

Infantile Beriberi

The child has symptoms like sleeplessness, restlessness, vomiting, convulsions, and death.

Cerebral beriberi (Wernicke-Korsakoff syndrome): There will be encephalopathy including ophthalmoplegia, nystagmus, cerebellar ataxia along with psychosis.

Polyneuritis: Seen in chronic alcoholic patients. Alcohol inhibits absorption of thiamine leading to thiamine deficiency. This causes impairment of conversion of pyruvate to acetyl-CoA resulting in accumulation of lactate leading to lactic acidosis.

8. **Vitamin B12 (extrinsic factor of castle) (Fig. 20).**

Chemistry

Vitamin B12 has got a corrin ring similar to porphyrin ring having 4 pyrrole rings with a cobalt atom

1. Cyanide—cyanocobalamin (oral preparation of B12)
2. Hydroxyl—hydroxycobalamin—(Injectable form)
3. Methyl—methylcobalamin. Major circulatory form and coenzyme form of cytosol
4. Deoxyadenosyl—deoxyadenosyl cobalamin—major storage form in liver coenzyme form in mitochondria.

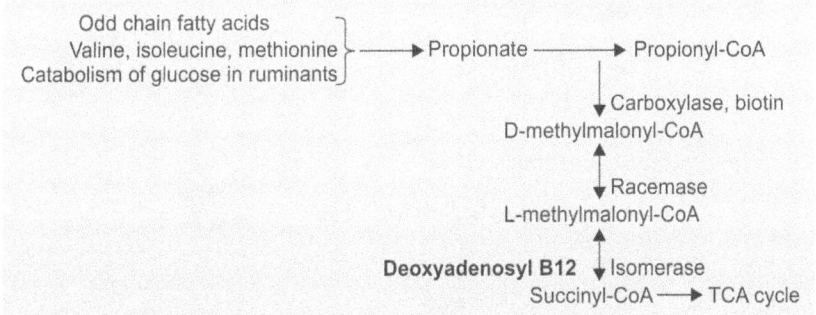

Fig. 20: Coenzyme function of deoxyadenosylcobalamin.

Sources
- Only **animal** sources—not present in vegetables
- Richest source—liver; good source—curd.

Daily Requirement
- Adults - 1 to 2 microg/day
- Pregnancy and lactation - 2 mg/day.

Absorption of B12 (Fig. 21)
- Absorption of B12 needs 2 binding proteins namely—intrinsic factor (IF) of Castle and cobalophilin secreted in the saliva
- B12 is otherwise known as extrinsic factor (EF) which has external sources
- IF is a glycoprotein secreted by gastric parietal cells.
- Cobalophilin, the second factor binds with B12 in the stomach
- In the duodenum cobalophilin is hydrolyzed by trypsin of pancreatic juice to release vitamin
- The vitamin then binds with intrinsic factor. One molecule of IF combines with 2 molecules of B12 to form IF-B12 complex. This is then internalized with specific receptors on mucosal cells and B12 is absorbed
- Then it is transported by a glycoprotein—transcobalamin
- In the liver it is stored as Ado-B12 with transcorrin.

BIOCHEMICAL FUNCTIONS: (COENZYME FUNCTIONS)

Deoxyadenosylcobalamin (Fig. 20)
- Deoxyadenosylcobalamin acts as a coenzyme for the isomerization reaction which isomerises L-methylmalonyl-CoA to succinyl-CoA
- During B12 deficiency, methylmalonyl-CoA is excreted in excess through urine and

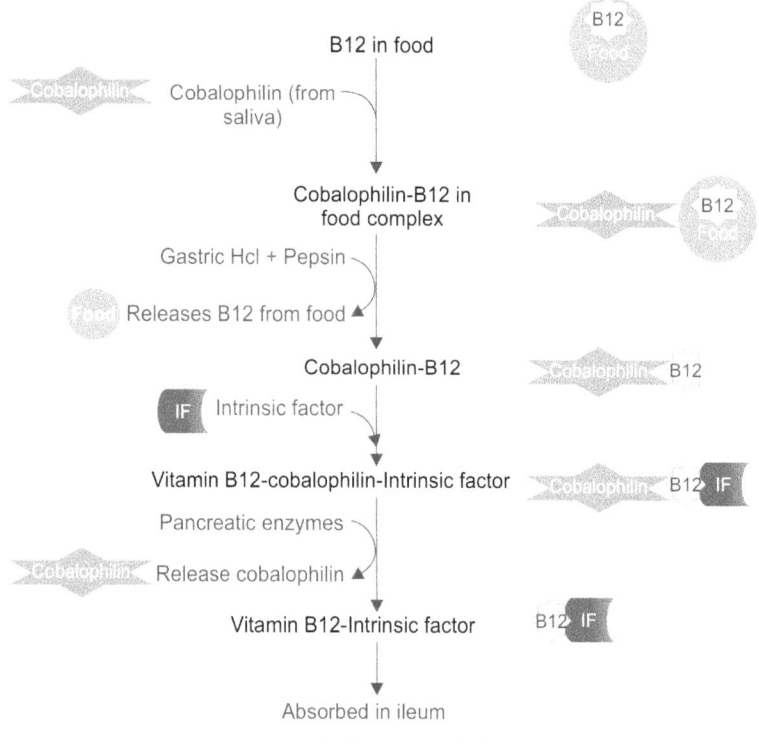

Fig. 21: Absorption of B12.

the condition is known as **Methylmalonic aciduria.**

Methylcobalamin (Fig. 22)

- It acts as the coenzyme in the conversion of homocysteine to methionine
- Folic acid also plays important role in it
- In the folic acid metabolism H4F is reversibily converted to N5, N10 methylene-tetrahydrofolate (THF) by serine hydroxymethyl transferase enzyme which is then irreversibly reduced to N5 methyl tetrahydrofolate
- This methyl THF donates its methyl group to cobalamin which is converted to methyl-cobalamine
- This methyl B12 then supplies the methyl group to homocysteine to form methionine
- In the case of B12 deficiency, this transfer of methyl group is not possible and so methyl THF is trapped inside the cells and there is no formation of methionine from homocysteine. This is called **folate trap.**

Deficiency Manifestations of B12

- Folate trap—this also manifests the deficiency manifestations of folic acid like inadequate DNA synthesis with macrocytic anemia
- Megaloblastic anemia—due to premature large RBCs
- Homocystinuria—due to the failure of conversion of homocysteine to methionine. Homocystine level gets elevated in blood leading to homocystinuria which is associated with ischemic heart diseases
- Methylmalonic aciduria—due to the deficiency of B12 there will be no isomerization of L-methylmalonyl-CoA to succinyl-CoA and so there is accumulation of methylmalonic acid in blood which leads to methylmalonic aciduria
- Demyelination of nerves—due to the failure of converting homocysteine to methionine, active methionine level is reduced and so methylation of phosphatidylcholine to phosphatidyl-ethanolamine will be inadequate and so demyelination occurs
- Subacute combined degeneration—demyelination of cerebral cortex, dorsal column and pyramidal tract of spinal cord occur causing sensory and motor tracts defective. So it is called combined degeneration. Positive Romberg's sign and Babinski signs are seen
- Achlorhydria is associated with B12 deficiency.

9. **Acute intermittent porphyria (AIP).**

- It is one of the inborn errors of metabolism in heme synthesis pathway
- It is an inherited autosomal dominant trait. Most common porphyria (1 in 10,000)
- The defective enzyme is porphobilinogen (PBG) deaminase which is involved in the conversion of porphobilinogen to uroporphyrinogen

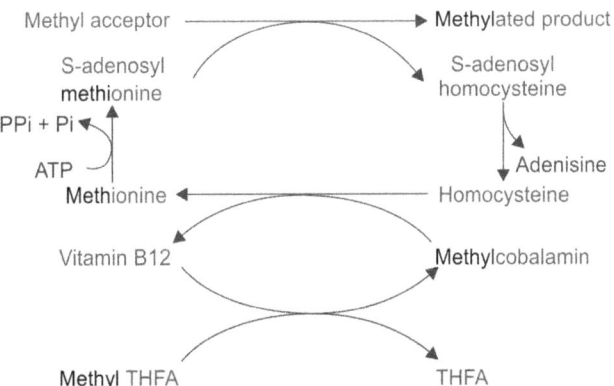

Fig. 22: Coenzyme function of methylcobamin.

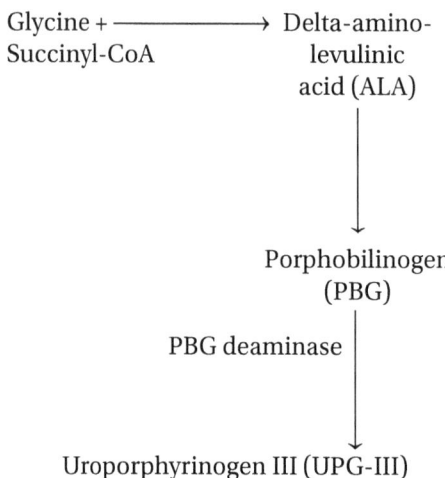

- The levels of ALA and PBG are elevated in blood and urine. Fresh urine is colorless, but on standing it become color due to photo-oxidation of PBG to porphobilin. Because of this reason urine sample should be collected freshly and transported in dark color bottle for analysis
- Patients have acute abdominal pain. In some cases neurological symptoms like sensory and motor disturbances, agitation ad confusion may be present. **No photosensitivity**
- Females have less severe manifestations than male, since female sex hormones have a stimulatory effect on ALA synthase
- Condition is precipitated by starvation and drugs like barbiturates. It is alleviated by carbohydrate rich diet.

10. Physiological jaundice (neonatal jaundice).

- Most infants develop visible jaundice during first few days (within a week) after birth and the most common condition is called physiological or neonatal jaundice.
- This is due to accelerated rate of hemolysis or due to immature enzyme system-UDP glucuronyltransferase which is needed for conjugation of bilirubin
- There will be elevation of unconjugated bilirubin concentration within 5 mg/dL
- This transient hyperbilirubinemia will disappear by the second week of life
- Phototherapy with blue light can be given to these children
- In some infants if the unconjugated bilirubin is very high (beyond 25 mg/dL), this bilirubin crosses blood-brain barrier resulting in toxic encephalopathy or kernicterus which may lead to mental retardation
- The drug phenobarbital can be given to induce bilirubin metabolizing enzymes in liver.

11. Isoelectric pH.

- It is the pH at which a particular molecule or surface carries no net electrical charge or contain electric charges negative as well as positive
- The pI is the pH value at which the amino acids exist as ampholytes or zwitterion in solution depending on the pH of the medium
- At this point there is no mobility in an electric field
- Solubility and buffering capacity will be minimum at this pH
- The net charge on the molecule is affected by pH of its surrounding environment and can become more positively or negatively charged due to the loss or gain of protons (H^+). In acidic solution they are cationic and in alkaline solutions they are anionic
- If we add hydrochloric acid to this solution drop by drop at a particular pH, 50% of the molecules are cations and 50% in zwitter- ionic form. pH at this position is $pK1$
- If we titrate the solution with NaOH, molecules become anions. When 50% of molecules are anions, that pH is known as $pK2$
- Isoelectric pH of monoamino-monocarboxylic acids (MAMC) can be calculated as:

$$\frac{pK1 + pK2}{2}, \text{ e.g. pI of glycine} = \frac{2.4 + 9.8}{2} = 6.1$$

- In amino acids with more than two ionizable groups, pK values are also more, e.g. aspartic acid has pK1, 2.1; pK2, 9.8 and pK3, 3.9. At physiological pH of 7.4, both the carboxyl and amino groups of amino acids are completely ionized.

12. Thin layer chromatography.

- This is liquid-liquid chromatography under partition
- A thin layer chromatography (TLC) plate is a sheet of glass, metal, or plastic which is coated with a thin layer of a solid adsorbent (usually silica or alumina)
- A small amount of the mixture to be analyzed is spotted near the bottom of this plate. The TLC plate is then placed in a shallow pool of a solvent in a developing chamber so that only the very bottom of the plate is in the liquid. This liquid, or the eluent is the mobile phase and it slowly rises up the TLC plate by capillary action
- As the solvent moves past the spot that was applied, the components in the mixture differ in solubility and in the strength of their adsorption to the adsorbent and some components will be carried further up the plate than others
- When the solvent has reached the top of the plate, the plate is removed from the developing chamber, dried, and the separated components of the mixture are visualized
- After the run is over, the paper or the plate is dried
- Location reagents, such as ninhydrin will be sprayed for amino acids and proteins; sulfuric acid sprayed for phospholipids and diphenylamine for sugars
- If the compounds are colored, visualization is straightforward. Usually the compounds are not colored, so a UV lamp is used to visualize the plates. (The plate itself contains a fluorescent dye which glows everywhere *except* where an organic compound is on the plate)
- Spots are identified and the distance traveled by the solute and solvent are marked and Rf value is calculated.

Importance of Rf Value

Rf value is the ratio of distance traveled by substance to distance traveled by the solvent. It is a constant for a particular solvent system.

$$Rf \text{ value} = \frac{\text{Distance traveled by solvent front}}{\text{Distance traveled by substance}}$$

The Rf values are strongly dependent upon the nature of the adsorbent and solvent.

13. Functions of plasma proteins.

- The total protein content of plasma is 6-8 g/dL
- Plasma proteins consist of albumin, globulins - ($\alpha1, \alpha2, \beta$ and γ) and fibrinogen
- Albumin—3.5-5 g/dL; Globulins—2.5-3.5 g/dL and fibrinogen—200-400 mg/dL
- Normal albumin: Globulin ratio is 1.2:1 to 1.5:1.

Albumin

It is produced by the liver and of 69,000 D molecular weight. It is a globular protein elliptical in shape and it has 585 amino acids arranged in one polypeptide chain.

Functions of Albumin

- Transport protein—it transports various substances like bilirubin, free fatty acid, drugs like aspirin, hormones like thyroxine, steroid hormones, minerals like calcium, copper, etc.
- Colloid osmotic pressure—it maintains colloid osmotic pressure in vascular and extravascular compartments. It contributes to plasma oncotic pressure. It cannot pass between intracellular and extracellular compartment. So exerts a net osmotic pressure. The osmotic pressure of plasma is about 278-305 mosm/kg which is necessary for the movement of water from ECF to ICF in arteriolar end and reverse in venular end of capillaries
- Buffer—albumin has the maximum buffering capacity. 16 histidine residues are present in albumin which can bind to H^+ and can function as a buffer
- Nutrition—liver takes up amino acids from diet and converts it into albumin. It is then released in blood and taken up by

other tissues by pinocytosis. So albumin is a source of aminoacids for the cells. PEM is characterized by hypoalbuminemia which results in growth retardation and edema. Human albumin is used in the treatment of liver diseases, hemorrhage, shock, and burns.

Globulin

Globulins are globular proteins bigger in size than albumin.

There are different fractions present with globulins. They are α_1 globulin, α_2 globulins, β-globulins and γ-globulin

- α_1 globulin—they include retinol binding protein (RBP), α_1- fetoprotein, α_1 - antitrypsin, α_1 acid glycoprotein (AAG), HDL and prothrombin
- α_2-globulins—they include ceruloplasmin, transcortin, haptoglobin, thyroxine binding protein (TBP), α_2-macroglobuliin (AMG)
- β-globulin—they include hemopexin, transferrin, β_2-microglobulin (BMG), C-reactive protein (CRP), low density lipoprotein (LDL)
- γ-globulins – IgG, IgM, IgA, IgD, IgE—they act as antibodies:
  - Most of them are transport proteins, e.g. thyroxine binding globulin (TBG), RBP, transcortin and transferrin
  - Haptoglobin binds with free Hb and prevents the loss of iron and hemopexin binds with free heme and prevents loss of iron.
- **Clotting factors**—there are 12 clotting factors–I, II, IV to XIII present along with plasma proteins. Except calcium (factor IV) all others are proteins produced by the liver. They are in the inactive zymogen form and activated when the coagulation process is initiated
- **Acute phase reactants**—CRP, ceruloplasmin, alpha-1 antitrypsin, alpha-2 macroglobulin are acute phase reactants. Their levels increase in the blood during acute conditions like fever, inflammations, etc.

14. Zinc.

- Total zinc content of body is 2 g, out of which 60% is in skeletal muscle and 30% in bones
- In liver, zinc is stored in combination with a specific protein, metallothionine
- More than 300 enzymes are zinc dependent
  - Example are carboxypeptidase— cleaves C-terminal ends of dietary proteins
  - Carbonic anhydrase—$H^+ + HCO_3^- \rightarrow H_2CO_3 \rightarrow H_2O + CO_2$
  - Alkaline phosphatase—needed for bone formation
  - Lactate dehydrogenase—pyruvate to lactate
  - Glutamate dehydrogenase—deamination process.

Functions of zinc

- It is a component of RNA polymerase. It is also needed for protein synthesis
- Superoxide dismutase contains Zn which is an antioxidant enzyme and so zinc is also an antioxidant
- Zinc stabilizes insulin. Insulin when stored in beta-cells of pancreas contains zinc which stabilizes the hormone
- Gusten is a salivary protein which contains zinc. It is needed for taste sensation.

15. Metabolic acidosis.

Refer 2004 Short Note 16.

16. Gamma-aminobutyric acid (Fig. 23).

- Glutamate on decarboxylation produces gamma-aminobutyric acid (GABA)
- It is produced in brain. It is an inhibitory neurotransmitter
- It inhibits nerve transmission in the brain, calming nervous activity by opening the chloride channel
- Glutamate and GABA are the most abundant neurotransmitters in the central nervous system, and especially in the cerebral cortex. GABA is an inhibitory neurotransmitter because it opens chloride channels in postsynaptic membranes in CNS

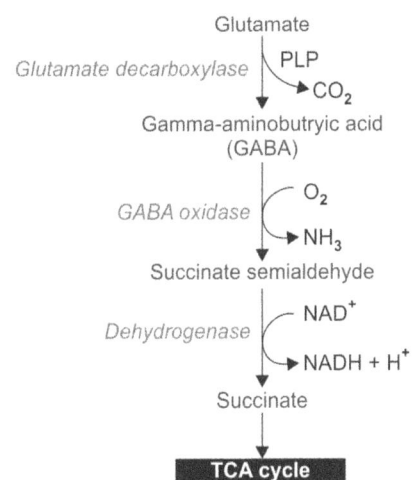

Fig. 23: Synthesis of GABA.

- Both formation and catabolism of GABA requires PLP. So in pyridoxine deficiency GABA will be deficient leading to convulsions. Sodium valproate inhibits GABA oxidase and is used for epilepsy treatment.

17. Methylmalonic aciduria (Fig. 24).

- Methylmalonic aciduria is an inherited disorder occurs due to the deficiency of B12
- There are 2 coenzymes of B12—methylcobalamin and deoxyadenosylcobalamine
- Deoxyadenosylcobalamine acts as a coenzyme for the isomerization reaction which isomerises L-methylmalonyl-CoA to succinyl-CoA
- There will be no isomerization of L-methylmalonyl-CoA to succinyl-CoA and so there is accumulation of methylmalonic acid in blood which leads to methylmalonic aciduria
- During B12 deficiency, methylmalonyl-CoA is excreted in excess through urine and the condition is known as **methylmalonic aciduria**.

18. Structure of tRNA.

Refer 2004 Short Note 12.

19. LAC operon.

Refer 2004 Short Note 19.

20. Insulin.

Hypoglycemic hormone.

Structure (Fig. 25)

- It is a peptide hormone with 2 polypeptide chains—A and B
  - A chain has 21 amino acids and B chain has 30 amino acids. So, total 51 amino acids
  - Two interchain disulfide bridges is between A7–B7 and A20–B19
  - One intrachain disulfide bridge in A chain is between A6–A11

Synthesis

- Insulin is synthesized and secreted by beta cells of islet of langerhans of pancreas
- It is synthesized as preproinsulin which has 109 amino acids
- It is converted to proinsulin in the endoplasmic reticulum by removal of leader sequence of 23 amino acids
- Proinsulin with 86 amino acids is cleaved by a protease enzyme in Golgi apparatus to produce insulin of 51 amino acids and

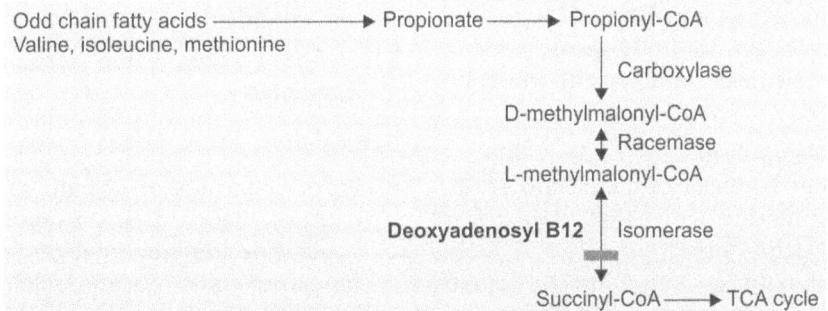

Fig. 24: Methylmalonic aciduria.

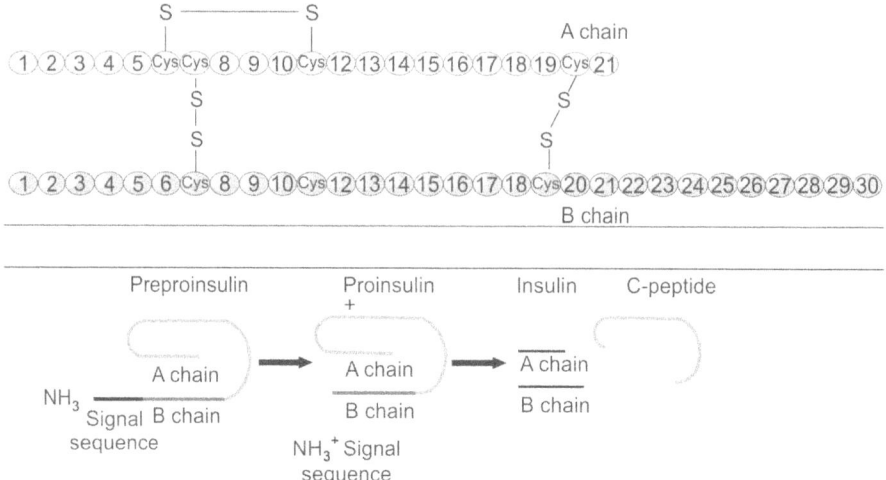

Fig. 25: Structure of insulin.

one C-peptide or connecting peptide of 33 amino acids.

Actions of Insulin

On Carbohydrate Metabolism

Hypoglycemic hormone
- Uptake of glucose by tissues—facilitates membrane transport of glucose
- Stimulates glycolysis by increasing the activity of glucokinase, phosphofructokinase and pyruvate kinase
- Promotes glycogenesis by activating glycogen synthase and favors glycogen storage
- It also inhibits glycogenolysis by inactivating glycogen phosphorylase
- Gluconeogenesis is inhibited by insulin by inhibiting the key enzymes—pyruvate carboxylase, phosphoenolpyruvate carboxykinase, fructose 1,6-bisphosphatase and glucose-6-phosphatase
- Stimulates glucose-6-phosphate dehydrogenase of HMP pathway and generates NADPH.

On Lipid Metabolism

- Promotes fatty acid synthesis (lipogenesis) by stimulating acetyl-CoA carboxylase, and glycerol kinase
- It inhibits lipolysis in adipose tissue by inhibiting hormone sensitive lipase
- It depresses HMG-CoA synthase and so ketogenesis is inactivated
- It stimulates HMG-CoA reductase thereby stimulating cholesterol synthesis.

On Protein Metabolism

- Promotes protein synthesis by promoting RNA polymerase and ribosome assembly
- It stimulates replication of cells
- It inhibits transamination and ornithine transcarbamoylase enzyme and inhibits protein catabolism
  - The metabolic disorder associated with insulin deficiency is diabetes mellitus (DM)
  - 2 types
    1. Type I—insulin dependent DM (IDDM)
    2. Type II—noninsulin dependent (NIDDM).

21. Define and classify polysaccharides with examples.

Definition

- Polysaccharides or glycans are carbohydrates made up of 10 or more monosaccharide units or their derivatives in repeating units. Monosaccharides are linked by glycosidic bonds.

Classification

- As per their sources:
  - Plant polysaccharides—e.g. starch, inulin, cellulose
  - Animal polysaccharides—e.g. glycogen.
- As per the monosaccharide units:
  - Homopolysaccharides (homoglycans)
    - Made up of same monosaccharide units, e.g. starch, glycogen made up of glucose; inulin made up of fructose.
  - Heteropolysaccharides (heteroglycans)
    - Made up of different types of sugars, e.g. agar, mucopolysaccharides (glycosaminoglycans)—hyaluronic acid, chondroitin sulfate, dermatan sulfate, keratan sulfate, heparin and heparan sulfate.

22. Define and classify enzymes with examples.

Definition

Enzymes are biocatalysts which are proteins in nature (except ribozymes). They are specific in their reaction. They are heat labile and colloidal which are required in small quantities for their action.

Classification

- **As per the site of location**
  - Intracellular enzymes within the cellular organelles, e.g. cytosol—enzymes of glycolysis, mitochondria—enzymes of TCA cycle
  - Extracellular enzymes—secreted from the cells but function outside the cells, e.g. digestive enzymes—pepsin, trypsin.
- **As per the diagnostic use—plasma enzymes**
  - Plasma specific or plasma functional enzymes—they have definite functions in plasma found in high concentration than in tissues mostly synthesized in liver, e.g. lipoprotein lipase, pseudocholinesterase
  - Plasma nonspecific or plasma nonfunctional enzymes—they have no definite function in plasma; they may be absent or present in low amounts in plasma. During the damage of tissues of its origin, its level is elevated in plasma—e.g. amylase, acid phosphatase.
- **As per the types of reaction catalyzed.**
  For example, dehydrogenases—removes hydrogen atom. Proteases—hydrolase proteins
- **IUB systems of classification- 6 classes**
  As per this system enzymes are represented as EC number with 4 digits (IUB system). First digit represent the class, second for the subclass, third for the sub-subclass, and fourth represents specific enzyme in list.

Classes: (OTHLIL)

- Oxidoreductases—these class of enzymes catalyze oxidations and reductions.
  - $AH_2 + B \rightarrow A + BH_2$

  For example, alcohol dehydrogenase, oxidases, reductases
- Transferases—these classes of enzymes catalyze transfer of moieties between substrate, such as amino acids, glycosyl, methyl, or phosphoryl group.
  - $A\text{-}R + B \rightarrow A + B\text{-}R$

  For example, hexokinase, transaminase
- Hydrolases—these classes of enzymes catalyze hydrolytic cleavage of C-C, C-O, C-N, and other bonds by adding of water.
  - $A\text{-}B + H_2O \rightarrow A\text{-}OH + B\text{-}H$

  For example, acetylcholine + $H_2O \rightarrow$ Choline + acetate catalyzed by acetylcholine esterase
- Lyases—these classes of enzymes catalyze cleavage of C-C, C-O, C-N, and other bonds by elimination, leaving double bonds without adding water

  For example, fructose-1, 6-bisphosphate $\xrightarrow{\text{Aldolase}}$ Glyceraldehyde -3-phosphate + DHAP
- Isomerases—these class of enzymes catalyze geometric or structural changes within a molecule.

  For example, recemases, epimerase, cis-trans isomerases

- Ligases—these class of enzymes catalyze the joining together of two molecules coupled to the hydrolysis of ATP.
  For example, acetyl-CoA + ATP → Malonyl-CoA + ADP + Pi.

23. Protein-energy malnutrition.

Disorders of malnutrition commonly manifested as protein-energy malnutrition (PEM). There are two major types of malnutritional diseases which are as follows:
1. **Marasmus:** This is due to severe deficiency of both dietary energy and proteins. Marasmus means "to waste"
2. **Kwashiorkor:** This is due to isolated deficiency of proteins with sufficient calorie intake. This is seen in the first child when the second child is born

The differences between these two malnutrition conditions are tabulated.

	Marasmus	Kwashiorkor
Age of onset	Below 1 year	1-5 years
Deficiency of	Calorie and proteins	Proteins alone
Cause	Early weaning and repeated infection	Starchy diet after weaning. Precipitated by acute infection
Growth retardation of child	Marked	Severe
Attitude	Irritable and fretful	Lethargic and apathetic
Appearance	Shrunken skin and bones, dehydrated	Looks plump due to edema of face and lower limbs
Appetite	Normal	Anorexia
Skin	Dry and atrophic	Crazy pavement dermatitis due to pealing and cracking of skin
Hair	No change	Sparse, soft and thin
Other features	Watery diarrhea, weakness and other nutritional deficiencies	Angular stomatitis, cheilosis, watery diarrhea, muscle wasting
Serum albumin	2-3 g/dL	<2 g/dL
Serum cortisol	Increased	Decreased

24. Acute intermittent porphyria.

Refer 2006 Short Note 9.

25. Role of cytochromes in ETC.

- Cytochromes present in ETC components are hemoproteins and they are cytochrome b, cytochrome C1 and cytochrome aa3 oxidase
- All except cytochrome oxidase are anaerobic dehydrogenases
- **Complex III/cytochrome reductase**—It is a cluster of iron sulfur proteins. It contains cytochrome b and cytochrome C1 and both contain heme as prosthetic group
- During the electron transfer, the iron in heme group shuttles between Fe_3^+ and Fe^{2+}. The free energy change is -10 kcal/mol and 4 protons are pumped out
- **Cytochrome C**—it contains one heme as prosthetic group. It collects electrons from complex II and transfers them to complex IV
- **Complex IV/cytochrome oxidase**— it is a cluster of proteins and contain cytochrome a and cytochrome a3 and both the proteins contain two heme and two copper ions. It is tightly bound to mitochondrial inner membrane. Four electrons are accepted from cytochrome C (cyt C) and passed on to molecular oxygen. And two protons are pumped out to the intermembrane space.

26. Comparison between prokaryotic and eukaryotic cells.

- Prokaryotic cells do not have typical nucleus, e.g. bacteria and algae
- Eukaryotic cells have nucleus surrounded by nuclear membrane
- The anatomical and physiological differences between prokaryotic and eukaryotic cells are showing following table:

S. No.	Characteristics	Prokaryotic cells	Eukaryotic cells
1.	Size	Small (1-10 μm)	Large (10-100 μm)
2.	Cell membrane	Rigid cell wall	Flexible plasma membrane
3.	Subcellular organelles	Absent	Distinct organelles seen (mitochondria, nucleus, lysosomes)
4.	Nucleus	Not well defined; no nuclear membrane	Well defined nucleus surrounded by nuclear membrane; DNA present with histones
5.	Mitochondria	Absent. Enzymes of energy metabolism bound to membrane	Present energy in the form of ATP synthesized in mitochondria
6.	Cytoplasm	Organelles and cytoskeletons absent	Contains organelles and cytoskeletons
7.	Cell division	By fission; no mitosis	Mitotic division
8.	Examples	Unicellular organisms — bacteria, algae	Multicellular organisms — higher animals and plant cells

27. Post-translational modifications with two examples.

Post-translational Modifications

Once the protein is synthesized by the process of translation by the ribosomes, it undergoes various modifications to become a fully functional protein. Those processes are called post-translational modification or post-translational processing of proteins. They are:
- Trimming
- Covalent modifications
  - Phosphorylation
  - Glycosylation
  - Hydroxylation
  - Carboxylation
  - Addition of groups—methyl, acetyl, farnesyl, amide
- Subunit aggregation
- Protein folding.

Cleaving of Large Precursor Molecules (Trimming)–ER/Golgi/Secretory Vescicles

- Proteins like insulin are secreted as preproprotein. Proteinases cleave the N terminal and C-terminal portions of preproinsulin. Then it undergoes disulfide bond creation to form mature insulin and get released
  - **Preproinsulin → Proinsulin → Insulin**
  - **Cleaved after secretion, e.g. collagen**
  - **Zymogens (inactive proenzymes) → active enzymes, e.g. trypsinogen → Trypsin**
- **Proteolytic cleavage**—of 'N' terminal methionine by hydrolysis
- **Removal of signal sequences**—signal peptides—endoplasmic reticulum.

Protein Folding

Chaperons—heat shock proteins facilitate and favor interactions on polypeptide surfaces to get specific confirmation of a protein. They irreversibly bind to hydrophobic regions of unfolded proteins and folding intermediates and stabilize them.

Covalent Modifications

- **Gamma-carboxylation**—the gamma carbon of glutamic acid in clotting factors (II,VII,IX,XI) under the influence of vitamin K is needed for them to become active clotting factors
- **Hydroxylation**—hydroxylation of lysine and proline in alpha chain of collagen is needed for making bonds between them to increase the strength of collagen. Vitamin C acts as a cofactor in this
- **Phosphorylation**—phosphorylation of ser, thr, tyr in many regulatory enzymes like phosphorylase are important for regulation of metabolic pathways
- **Glycosylation**—many proteins are glycoproteins. Carbohydrates are attached to ser/thr residues to the OH group or to the amide N of asparagine, e.g. proteins of plasma membrane and lysosomes occurs in ER/Golgi
  - Used to target proteins in specific organelles, e.g. lysosomal enzymes—modified by addition of mannose 6-phosphate

- **Methylation**—methylation of lysine/histidine/arginine, e.g. histones
- **Acylation**—myelin proteolipids or transferrin receptor help in stable anchorage of protein in lipid bilayer of membranes.

Subunit Aggregation

Occurs in:
- Immunoglobulin
- Hemoglobin
- Maturation of collagen.

Clinical Applications
- Defective hydroxylation in collagen leads to collagen disorders like Ehlers-Danlos syndrome
- Defective protein folding may lead to dangerous prion diseases like bovine spongiform encephalopathy and crueztfolt Jakob disease.

28. Alpha-helical structure of a peptide/secondary structure of proteins.

- Proteins contain primary, secondary, tertiary and sometimes quaternary structure
- **Secondary structure** of protein denotes the relationship between residues (amino acids) which are 3-4 residues apart in linear structure
- Secondary structure of proteins is stabilized by noncovalent bonds such as:
  - Hydrogen bond—weak
  - Electrostatic bonds—ionic bonds (salt bridges)
  - Hydrophobic bonds—weak
  - Vander Waal's forces
- **Types of secondary structures**—the types of secondary structure are: (i) Alpha helix, e.g. alpha-keratin, (ii) Beta-pleated sheet, beta bends (reverse turns, beta turns), (iii) Nonrepetitive secondary structure and supersecondary motifs.

α-helix (Fig. 26)

Structures of Proteins
- Alpha helix is one type of secondary structure of proteins
- It was the first structure found out by Pauling and Corey
- It is the most common and stable confirmation in a polypeptide chain. It is

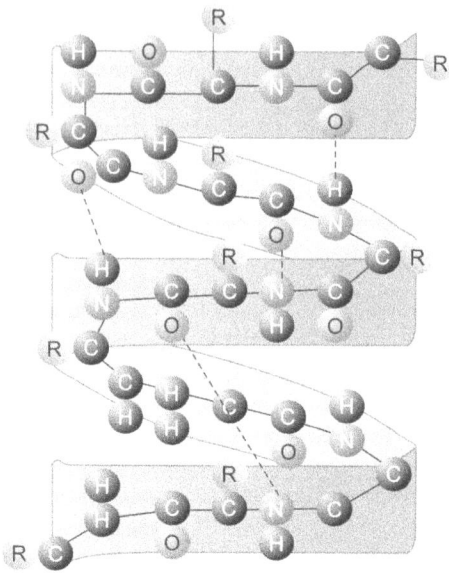

Fig. 26: Alpha helix.

seen in Hb, myoglobin and collagen and absent in chymotrypsin
- It has a spiral structure which is stabilized by hydrogen bond between NH and CO groups of amino acids
- The alpha helix is mostly right handed since amino acids are usually L variety
- Polypeptide bonds form the backbone of the helix and the side chains of amino acids extend outward
- Each turn of helix contain about 3.6 residues. The distance between each amino acids is about 1.5 Å apart
- Proline and hydroxy proline will not allow α-helix formation
- Alpha helix is seen in alpha-keratin, Hb.

29. Buffer system in the body.

- Buffers resist changes in pH when small quantities of an acid or an alkali are added. Various buffers in blood are:

Bicarbonate Buffer System
- It is also known as bicarbonate - carbonic acid buffer system ($NaHCO_3/H_2CO_3$)
- It is the most important buffer in plasma and is formed by ($NaHCO_3/H_2CO_3$)
- It accounts for 40% in whole body and 65% in plasma

- The base HCO_3^- is the **metabolic component** and it is regulated by kidney and carbonic acid (H_2CO_3) is called **respiratory component** since it is regulated by the lungs
  - The **normal bicarbonate level** in plasma is 24 mmol/L.
  - The **normal pCO_2** of arterial blood is 40 mm Hg.
  - The **normal carbonic acid concentration** in blood is 1.2 mmol/L
- Carbonic acid has a pKa of 6.1 so it is a poor buffer. But the high blood concentration and the ratio of base to salt is high (20:1) which makes it an effective buffer.
- Under physiological conditions with pH 7.4 the ratio of bicarbonate to carbonic acid is **20: 1.**

Phosphate Buffer System

- It is an intracellular buffer with low concentration in plasma
- It is made of Na_2HPO_4/NaH_2PO_4. It has a pK_a of 6.8. It is an effective buffer system because its pKa value 6.7 is nearer to physiological pH
- **The ratio of $HPO_4 : H_2PO_4 = 4:1$.**

Protein Buffer System

Extracellular – (Na Protein/H protein)

- Buffering capacity of proteins depend on the pKa value of ionisable side chains
- The most effective buffer is imidazole group of **histidine** molecules with a pKa value of 6.1
- Albumin contains 16 histidine residues and so albumin accounts for the non-bicarbonate buffer system.

Intracellular – Hb buffer system (KHb/HHb)

- Hb is the major blood buffer in RBCs and it acts along with bicarbonate system.
- It has 38 histidine residues.
- **In the lungs:** OxyHb releases H⁺ which is buffered by bicarbonate to form carbonic acid which is converted by carbonic anhydrase to CO_2 and water which get eliminated by ventilation **(Fig. 27)**.
- **In the RBC:** CO_2 is converted to carbonic acid by carbonic anhydrase resulting in decrease in pH and the Hb becomes deoxy-Hb.
- **In the tissue level:** The oxyHb releases O_2 to the tissues which is facilitated by low pO_2, low pH and high pCO_2 and CO_2 produced is returned to the lungs, carried by Hb where CO_2 is eliminated in expired air **(Fig. 28)**
- DeoxyHb neutralizes carbonic acid to increase the pH and there will be increase in bicarbonate and decrease in pCO_2
- To maintain electroneutrality chloride ions enter into RBC for each bicarbonate leaves. This is called **chloride shift**

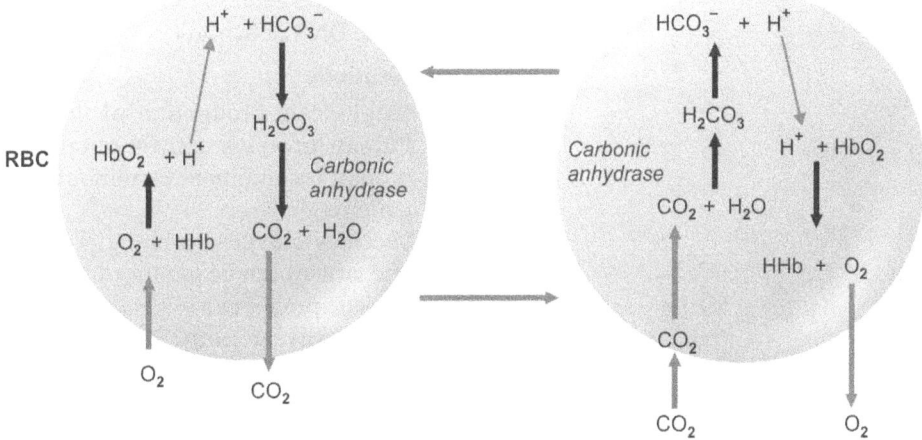

Fig. 27: Hemoglobin action in lungs.   **Fig. 28:** Hemoglobin action in tissues.

30. Principles of electrophoresis and its clinical applications.

Principle

The term electrophoresis refers to the movement of charged particles through an electrolyte when subjected to an electric field.
- Cations (positively charged ions) move towards cathode and anions (negative) to anode
- When a biological mixture is subjected to electrophoresis, the compounds in the mixture move in relation to their net charge, size, molecular weight and mass and gets separated according to these characteristics so that the desired compound can be identified and isolated.

Clinical Applications

Separation of serum proteins, lipoproteins and other classes of macromolecules. Electrophoretic pattern of plasma proteins — normal and abnormal **(Fig. 29)**.

Normal Bands

- 5 bands—albumin (55-65%), alpha-1-globulin (2-4%), alpha-2 globulin (6-12%), beta globulin (8-12%) and gamma globulin (12-22%)
- Albumin has maximum and gamma globulin has minimum mobility.

Abnormal Bands

- Nephrotic syndrome—globulin is produced more by liver in compensation of renal loss of albumin. So alpha-2 band is prominent
- Cirrhosis—albumin synthesized in liver is decreased due to cirrhosis and so albumin band is thin and less prominent
- Multiple myeloma—light chain immunoglobulins are produced more so there will be a prominence in gamma globulin region (M band).

Hemoglobin Electrophoresis

- S band is seen in sickle cell anemia
- Various hemoglobinopathies and thalassemias can be diagnosed
- **Immunoelectrophoresis**—to separate various classes of immunoglobulins
- **Blotting techniques**—electrophoresis is an integral part of blotting techniques.

31. Applications of genetic engineering.

Recombinant DNA Technology

When a gene of one species is transferred to another gene of different species, it is called recombinant DNA technology or genetic engineering. Usually there will be combination of human DNA and bacterial DNA. The DNA thus formed is called as recombinant DNA or chimeric DNA or hybrid DNA.

Applications

- Large scale production of therapeutic human proteins can be obtained, e.g. human recombinant insulin for diabetic patients
- Vaccines with genetic material of bacteria and viruses can be produced
- Genetic probes can be produced to:
  - Identify genetic diseases during antenatal period
  - Diagnosis of virus and bacteria in blood using their DNA

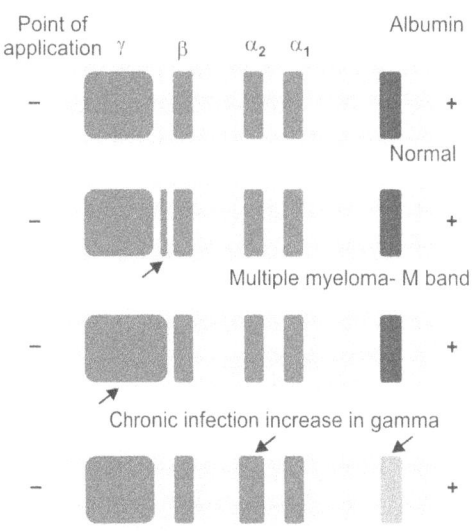

Fig. 29: Serum protein electrophoresis in health and disease.

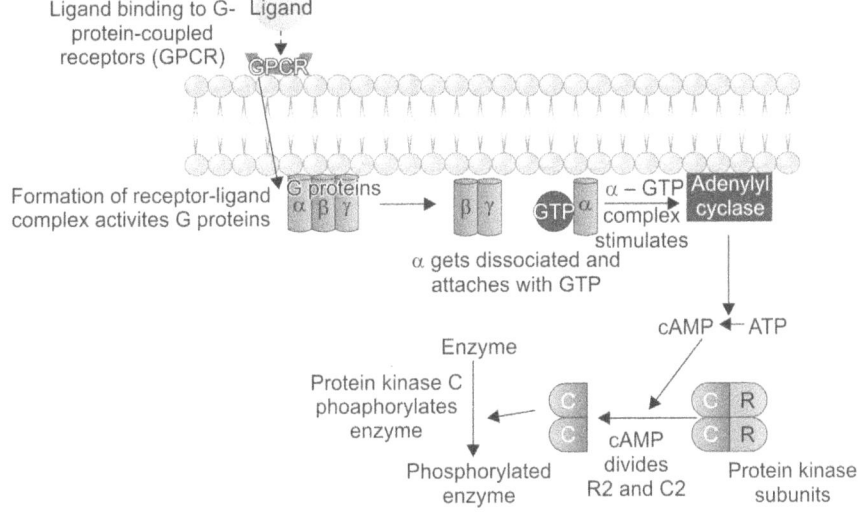

Fig. 30: G protein in signal transduction.

- To pinpoint location of a gene in chromosome
- To identify mutations in genes
- To detect activation of oncogenes
- Gene therapy—normal genes could be inserted into the patient's cells where it is defective, e.g. adenosine deaminase deficiency
  - Prenatal diagnosis by amniocentesis.

32. G proteins.

- G proteins are signaling transducing molecules attached to the cell membrane receptors
- It is a heteromeric GTP binding protein for group II hormones, e.g. catecholamines, glucagon, etc.
- It has 3 subunits- α, β and γ
- They G proteins are named such because of its ability to bind GTP
- Receptors that couple to effectors through G proteins [G protein-coupled receptors (GPCR)] have seven helical membrane spanning domains that loop in and out of cell membrane
- **In the absence** of hormone, G protein complex (α, β, γ) is in an inactive GDP bound form and not associated with the receptor. This complex is anchored to the plasma membrane through prenylated groups on the $\beta\gamma$ subunits
- **On binding of hormone** (H) to the receptor, there is a conformational change of the receptor and activation of the G-protein complex
- This results from the exchange of GDP with guanosine triphosphate (GTP) on the α-subunit, after which α and $\beta\gamma$ dissociate. The α-subunit binds to and activates the effector (E)
- Effector can be any of the further pathways or second messengers:
  - Adenylyl cyclase—which converts ATP to cAMP which is a second messenger
  - Ca^{2+}, Na^+, Cl^- channels, K^+ channel, PIP.
- The G protein is inactivated when GTP is hydrolyzed by GTPase to GDP which is a part of alpha subunit. This α-subunit once again combines with β and γ subunits to form inactive trimeric G protein **(Fig. 30)**
- Defects in G protein can cause diseases like cholera and whooping cough.

MBBS Examination 2007

ANSWER ALL QUESTIONS

I. **Essay questions**   (10 Marks each)

1. Write in detail about gluconeogenesis and mention its significance. Write about glucose alanine cycle.
2. What are isoenzymes? Write about different isoenzymes and their importance.
3. Describe the chemistry, source, RDA, biochemical functions and deficiency manifestation of folic acid.
4. What is the active form of methionine? How it is formed? What are its functions? Enumerate the steps of methionine metabolism and write the disorders associated with its metabolism.
5. What is the normal pH of blood. Discuss the mechanism involved in its regulation.
6. Mention the sources, daily requirement, functions and deficiency symptoms of calcium. Explain how serum level of calcium is regulated.
7. Define biological oxidation. Mention the components and organization of ETC. Describe the mechanism of ATP synthesis. Add a note on uncouplers.
8. Describe the chemistry, sources, RDA, and functions of thiamine. Add a note on beriberi.
9. Describe the mechanism of DNA replication. Add a note on DNA repair mechanism.
10. Name the branched-chain amino acids. Describe the pathway for the metabolism of branched-chain amino acids. Add a note on maple syrup urine disease.

II. **Short notes**   (5 Marks each)

1. Phospholipids.
2. Congenital hyperbilirubinemias.
3. Formation of ketone bodies and their significance.
4. Basal metabolic rate.
5. HMP shunt pathway.
6. Oxidative phosphorylation.
7. Oncogenes.
8. Electrophoresis.
9. Genetic code.
10. Insulin.
11. Gout.
12. Detoxification.
13. Polyunsaturated fatty acids (PUFA).
14. Balanced diet.
15. Glycosylated hemoglobin.
16. Chondroitin sulphate.
17. Synthesis and utilization of ketone bodies.
18. Rapoport-Luebering cycle (glycolysis in RBC) (2,3-Bisphosphoglycerate cycle/2,3 BPG shunt).
19. Folate trap.
20. Glycosides.
21. Apolipoproteins and their significance.
22. Renal glycosuria.
23. Recombinant DNA technology.
24. Wilson's disease.
25. Secondary structure of proteins.
26. Polyamines.
27. Metabolic acidosis.
28. Restriction endonucleases.
29. Functions of phosphorous.
30. Purine salvage pathway.
31. Post-translational modification.
32. Role of lungs in acid-base balance.

I. ESSAY QUESTIONS

1. Write in detail about gluconeogenesis and mention its significance. Write about glucose alanine cycle.

Definition: Synthesis of glucose from non-carbohydrate substrates
- Organs—liver and kidney (cortex)
- Substrates—pyruvate, lactate, amino acids (glucogenic), propionate, glycerol.

Key Enzymes in Gluconeogenesis

- **Pyruvate carboxylase**—pyruvate in the cytoplasm enters the mitochondria. Then carboxylation of pyruvate to oxaloacetate is catalyzed by pyruvate carboxylase. It needs biotin and ATP
- **Phosphoenolpyruvate carboxykinase** —(PEPCK) it converts oxaloacetate to phosphoenolpyruvate by removing CO_2. GTP donates the phosphate
- **Fructose 1,6-bisphosphatase**
  Fructose 1, 6-bisphosphate → Fructose 6-phosphate + Pi
  This step will bypass phosphofructokinase (PFK) step
- **Glucose-6-phosphatase**—it is active in liver and absent in muscle.
  Glucose-6-phosphate + H_2O → Glucose + Pi.

Steps of Gluconeogenesis

It involves glycolysis (not a reversal), TCA cycle and some reactions like transamination.
- **Conversion of pyruvate to glucose (mitochondria + cytosol)**
  - Carboxylation of pyruvate to oxaloacetate by pyruvate carboxylase enzyme, and the coenzyme biotin and ATP
  - Transport of oxaloacetate to cytosol through malate aspartate shuttle **(Fig. 1)**. Oxaloacetate cannot cross the inner mitochondrial membrane. So it is reduced to malate which can be transported across the mitochondrial membrane to cytosol. In the cytosol, malate is re-oxidised to oxaloacetate by malate dehydrogenase of cytosol
  - Decarboxylation of cytosolic oxaloacetate to phosphoenolpyruvate (PEP) by phosphoenolpyruvate carboxykinase. One GTP is required for this step
  - Phosphoenolpyruvate—by reversal of glycolysis forms fructose 1, 6-bisphosphate
  - Dephosphorylation of fructose 1, 6-bisphosphate to fructose 6 phosphate by fructose 1, 6-bisphosphatase (allosteric enzyme). Fructose 6-phosphatase is isomerised to glucose-6-phosphatase

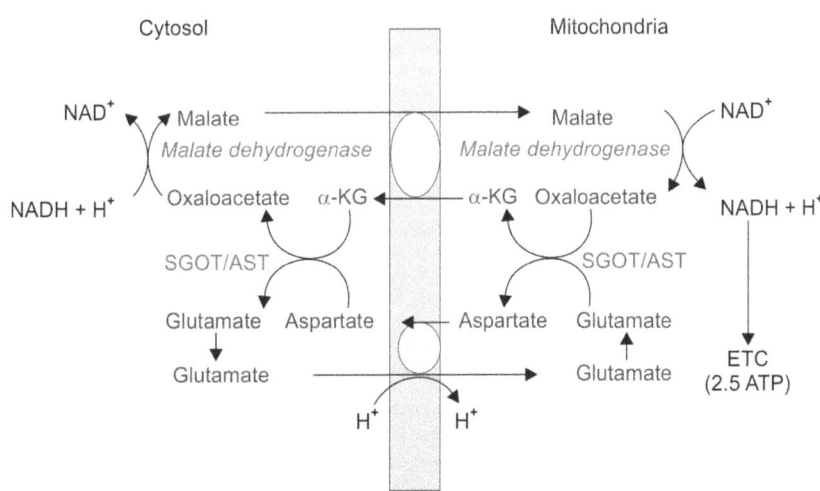

Fig. 1: Malate aspartate shuttle.

- Dephosphorylation of glucose-6 phosphate to glucose by glucose-6-phosphatase enzyme which is not present in muscles but present only in liver and kidney.
- **Lactate to glucose (Cori cycle):** Lactate dehydrogenase converts lactate to pyruvate. Pyruvate enters neoglucogenic pathway to form glucose.
  Lactate → Liver, Kidney → Pyruvate → Gluconeogenic pathway → Glucose.
- **Glycerol to glucose (Fig. 2):** From adipose tissue the hydrolytic product of TAG—glycerol is shifted to liver by blood where it gets phosphorylated to form glucose-3-phosphate. This is then dehydrogenated to form DHAP which by reversal of glycolysis produces glucose.
- **Glucogenic amino acids**
  - Alaninme—released from muscle is taken to liver by glucose-alanine cycle

  $$\text{Alanine} \xrightarrow[\text{Transamination}]{\text{ALT}} \text{Pyruvate} \longrightarrow \longrightarrow \longrightarrow \text{Glucose}$$

  - Other glucogenic amino acids—transaminated to keto acids to enter into TCA cycle to form oxaloacetate/pyruvate

  $$\text{Aspartate/ASN} \xrightarrow[\text{Transamination}]{\text{AST}}$$

  Oxaloacetate ⟶ TCA cycle
  Valine, isoleucine, methionine ⟶
  Oxaloacetate ⟶ TCA cycle
  Phenylalanine, tyrosine ⟶ Fumarate ⟶ TCA cycle

  All of them then enter into neoglucogenic pathway to get converted to glucose.
- **Propionate to glucose (Fig. 3):** Propionate is formed by the oxidation of odd chain fatty acids and also from certain glucogenic amino acids and by glycolysis in ruminants. Propionate is converted to succinyl-CoA which then enters into TCA cycle.

Significance of Gluconeogenesis

- Whenever carbohydrate source is insufficient, gluconeogenesis meet the needs of the body to maintain blood glucose homeostasis
- It is a continuous source of glucose to tissues like brain, RBC, lens, cornea of eyes, and renal medulla.

Reciprocal Regulation

Gluconeogenesis and glycolysis are reciprocally regulated so that one pathway is relatively inactive when the other is active.

- **Pyruvate carboxylase**—acetyl-CoA is an activator of pyruvate carboxylase which is an allosteric enzyme
- **Fructose 1, 6-bisphosphatase**—citrate is an activator of fructose 1, 6-bisphosphatase; fructose 2, 6-bisphosphate and AMP are inhibitors
- **ATP**—gluconeogenesis is enhanced by ATP.

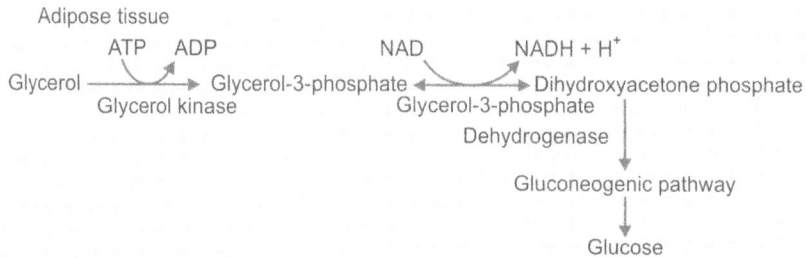

Fig. 2: Conversion of glycerol to glucose.

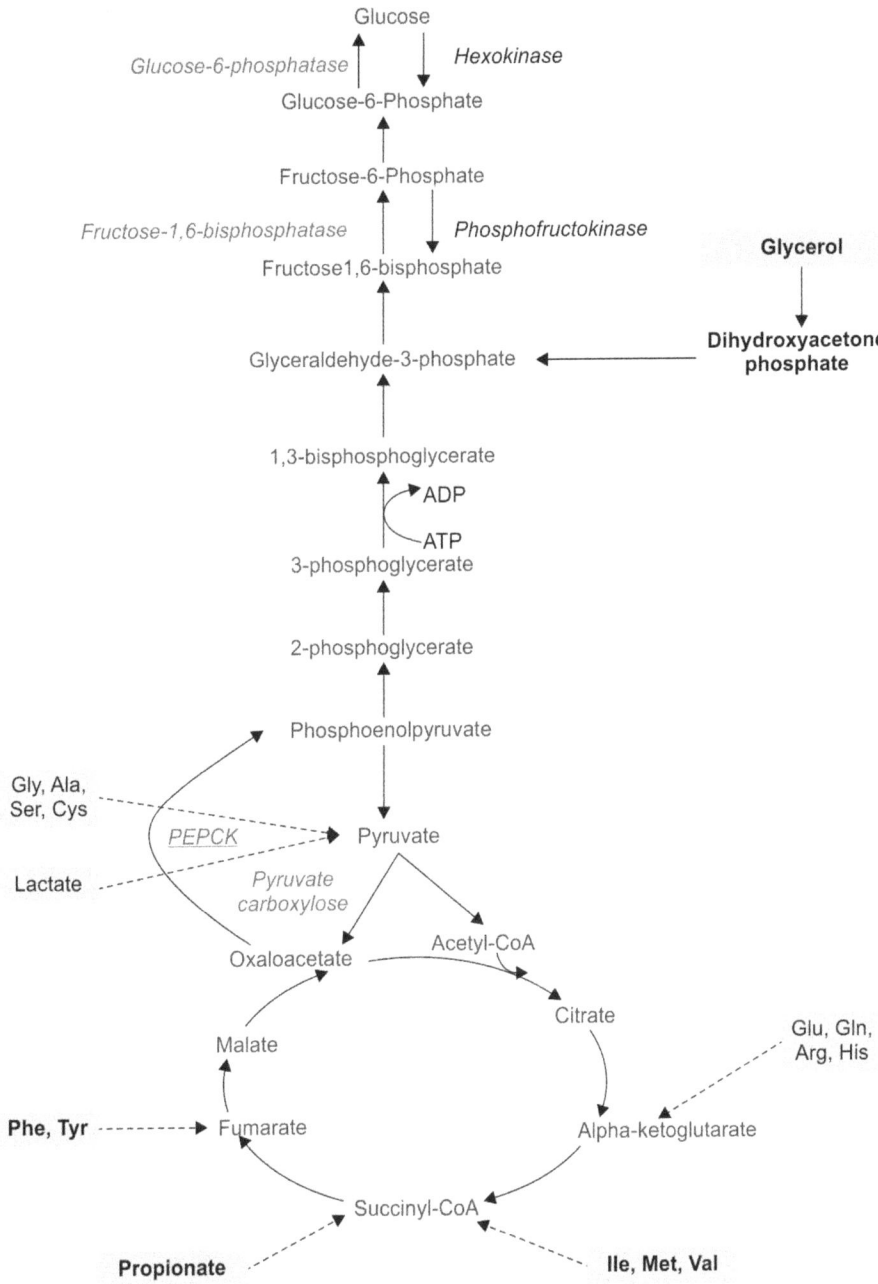

Fig. 3: Conversion of propionate to glucose.
(PEPCK: Phosphoenolpyruvate carboxykinase)

Glucose-Alanine Cycle (CAHILL Cycle) (Fig. 4)

Alanine synthesized in muscle is transported to liver where it is converted to glucose.

Transamination Gluconeogenesis
Muscle protein→ Alanine ⟶ Pyruvate ⟶ Glucose.

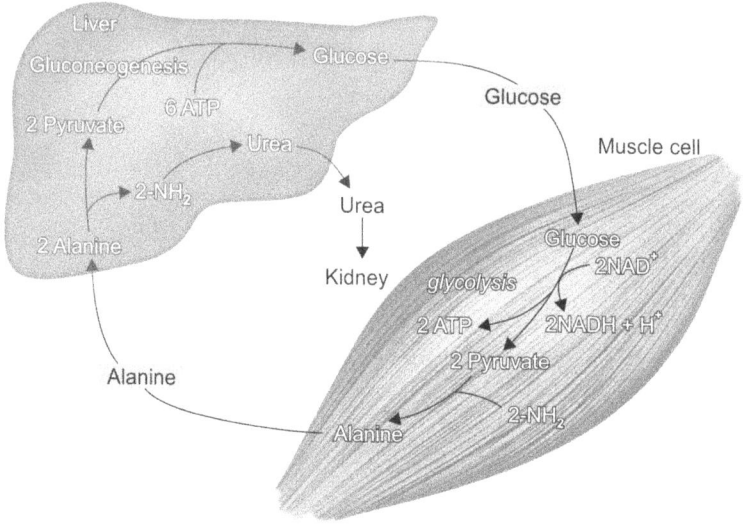

Fig. 4: Glucose-alanine cycle.

Significance
- Liver maintains glucose output by gluconeogenesis of alanine
- It also maintains nitrogen balance.

2. What are isoenzymes? Write about different isoenzymes and their importance.

Refer 2003 Short Notes 5.

- Multiple molecular forms of an enzyme catalyzing the same reaction are isoenzymes or isozymes, e.g. lactate dehydrogenase—5 isoenzymes (LDH 1, 2, 3, 4 and 5), creatine kinase—3 isoenzymes (CK-1, 2, 3) and alkaline phosphatase
- They are physically distinct forms of the same enzyme activity
- They are synthesized from various tissues and hence useful to study the disorders of those organs
- They are made up of different subunits. If the subunits are the same they are known as homomultimer. They are represented by same gene. If the subunits are different they are known as heteromultimer produced by different gene.

Separation and Identification of Isoenzymes
- Electrophoresis—depends upon the mobility in electrical field
- Heat stability—some gets denatured by heat, e.g. bone isoenzyme of ALP
- Inhibitors—tartrate labile ACP
- Substrate specificity or K_m value—different for each isoenzyme, e.g. glucokinase and hexokinase
- Localization—LDH-H4 form is present in heart; LDH-M4 in skeletal muscle.

Lactate Dehydrogenase
- LDL catalyses the conversion of pyruvate to lactate and vice versa. LDL is concentrated in RBC cell; therefore minor hemolysis causes the false value. Normal values ranges from 100-200 U/L
- Elevation of LDH is seen in hemolytic anemia, hepatocellular damage, muscular dystrophy, cancer, etc.
- LDH is tetramer made up of two H (heart) bands and two M (muscle) bands. Both of these are same molecular weight and with minor amino acid variations
- There are 5 isoenzymes. They are LDH1, LDH2, LDH3, LDH4, and LDH5

- With two different polypeptide chains therefore 5 combinations of H and M are possible namely H4, H3M, H2M2, M3H, M4. The tissue specificity and diagnostic importance of these 5 isoenzymes is as follows:
  - H4 form found in heart which is useful for diagnosing heart disease
  - M4 form found in muscle hence it is useful in diagnosing muscle diseases
  - Isoenzymes of LDH help in the diagnosis of heart and liver diseases
  - Flipped pattern is observed in myocardial infarction (LDH-1 > LDH-2)
  - Increased activity of LDH-5 is an indicator of liver diseases.

Creatine Kinase

- It catalysis the synthesis of creatine phosphate from creatine and ATP
- Normal blood ranges from 15-100 IU/L
- It is made up of two polypeptides namely M and B, therefore three combinations of isoenzymes are possible. They are MM found in skeletal muscle, MB found in heart and BB found in brain
- Creatine kinase (CK) subform is highly elevated in muscular dystrophies, acute cerebrovascular injuries. It is most reliable factor in diagnosing AMI
- Three isoenzymes—CK BB(1), CK MB(2), CK MM(3)
  1. CK BB(1)—present in brain
  2. CK MB(2)—it is the earliest reliable marker of myocardial infarction
  3. CK MM(3)—it is elevated in muscle diseases.

Alkaline Phosphatase

- It is nonspecific enzyme which hydrolyses aliphatic, aromatic and heterocyclic compounds at pH 9-10 in the presence of Mn and Mg. Zinc is a constituent ion of ALP
- ALP produced by osteoblasts for the calcification process
- Normal serum levels are 40-125 U/L. Moderate increase seen in hepatic diseases, and very high levels are seen in extrahepatic obstruction or intrahepatic obstructions, and very high levels are seen in bone diseases
- ALP has nearly 6 types of Iso-enzymes are: Alpha-1 ALP, Alpha-2 heat labile ALP, Alpha-2 heat stable ALP, Pre-beta ALP, Gamma-ALP, Leucocyte ALP (LAP)
- They are due to the difference in the carbohydrate content
- Alpha-1 ALP—it is about 10% total ALP, and is increased in obstructive jaundice
- Alpha-2 ALP—it is about 20% of total ALP—increased in hepatitis
- Alpha-2 heat stable ALP—it is about 1% of total ALP. It is heat stable above 65°C
- Pre-beta ALP—it is about 50% of total ALP. It is elevated in bone diseases
- Gamma-ALP—it is about 10%, it is increased in ulcerative colitis
- Leucocyte-ALP (LAP)—it is increased in lymphomas and decreased in chronic myeloid leukemia.

Acid Phosphatase

- It acts at a pH between 4 and 6
- Normal value in serum is 2.5 to 12 U/L
- Secreted by prostate cells, RBCs, WBCs and platelets
- The value of acid phosphate (ACP) is increased in prostate cancer and it is an important tumor marker for prostate cancer
- It has got a tartrate labile isoenzyme which is helpful in follow-up of prostate cancer. Its normal level is 1 U/L.

3. **Describe the chemistry, source, RDA, biochemical functions and deficiency manifestation of folic acid.**

- The latin word folium means **leafy vegetables.**

Chemistry: It is composed of pteridine, para-aminobenzoic acid (PABA) and glutamic acid.

Pteridine + PABA + glutamic acid → pteroylglutamic acid or folic acid

Source:
- Rich—yeast, green leafy vegetables (folium).
- Moderate—cereals, pulses, oil, seeds and eggs.

RDA:
- Adult: 200 µg/day
- Pregnancy: 400 µg/day

Biochemical functions: Coenzyme form of folic acid—tetrahydrofolate **(Fig. 5)**
- Folic acid is first reduced to 7, 8 dihydrofolic acid and further reduced to 5, 6, 7, 8 tetrahydrofolic acid (THFA) by folate reductase enzyme
- THFA is a carrier of one-carbon groups. One-carbon groups play a vital role in donating carbon atoms for the synthesis of different types of compounds
- **Different One-Carbon Compounds**

Group	Structure
Formimino	HN=CH-
Formyl	HCO
Methyl	CH_3
Methylene	CH_2-
Methenyl	=CH

[N^5 and N^{10} atoms of THFA carry the one-carbon groups]

- Except methyl group, other one-carbon groups are carried by THFP.

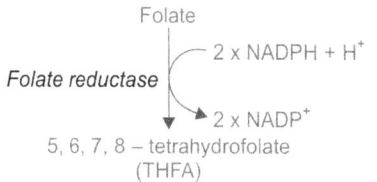

Fig. 5: Formation of tetrahydrofolate.

S. No.	Folic acid derivative	One-carbon group transferred	Compounds produced
1.	N^5, N^{10} methylene-THFA	Methylene (CH_2)	Serine- glycine interconversion - dTMP Glycine cleavage system
2.	N^5, N^{10} methenyl THFA	Methenyl (=CH)	C_8 of purine ring
3.	Formyl THFA	Formyl	C_2 of purine ring
4.	N^5, N^{10}-methylene THFA	Methylene (CH_2)	dTMP in DNA
5.	N^5-methyl-THFA	Methyl (CH_3)	N_5-methyl –H4F-methyl Cobalamin Homocysteine to methionine
6.	N^5-formimino THFA	Formimino (-CH=NH)	Histidine –FIGLU

Causes of Folate Deficiency
- Pregnancy
- Dietary deficiency
- Defective absorption
- Hemolytic anemia
- **Folate trap:** When vitamin B12 is deficient, methyl tetrahydrofolate (THFA) cannot be converted to THFA B12 takes up this methyl group to form methylcobalamine to supply the methyl group to homocysteine to form methionine. So methyl-THFA gets trapped inside the cell in B12 deficiency the following reaction cannot take place, leads to folate deficiency **(Figs. 6 and 7)**.

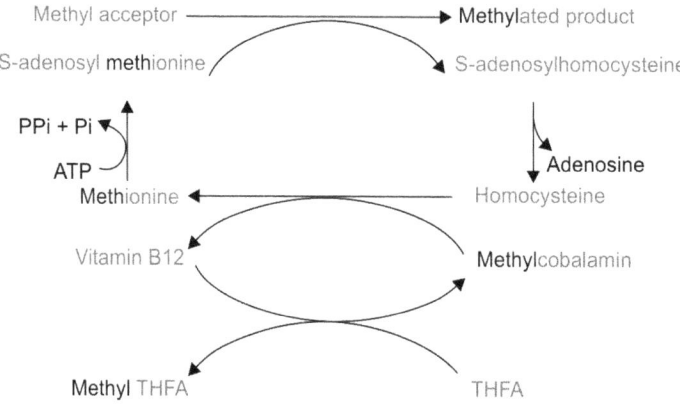

Fig. 6: Folate trap.

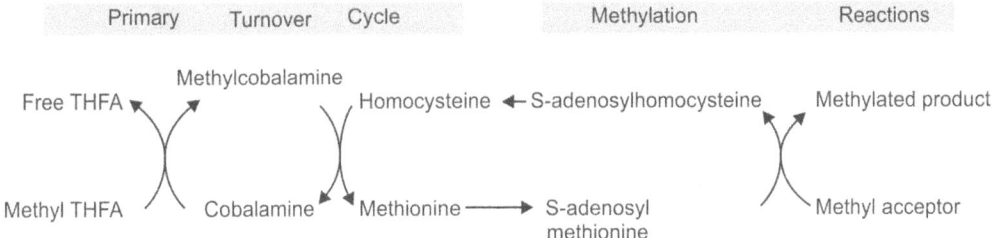

Fig. 7: Role of methyl H4F as methyl donor.

Deficiency Manifestations
- Reduced DNA synthesis
- Macrocytic anemia
- Hyperhomocysteinemia
- Birth defects—neural tube defects in fetus
- Cancer.

Assessment of Folate Deficiency

FIGLU Excretion Test or Histidine Load Test

Histidine is metabolized to formimino glutamic acid from which formimino group is removed by THFA. Therefore, in folate deficiency, formiminoglutamic acid (FIGLU) is excreted in urine.

Folate Antagonists
- Sulphonamides
- Aminopterine
- Primethamine.

---

4. **What is the active form of methionine? How it is formed? What are its functions? Enumerate the steps of methionine metabolism and write the disorders associated with its metabolism.**

METHIONINE METABOLISM

- Methionine is a sulfur containing amino acid; it is an essential, glucogenic amino acid
- From methionine the other sulfur containing amino acid—cysteine is produced
- The active form of methionine is S-adenosyl methionine (SAM).

STEPS OF METHIONINE METABOLISM (FIG. 8)

- **Activation of methionine to S-adenosyl methionine (SAM) (Fig. 9)**
  – Methionine adenosyltransferase enzyme transfers the adenosyl group to the sulfur atom of methionine to form the active methionine—S-adenosyl methionine
- **Transfer of methyl group to other acceptors (transmethylation):** SAM donates methyl group to methyl acceptors by methyltransferases to form S-adenosyl-homocysteine (SAH)
- **Formation of homocysteine:** From S-adenosyl homocysteine adenosine group is removed by adenosine homocysteinase to form homocysteine **(Fig. 9)**
- **Resynthesis of methionine:** Homocysteine forms methionine by homocysteine methyltransferase. This step uses methyltetrahydrofolate which becomes THFA in the presence of B12
- **Formation of cysteine:** Homocysteine combines with serine to form cystathionine using cystathionine synthase in the presence of PLP. Cystathionine is hydrolyzed to cysteine and homoserine by cystathioninase. PLP acts as a coenzyme for this step also. This is trans-sulfuration reaction
- **Final oxidation of homoserine:** Homoserine is deaminated and decarboxylated to propionyl-CoA which is converted to methylmalonyl-CoA and then to succinyl CoA with the help of deoxyadenosyl cobalamin. Succinyl-CoA enters into TCA cycle and hence methionine is a glucogenic amino acid

Transmethylation reaction

It is an acceptance of a methyl group from a donor like S-adenosyl methionine—by

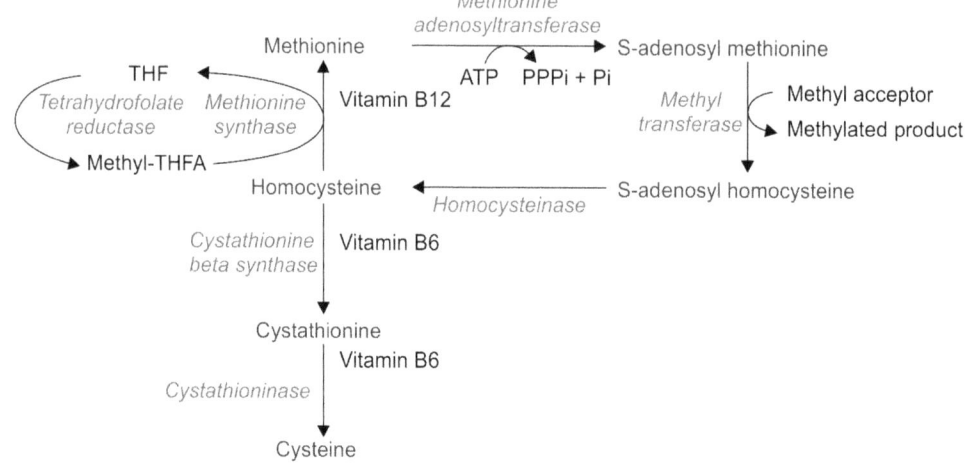

Fig. 8: Methionine metabolism.

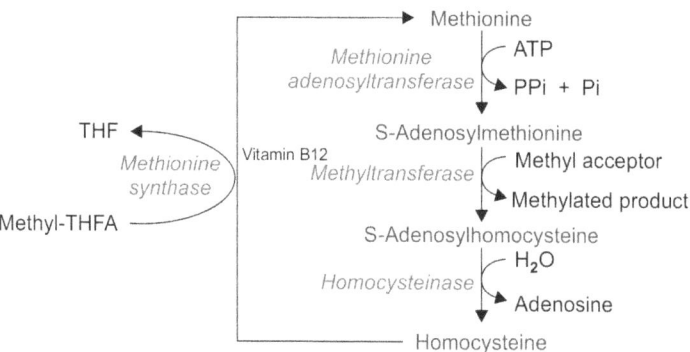

Fig. 9: S-adenosyl methionine cycle.

an acceptor resulting in the formation of a methylated compound

- Transmethylation reaction requires SAM which is obtained by accepting adenosyl group from ATP by methionine by methionine adenosyltransferase.

Methionine $\xrightarrow{\text{ATP} \quad \text{PPi + Pi}}$ S-Adenosyl methionine

The examples for transmethylation reactions are:

Methyl acceptor	Methylated product
Guanidinoacetic acid	Creatine
Serine	Choline
Epinephrine	Metanephrine
Norepinephrine	Epinephrine
TRNA	Methylated tRNA

DISORDERS IN METHIONINE METABOLISM (FIG. 10)

Homocystinurias

- These are autosomal recessive disorders of about 1:200,000 child births
- Normal homocysteine level in blood is 5 to 15 µmol/L. This is increased to 50 to 100 times in homocystinurias
- Hyperhomocysteinemia is a risk factor for coronary heart disease. It is seen in smokers, alcoholics, and hypothyroidism
- Other disorders associated with this are neurological disorders, pre-eclampsia of pregnancy, chronic pancreatitis.

Homocystinurias are due to the following conditions:

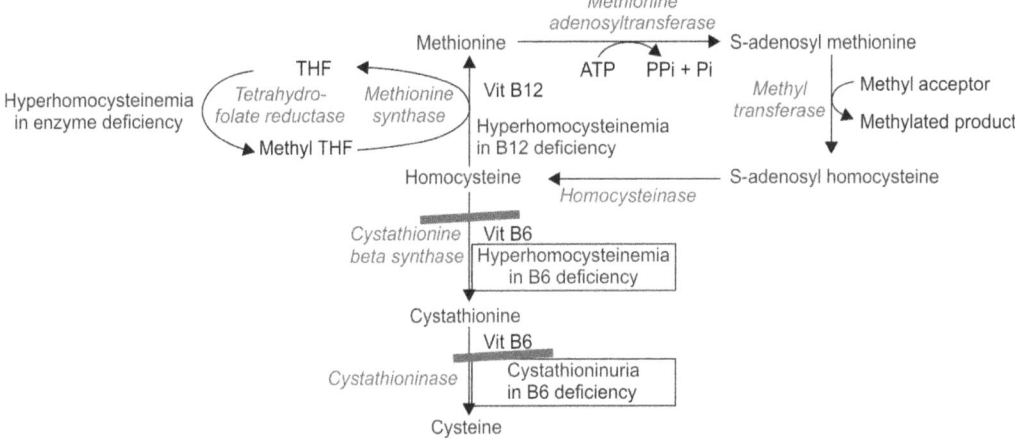

Fig. 10: Disorders in methionine metabolism.

- **Cystathionine beta synthase deficiency**
  - Methionine and homocysteine levels are increased in blood and in urine
  - Marked decrease in plasma cysteine level
  - **Clinical features:** Mental retardation, Charlie Chaplin gait, skeletal deformities and ectopia lentis in eyes are seen
  - Homocysteine activates Hageman's factor causing platelet aggregation leading to intravascular thrombosis
  - Cyanide-nitroprusside test will be positive. Urinary homocysteine levels are elevated
  - Treatment is a diet low in methionine and rich in cysteine.
- **Cobalamine deficiency:** N^5 methyl-THFA homocysteine methyltransferase is dependent on B12. Hyperhomocysteinemia occurs
- **Deficient N^5, N^{10} methylene-THFA reductase**
  - This leads to reduced methionine synthesis with increase in homocysteine level in urine
  - There will be behavioral changes and vascular abnormalities.
- **Acquired hyperhomocysteinemia**
  - Nutritional deficiency of vitamins like cobalamine, folic acid and pyridoxine
  - Metabolic: Chronic renal diseases, hypothyroidism
  - Drug induced: Folate agonists, vitamin B12 antagonists, pyridoxine agonists, estrogen antagonists and nitric oxide antagonist.

Cystathioninuria
- It is due to cystathioninase deficiency
- It is an autosomal recessive disorder
- **Clinical features:** Mental retardation, anemia, thrombocytopenia and endocrinopathies
- In B12 deficiency and in impaired folate metabolism there will be less severe form of cystathioninuria
- Acquired cystathioninuria is seen in pyridoxine deficiency.

5. **What is the normal pH of blood? Discuss the mechanism involved in its regulation.**

Refer 2005 Essay Question 4.

6. **Mention the sources, daily requirement, functions and deficiency symptoms of calcium. Explain how serum level of calcium is regulated.**

Refer 2004 Essay Question 4.

CALCIUM

Calcium is one of the major mineral needed for the body.

Sources

Good source—milk; medium sources—egg, fish, vegetables; cereals—rice, wheat contain small amounts of calcium but they are the good source of calcium in India.

Daily Requirement

- Adult — 500 mg
- Children — 1200 mg
- Pregnancy and lactation — 1500 mg
- Above 50 years — 1500 mg + vitamin D (20 mg)

Functions of Calcium

Activation of Enzymes

- Through calmodulin—calcium binding regulatory protein of molecular weight—17,000 daltons
  - Calcium + calmodulin → calcium bound calmodulin
  - Calcium bound calmodulin activates kinases to phosphorylated enzymes for active biological effects, e.g. adenyl cyclase.
- Activation of enzymes directly by calcium without calmodulin, e.g. pancreatic lipase, enzymes of coagulation pathway, rennin - to clot milk.

Muscle Contraction and Excitation

- Mediated by calcium—calcium channels
- Calcium released from sarcoplasmic reticulum activates ATPase and increases the action of actin and myosin and facilitates excitation-contraction coupling
- Interaction of calcium + troponin C triggers muscle contraction
- Active transport system uses calcium binding protein called calsequestrin
- Calcium decreases neuromuscular irritability.

Nerve Conduction

Transmit nerve impulses from pre-synaptic to postsynaptic region.

Hormone Secretion

Secretion of hormones like insulin, PTH, calcitonin, vasopressin are mediated by calcium.

Second Messenger

- Ca and cyclic AMP are the II messengers in hormone action, e.g. glucagon
- It acts as a II messenger in mechanisms involving G proteins and inositol triphosphate.

Vascular Permeability

Calcium decreases passage of serum through capillaries and so used to reduce allergic exudates.

Myocardium

Calcium prolongs systole and so in hypocalcemia—cardiac arrest occurs in systole.

Bone and Teeth

- Calcium is used in bone and teeth formation; bones act as reservoir of calcium
- Osteoblasts—induce bone deposition and osteoclasts induce bone demineralization.

Maintenance/Regulation of Calcium Level

Normal Blood Level of Calcium

- Total calcium level—9-11 mg/dL
- Three forms of calcium in blood:
  1. Ionized calcium (active form)—5 mg/dL
  2. Protein bound calcium—4 mg/dL
  3. Protein complexed with phosphate, HCO_3^-, citrate—1 mg/dL.

Factors Regulating Calcium Level

- Hormones: A. Vitamin D—calcitriol
             B. Parathyroid hormone (PTH)
             C. Calcitonin—thyroid
- Phosphorus
- Serum proteins
- Alkalosis and acidosis
- Renal threshold
- Ionic product of calcium and phosphorus in children.

Hormonal Regulation

Vitamin D (Calcitriol- 1,25 dihydroxycholecalciferol): The active vitamin D (calcitriol) acts as a steroid hormone. It is synthesized in kidney

- **Effect on intestine:** Calcitriol binds to specific cytoplasmic receptors which interacts with DNA and induces the synthesis of mRNA for specific proteins.

Calbindin which is a calcium binding protein which helps in the absorption of calcium and phosphorus from the intestines
- **Effects on bone:** Calcitriol stimulates the activity of osteoblasts which help in mineralization of bones. They secrete alkaline phosphatase enzyme which in turn increases the ionic concentration of phosphate and calcium
- **Effects on kidney:** Calcitriol increases the reabsorption of calcium and phosphorous from the renal tubules thereby conserving both minerals.

Parathyroid hormone

- Parathyroid hormone (PTH) is secreted by four parathyroid glands present at the posterior aspect of thyroid gland
- Decreased serum calcium level leads to release of PTH from parathyroids. PTH activates the enzyme adenyl cyclase in target cells and increases intracellular calcium concentration
- **PTH and bones**—PTH causes demineralization of bones. It activates pyrophosphatase in osteoclasts leading to bone resorption and decalcification. Calcium is released into the bloodstream and increases blood calcium level. This leads to loss of bone matrix
- **PTH and kidneys**—PTH causes decreased renal excretion of calcium and increased excretion of phosphates and increased reabsorption of calcium leading to increased blood calcium level
- **PTH and intestines**—PTH stimulates increased production of calcitriol which acts on intestine to absorb more calcium leading to increased calcium level in blood.

Calcitonin

- Secreted by parafollicular cells of thyroid gland
- It is a polypeptide of 32–34 amino acids and its secretion is stimulated by serum calcium, gastrin, glucagon and biological amines
- It decreases serum calcium level by inhibiting resorption of bone and decreases the activity of osteoclasts and increases the activity of osteoblasts
- Calcitonin and PTH are antagonistic to each other but both together promote growth and remodeling of bone
- In kidney—calcitonin increases excretion of phosphates in urine like PTH.

Phosphorus

- There is a reciprocal relationship of calcium (Ca) with phosphorus (p)
- Ionic product of Ca x P is kept as a constant
- Normally—(Ca) 10 mg/dL x (P) 4 mg/dL = 40; ionic product is 40.

Serum Proteins

- Total calcium level is decreased in hypoalbuminemia for reduction of each 1 g/dL of albumin there will be reduction of 0.8 mg/dL of calcium
- Ionized calcium level will be normal and so no deficiency manifestations will be present.

Alkalosis and Acidosis

- Alkalosis favors binding of more calcium with proteins by lowering of ionized calcium but the total calcium level is normal. Calcium deficiency is manifested
- Acidosis favors ionization of calcium.

Renal Threshold for Calcium

Renal threshold for calcium is 10 mg/dL and calcium gets excreted at this level

Ionic Product of calcium and phosphorus in children

In children the normal calcium level will be near the upper limit and the ionic product of calcium x P = 50 (adult -40)

Disorders of Calcium Homeostasis

Deficiency manifestations of calcium—hypocalcemia.

Causes of Hypocalcemia

- Deficiency of vitamin D
- Deficiency of parathyroid hormone
- Increased calcitonin—as in medullary carcinoma of thyroid
- Deficiency of calcium
- Deficiency of magnesium

- Increase in phosphorus level—as in renal failure and in renal tubular acidosis
- Hypoalbuminemia.

Symptoms of Hypocalcemia
- Muscle cramps
- Paresthesia in fingers
- Neuromuscular irritability, twitching
- Tetany (Chvostek's sign, Trousseau's sign)
- Seizures
- Bradycardia
- Prolonged QT interval in ECG.

Tetany
- When serum calcium level is less then 8.8 mg/dL is hypocalemia
- Serum calcium level is less than 8.5 mg/dL there will be mild tremors
- Serum calcium level is less than 7.5 mg/dL it leads to tetany
- It may be due to accidental surgical removal of parathyroid gland or by autoimmune disease
- In this condition neuromuscular irritability is increased
- Increased Q-T interval in ECG is seen. Serum calcium is low and there is increase in phosphate level. Calcium and phosphate excretion in urine is decreased
- Clinical signs are Chvostek (tapping over 5th cranial nerve causes facial contraction) and Trousseau's sign.

7. Define biological oxidation. Mention the components and organization of ETC. Describe the mechanism of ATP synthesis. Add a note on uncouplers.

Biological Oxidation

Oxidation which occurs in living systems is known as biological oxidation. It is an endergonic reaction. Heat energy released is converted to chemical energy. Oxidation of a molecule (electron donor) is accompanied by reduction of a second molecule (electron acceptor).

Electron Transport Chain (ETC)
- Located in the inner mitochondrial membrane
- Electrons are transferred from more negative components to more electropositive components.

Components of ETC (Figs. 11 and 12)
- Mutiprotein complexes—complex I, II, III, and IV which are connected by 2 mobile carriers—coenzyme Q and cytochrome C (**Figs. 11 and 12**)
  - Complex I—NADH dehydrogenase complex/NADH coenzyme Q reductase
  - Complex II—Succinate - coenzyme Q reductase
  - Complex III—Coenzyme Q-Cytochrome c reductase
  - Complex IV - Cytochrome oxidase.

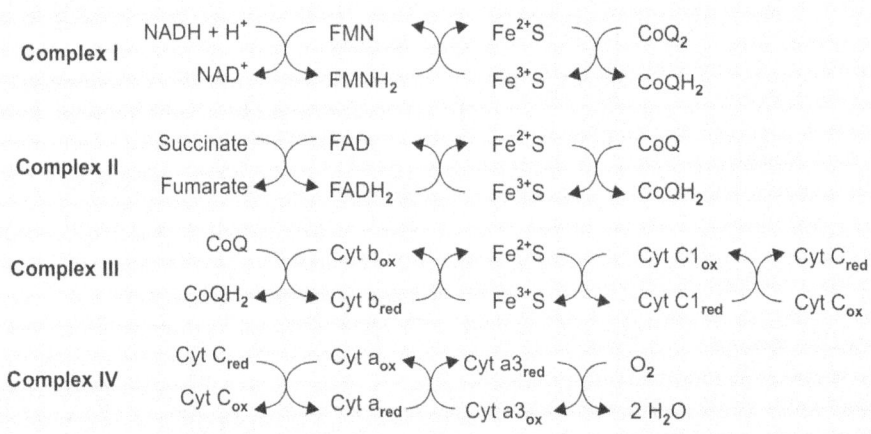

Fig. 11: Complexes of ETC.

- Complexes I, III, and IV are proton pumps
- Complex II is part of the Kreb's cycle and does not pump protons
- Complex IV is the terminus of the electron transfer chain, consuming oxygen and making water.

ETC Complex I: NADH Dehydrogenase Complex/NADH Coenzyme Q Reductase (Proton Pump)

- It contains flavoprotein (Fp) consisting of FMN and iron sulfur (FeS) protein
- NADH donates electrons and FMC accepts it and get reduced to $FMNH_2$
- Electrons are then transferred to FeS and then to coenzyme Q
- Net energy released is 12 kcal/mol which is used to drive 4 protons.

ETC Complex II - Succinate - Coenzyme Q Reductase

Electrons from FADH2 enter ETC at the level of coenzyme Q. No energy is liberated in this complex to act as proton pump. Substrates oxidized by FAD linked enzyme bypass complex-I

Three main enzymes which transfer electrons directly to ubiquinone from FAD group are:
1. Succinate dehydrogenase (TCA cycle)
2. Fatty acyl-CoA dehydrogenase
3. Mitochondrial glycerol phosphate dehydrogenase.

Coenzyme Q (Ubiquinone)

- Coenzyme Q is a quinone derivative with a long isoprenoid tail
- Ubiquinone is reduced to semiquinone and reduced finally to quinol
- It accepts a pair of electrons from NADH or $FADH_2$ through complex I or complex II
- Q cycle facilitates changing from 2 electron carrier ubiquinol to single electron carrier—cytochrome C.

ETC Complex III - Coenzyme Q - Cytochrome C reductase (Proton Pump)

- Contains FeS, and heme containing cytochrome b and cytochrome C1
- Iron in the heme group shuttles between ferric to ferrous forms
- Free energy changes is 10 kcal/mol
- Four protons are pumped out.

Cytochrome C

- It collects electrons from complex III and delivers them to complex IV
- Cytochrome C is a peripheral membrane protein having one heme group.

Complex IV – Cytochrome Oxidase (Proton Pump)

- This complex is tightly bound to mitochondrial membrane
- Contains 2 heme groups—cytochrome-a and a3 and two copper ions. Functional unit is referred to as cytochrome a-a3
- Two protons pumped out to the space in between both mitochondrial membranes
- Four electrons are transferred from cytochrome C and passed on to molecular oxygen
- P:O Ratio: Number of inorganic phosphates incorporated into ATP for every atom of oxygen consumed. Oxidation of NADH generates 2.5 ATP (Old – 3 ATP) and FADH generates 1.5 ATP.

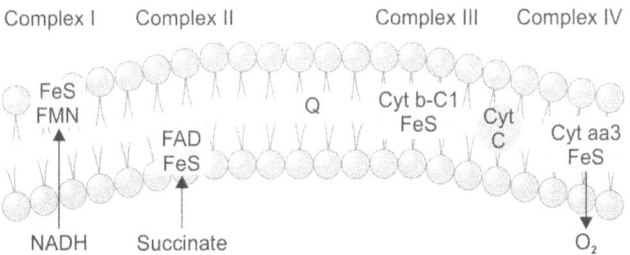

Fig. 12: I, II, III and IV complexes of METC and their reactions.

OXIDATIVE PHOSPHORYLATION-CHEMIOSMOTIC THEORY

- Coupling of oxidation with phosphorylation is known as oxidative phosphorylation. Oxidative phosphorylation is explained by chemiosmotic theory by Peter Mitchell
- The transport of protons from inside to outside of inner mitochondrial membrane is accompanied by the generation of proton gradient across the membrane
- Protons (H^+ ions) accumulate outside the membrane to create an electrochemical potential difference and this force drives the synthesis of ATP by ATP synthase (V) complex. There is also the creation of pH gradient on either side of membrane.

COMPLEX V–ATP SYNTHASE (FIG. 13)

- It is a proton assembly in the inner mitochondrial membrane
- It has 2 functional subunits—F_1 and F_0 and looks like a lollipop. F_0 is embedded in the membrane and water insoluble. Both F_0 and F_1 are connected by a protein stalk. Protons enter through F_0 subunit and it acts as a proton channel. F_1 unit projects into the matrix and catalyses ATP synthesis
- As per Boyer's hypothesis, there will be a conformational change in the mitochondrial membrane proteins which leads to ATP synthesis. This is considered as rotary motor or energy driving model or binding-change model
- ATP synthase enzyme has a central gamma unit surrounded by alternating $\alpha 3$ and $\beta 3$ subunits. Due to the proton flux γ subunit rotates and that induces conformational changes in the $\beta 3$ subunits which releases ATP. One β subunit has open (O) conformation, the second has loose (L) conformation and the third has tight (T) conformation
- Protons induce the rotation of γ subunit which in turn induces conformation changes in β subunits. ADP and Pi bind to β subunits in L conformation to form ATP by changing O site to L conformation and then T to O conformation and 3 ATPs are generated for each revolution. So ATP synthase is considered as world's smallest molecular motor.

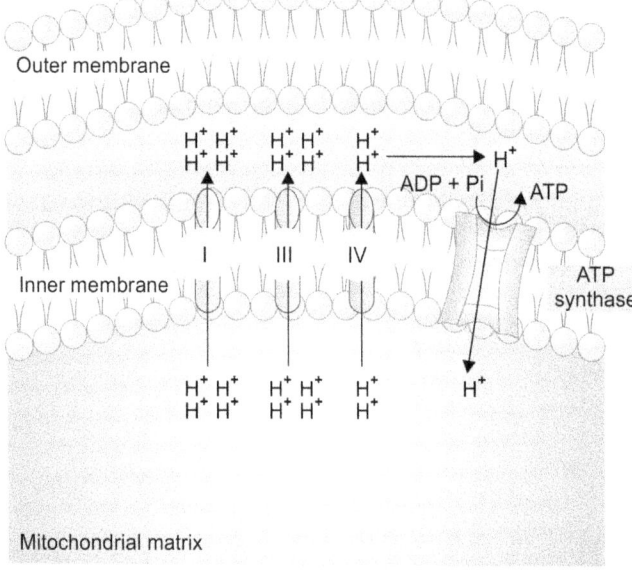

Fig. 13: Complexes of ETC and synthesis of ATP (complex V).

Regulation of ATP Synthesis

- Availability of ADP—respiratory or acceptor control
- Source of NADH and FADH$_2$ from TCA cycle
  - **Inhibitors of oxidative phosphorylation**
    - Atractyloside—inhibits translocase
    - Oligomycin—inhibits flow of protons through F$_O$
    - Ionophores, e.g. valinomycin mobile ion carriers—allows potassium (K) to permeate mitochondria; gramicidin—channel former.
  - **Uncouplers of oxidative phosphorylation**
    - 2, 4-Dinitrophenol (2, 4-DNP)
    - 2, 4-Dinitrocresol (2, 4-DNC)
    - Chlorocarbonyl cyanide phenylhydrazone (CCCP).
  - **Physiological Uncouplers**
    - Thyroxine
    - Thermogenin in brown adipose tissue.

8. **Describe the chemistry, sources, RDA, and functions of thiamine. Add a note on beriberi.**

Refer 2003 Essay Question 1.

9. **Describe the mechanism of DNA replication. Add a note on DNA repair mechanism.**

DNA REPLICATION

- During cell division each daughter cell receives an exact copy of genetic information of the mother cell. The synthesis of DNA or duplication is called replication
- In daughter DNA, one strand is derived from mother and the other is newly synthesized. This is called semiconservative method of replication.

Requirements

- Four deoxyribonucleotides—A, G, C and T
- Template strand—separated single strand from double helical DNA.

Enzymes

- DNA dependent DNA polymerase—different in bacteria and mammals
  - Bacterial (prokaryotic) DNA polymerase
    - DNAP-I (Pol I) (Kornberg enzyme)—repair enzyme
    - DNAP-II (Pol II)—proofreading and repair
    - DNAP-III (Pol III)—synthesizing leading and lagging strands.
  - Mammalian (Eukaryotic) DNA Polymerase-5 types—α, β, γ, δ and ε. Alpha—gap filling, Beta—DNA repair, Gamma—mitochondrial DNA synthesis, Delta—synthesis of leading and lagging strand and Epsilon—proof-reading and DNA repair.
- Primase
- DNA topoisomerase—Type I and II
- Helicase
- DNA gyrase—Type II topoisomerase.

Steps of Replication: 3 Steps—Initiation, Elongation and Termination (Fig. 14)

Each strand serves as template for new complementary strand synthesis. The base pairing rule is always followed.

Initiation

- At the **origin of replication (ORI)**, there is an association of sequence-specific (double-stranded DNA) dsDNA-binding proteins with a series of direct repeat DNA sequences. This leads to the local denaturation and unwinding of an adjacent A + T rich region of DNA
- **Unwinding of DNA**: The interaction of proteins with ORI defines the start site of replication and provides a short region of (single-stranded DNA) ssDNA essential for initiation of synthesis of the nascent DNA strand. A critical step is provided by a DNA helicase that allows for unwinding of DNA. Single-stranded DNA-binding proteins (SSB) stabilize this complex
- **Formation of replication fork**: A replication fork consists of:

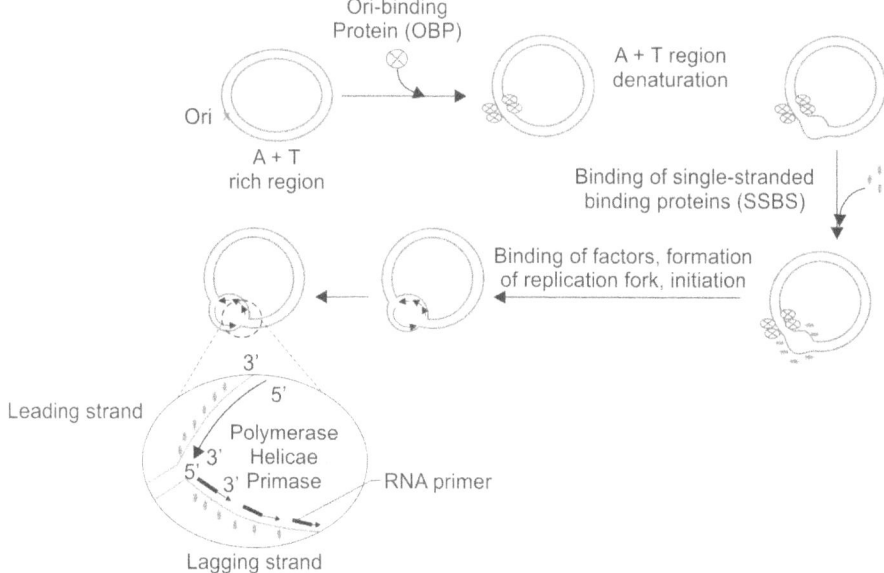

Fig. 14: Steps of DNA replication.

1. DNA helicase which unwinds a short segment of parental duplex DNA
2. A DNA dependent RNA primase which synthesises RNA primer—a short length of RNA molecule of 10–200 nucleotides. This priming process involves the nucleophilic attack by the 3'-hydroxyl group of the RNA primer on the α–phosphate of the first entering deoxynucleoside triphosphate with the splitting off of pyrophosphate. The 3'-hydroxyl group of the recently attached deoxyribonucleoside monophosphate is then free to carry out a nucleophilic attack on the next entering deoxyribonucleoside triphosphate again at its α-phosphate moiety with the splitting off of pyrophosphate.

Elongation

The polymerase III holoenzyme binds to template DNA and synthesizes DNA in the 5' to 3' direction because the DNA strands are antiparallel, the polymerase functions asymmetrically. On the leading (forward) strand, the DNA is synthesized continuously. On the lagging (retrograde) strand, the DNA

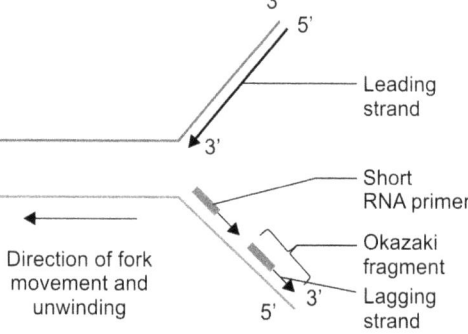

Fig. 15: Okasaki fragments.

is synthesized in short (1–5 kb) fragments, the so-called **Okazaki fragments (Fig. 15)**

Gap filling: In mammals, after many Okazaki fragments are generated, the replication complex begins to remove the RNA primers to fill in the gaps by their removal with the proper base paired deoxynucleotide, and then to seal the fragments of newly synthesized DNA by enzymes referred to as **DNA ligases.**

Termination

- Termination of replication is done by termination sequence-ter. A specific binding protein ter-binding protein binds

these sequences and prevents helicase from further unwinding of DNA and facilitated termination of replication
- **Proofreading:** Done by Pol I and Pol II to remove erroneous nucleotides.

Inhibitors of Replication

- Topoisomerase II DNA gyrase—inhibited by antibacterial drugs like novobiocin, nalidixic acid and ciprofloxacin (used for treating urinary tract infection)
- Topoisomerase I—inhibited by antitumor drug—camptothecin in humans

Elongation of DNA chain by incorporating nucleotide analogues such as cytarabine, ara-C, 2,3-dideoxyinosine.

DNA REPAIR

- The process of replication occurs with high fidelity. Proofreading is done after replication to correct mistakes in arrangement of bases and base pairs
- Inspite of all these things alterations in base arrangements may occur due to various physical and chemical agents causing damage in DNA which can be corrected by the following mechanisms:
    - Mismatch repair
    - Base excision repair
    - Nucleotide excision repair (NER)
    - Double strand break.

Mismatch Repair (Fig. 16)

- This may occur due to copying error
- During replication one to few bases may be unpaired in a DNA strand causing mismatch
- Mut proteins identify the mismatched nucleotides based on the degree of methylation
- GATC sequences which are present 1/1,000 nucleotides approximately are methylated on the adenine residue on the parent strand (not on the newly synthesized strand)
- GATC endonuclease cuts the strand bearing the mismatch and the mismatched

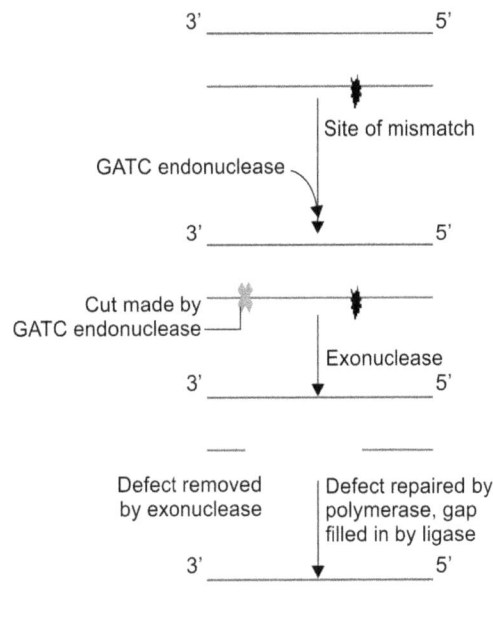

Fig. 16: Mismatch repair.

nucleotide(s) is/are removed by an exonuclease
- The gap left is then filled in by DNA polymerase enzyme and the ends are joined to the 5'phosphate of the remaining original strand by DNA ligase enzyme.

Base Excision Repair (Fig. 17)

- **Depurination of DNA** which happens spontaneously owing to the thermal lability of the purine N-glycosidic bond occurs at a rate of 5,000–10,000/cell/day at 37°C causing base alterations. Spontaneous deamination of cytosine to uracil may occur or by alkylating or deaminating compounds which will be repaired by this process
- **Specific glycosylases** can recognize these abnormal bases and remove the base from the deoxyribose phosphate backbone of DNA. This will produce an apyrimidinic or apurinic site as per the base is removed
- **Specific endonucleases** do the excision and a lyase enzyme removes it. The gap is then filled in by DNA polymerase and ligase enzymes.

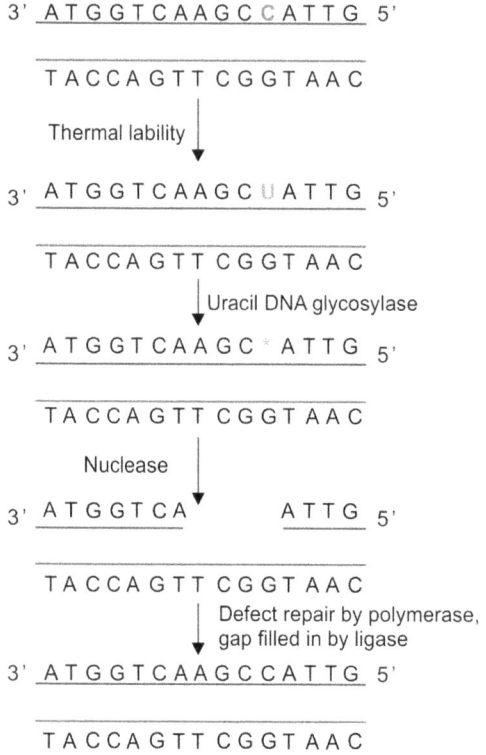

Fig. 17: Base excision repair.

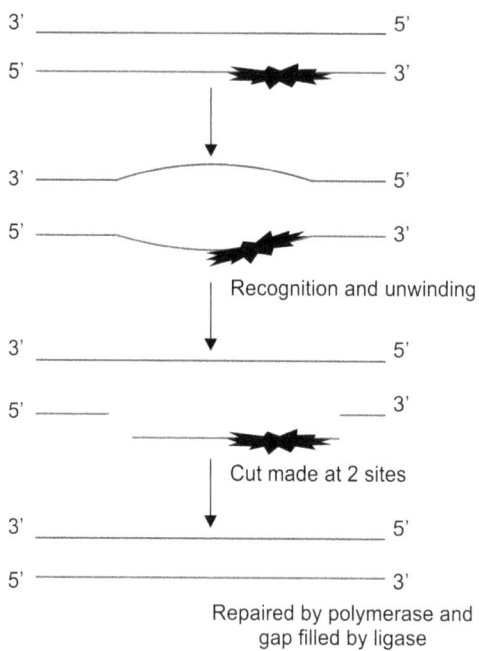

Fig. 18: Nucleotide excision repair.

Nucleotide Excision Repair (For Thymine-Thymine Dimer) (Fig. 18)

- This mechanism is used to repair and replace regions of damaged DNA up to 30 bases in length due to damage by ultraviolet (UV) light causing joining of adjacent pyrimidines usually thymines producing dimers
- A special UV-specific endonuclease (UvrABC excinuclease) recognizes the dimer and cleaves the damaged strand on either side of the dimer releasing a short oligonucleotide leaving a gap
- This gap is then filled by normal cellular enzymes like DNA polymerase and ligase.

Double-strand (ds) DNA Break Repair (Fig. 19)

- Double-strands breaks can occur in DNA as a result of ionizing radiation or oxidative free radical generation. Some chemotherapeutic agents can destroy cells by causing ds breaks or preventing their repair

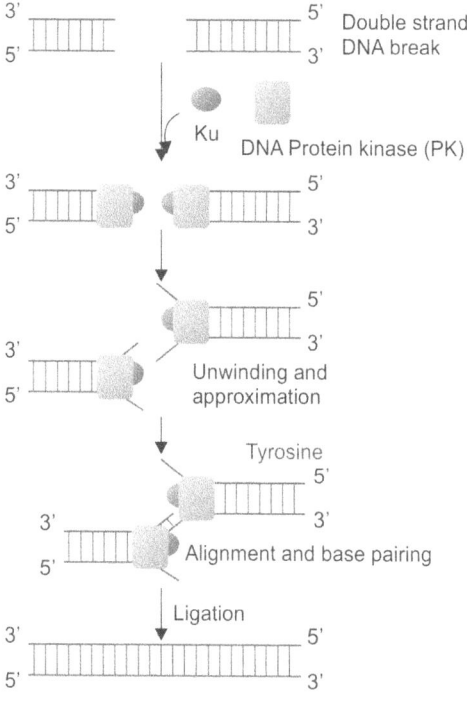

Fig. 19: dsDNA break repair.

- DNA protein kinase (PK) has one binding site for the free ends of the DNA and another for dsDNA just inside these ends. Therefore allows for the approximation of these two separated ends
- The unwound approximated DNA forms base pairs
- The extra nucleotide tails are removed by an exonuclease; and the gaps are filled and closed by DNA ligase.

Biomedical Importance

Xeroderma Pigmentosum (XP)
- It is an autosomal recessive condition in which there is defect in nucleotide excision repair mechanism
- Pyrimidine dimers are formed in the skin cells which are exposed to UV light. The patient becomes highly sensitive to UV rays. Sunlight causes blisters in the skin
- Because of the defective repair system, the cells cannot repair the damaged DNA resulting in skin cancer. Death occurs in second decade due to skin cancer
- This is also caused by defects in the genes coding for any of the XP proteins required for the repair.

Ataxia Telengiectasia
- Autosomal recessive disease due to mutated *ATM* gene
- It is associated with DNA repair mechanisms
- Caused due to UV sensitivity
- Associated with cerebellar ataxia, telengiectasia in eyes, lymphoreticular neoplasms. It is present in 1:40,000 persons.

Other diseases of defective DNA repair are: Fanconi's anemia, Bloom's syndrome, Lynch syndrome, Cockayne syndrome and hereditary polyposis, colon cancer.

---

10. Name the branched chain amino acids. Describe the pathway for the metabolism of branched chain amino acids. Add a note on maple syrup urine disease.

- Branched-chain amino acids are valine, leucine and isoleucine
- Valine is glucogenic, leucine is ketogenic and isoleucine is both ketogenic and glucogenic. All three are essential amino acids
- During starvation these amino acids act as fuel for the brain.

METABOLISM OF BRANCHED CHAIN AMINO ACIDS (FIG. 20)

First 3 steps are same for all 3 amino acids.

Step 1: Transamination—all three are transaminated to corresponding keto acids using PLP.

Step 2: Oxidative decarboxylation of keto acids with the help of CoA, NAD, FAD, TPP and Lipoic acid by alpha-ketoacid dehydrogenase to form isovaleryl-CoA, isobutryl-CoA, methylbutyryl-CoA from leucine, valine and isoleucine.

Step 3: Dehydrogenation by FAD-dependent dehydrogenation results in methylcrotonyl-CoA, methylacrylyl-CoA and tiglyl-CoA from leucine, valine and isoleucine, respectively.

Step 4: Individual reactions

Valine
- Methylacrylyl-CoA with the removal of one molecule of water and CoA to form beta hydroxyisobutyrate
- Formation of methylmalonyl-CoA by NAD dependent dehydrogenation
- Methylmalonyl-CoA is converted to succinyl-CoA by adenosyl B12.

Leucine
- Beta methylcrotonyl-CoA forms beta-methylglutaconyl-CoA by carboxylation in the presence of biotin.
- Hydrolysis of beta methylglutaconyl-CoA produces HMG CoA—beta hydroxy, beta methylglutaryl-CoA.
- This is acted by a lyase enzyme to form acetoacetate and acetyl-CoA.

Isoleucine
- Formation of alpha methyl-beta hydroxy butyryl-CoA by addition of water to Tigyl-CoA

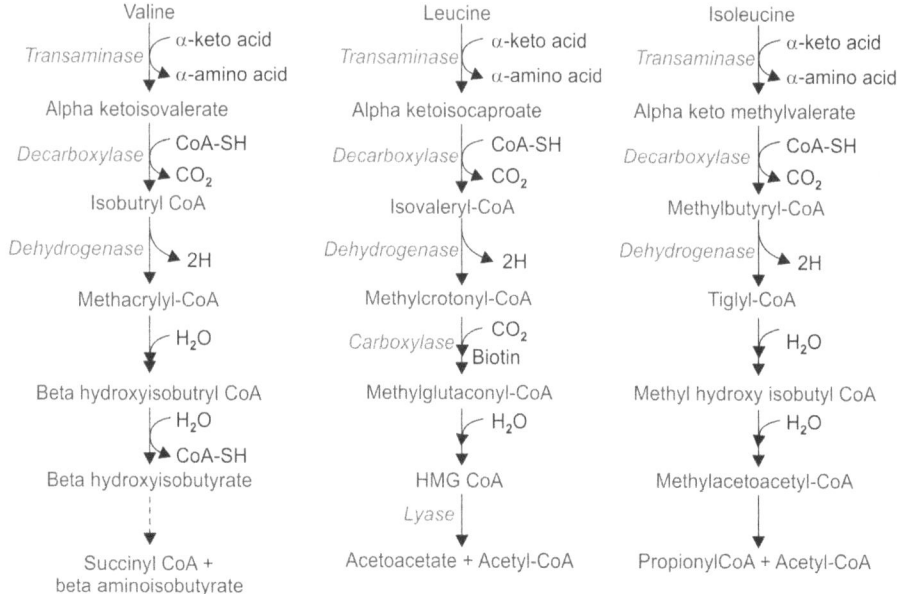

Fig. 20: Metabolism of branched-chain amino acids.

- NAD dependent dehydrogenation forms alpha-methylacetoacetyl-CoA
- Cleavage of methylacetoacetyl-CoA forms acetyl-CoA to enter ketogenic pathway and propionyl-CoA to enter glucogenic pathway.

Maple Syrup Urine Disease (MSUD) (Fig. 21)

Refer 2009 Short Notes 31
- This is also known as branched-chain ketonuria
- This is due to the deficiency of the enzyme branched-chain ketoacid dehydrogenase the second enzyme in the catabolism of branched-chain amino acids, such as valine, leucine and isoleucine. It is a complex of decarboxylase, transacylase and dihydrolipoyl dehydrogenase
- The incidence is 1:100,000
- **Clinical features:** Symptoms start from the first week of birth. It is characterized by mental retardation, convulsions, vomiting, acidosis, coma and death within first year of life
- The urine smells like burnt sugar or maple syrup. Urine contains branched-chain keto, such as acids, valine, leucine or isoleucine
- Rothera's test—positive.

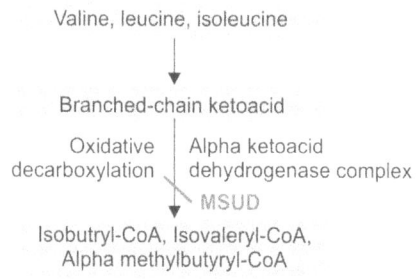

Fig. 21: Maple syrup urine disease.

Diet deficient in branched chain-amino acids should be given. Thiamine is helpful in some patients. Liver transplantation can be done.

II. SHORT NOTES

1. Phospholipids.

Refer 2004 Short Notes 1.

2. Congenital hyperbilirubinemias.
- Bilirubin is the end product of catabolism of heme. Normal value of total bilirubin is 0.2 to 0.8 mg/dL; unconjugated bilirubin is 0.2 to 0.6 mg/dL and conjugated bilirubin is 0 to 0.2 mg/dL

- If the bilirubin level is elevated it is known as **hyperbilirubinemia.** Depending upon the type of bilirubin raised it is grouped as conjugated or unconjugated hyperbilirubinemia
- **Hyperbilirubinemia** may be:
  - **Congenital** due to inherited defects—enzyme deficiency
  - **Acquired** due to hemolysis or hepatic diseases.

Congenital Hyperbilirubinemia

It results from abnormal uptake, conjugation or excretion of bilirubin due to inherited defects.

Congenital Unconjugated Hyperbilirubinemia

- **Crigler-Najjar syndrome Type I**
  - **Deficiency:** UDP Glucuronyl-transferase
  - **Characteristic feature:** Defect in the conjugation of bilirubin. Jaundice appears within first 24 hours of birth. Kernicterus occurs due to increased unconjugated bilirubin (more than 20 mg/dL) and early death will occur.
- **Crigler-Najjar syndrome Type II—milder form**
  - Enzyme deficiency is partial and survival rate is prolonged
  - Bilirubin level does not exceed 20 mg/dL.
- **Gilbert's syndrome**
  - Autosomal dominant trait
  - **Defect:** In the uptake of bilirubin by the liver. Bilirubin level is around 3 mg/dL
  - Patient is asymptomatic, except for the presence of mild jaundice.

Congenital Conjugated Hyperbilirubinemia

- **Dubin Johnson syndrome**—autosomal recessive trait
- **Defect:** Defective ATP dependent anion transport in bile canaliculi due to mutation in MRP2 protein which is responsible for the transport of conjugated bilirubin
- Defective excretion of conjugated bilirubin and so its level increased in blood
- Bilirubin gets deposited in the liver and the liver appears black—black liver jaundice
- **Rotor Syndrome**
  - It is inherited autosomal recessive. The exact cause is not identified
  - Bilirubin excretion is defective, but there is no deposit in the liver.

3. **Formation of ketone bodies and their significance.**

Refer 2005 Essay Questions 2 and 2005 Short Notes 14.

4. **Basal metabolic rate.**

Refer 2005 Short Notes 26.

5. **HMP shunt pathway.**

- **HMP**- Hexose monophosphate shunt is an alternate pathway for oxidation of glucose
- **Other name**: Pentose phosphate pathway Warburg-Dickens-Horecker pathway, phospogluconate oxidative pathway
- **Occurrence**: Liver, adipose tissue, RBC, mammary glands, testes, adrenal gland.

Steps of HMP Pathway (Reactions)

There are two phases **(Fig. 22)**
1. Phase I oxidative phase (irreversible phase)
2. Phase II nonoxidative phase (reversible phase).

Oxidative Phase

Rate-limiting step—catalyzed by glucose-6-phosphate dehydrogenase enzyme which is NADP dependent. One NADPH is produced

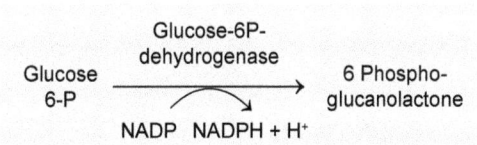

- Hydrolysis of 6-phosphoglucanolactone to 6-phosphogluconate by hydrolase enzymes
- Oxidation and decarboxylation of 6-phosphogluconate to form ribulose-5-phosphate by phosphogluconate dehydrogenase.

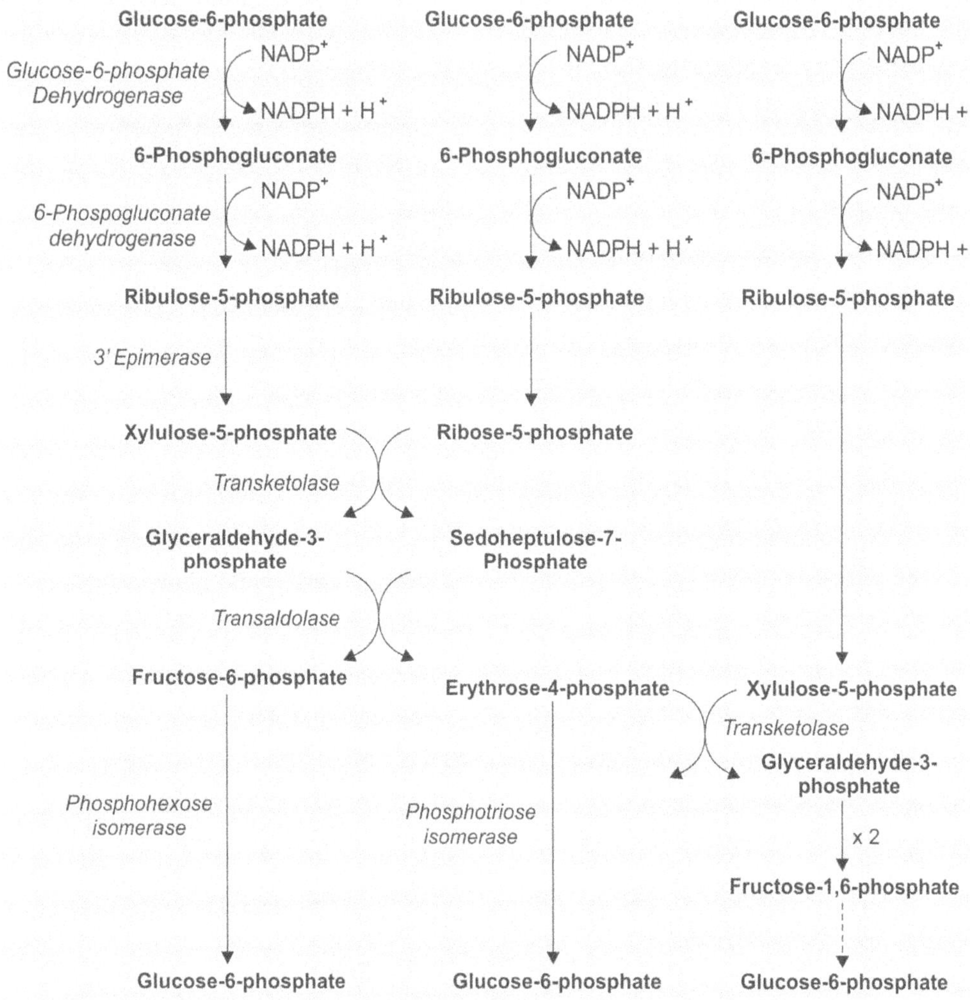

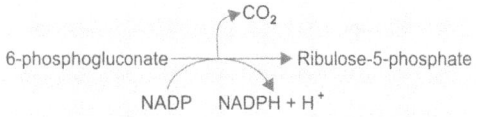

Fig. 22: HMP shunt.

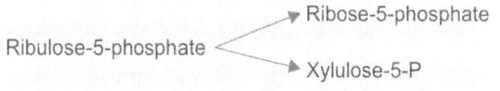

Nonoxidative Phase
- Isomerization—Ribulose-5-phosphate is isomerized to ribose-5-phosphate by keto-isomerase or epimerised to xylulose-5P by epimerase

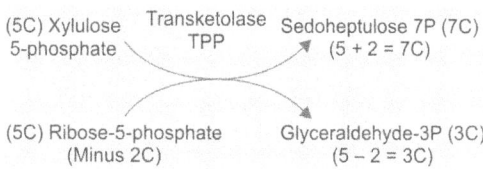

- **Transketolase reaction:** TPP dependent reaction

  (5C) Xylulose 5-phosphate → Transketolase TPP → Sedoheptulose 7P (7C) (5 + 2 = 7C)

  (5C) Ribose-5-phosphate (Minus 2C) → Glyceraldehyde-3P (3C) (5 – 2 = 3C)

  7C—ketose sedoheptulose and 3C—aldose glyceraldehyde-3-P are generated
- **Transaldolase reaction:**
  3C-from sedoheptulose 7P-are removed and joined with glyceraldehyde 3-phosphate to form 6C ketose fructose 6-phosphate

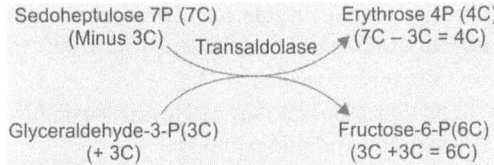

- Second transketolase reaction—TPP dependent

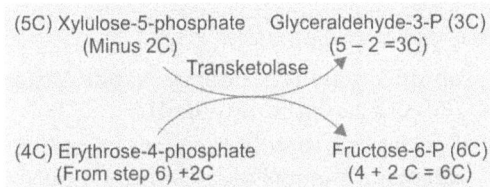

- Regeneration of glucose-6-phosphate: Two molecules of glyceraldehyde-3-phosphate from above point are condensed to form fructose 6-phosphate (3 × 2 = 6C). This is then converted to glucose-6-p by reversal of glycolysis by fructose 1-6-bisphosphatase.

Significance of HMP Shunt

- Production of NADPH which serves as hydrogen and electron donor in reductive biosynthesis of fatty acids, cholesterol and bile acids
- Production of 5 carbon sugars—ribose which is a component of DNA, RNA, ATP, NAD, FAD.

Regulation of HMP Shunt

- Rate-limiting enzyme—glucose 6-phosphate dehydrogenase is regulated by NADPH by competitive inhibition. Oxidative phase is controlled by NADPH.
- Insulin induces G6PD enzyme and increase the overall pathway
- Nonoxidative phase is controlled by the requirement of pentoses.

Significance of HMP Pathway

Biochemical Significance (Oxidative Phase)

- Biosynthesis of pentoses—ribose-5-phosphate for the synthesis of nucleotides and nucleic acids
- Provides way for interconversion of pentoses and hexoses (both phases)

- Generation of NADPH reducing equivalents for:
  - Reductive synthesis of fatty acids, bile acids, cholesterol
  - NADPH is needed for the integrity of RBC membrane
  - Antioxidant—free radical scavenger
  - Helps to prevent metHb
  - Detoxifies drugs by liver microsomes P450 enzymes.

Clinical Significance

Glucose-6-phosphate dehydrogenase deficiency
- X-linked recessive trait
- Cells having the deficient enzyme have lower rate of NADPH production and deficiency of reduced glutathione leading to hemolysis
- This deficiency is manifested only when exposed to certain drugs such as primaquine (antimalarial)
- Fava beans consumption and sulfa drugs also precipitate hemolysis
- Methemoglobinemia will be seen in circulation in glucose-6-phosphate deficiency. There is no cyanosis
- Transketolase activity of RBC is used to measure the deficiency level of thiamine
- Genetic defect in transketolase enzyme will lead to Wernick-Korsakoff syndrome (encephalopathy) seen in alcoholics.

Disorder: Glucose-6-phosphate Dehydrogenase Deficiency

- It is the most common inborn error of metabolism. It is X-linked recessive trait
- This will lead to drug induced hemolytic anemia
- The deficiency is manifested only when exposed to certain oxidant drugs or toxins like primaquine for malaria or ingestion of toxic glycosides in Fava beans
- Sulfa drugs may also precipitate hemolysis
- This disease offers resistance to plasmodium infection and protects the individual from malaria since the parasite requires reduced glutathione which is not available in the G6PD deficiency.

6. Oxidative phosphorylation.
Refer 2006 Short Notes 5.

7. Oncogenes.
Refer 2005 Short Notes 20.

8. Electrophoresis.
Refer 2006 Short Notes 30.

9. Genetic code.
Refer 2005 Short Notes 19.

10. Insulin.
Refer 2006 Short Notes 20.

11. Gout.
Refer 2005 Short Notes 17.

12. Detoxification.
Refer 2005 Short Notes 16.

13. Polyunsaturated fatty acid.
- Polyunsaturated fatty acid (PUFA) are having more than one double bond. They exhibit cis configuration.
- The important PUFA are:
  - Linoleic acid
  - Linolenic acid
  - Arachidonic acid

They are present in vegetable oils and fish oils.

Significance of PUFA

- Used for esterification and excretion of cholesterol
- They are **essential fatty acids**.
- It increases the fluidity of membranes
- Eicosanoids (prostaglandins, prostacycline and thromboxanes) are derived from arachidonic acid
- Antiatherogenic.

PUFA	Carbon atom	Double Bond	Family
Linoleic acid	18	2	Omega 3
Linolenic acid	18	3	Omega 6
Arachidonic acid	20	4	Omega 6

14. Balanced diet.

Definition—it is defined as the diet which contains all the necessary food materials like carbohydrates, proteins, and lipids along with vitamins, minerals in adequate proportions to meet the body's need.

- The diet should be simple, locally available, palatable and digestible
- Adequate protein content with essential amino acids should be supplied. This is achieved by cereal, pulses, mixture with additional animal proteins
- Calorie intake should be correct and should balance energy expenditure (30-35 k cal/kg body weight)
- Special care should be taken to see that adequate quantity of calcium and iron are obtained from the diet
- Should provide adequate roughage
- Cereals, pulses ratio is maintained at 5:1
- Daily requirement of protein is 60 g, fat—45 g, calories—2000 kcal, calcium—400 mg, iron—25 mg
- Diet is divided into 3 meals per day, breakfast, lunch, supper
- **Balanced diet should contain calories from carbohydrates, protein and fat in the ratio 60:20:20.**

15. Glycosylated hemoglobin.

- The best index of long-term control of blood glucose level is measurement of glycated hemoglobin or glycosylated Hb (HbA1c)
- When there is excess glucose in blood, it goes and binds with proteins especially Hb
- When once attached, glucose is not removed from Hb. Therefore, it remains inside the RBC throughout the lifespan of RBC (120 days).

Interpretation

- It is used for monitoring the response to treatment
- Normal level: 4-7%
- Diabetes: 8-15%
- HbA1c level reveals the mean glucose level over previous 10-12 weeks
- It is not affected by recent food intake or recent changes in sugar level

- Elevated HbA1c indicates poor control of diabetes
- The risk of retinopathy and nephropathy are directly proportional to elevated HbA1c level.

16. Chondroitin sulfate (Fig. 23).

- It is one of the glycosaminoglycans/mucopolysaccharides/heteropolysaccharides
- It consists of repeating units of L-iduronic acid and N-acetylgalactosamine
- It is an important structural component of cartilage and it is also present in bone, tendons, cornea and skin
- Usually it is attached to proteins as part of proteoglycans.

Uses

- It provides an endoskeletal structure to maintain the structure and shape of the tissues like cartilage
  - **Therapeutic Uses:** It is used to treat osteoarthritis as anti-inflammatory agent, stimulating the synthesis of proteoglycans.

17. Synthesis and utilization of ketone bodies.

Refer 2005 Essay Question 2.

18. Rapoport-Luebering cycle (glycolysis in RBC), (2,3-bisphosphoglycerate cycle/ 2,3 BPG shunt) (Fig. 24).

- Glycolysis in RBC is explained as Rapoport-Luebering cycle or 2,3-BPG cycle
- Other name: Bisphosphoglycerate shunt (BPG shunt)
- Mature RBCs do not contain mitochondria and they depend on glycolysis for ATP
- In RBC, reaction catalyzed by 1, 3 bisphosphoglycerate kinase is bypassed
- In turn, bisphosphoglycerate mutase converts 1,3-BPG to 2,3-BPG and then converted to 3 phosphoglycerate by phosphatase enzyme **(Fig. 24)**.

Significance

- No release of energy/ATP
- 2,3-BPG combines with Hb and reduces the affinity towards oxygen. So, in the presence of 2,3-BPG OXYHb will unload more O_2 so that the tissues get more O_2. There is shift of oxygen dissociation curve to the right
- In hypoxia and in high altitude 2,3-BPG level increases in RBCs and favors the release of oxygen to tissues even when pCO_2 is low
- 2,3-BPG level is increased in fetal circulation.

19. Folate trap (Fig. 25).

- B12 coenzyme methylcobalamin acts as the coenzyme in the conversion of homocysteine to methionine
- Folic acid also plays important role in it. In the folic acid metabolism H4F is reversibily converted to N5, N10-methylenetetrahydrofolate by serine hydroxy methyltransferase enzyme which is then irreversibly reduced to N5 methyltetrahydrofolate
- This methyltetrahydrofolate donates its methyl group to cobalamin which is converted to methylcobalamin
- This methyl B12 then supplies the methyl group to homocysteine to form methionine

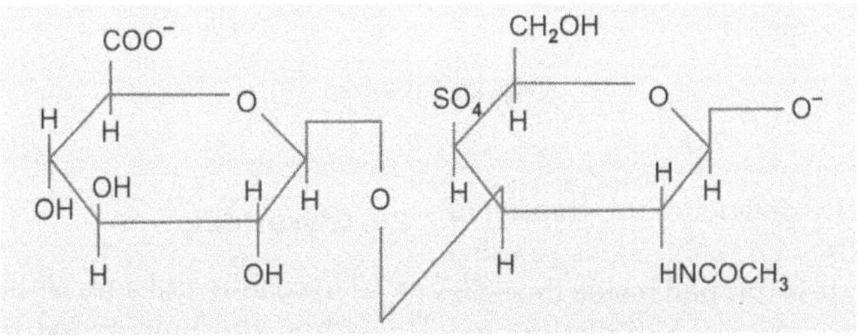

Fig. 23: Chondroitin sulfate.

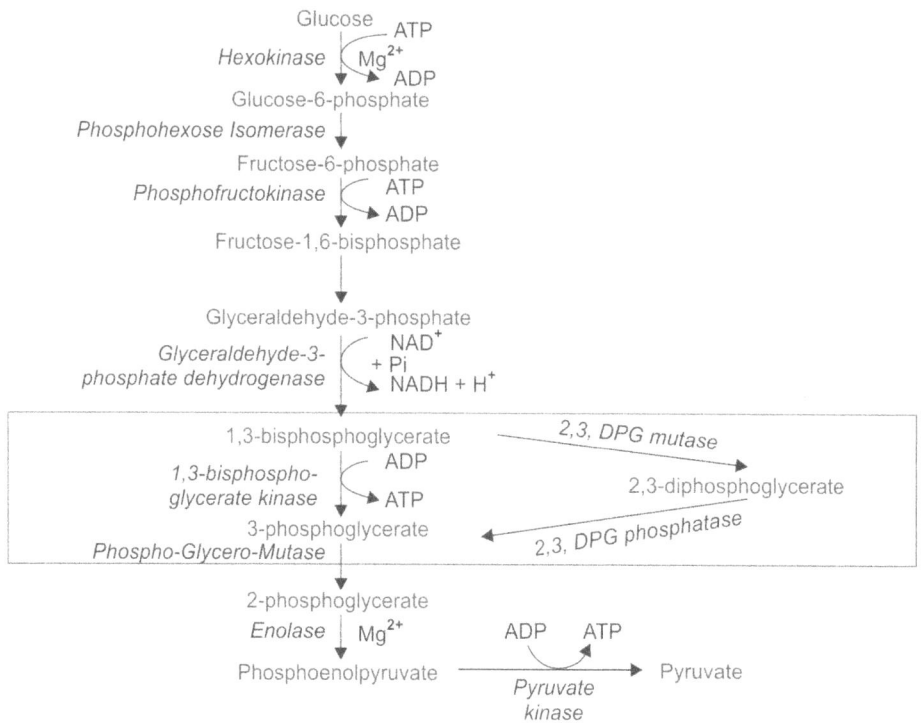

Fig. 24: 2,3 BPG Shunt.

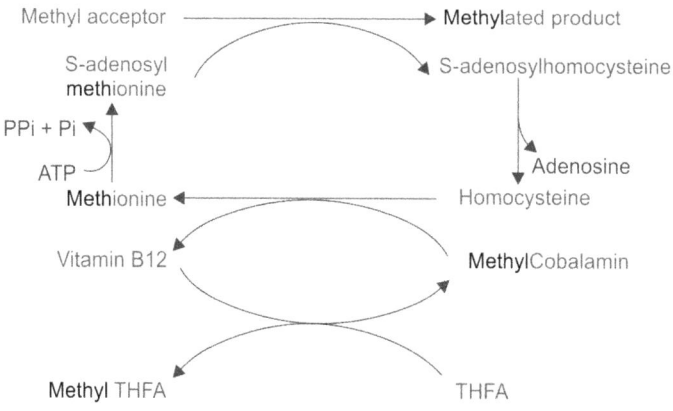

Fig. 25: Folate trap.

- In the case of B12 deficiency this transfer of methyl group is not possible and so methyl tetrahydrofolate is trapped inside the cells and there is no formation of methionine from homocysteine, this is called **folate trap.**

20. Glycosides.

- Glycosidic linkages or bonds are formed when the hemiacetal or hemiketal OH group of anomeric carbon (C-1) reacts with a hydroxyl group of another carbohydrate

or noncarbohydrate (like methyl alcohol or glycerol or phenol)
- Noncarbohydrate units are called aglycones. The bonds may be O-glycosidic if they form disaccharides, oligosaccharides or polysaccharides
- The bonds may be N-glycosidic which are found in nucleotides, e.g. ATP
- The resulting compounds are called glycosides. If the sugar is glucose the compound is called glucosides
- Glycosides do not reduce Benedict's reagent as there is no free aldehyde or keto group but they may be hydrolysed with boiling with dilute acids to release free sugar to reduce Benedict's reagent.

Glycosides of Medical Importance (All are of Plant Origin)

- Antibiotics like streptomycin is a glycoside
- Cardiac glycosides like ouabain and digoxin which increase the heart muscle contraction and used in the treatment of congestive heart failure. They inhibit Na^+/K^+ ATPase system
- Anticancer drugs such as daunorubicin and doxirubicin are anthracycline glycosides.

21. Apolipoproteins and their significance.

- The protein part of lipoprotein is called apolipoprotein
- Apolipoproteins are synthesized in liver
- ApoA is from intestinal cells.

Types: ApoA1, ApoB48, ApoB100, ApoC, ApoE

ApoA1
- It activates lecithin-cholesterol acyltransferase (LCAT) enzyme
- It is a ligand for HDL
- It is antiatherogenic.

ApoB48
- It is present in chylomicrons
- Synthesized in the intestinal cells
- ApoB100 and ApoB48 are the products of the same gene, but in the intestine, the mRNA undergoes editing, so as to produce the B48. B48 is so named because it is only 48% of the size of B100.

ApoB100
- It is present in LDL
- It binds to LDL receptors
- Biggest protein
- Synthesized in the liver.

ApoCII
- It activates lipoprotein lipase.

ApoE
- It is rich in arginine
- It is present in chylomicrons, LDL, VLDL
- ApoE is present in astrocytes also which is involved in cellular transport of lipids in CNS
- Implicated in the development of senile dementia and Alzheimer's disease.

Apoproteins	Blood level mg/dL	Site of production	Component of	Functions
ApoAI	150	Intestine, liver	HDL2	Activation of LCAT
ApoAII		Intestine, liver	HDL	Inhibits LCAT; Stimulates lipase
ApoB48	-	Intestines	Chylomicrons (Chylo)	48% of B100
ApoB100	100	Liver	LDL, VLDL	Binds LDL receptor
ApoE	2	Liver Rich in arginine	LDL, VLDL, chylomicron	Ligand for hepatic uptake
ApoCI	10	Liver	Chylo, VLDL	Activates LCAT Antiatherogenic
ApoCII	5	Liver	Chylo, VLDL	Clearance of TG
ApoCIII	10	Liver	Chylo, VLDL	Antiatherogenic
ApoLp(a)		Liver	Lp(a)	Attached to B100 Highly atherogenic

22. Renal glycosuria.

- Normal renal threshold for glucose is 175-180 mg/dL
- If blood glucose level rises above this level, glucose starts appearing in urine
- When renal threshold is lowered, glucose is excreted in urine. This is known as renal glycosuria
- **Physiological cause**—pregnancy
- **Pathological cause**—renal tubular transport, e.g. Fanconi syndrome along with glucosuria there will be amino aciduria and phosphaturia.

23. Recombinant DNA technology.

When a gene of one species is transferred to another gene of different species, it is called recombinant DNA technology or genetic engineering. Usually there will be combination of human DNA and bacterial DNA. The DNA thus formed is called as recombinant DNA or chimeric DNA or hybrid DNA.

Preparation of Specific Human Gene

The mRNA of the desired gene is extracted and by using reverse transcriptase enzyme complementary copy of that mRNA called complementary DNA (cDNA) is produced.

Preparation of Chimeric DNA Molecules

Vectors are hosts like bacteria in which the desired gene is inserted into their genome. Restriction endonuclease is the enzyme which cuts DNA at specific sites. Using a restriction enzyme like EcoRI both the human DNA and plasmid DNA of the vector are cut. They are cut in such a way that the ends of both the DNA are sticky and anneal with each other. DNA ligase forms phosphodiester linkages between both ends and joins them. The resulting hybrid DNA with the desired gene is called chimeric DNA **(Fig. 26)**.

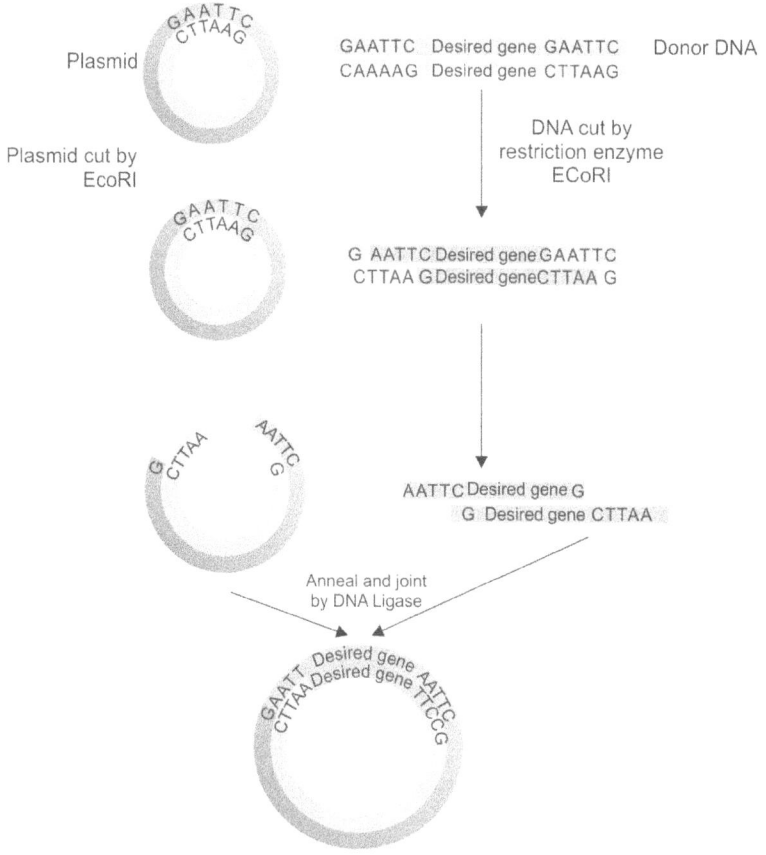

Fig. 26: Preparation of chimeric DNA molecules.

Cloning of Chimeric DNA

Transfection: The plasmid is introduced into the host cell by a process called transfection. Host *E coli* cells are incubated with plasmid vectors in a hypertonic medium containing calcium. The calcium ion channels are opened through which the plasmid is imbibed into the host cell.

Cloning: Clone is a large population of identical cells arising from a common ancestor molecule. The cells are allowed to divide so that a large population of cells with the chimeric DNA is obtained (**Fig. 27**).

Checking the Viability of the Process

Plasmid pBR-325 contains *chloromphenicol resistance* gene (Cmr), *Ampicillin* (Apr) resistance and - *tetracycline resistance* (Tcr) genes. When this plasmid is cut by the EcoRI enzyme it will cut in the middle of *Cmr* gene. When the foreign DNA is inserted, the chloramphenicol resistance will be lost. This process functions as a marker for hybrid DNA.

Selection of Colony with the Desired Gene

After the transfection, the bacteria are cultured in a medium containing ampicillin and tetracycline. Wild bacteria are killed in that medium and the bacteria containing the cloned plasmids will grow. To check whether the colony contains the desired plasmid, a part of the colony is subjected to chloramphenicol media. If the bacterium dies, then it is the colony that contains the hybrid DNA plasmid.

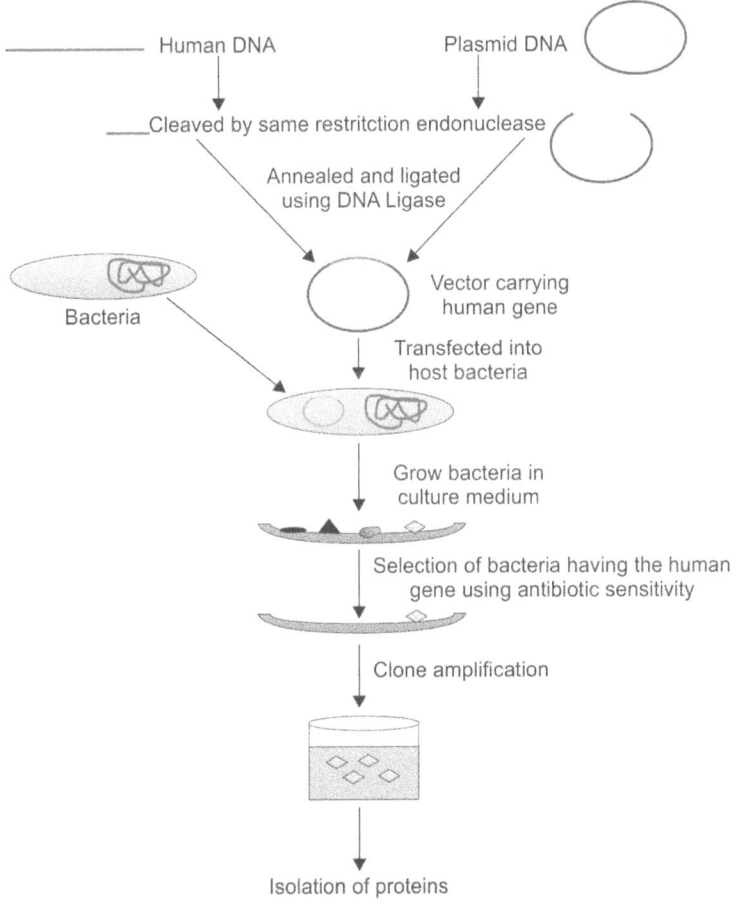

Fig. 27: Cloning.

Expression Vectors

Vector carrying a foreign gene which can produce the desired protein is called expression vector. Thus the human proteins like insulin can be harvested from such cultures.

Applications

- Large scale production of therapeutic human proteins can be obtained, e.g. human recombinant insulin for diabetic patients
- Vaccines with genetic material of bacteria and viruses can be produced.
- Genetic probes can be produced to:
  - Identify genetic diseases during antenatal period
  - Diagnosis of virus and bacteria in blood using their DNA
  - To pinpoint location of a gene in chromosome
  - To identify mutations in genes
  - To detect activation of oncogenes
- Gene therapy—normal genes could be inserted into the patient's cells where it is defective, e.g. adenosine deaminase deficiency
- Prenatal diagnosis by amniocentesis.

24. Wilson's disease.

- Normal blood level of ceruloplasmin is 25-50 mg/dL. This level is reduced to less than 20 mg/dL in Wilson's hepatolenticular degeneration
- It is an inherited autosomal recessive disease. Incidence is 1 in 50,000
- The basic defect is a mutation in a gene encoding a copper binding ATPase in cells required for excretion of copper (Cu) from cells. Hence Cu gets accumulated to produce Cu toxicity
- Increased copper content in hepatocytes inhibits the incorporation of copper to apoceruloplasmin.

Clinical Features

- Accumulation of Cu in liver causing hepatocellular degeneration and cirrhosis
- Deposition of copper in basal ganglia of brain leads to lenticular degeneration and neurological symptoms
- Copper deposits around the cornea as green or golden pigmented ring called Kayser-Fleischer ring
- Treatment consists of diet containing low copper and injection of D-pencillamine. Zinc is also given as treatment as it decreases Cu absorption.

25. Secondary structure of proteins.

Alpha Helix (Fig. 28)

- Proteins contain primary, secondary, tertiary and sometimes quaternary structure
- **Secondary structure** of protein denotes the relationship between residues (amino acids) which are 3-4 residues apart in linear structure
- Secondary structure of proteins is stabilized by noncovalent bonds such as:
  - Hydrogen bond—weak
  - Electrostatic bonds—ionic bonds (salt bridges)
  - Hydrophobic bonds—weak
  - Van der Waals forces.

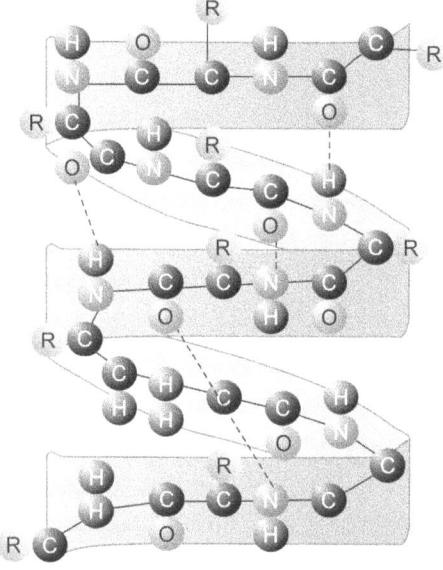

Fig. 28: Alpha helix.

- **Types of secondary structures:** The types of secondary structure are:
  - Alpha helix, e.g. alpha keratin
  - Beta pleated sheet, Beta bends (reverse turns, beta turns)
  - Nonrepetitive secondary structure and supersecondary motifs.

α-helix

- Alpha helix is one type of secondary structure of proteins
- It was the first structure found out by Pauling and Corey
- It is the most common and stable confirmation in a polypeptide chain. It is seen in Hb, myoglobin and collagen and absent in chymotrypsin
- It has a spiral structure which is stabilized by hydrogen bond between NH and CO groups of amino acids
- Alpha helix is mostly right handed since amino acids are usually L variety
- Polypeptide bonds form the backbone of the helix and the side chains of amino acids extend outward
- Each turn of helix contain about 3.6 residues. The distance between each amino acids is about 1.5 Å apart
- Proline and hydroxy proline will not allow α-helix formation
- Alpha helix is seen in alpha keratin, Hb.

β-pleated Sheet (Fig. 29)

- Second structure found out by Pauling and Corey
- Here the polypeptide chain is fully extended
- The distance between each residue is about 3.5 Å
- It is stabilized by hydrogen bonds between NH and C=O groups of neighboring polypeptide segments
- The beta bends formed by the U turn folding is stabilized by intrachain disulfide bonds
- Adjacent strands in a sheet can run in same direction (parallel) or in opposite fashion (antiparallel)
- It is found in silk fibroin (antiparallel), flavidoxin (parallel) and carbonic anhydrase (both).

β-Bends (β-Turns) and loops

- Globular proteins contain beta bends
- Bends are made up of 4 amino acids where the 1st and 4th are connected by hydrogen bonds making a U turn. Here the polypeptide chain abruptly reverse the direction and connects the ends of beta pleated sheets. It is known as reverse turn or hairpin turn
- Loops are made of many amino acids and it functions in connecting two strands of beta sheet or alpha and beta sheets. It also takes part in the formation of active site in many enzymes.

Supersecondary Structure

It is a combination of secondary structural characters like α-helix, β-pleated sheets of

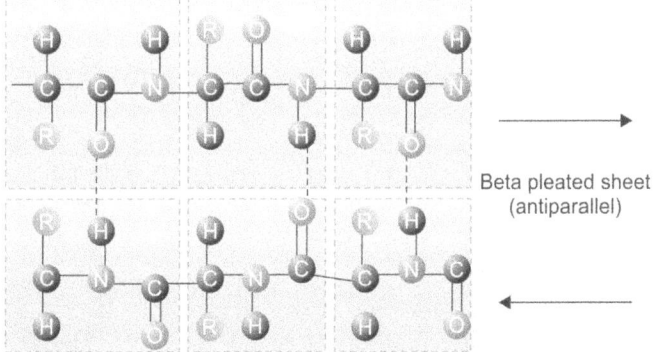

Beta pleated sheet (antiparallel)

Fig. 29: β-pleated sheet.

both parallel and anti-parallel regions with intervening β-turns, loop regions, etc.

26. Polyamines.

- A polyamine is an organic compound having two or more primary amino groups ($-NH_2$)
- Polyamines are putrescine, spermidine and spermine
- They are aliphatic amines synthesized from ornithine (arginine) **(Fig. 30)**

Functions

- The polyamines help in protein synthesis
- Polyamines are involved in cell proliferation, stabilization of ribosomes and DNA, synthesis of DNA and RNA, protection of DNA against deprivation
- Polyamine concentration is increased in cancer cells
- Polyamines are growth factors in cell culture systems.

Inhibitors

- Difluromethyl ornithine (DFMO) is a powerful inhibitor of polyamine synthesis by suicidal inhibition. Trypanosomes are parasites that are destroyed by DFMO since polyamines are needed for their reproduction.

27. Metabolic acidosis.

Refer 2004 Short Notes 16.

28. Restriction endonucleases.

- They are known as molecular scissors
- Restriction endonucleases **(Fig. 31)** are enzymes which are very important for recombinant DNA technology. They are derived mostly from bacteria. They can cut nucleic acid at specific sites called restriction sites
- They are named after the species and strains of bacteria and the order of discovery. For examples the enzyme EcoRI is isolated from *Escherichia coli* RY 13 strain. The roman numeral-one indicates the order of discovery
- Restriction enzymes cut DNA of any source into short pieces in a sequence-specific manner. These defensive enzymes (hundreds have been discovered) protect the host bacterial DNA from DNA of foreign organisms
- However, they are present only in cells that also have a companion enzyme which methylates the host DNA rendering it an unsuitable substrate for digestion by the restriction enzyme. Thus site-specific DNA methylases and restriction enzymes always exist in pairs in a bacterium

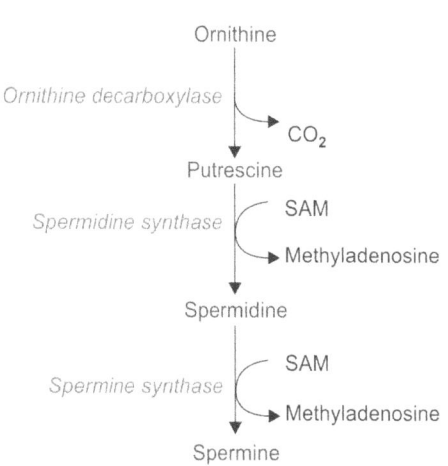

Fig. 30: Polyamines.

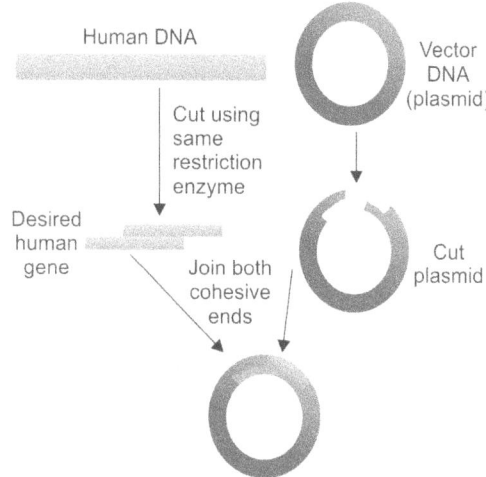

Fig. 31: Action of restriction endonucleases.

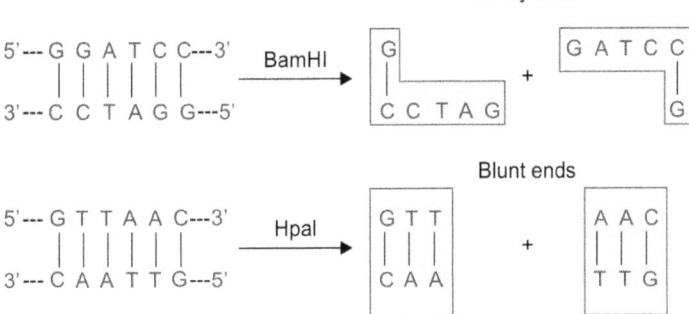

Fig. 32: Cleavage of DNA by gestriction endonucleases.

- Each enzyme recognizes and cleaves a specific double-stranded DNA sequence that is 4-7 bp long. They recognize the areas of palindromes (reading front and back in same sequences) and cut the DNA
- These DNA cuts result in **blunt ends** (e.g. HpaI) or overlapping **(sticky) ends** (e.g. BamHI). Sticky ends are particularly useful in constructing hybrid or chimeric DNA molecules **(Fig. 32)**
- When DNA is digested with a given enzyme, the ends of all the fragments have the same DNA sequence
- The fragments produced can be isolated by electrophoresis on agarose or polyacrylamide gels. This is an essential step in cloning and a major use of these enzymes
- A given piece of DNA has a characteristic linear array of sites for the various enzymes dictated by the linear sequence of its bases; hence, a **restriction map** can be constructed.

29. Functions of phosphorous.

Formation of Bone and Teeth

Vitamin D stimulates osteoblasts to produce alkaline phosphatase which leads to the formation of calcium phosphate hydroxyapatite crystals which is deposited on the bone causing mineralization.

- **Production of high energy phosphates** like:
  - ATP—energy currency of the cell
  - CTP—needed for phosphatidylcholine and other compound synthesis
  - GTP—is needed for G proteins
  - UTP—bilirubin conjugation and glycogen metabolism.
- Synthesis of coenzymes like NAD and NADP
- DNA and RNA synthesis—phosphodiester bond links the sugar units which forms backbone of nucleic acids
- Esters—formation of G6P, F6P, etc
- Phospholipids like lecithin formation
- Formation of phosphoproteins like casein
- Activation of enzymes by phosphorylation
- Phosphate buffer—it is made of Na_2HPO_4/NaH_2PO_4. It has a pKa of 6.8.

30. Purine salvage pathway.

Refer 2004 Short Note 15.

31. Post-translational modification.

Refer 2006 Short Note 27.

32. Role of lungs in acid-base balance.

It is the second line of defence to maintain acid-base balance.

- When there is fall in pH (acidosis) the respiratory rate is stimulated resulting in hyperventilation. This would eliminate more CO_2 thereby lowering H_2CO_3
- In the lungs, H^+ combines with HCO_3^- to form H_2CO_3 which becomes H_2O and CO_2. This CO_2 is released into the lungs. So lungs reduce the acid load of H_2CO_3 by the excretion of CO_2 **(Fig. 33)**

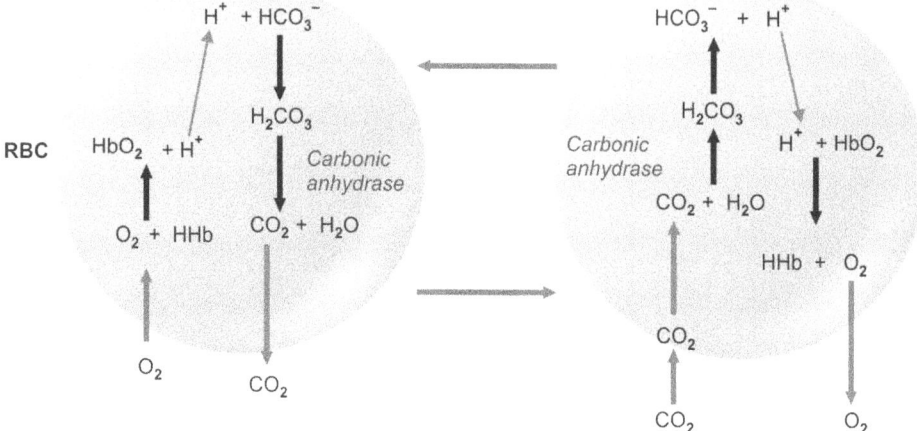

Fig. 33: Reactions in lungs. **Fig. 34:** Reaction in tissues.

- In tissues, pCO$_2$ is high and pH is low to the formation of acids by the cells like lactate and production of CO$_2$ by cells. CO$_2$ diffuses into RBC. It combines with water to form carbonic acid by carbonic anhydrase. And dissociates into H$^+$ and HCO$_3^-$. So RBC traps H$^+$ from the tissues. Some of the HCO$_3^-$ diffuses out of the cell in exchange for chloride **(Fig. 34)**

- In metabolic acidosis lungs hyperventilate to excrete more acid. In metabolic alkalosis the reverse happens.

MBBS Examination 2008

ANSWER ALL QUESTIONS

I. Essay questions (10/15 Marks each)

1. Describe the site, process of β-oxidation of fatty acid and add a note on role of carnitine. Write the energetics.
2. Describe the synthesis of HEME. What is porphyria? Classify the different types of porphyrias. Give the enzyme defect and biochemical findings.
3. What is the normal blood glucose level? Describe the regulation of blood glucose.
4. Write in detail about how ammonia is formed from amino acids transported and connected to urea.
5. Explain the steps of beta oxidation of palmitic acid. Add a note on energetics.
6. What is gluconeogenesis? Describe the pathway involved in gluconeogenesis. Add a note on regulation of gluconeogenesis.
7. Describe the pathways of methionine metabolism. Add a note on metabolic functions of methionine and cysteine.
8. Describe the biosynthesis of purine nucleotide. Add a note on regulation.

II. Short notes (5 Marks each)

1. Biotin.
2. Enzymes for myocardial infarction.
3. Protein-energy malnutrition.
4. Oxidative phosphorylation (chemiosmotic theory).
5. Structure of cell membrane.
6. How glucose is absorbed from small intestine?
7. Catabolism of cholesterol.
8. Wald's visual cycle.
9. Glycogen storage diseases.
10. Fiber diet.
11. Give the structure of immunoglobulin and their functions.
12. Functions of zinc and selenium.
13. Storage and transport of iron in the body.
14. Transamination reaction.
15. Renal regulation of pH of blood.
16. Van den Bergh reaction.
17. Fluorometry.
18. Hyperuricemia.
19. Secondary structure of proteins.
20. Transmethylation.
21. Functions of vitamin C.
22. Digestion and absorption of lipids (TAG).
23. Hemoglobin S.
24. Isoenzymes.
25. Structure of cell membrane.
26. Define BMR. What are the factors that can affect BMR?
27. Define oxidative phosphorylation. Explain chemiosmotic theory.
28. Galactosemia.
29. Ketogenesis.
30. Glucose tolerance test.
31. Transamination reactions.
32. Renal regulation of pH.
33. Gout.
34. Mutation.
35. Differences between DNA and RNA.
36. Oncogenes.
37. Post-translational modification.
38. Formation of creatine.
39. Alkaptonuria.
40. Southern blotting.

III. Short answer questions

(2/3 Marks each)

1. Name the essential fatty acids.
2. Significance of HMP shunt pathway.
3. Benedict's test.
4. Inhibitors of citric acid cycle.
5. Chloride shift.
6. Functions of calcium.
7. Lipotropic factors.
8. Normal blood levels of: 1. Cholesterol, 2. Bilirubin, 3. Sodium, 4. Potassium
9. Phospholipids.
10. Fluorosis.
11. Name the buffer systems of blood.
12. Sources of carbon and nitrogen in purine ring.
13. Wobble hypothesis.
14. Write the enzyme defect in: (1) Lesch-Nyhan syndrome, (2) Orotic aciduria.
15. Okazaki fragments.
16. What are xenobiotics?
17. Causes of metabolic acidosis.
18. Name the important compounds formed from glycine.
19. Inhibitors of protein biosynthesis.
20. Apoptosis.

I. ESSAY QUESTIONS

1. **Describe the site, process of β-oxidation of fatty acid and add a note on role of carnitine. Write the energetics.**

Refer 2006 Essay Question 5.

2. **Describe the synthesis of HEME. What is porphyria? Classify the different types of porphyrias. Give the enzyme defect and biochemical findings.**

Heme is the prosthetic group of proteins like Hb, myoglobin, cytochrome. It is synthesized from porphyrin and iron.

Biosynthesis of Heme

Site: All cells especially in bone marrow and liver partly in mitochondria and partly in cytoplasm.

Stages of Heme Synthesis (Fig. 1)

- **Synthesis of aminolevulinic acid (ALA): Mitochondria (Fig. 2)**
  - Condensation of succinyl-CoA and glycine in the presence of PLP to form alpha amino beta ketoadipic acid by the rate-limiting enzyme ALA synthase. One CoA SH is removed
  - Alpha amino beta ketoadipic acid is again acted by the same ALA synthase to form δ-aminolevulinic acid.
- **Formation of porphobilinogen: Cytoplasm**

In the cytoplasm two molecules of ALA are condensed to form porphobilinogen (PBG) by the removal of two molecules of water by the enzyme ALA dehydratase.

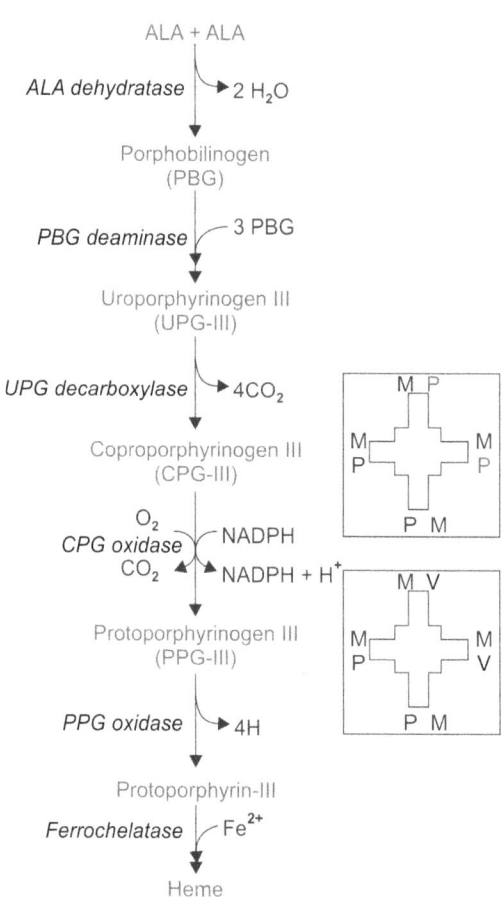

Fig. 1: Steps of heme synthesis.

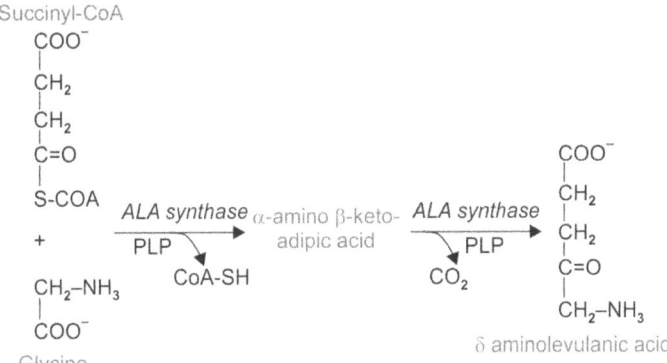

Fig. 2: Synthesis of aminolevulinic acid.

This enzyme contains zinc (Zn) and it is inhibited by lead.

- **Formation of uroporphyrinogen (UPG): Cytoplasm**
  - Condensation of four molecules of PBG to form hydroxymethylbilane (HMB) by PBG deaminase or uroporphyrinogen-I synthase or HMB synthase
  - HMB cyclizes spontaneously to form uroporphyrinogen-I which is the first porphyrin of the pathway
  - UPG-I is converted to uroporphyrinogen III by the synthase enzyme.
- **Synthesis of coproporphyrinogen (CPG): Cytoplasm**
  Uroporphyrinogen decarboxylase enzyme decarboxylates UPG-III to form coproporphyrinogen III after the removal of four molecules of CO_2. Acetate groups are decarboxylated to methyl groups.
- **Synthesis of protoporphyrinogen (PPG): Mitochondria**
  CPG enters into the mitochondria where it is oxidized by an oxidase enzyme specific for type III series to form protoporphyrinogen-III (PPG–III) with the help of molecular oxygen
- **Synthesis of protoporphyrin-III (PP): Mitochondria**
  - In the mitochondria, protoporphyrinogen oxidase enzyme oxidises PPG-III to protoporphyrin-III (PP-III) – (PP-9)
  - This requires molecular oxygen.
- **Generation of heme:**
  - Attachment of ferrous iron to protoporphyrin-III leads to the formation of heme by the enzyme heme synthase or ferrochelatase in the mitochondria
  - When the ferrous iron is oxidized to ferric form, **hematin** is formed.

Regulation of Heme Synthesis

- **Rate-limiting enzyme ALA synthase is regulated:**
  - By repression. Heme inhibits the synthesis of ALA synthase enzyme as a co-repressor
  - By allosteric inhibition by hematin.
- **Compartmentalization of the enzymes:** Rate-limiting enzyme is in mitochondria. Steps 1, 5, 6 and 7 take place in mitochondria and steps 2, 3 and 4 occur in cytoplasm.
- **Drugs/poisons**
  - Barbiturates induce heme synthesis
  - Isoniazide decreases the availability of PLP and so decreases heme synthesis
  - Lead inhibits ferrochelatase and ALA dehydratase.
- **Glucose:** High cellular concentration of glucose in the cells prevent induction of ALA synthase.

Disorders of Heme Synthesis

Porphyrias: Porphyrias are a group of inborn errors of metabolism associated with the biosynthesis of heme. These are characterized by increased production and excretion of porphyrins and/or their precursors. They may be: a. congenital and b. acquired.

- Congenital porphyrias are classified into: a. Hepatic b. Erythropoietic c. Hepato-erythropoietic
- **a. Hepatic porphyria:**
  - *Acute intermittent porphyria*: Uroporphyrinogen-I synthase deficiency (AD). This leads to secondary increase in activity of ALA. The levels of ALA and PBG are elevated in blood and urine. Urine is dark on voiding due to photo-oxidation of PBG to porphobilin. Symptoms appear intermittently. Patients will have acute abdominal pain. An attack is precipitated by starvation and symptoms are relieved by glucose infusion. Patients may have neurological abnormality like sensory and motor disturbances, agitation and confusion. Patients may have neuropsychiatric problems.
  - *Variegate porphyria*: Protoporphyrinogen oxidase deficiency (AD)
    * Acute hepatic - 1/100,000
    * Deficiency—protoporphyrinogen oxidase
    * Accumulation—urinary ALA, protoporphyrinogen IX, coproporphyrin-III
    * Scarring following photosensitive eruption
    * Photosensitivity, abdominal pain, neuropsychiatric **symptoms.**
  - *Hereditary coproporphyria*: Due to coproporphyrinogen-III oxidase deficiency
    * It is an autosomal dominant (AD) condition
    * Uroporphyrin and copropor-phyrin are excreted in urine and in feces. Urine is colored
    * Symptoms are similar to acute intermittent porphyria but milder
    * Photosensitivity, abdominal pain, neuropsychiatric symptoms are present.
  - *ALA dehydratase deficiency*:
    * Abdominal pain, neuropsychiatric symptoms present
    * Increased excretion of urinary ALA, coproporphyrin-III.
  - *Porphyria cutanea tarda (AD):*
    * Uroporphyrinogen decarboxylase deficiency
    * Here patients are more prone for photosensitivity. The urobilinogens get accumulated and when patients come under light they spontaneously form urobilin which is a potent oxidant and destroys skin cells and causes scarring
    * Patients have gross skin malformations leading to monster like appearance, and they prefer night. Sunscreens are mildly effective
    * Uroporphyrins are colored and excreted in urine.
- **b. Erythropoietic:**
  - *Erythropoietic protoporphyria (AD) hereditary protoporphyria:*
    * Due to ferrochelatase deficiency or heme synthase
    * Autosomal dominant condition
    * Photosensitivity++
    * Porphyrins or their precursors are not excreted in urine
    * Protoporphyrin level—increased in plasma, RBCs and feces. RBCs show fluorescence
  - *Congenital erythropoietic porphyria - AR*
    * Uroporphyrinogen-III synthase deficiency
    * Autosomal recessive disorder
    * Photosensitivity++
    * Dark urine—uroporphyrinogen I and coproporphyrinogen I— urine—portwine appearance
    * Dermatitis and scarring - monkey faces, mutilation of nose, ear and cartilage
    * Erythrodontia.

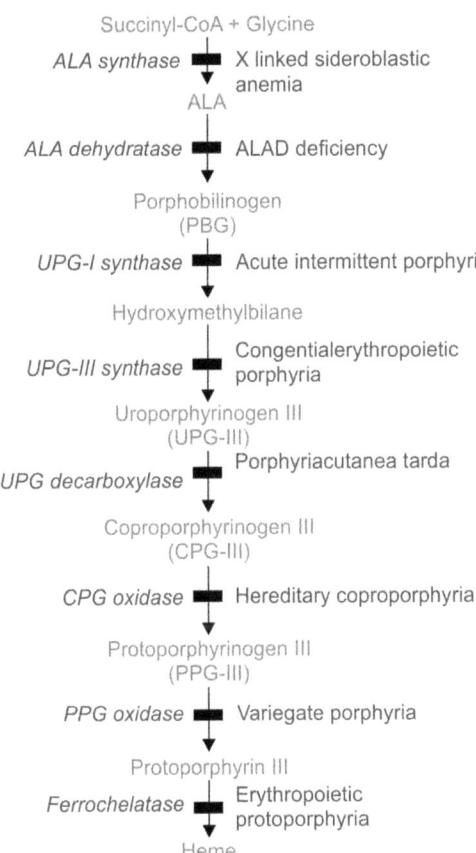

Fig. 3: Enzyme deficiency in porphyrias.

- *ALA synthase deficiency (Fig. 3)*
  * Erythroid form
  * X-linked sideroblastic anemia
  * RBC count and Hb—decreased.
- Protoporphyria.
c. **Hepatoerythropoietic porphyria:**
  - *Chronic – porphyria cutanea tarda*
  - *Hepatoerythropoietic porphyria.*
- Acquired porphyria:
  - Due to lead poisoning
  - Drug induced—barbiturates, antifungal—grisofulvin
  - Due to inhibition of ferrochelatase
  - Associated anemia.

3. **What is the normal blood glucose level? Describe the regulation of blood glucose.**

Refer 2003 Essay Question 2.

4. **Write in detail about how ammonia is formed from amino acids transported and connected to urea.**

Refer 2005 Essay Question 7.

Formation of Ammonia

- Ammonia is produced in human body mostly by the catabolism of amino acids and by other nitrogenous substances like amino sugars, purines, pyrimidines and biological amines
- **Ammonia is toxic to the body and so it should be eliminated or detoxified. Very minute amount of ammonia may produce toxicity in CNS**
- Production of ammonia from amino acids are done by the following steps:
  - Transamination
  - Transdeamination (oxidative deamination)
  - Nonoxidative deamination.

Transamination (Fig. 4)

- Transamination is the exchange of the alpha amino group between one alpha amino acid and another alpha-keto acid forming a new alpha amino acid (II) and

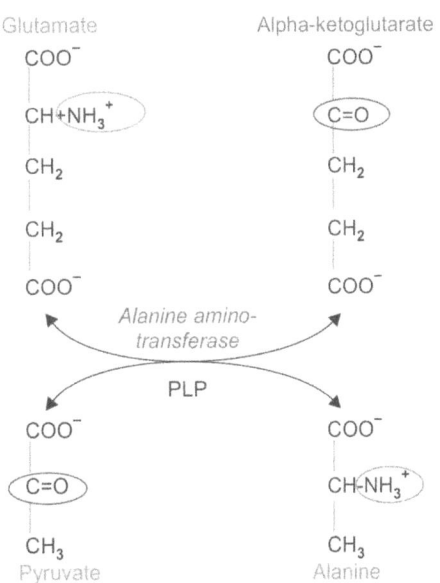

Fig. 4: Transamination.

a new keto acid (II). This is catalyzed by a group of enzymes known as transferases or aminotransferases with pyridoxal phosphate (PLP) as its coenzyme
- It is a reversible reaction
- **Reaction sequence:**
Amino acid 1 + keto acid 1 → amino acid 2 + keto acid 2
E.g. Alanine + Alpha-ketoglutarate →
 (1AA)   (1KA)
Glutamate + Pyruvate (Alanine aminotransferase, PLP)
(II AA)   (II KA)
PLP acts as an acceptor of amino group forming a Schiff's base. In the above example, first the amino group from alanine (amino acid 1) is removed to form pyruvate (keto acid 2). Then this amino group is taken up by alpha ketoglutarate (keto acid 1) to form glutamate (amino acid 2)
- **Exception:** Transamination will not occur in lysine, threonine, proline and hydroxyproline.

Transdeamination (Fig. 5)
a. Oxidative deamination of glutamate:
   - Transamination is followed by deamination is known as transdeamination.
   - Transamination takes place in the cytoplasm of all the cells of the body. After transamination, the amino group is transported to liver as glutamic acid
   - In the liver mitochondria, glutamate dehydrogenase enzyme which deaminates glutamate to form ammonia and alpha-ketoglutarate with the help of NAD.

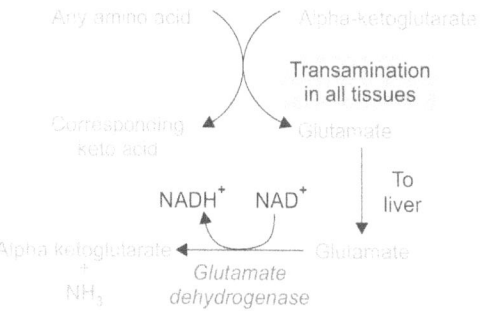

Fig. 5: Transdeamination.

b. Other pathways of deamination:
   - This is done by L- and D amino acid oxidases and monoamine oxidase
   - **L-amino acid oxidase:** Acts on all amino acids except hydroxyl group containing amino acids and acidic amino acids with FMN as coenzyme to form keto acid and peroxides which is acted by catalase enzymes in peroxisomes
   - **D-amino acid oxidase:** This oxidises glycine and all D-amino acids (bacterial metabolism) using FAD as coenzyme to liberate ammonia and keto acids
   - **Monoamine oxidases:** Oxidation of monoamines mainly in tyrosine metabolism.

Nonoxidative Deamination
Done by:
a. Dehydratase—acts on hydroxy amino acids, e.g. serine → pyruvate + ammonia. Threonine → α-ketobutyric acid + ammonia
b. Desulfhydratase—deamination + transsulfuration, e.g. cysteine → H_2S + pyruvate + ammonia (thro' imino acid)
c. Histidase—histidine → urocanate + NH_3
d. GIT—NH_3 formed by bacterial putrefaction.

Transport of Ammonia
- Ammonia is toxic to brain, so it has to be eliminated or detoxified quickly
- So it combines with glutamate to form glutamine especially in brain cells
- This glutamine is taken into liver and by glutaminase; it is converted back to ammonia
- Glutamic acid acts as a link between amino groups of amino acids and ammonia
- Concentration of glutamic acid is 10 times more than other amino acids in blood
- Major form of transport of ammonia is glutamine from brain and intestines to liver
- Alanine is the transport form of ammonia from muscles.

Final Disposal of Ammonia/Formation of Urea

- First line of defence against ammonia is done by trapping of NH_3 by glutamic acid to form glutamine brain cells
- Second line of defence is by the formation of urea which is the end product of protein metabolism in liver.

Steps of Urea Formation

The urea cycle is the first metabolic pathway to be elucidated in 1932. This cycle is also called as Krebs-Henseleit urea cycle or ornithine cycle (**Fig. 6**).

Site: In **LIVER**. First two steps of urea cycle are taken place in liver mitochondria and other steps are taken place in cytosol.

The two nitrogen atoms of urea derived from two different sources, one from ammonia and other directly from aspartic acid (α amino group).

STEP 1: Formation of carbamoyl phosphate

- One molecule of ammonia condenses with CO_2 in the presence of two molecules of ATP to form carbamoylphosphate by the enzyme carbamoylphosphate synthetase-I (CPS-1). This occurs in liver mitochondria
- This is the rate-limiting step. It is an irreversible step and regulated allosterically by N-acetylglutamate (NAG).

STEP 2: Formation of citrulline: Mitochondria

- The carbamoyl group is transferred to the NH_2 group of ornithine by ornithine transcarbamoylase (OTC)
- Citrulline enters into the cytoplasm to continue further reactions.

STEP 3: Formation of arginino-succinate

- One molecule of aspartic acid adds to citrulline forming a carbon to nitrogen bond which provides second nitrogen of urea by argininosuccinate synthetase
- Two high energy phosphate bonds are utilized.

STEP 4: Formation of arginine

- Argininosuccinate is cleaved by argininosuccinate lyase argininosuccinase to arginine and fumarate. Fumarate inhibits this step
- Fumarate enters into TCA cycle to be converted to malate which is then converted to oxaloacetate
- Oxaloacetate is transaminated to aspartate. This is a link between TCA cycle and urea cycle.

STEP 5: Formation of urea

- Hydrolysis of arginine gives rise to urea and ornithine by the enzyme arginase
- Ornithine returns to the mitochondria to react with another molecule of carbamoyl phosphate to proceed the next cycle.

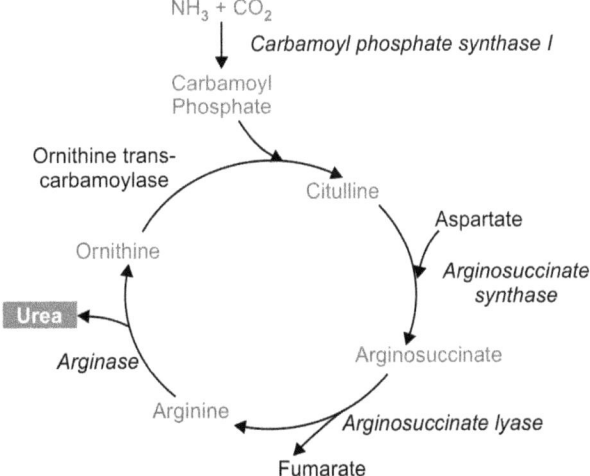

Fig. 6: Steps of urea cycle.

5. **Explain the steps of β-oxidation of palmitic acid. Add a note on energetics.**

Refer 2006 Essay Question 5.

6. **What is gluconeogenesis? Describe the pathway involved in gluconeogenesis. Add a note on regulation of gluconeogenesis.**

Refer 2007 Essay Question 1.

Definition: Synthesis of glucose from non-carbohydrate substrates.
- **Organs:** Liver and kidney (cortex)
- **Substrates:** Pyruvate, lactate, amino acids (glucogenic), propionate, glycerol.

Key Enzymes in Gluconeogenesis

- **Pyruvate carboxylase:** Pyruvate in the cytoplasm enters the mitochondria. Then, carboxylation of pyruvate to oxaloacetate is catalyzed by pyruvate carboxylase. It needs-biotin and ATP
- **Phosphoenolpyruvate carboxykinase (PEPCK):** It converts oxaloacetate to phosphoenolpyruvate by removing CO_2. GTP donates the phosphate
- **Fructose 1, 6-bisphosphatase**
  Fructose 1, 6-bisphosphate → Fructose 6 phosphate + Pi.
  This step will bypass PFK step.
- **Glucose-6-phosphatase:** it is active in liver and absent in muscle.
  Glucose-6-phosphate + H_2O → Glucose + Pi

Steps of Gluconeogenesis

It involves glycolysis (not a reversal), TCA cycle and some reactions like transamination.

I. **Conversion of pyruvate to glucose (mitochondria + cytosol)**
   – Carboxylation of pyruvate to oxaloacetate by pyruvate carboxylase enzyme, and the coenzyme biotin and ATP
   – Transport of oxaloacetate to cytosol through malate-aspartate shuttle **(Fig. 7)**.
   Oxaloacetate cannot cross the inner mitochondrial membrane. So it is reduced to malate which can be transported across the mitochondrial membrane to cytosol. In the cytosol, malate is re-oxidised to oxaloacetate by malate dehydrogenase of cytosol
   – Decarboxylation of cytosolic oxaloacetate to phosphoenolpyruvate (PEP) by phosphoenolpyruvate carboxykinase. 1 GTP is required for this step
   – Phosphoenol pyruvate—by reversal of glycolysis forms fructose 1, 6-bisphosphate

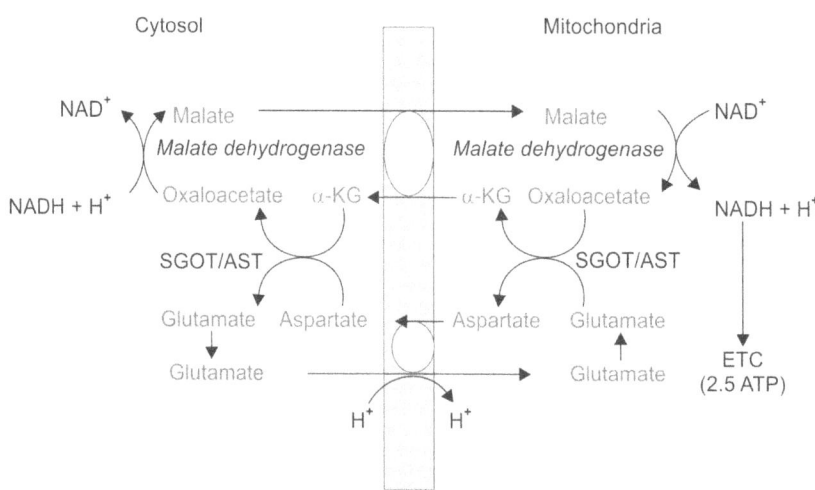

Fig. 7: Malate-aspartate shuttle.

- Dephosphorylation of fructose 1, 6-bisphosphate to fructose 6-phosphate by fructose 1, 6-bisphosphatase (allosteric enzyme). Fructose-6-phosphate is isomerized to glucose-6-phosphate
- Dephosphorylation of glucose-6-phosphate to glucose by glucose-6-phosphatase enzyme which is not present in muscles but present only in liver and kidney.

II. **Lactate to glucose (Cori cycle):** Lactate dehydrogenase converts lactate to pyruvate. Pyruvate enters neoglucogenic pathway to form glucose.

Lactate → Liver, Kidney → Pyruvate → Gluconeogenic pathway → Glucose

III. **Glycerol to glucose (Fig. 8):** From adipose tissue the hydrolytic product of TAG - Glycerol is shifted to liver by blood where it gets phosphorylated to form Glycerol-3-phosphate. This is then dehydrogenated to form DHAP which by reversal of glycolysis produces glucose.

IV. **Glucogenic amino acids**
 i. Alanine—released from muscle is taken to liver by glucose alanine cycle.

Alanine $\xrightarrow[\text{Transamination}]{\text{ALT}}$ Pyruvate $\longrightarrow$ Glucose

 ii. Other glucogenic amino acids transaminated to keto acids to enter into TCA cycle to form oxaloacetate/pyruvate.

Aspartate/ASN $\xrightarrow[\text{Transamination}]{\text{AST}}$ Oxaloacetate $\longrightarrow$ TCA cycle

Valine, isoleucine, methionine → Oxaloacetate → TCA cycle
Phenylalanine, tyrosine → fumarate → TCA cycle
All of them then enter into neoglucogenic pathway to get converted to glucose.

V. **Propionate to glucose:** Propionate is formed by the oxidation of odd chain fatty acids and also from certain glucogenic amino acids and by glycolysis in ruminants. Propionate is converted to succinyl-CoA which then enters into TCA cycle **(Fig. 9)**.

Significance of Gluconeogenesis

- Whenever carbohydrate source is insufficient, gluconeogenesis meet the needs of the body to maintain blood glucose homeostasis
- It is a continuous source of glucose to tissues like brain, RBC, lens, cornea, etc.

7. **Describe the pathways of methionine metabolism. Add a note on metabolic functions of methionine and cysteine.**

Refer 2007 Essay Question 4.

Methionine Metabolism

- Methionine is a sulfur containing amino acid; it is an essential, glucogenic amino acid
- Methionine gives rise to the other sulphur containing amino acid—it cysteine.

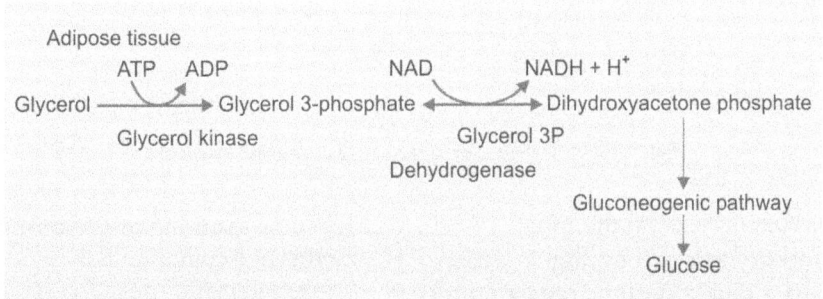

Fig. 8: Conversion of glycerol to glucose.

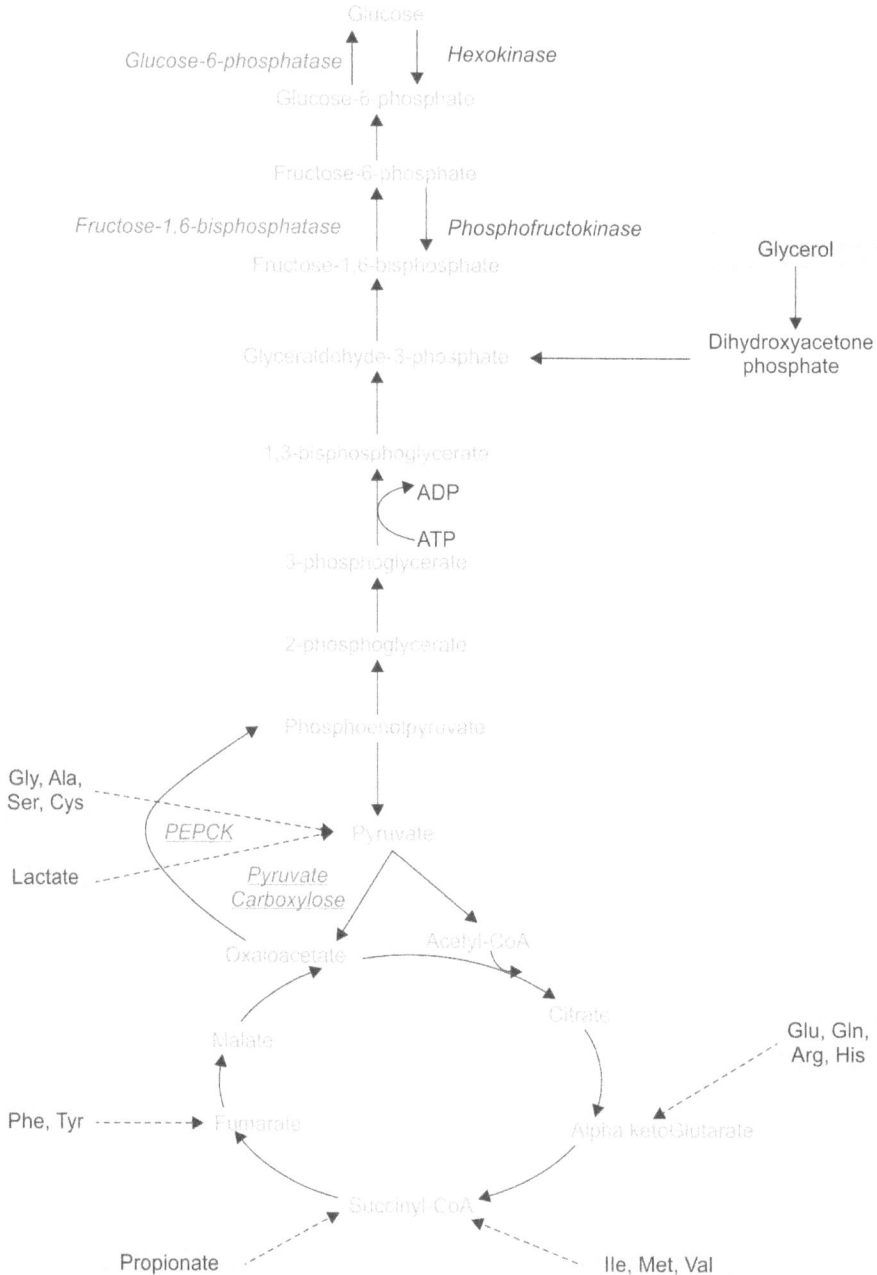

Fig. 9: Gluconeogenesis—conversion of propionate to glucose.

Metabolic Functions of Methionine
- **Transmethylation reaction** is acceptance of a methyl group from a donor like S-adenosyl methionine (SAM) by an acceptor resulting in the formation of a methylated compound
- Transmethylation reaction requires SAM which is obtained by accepting adenosyl

group from ATP by methionine by methionine adenosyltransferase.

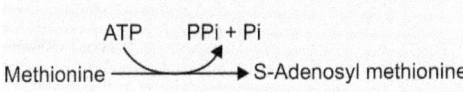

The examples for transmethylation reactions are shown in following table.

Methyl acceptor	Methylated product
Guanidoacetic acid	Creatine
Serine	Choline
Epinephrine	Metanephrine
Norepinephrine	Epinephrine
tRNA	Methylated tRNA

Metabolic Functions of Cysteine

Cysteine is formed from methionine catabolism.

Functions of Cysteine

- Formation of glutathione
  - Glutathione is involved in Meister cycle which is needed for amino acid transport
  - It is needed as a cofactor in maleyl-acetoacetate isomerase
  - Cysteic acid → taurine, iodine to hydrogen iodide
  - It is needed for glutathione peroxidase, glutathione reductase to protect RBCs from free radical induced damage
  - Conversion of metHb to normal Hb
  - It is involved in conjugation reactions in detoxification reactions.
- Disulfide bridges are formed by cysteine residues in proteins and are needed to stabilize the structure of proteins
- Cysteine is having SH groups which are involved in the active centers of many enzymes.

8. **Describe the biosynthesis of purine nucleotide. Add a note on regulation.**

Refer 2006 Essay Question 4.

II. SHORT NOTES

1. Biotin.

Other name: Egg white injury factor

Source

- Normal bacterial flora of gut will provide adequate quantities of biotin.
- Other sources are liver, yeast, soyabean, egg yolk.

RDA: 200–300 mg

Biochemical Functions

- Biotin acts as coenzymes for carboxylation reactions.
- CO_2 fixation reactions:
  i. Acetyl-CoA carboxylase:
     Acetyl-CoA + CO_2 + ATP → malonyl-CoA + ADP + PI
  ii. Propionyl-CoA carboxylase:
     Propionyl-CoA + CO_2 + ATP → methylmalonyl-CoA + ADP + PI
  iii. Pyruvate-CoA carboxylase:
     Pyruvate + CO_2 + ATP → oxaloacetate + ADP + PI

Deficiency Symptoms

- Dermatitis
- Muscle pain
- Anorexia
- Glossitis.

Treatment

Injection of biotin 100-300 mg.

2. Enzymes for myocardial infarction.

Creatine kinase (CK): Normal level 15-100 U/L in myocardial infarction (MI), CK starts to rise within 3-6 hours of infarction. First enzyme to be elevated.

Advantage

- It is useful to detect early cases where ECG changes may be ambiguous
- It is not increased in hemolysis or in congestive heart failure. Therefore, CK has an advantage over LDH.

Lactate dehydrogenase (LDH): Normal level—100-200 U/L. It will convert pyruvte to lactate.

Isoenzymes of LDH

Isoenzyme	Origin
LDH-1	Heart
LDH-2	RBC
LDH-3	Brain
LDH-4	Liver
LDH-5	Skeletal muscle

[In MI, total LDH activity is increased, where LDH-1 is increased 5-10 times. Normally, LDH-2 concentration in blood is greater than LDH-1; but this pattern is reversed in MI. This is called **flipped pattern.**]

Aspartate amino transferase (AST): Normal level—8-20 U/L. It is increased significantly in MI.

Cardiac troponin I and T: Not enzymes
- **Troponin I**—it is increased in blood within 4 hours after onset of symptoms, peaks at 14-24 hours and remains elevated for 3-5 days
- **Troponin T**—it is increases after 6 hours of MI, peaks at 72 hours and then remains elevated up to 7-10 days.

3. Protein-energy malnutrition.
Refer 2006 Short Note 23.

4. Oxidative phosphorylation (chemiosmotic theory).
Refer 2006 Short Note 5.

5. Structure of cell membrane.
- Cell membrane is also called as plasma membrane
- It protects the intracellular organelles from outer environment and provides selective permeability for cell function
- The structure of cell membrane was described by **Singer and Nicolson as fluid mosaic model**.

Structure of Cell Membrane (Fig. 10)
- Cell membrane has selective permeability

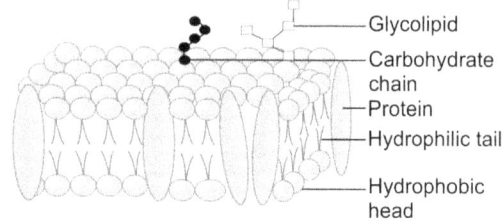

Fig. 10: Structure of cell membrane.

- Outer cell membrane has ectoenzymes, such as 5'nucleotidase and alkaline phosphatase
- Plasma membranes are made up of lipids, proteins and small amount of carbohydrates present as glycoproteins and glycolipids
- The **matrix** of a membrane is a polar bilipid layer
- **Fluid mosaic model**—the lipid bilayer shows free lateral movement and so it is said to be fluid in nature (flip flop movement is restricted)
- **The fluidity of the membrane depends upon:**
  - The cholesterol content of the membrane alters fluidity. Fluidity is less when cholesterol level is high.
  - This also depends upon the temperature (Tm) which is inversely proportional.
  - The nature of fatty acids—fluidity increases when there is more unsaturated fatty acids.
- **Phospholipids**—these are arranged in bilayers the with polar head oriented towards extracellular side and a hydrophobic nonpolar tail towards cytoplasmic side. Choline containing phospholipids are found in the external layer. Ethanolamine and serine containing phospholipids are in the inner layer
- **Thickness**—single layer thickness of 25Å thick. Head portion—10 Å and tail—15Å thick. Total thickness—50-80 Å

- **Membrane proteins**
  a. Peripheral proteins—present on the surfaces of the bilayer. They are attached by ionic and polar bonds to polar heads of lipids. They anchor proteins to lipid bilayer
  b. Integral membrane proteins deeply embedded in the bilayer and attached by hydrophobic bonds or van der Waals forces
  c. Transmembrane proteins—they span the whole bilayer. They serve as receptors for hormones, ion channels, etc.

6. **How glucose is absorbed from small intestine?**

Refer 2004 Short Note 7.

7. **Catabolism of cholesterol.**

Cholesterol is catabolized to bile acids (BA) and salts, vitamin D, sex and steroid hormones.

Bile Acids and Bile Salts

Primary BA—cholic acid and chenodeoxycholic acids; secondary bile acids—lithocholic acid and deoxycholic acid and their conjugated sodium and potassium salts.

Steps

- Cholesterol is hydroxylated at 7th position by 7 α hydroxylase enzyme which is the **rate-limiting enzyme** which needs NADPH and vitamin C and converted into 7 α hydroxycholesterol
- This in turn is acted by 12 α hydroxylase with the addition of CoA-SH in the presence of NADPH to form Cholyl-CoA and chenodeoxy cholyl-CoA with the removal of 3C propionate. This forms 24 carbon cholic acid or chenodeoxycholic acid
- The so formed 24C bile acids conjugated with glycine/taurine to produce glycocholic acid or taurocholic acid
- They are the sodium or potassium salts of primary and secondary bile acids.

Functions of Bile Salts

- They facilitate the lipid digestion
- They act as detergent in the formation of lipid micelle.

Vitamin D and Calcitriol

- Cholecalciferol is 7-dehydrocholesterol (7-DHC) which is an intermediate of cholesterol metabolism
- 7-DHC is rich in malphigian layer of epidermis. The bond between 9 and 10 of 7-DHC is cleaved and converted into cholecalciferol by the action of UV light.

$$7\text{-Dehydrocholesterol} \xrightarrow{\text{Light}} \text{Provitamin D} \xrightarrow[\text{Isomerization}]{\text{Thermal}} \text{Cholecalciferol}$$

Activation of provitamin D (cholecalciferol) into active vitamin D (calcitriol) takes place in two different sites—liver and kidney.

Biochemical Functions of Calcitriol

- Vitamin D acts as steroid hormone. It binds to specific cytoplasmic receptors which interacts with DNA and induces the synthesis of mRNA for specific proteins calbindin which is a calcium-binding protein will lead to biological action
- **Effect on intestine**—calcitriol induces the synthesis of calbindin and helps in the absorption of calcium and phosphorus from the intestines
- **Effects on bone**—calcitriol stimulates the activity of osteoblasts which help in mineralization of bones. They secrete alkaline phosphatase enzyme which in turn increases the ionic concentration of phosphate and calcium
- **Effects on kidney**—calcitriol increases the reabsorption of calcium and phosphorous from the renal tubules thereby conserving both minerals.

Steroid and Sex Hormones:

- Steroid hormones—glucocorticoids and mineralocorticoids from adrenal cortex.

Glucocorticoids mainly affect glucose metabolism
- Mineralocorticoids—mainly aldosterone increases sodium reabsorption from renal tubules leading to sodium retention.

Sex hormones—from gonads and sex organs (Fig. 11)

i. Ovarian hormones from pregnenolone-estrogens: Progesterone—maintains pregnancy and they help in maturation and function of female secondary sex organs
ii. Testicular hormones—androgens—testosterone and estrogens maturation of male secondary sexual characters.

8. Wald's visual cycle.

Refer 2006 Essay Question 7.
- Rhodopsin plays the pivotal role in vision. It is the membrane protein found in the photoreceptor cells of the retina
- Rhodopsin is made up of the protein opsin and 11-cis-retinal
- When light falls on the retina, 11-cis-retinal isomerizes to all-trans-retinal
- A single photon can excite the rod cell. The photon produces immediate conformational changes
- The unstable intermediates produced are: Rhodopsin → bathorhodopsin → lumirhodopsin → metarhodopsin → and finally opsin + all-trans-retinal
- The all-trans-retinal is then released from the protein and transported out of the retinal epithelium by an ABC protein. The all-trans-retinal is isomerized to 11-cis-retinal in the retina itself in the dark by the enzyme **retinal isomerase.** This reaction takes place in the retinal pigment epithelium
- The 11-cis–retinal combines with opsin to generate **Rhodopsin.** Alternatively the all-trans-retinal is transported to the liver and then reduced to all–trans-retinol by alcohol dehydrogenase (ADH)
- The all-trans-retinol is isomerized to 11-cis-retinol and then oxidised to 11-cis-retinal in liver. This is then transported to retina. This completes the Wald's visual cycle **(Fig. 12)**
- Visual pigments are G protein coupled receptors. 11-cis-retinal keeps it in an inactive form which gets activated by photoexcitation. Cyclic GMP is also

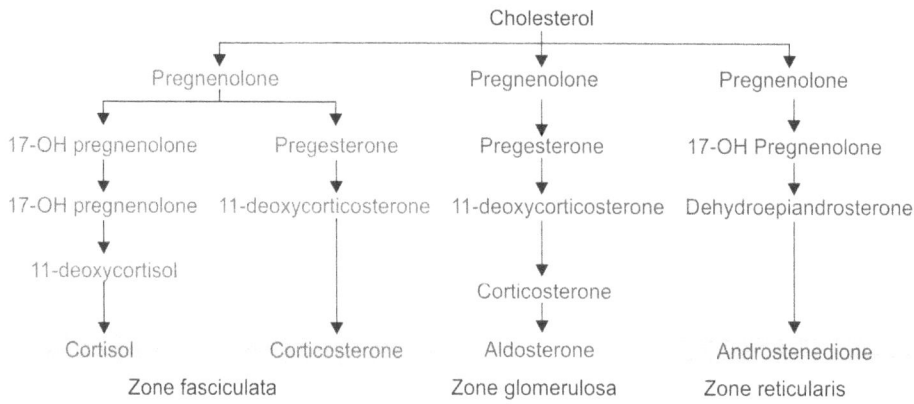

Fig. 11: Synthesis of sex hormones.

generated at the same time and it acts as a gate for cation specific channels
- G protein of retina is transducin
- Nerve impulse thus generated is transmitted to visual centers in brain **(Fig. 13)**.

9. Glycogen storage diseases.

They are inborn errors of metabolism in glycogen metabolism. There are about 10 types of glycogen storage diseases.

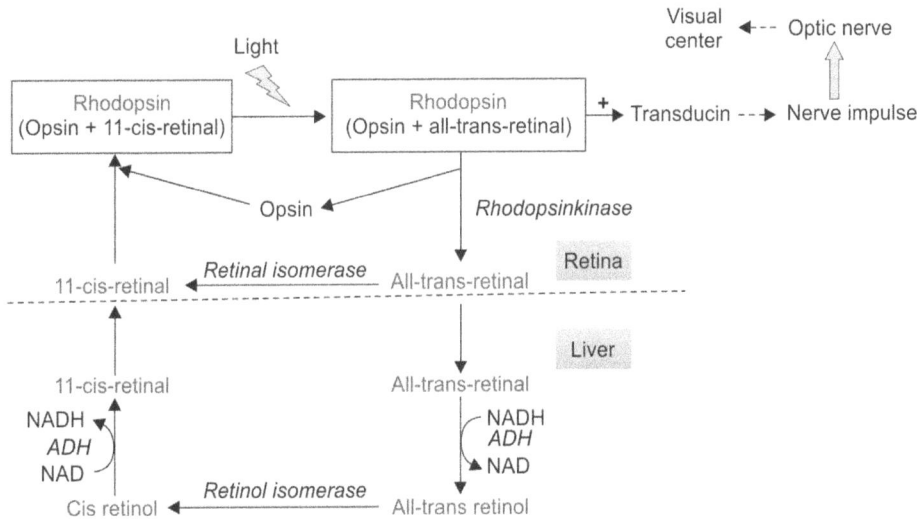

Fig. 12: Wald's visual cycle.

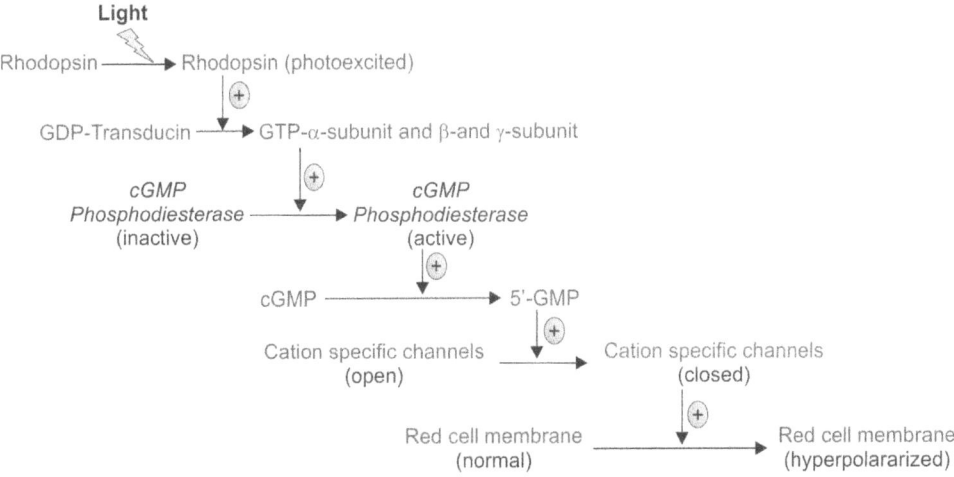

Fig. 13: Role of cGMP in visual cycle.

Type	Name	Defective enzyme	Clinical features
Type IA	Von Gierke's disease	Glucose-6-phosphatase	Hypoglycemia; hepatomegaly; ketosis, lactic acidosis, hyperlipidemia, hyperuricemia
Type IB	—	Glucose transporter in endoplasmic reticulum	Same as type IA + neutropenia and recurrent infections
Type II	Pompe disease	Lysosomal maltase	Accumulation of abnormal glycogen in lysosomes of liver, heart and muscles; infantile form—early death
Type III	Limit dextrinosis/ Forbe's/Cori's disease	Debranching enzyme	Accumulation of abnormal highly branched glycogen; hypoglycemia; hepatomegaly
Type IV	Amylopectinosis; Anderson's disease	Branching enzyme	Accumulation of abnormal few branched glycogen; mild hypoglycemia; early death by the age of 5
Type V	McArdle's disease	Muscle phosphorylase	Accumulation of glycogen in muscles; exercise intolerance
Type VI	Her's disease	Liver phosphorylase	Mild hypoglycemia, hepatomegaly, ketosis—good prognosis
Type VII	Tauri's disease	Muscle phosphofructo kinase	Mild hypoglycemia, prognosis—better
Type VIII	-----	Liver phosphorylase kinase	Mild hypoglycemia; better—prognosis
Type IX	-----	Muscle phosphorylase kinase	Mild exercise intolerance; better—prognosis
Type X	-----	Protein kinase A	Hepatomegaly

10. Fiber diet.

- The indigestible or unavailable carbohydrate in the diet is called dietary fiber
- For example, cellulose, hemicellulose, lignin, pectin
- RDA—about 30 g/day
- **Biochemical effects**
  - Necessary to maintain the normal motility of GI tract
  - It gives satiety effect thereby the quantity of food intake is reduced and helps in weight reduction
  - It prevents constipation
  - It decreases the reabsorption of bile acids and thus lowers cholesterol
  - It improves glucose tolerance
  - It prevents the incidence of cancers in gastrointestinal tract.

Fiber	Chemical nature	Uses
Cellulose	Polymer of glucose	Promotes peristalsis
Hemicellulose	Pentoses	Retains water in feces
Lignin	Aromatic alcohol	Antioxidant, hypocholesterolemic
Pectin	Partially esterified rhamnogalacturans	Slows gastric emptying

11. Give the structure of immunoglobulin and their functions.

Immunoglobulins are gamma globulins which act as antibodies. The antibody has a high specificity for a particular antigen only. The antibody's structure is complementary to that specific antigen.

Classification and Structure

- The different classes of Ig are IgG, IgM, IgA, IgD and IgE, IgG depending on the type of heavy chains. Gamma (γ), IgM - Mu (μ), IgA - Alpha (α), IgD -Delta (δ), IgE - Epsilon (ε)
- The light chains of immunoglobulins are either kappa (κ) or lambda (λ).

IgG (Fig. 14)

- IgG consists of two heavy chains and two light chains. Heavy chains are of gamma type
- Variable and constant regions are seen in both light and heavy chains. VL and VH are variable and constant regions in light chains and VH and CH are in heavy chains

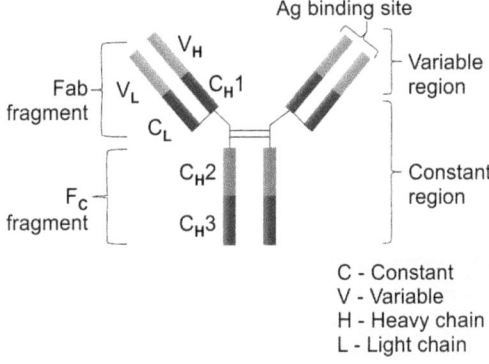

Fig. 14: Immunoglobulin G.

- The variable regions are important for antigen binding and recognition
- IgG is the major antibody (75-80%)
- They are produced by B cells and are involved in secondary immune response.
- It crosses placenta and is a reason for Rh isoimmunization.

IgM (Fig. 15)

- They are macroglobulins having five subunits. Each subunit has four peptide chains joined by J chain polypeptide
- They are involved in primary response
- Natural antibodies are IgM in nature.

IgA (Fig. 16)

- They are dimers (total four heavy chains and four light chains) connected by J chain
- These are secretory antibodies and gives protection to skin, intestine, eyes,

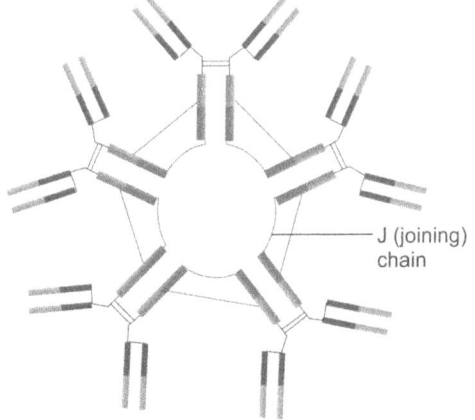

Fig. 15: IgM.

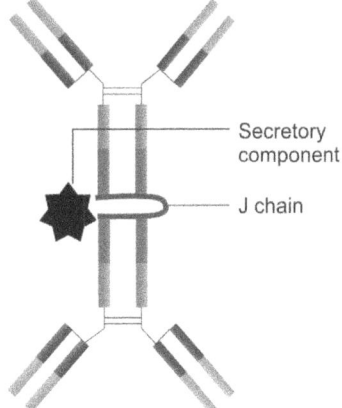

Fig. 16: IgA.

urogenital tract. It is also secreted in breast milk protecting the baby against intestinal infections.

IgE

- They are cytophilic antibodies. They mediate allergy
- They are produced by mast cells and are the cause for allergy and anaphylaxis by releasing histamine
- They lead to vasodilatation, hypotension and bronchiolar constriction
- Level of IgE is increased in helminthic infection.

IgD

- They are monomers having labile molecules
- Functions are not known.

12. Functions of zinc and selenium.

Zinc

- Total zinc content of body is 2 g, out of which 60% is in skeletal muscle and 30% in bones
- In liver, zinc is stored in combination with a specific protein, metallothionine
- More than 300 enzymes are zinc dependent
  - For example, carboxypeptidase cleaves, C-terminal ends of dietary proteins
  - Carbonic anhydrase— $H^+ + HCO_3^- \rightarrow H_2CO_3 \rightarrow H_2O + CO_2$

- Alkaline phosphatase—needed for bone formation
- Lactate dehydrogenase—pyruvate to lactate
- Glutamate dehydrogenase—deamination process.

Functions of Zinc

- It is a component of RNA polymerase. It is also needed for protein synthesis
- Superoxide dismutase contains Zn which is an antioxidant enzyme and so zinc is also an antioxidant
- Zinc stabilizes insulin. Insulin when stored in beta cells of pancreas contains zinc which stabilizes the hormone
- Gusten is a salivary protein which contains zinc. It is needed for taste sensation.

Selenium

- Selenium intake is dependent on the nature of soil in which food crops are growing
- Requirement is 50–100 µg/day
- In mammals, glutathione peroxidase is the important selenium containing enzyme. RBC contains large quantity of glutathione peroxidase
- 5-deiodinase enzyme which is involved in the synthesis of thyroid hormone in the conversion of thyroxin to T3 depends on selenium. Selenium deficiency leads to hypothyroidism
- Selenium concentration in testis is the highest in adult tissue. It is necessary for the development of spermatozoa
- It acts as nonspecific intracellular antioxidant
- Selenocysteine is considered as 21st amino acid which is genetically coded with UGA as codon.

Functions of Selenium

- Antioxidant function—the requirement of vitamin E reduces with increase in selenium intake. Both spare the action of one another
- Glutathione peroxidase antioxidant enzyme which protects RBC from free radicals
- 5'-deiodinase (thyroid metabolism)
- It is necessary for spermatogenesis
- Selenium is a constituent of selenocysteine, the 21st amino acid.

13. Storage and transport of iron in the body.

Storage

The storage form of iron is ferritin.
- Apoferritin combines with iron to form ferritin. It is seen in intestinal mucosal cells, liver cells, bone marrow and spleen. In mucosal cell iron is stored as ferritin. If body needs iron, ferritin is taken up; otherwise, the mucosal cell gets desquamated. In iron deficiency anemia ferritin content is reduced. After iron administration the ferritin content increases. It is the temporary storage form of iron
- Hemosiderin is also a storage protein for iron which can hold 15% of iron by weight. It is accumulated in spleen, liver when the supply of iron is in excess.

Transport
- Transport form of iron is transferrin or siderophilin which is synthesized in liver
- Normal plasma transferrin is 250 mg/100 mL
- From the intestinal cells, iron in the ferrous state is taken up by transferrin and transported in plasma. Here ceruloplasmin, a ferroxidase converts ferrous iron to ferric iron. One molecule of transferrin can transport 2 ferric atoms
- Total iron binding capacity (TIBC) is 400 mg/100 mL
- TIBC is provided by the transferrin. It increases in iron deficiency anemia. Soluble transferrin receptor levels also increased
- Transferrin receptors are present in most of the body cells. The iron-transferrin complex is taken up by these receptors and iron is utilized by the cell.

14. Transamination reaction.

- Transamination is the exchange of the alpha amino group between one alpha amino acid and another alpha keto acid forming a new alpha amino acid (II) and

a new keto acid (II). This is catalyzed by a group of enzymes known as transferases or aminotransferases with pyridoxal phosphate as its coenzyme (**Fig. 17**)
- It is a reversible reaction.

Reaction Sequence/Mechanism of Transamination

```
Alanine + alpha-ketoglutarate → Glutamate +
(1AA)         (1KA)                      (II AA)
pyruvate (alanine amino transferase, PLP)
(II KA)
```

PLP acts as an acceptor of amino group, forming a Schiff's base. In the above example, first the amino group from alanine (amino acid1) is removed to form pyruvate (keto acid 2). Then this amino group is taken up by alpha-ketoglutarate (keto acid 1) to form glutamate (amino acid 2)

Exception: Transamination will not occur in lysine, threonine, proline and hydroxyproline.

Salient features or Biological Importance of Transamination

- First step of catabolism of amino acids—ammonia is removed from the amino acids and the carbon skeleton enters into catabolic pathway
- It is a reversible reaction
- There are specific transaminases for each pair of amino acid and keto acid but there are mainly two important transaminases—alanine aminotransferase and aspartate aminotransferase
- Synthesis of nonessential amino acids—pyruvate can be transaminated for the synthesis of alanine; oxaloacetate is transaminated to produce aspartate and alpha-ketoglutarate is transaminated to form glutamate
- Interconversion of amino acids—if amino acid 1 is low and amino acid 2 is high the amino group from 2 is transferred to a keto acid to form the amino acid 1 to equalize the quantities of amino acids in the body.

Clinical Importance of Transaminases

- ALT is elevated in liver diseases; ALT and AST are markers for liver diseases
- AST is elevated in heart diseases along with CPK and LDH
- AST and ALT are induced by glucocorticoids and favor gluconeogenesis.

15. Renal regulation of pH of blood.

Refer 2005 Essay Question 4

16. Van den Bergh reaction.

- The serum bilirubin estimation is based on Van den Bergh reaction, where diazotised sulfanilic acid reacts with bilirubin to form a purple colored complex, azobilirubin. Normal serum does not give a positive Van den Bergh test
- When bilirubin is conjugated, the purple color is produced immediately on mixing with the reagent, the response is said to be Van den Bergh direct positive
- When the bilirubin is unconjugated, the color appears only after addition of alcohol, so it is said to be Van den Bergh indirect positive
- When both conjugated and unconjugated bilirubin are present, they produce an immediate color which intensifies

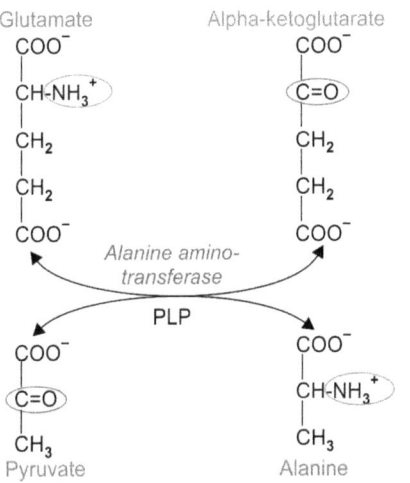

Fig. 17: Transamination.

on adding alcohol. It is then said to be biphasic
- In hemolytic jaundice unconjugated bilirubin elevated so indirect positive
- In obstructive jaundice conjugated bilirubin elevated so direct positive
- In hepatic jaundice both conjugated and unconjugated.

17. Fluorometry.

- An analytical technique for identifying and characterizing minute amounts of a substance by excitation of the substance with a beam of ultraviolet light and detection and measurement of the characteristic wavelength of fluorescent light emitted
- When a substance in excited it reaches the excited singlet stage. When it comes back to ground state after coming to triplet stage (lower energy state than singlet stage), it emits fluorescence. If it reaches further lower stages and comes to ground state it emits fluorescence
- Fluorescence is measured by using fluorometer (Fig. 18). It is similar to colorimeter except it contains an excitation and emission monochromator (whereas only one monochromator in colorimeter)
- And the fluorescence is detected by the detector placed right angles to the sample cuvette

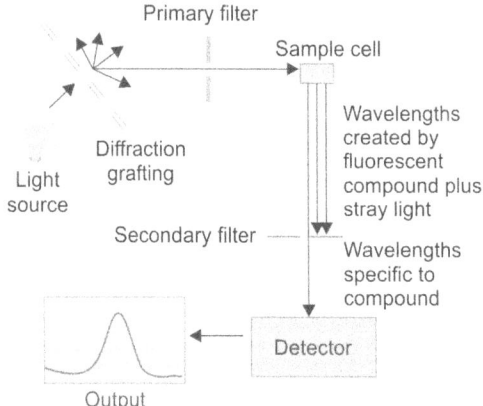

Fig. 18: Fluorometer.

- Fluorescence can be emitted by some analytes, but usually a fluorophore (e.g. fluorescien) is added to the sample which will combine with analyte to produce fluorescence according to the concentration of the analyte. This procedure is very sensitive and gives accurate results.

18. Hyperuricemia.

- Uric acid (UA) is the catabolic end product of purine nucleotides
- When uric acid level is increased in blood it is known as hyperuricemia.

Causes of Hyperuricemia

1. Normal production and excretion of urates due to renal disorders
2. Increased production and excretion of UA
   - Primary causes—enzyme defects
   - Secondary to other diseases—cancer, trauma, psoriasis, pre-eclamptic toxemia (PET), renal insufficiency
   - Unrecognized defects.
3. Decreased excretion of uric acid mostly due to secondary causes.

Hyperuricemia due to Increased Production of Uric Acid

Primary causes: Due to inherited enzyme defects gout

1. Due to abnormal PRPP synthetase enzyme—X-linked recessive: There will be increased production of PRPP due to:
   - Resistance to feedback regulation of PRPP synthetase
   - Superactive PRPP synthetase
2. Due to defective PRPP glutamyl amidotransferase enzyme—X-linked recessive: There will be increased production of purines due to absence of regulation on this rate limiting enzyme
3. Due to partial deficiency of HGPRTase enzyme—X-linked recessive: There would be more availability of PRPP leading to production of purines à uric acid
4. Von Gierke disease—due to glucose-6-phosphatase deficiency. Because of this glucose-6-phosphate is not converted to

glucose. So it goes through HMP shunt resulting in more nucleotide bases, increasing in more urate production

5. Lesch-Nyhan syndrome—it is an X-linked inborn error of purine metabolism and is due to complete deficiency of HGPRTase which is an enzyme of purine salvage pathway.

Secondary Causes: Secondary to other diseases

This may be seen in:
- Increased diet intake, alcohol consumption
- Increased production of uric acid due to increased turnover of cells as in malignancy lymphomas, leukemia, polycythemia, psoriasis, after the treatment of cancer, trauma and starvation
- Reduced excretion of uric acid—renal failure, thiazide diuretics, lactic acidosis and ketoacidosis

Clinical Features of Gout

- Hyperuricemia is manifested mostly as gout
- Uric acid gets deposited in the cooler areas of body like distal joints to form tophi
- There will be inflammatory reactions of joints due to tophi causing acute gouty arthritis which will be progressing to secondary arthritis
- Synovial fluid examination under microscopic examination shows needle shaped birefringent crystals of sodium urate
- Hyperuricemia leads to increased excretion of uric acid through the kidneys, so uric acid crystals gets deposited in the urinary tract leading to renal calculi.

Treatment

- Dietary purine intake should be reduced, alcohol should be restricted
- Uricosuric drugs which increases the excretion of uric acid like probenecid should be used
- For calculi allopurinol can be used. It inhibits xanthine oxidase and reduces the formation of uric acid. It is a type of suicide inhibition where the enzyme becomes completely functionless
- Colchicine, an anti-inflammatory drug used in RA can be used to reduce inflammation in joints.

Lesch-Nyhan Syndrome

- It is an X-linked inborn error of purine metabolism. Incidence 1:10,000
- Due to complete deficiency of HGPRTase which is a purine salvage pathway enzyme
- So the salvage pathway is stopped and PRPP accumulates which will go for increased purine synthesis and catabolism of purines to uric acid
- Hyperuricemia leads to nephrolithiasis and gout develops in later life.

It is also characterized by self-mutilation, mental retardation.

19. Secondary structure of proteins.

Refer 2007 Shor Note 25.

20. Transmethylation.

Refer 2007 Essay Question 4.

21. Functions of vitamin C.

Refer 2005 Essay Question 5.

22. Digestion and absorption of lipids (TAG).

Stomach

a. Lingual lipase—it acts on short chain TAG present in milk, butter and ghee
b. Gastric lipase—it is acid stable. pH is 5.4 and it digests 30% of TAG.

Intestine

a. Pancreatic lipase with colipase hydrolyses the fatty acids in 1st and 3rd carbon atoms of glycerol forming 2 monoacylglycerol and 2 fatty acids **(Fig. 19)**
b. Colipase is secreted from pancreas. It binds to TAG at the oil water interface.

Absorption of TAG (Bergstorm Theory)

- Digestory products of lipids, such as 2 monoacylglycerol, long chain fatty acids, cholesterol and phospholipid are incorporated to form mixed micelle with

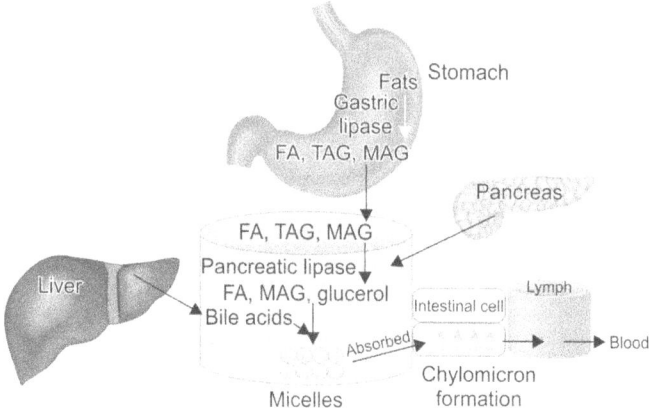

Fig. 19: Digestion of lipids.

the help of bile salts. Micelles are spherical particles with hydrophilic exterior and hydrophobic interior
- Micelles are aligned at the microvillous surface of jejunal mucosa and they diffuse passively into the mucosal cells
- Bile salts are reabsorbed from ileum and returned to liver for re-excretion— enterohepatic circulation
- Inside the mucosal cells long chain fatty acids are re-esterified to form TAG (Fig. 20).

Formation of Chylomicrons

- TAG, cholesterol ester and phospholipid molecules along with apoB48 and apoA are incorporated into chylomicrons and transported through lacteals to enter into lymphatic circulation via thoracic duct
- Chylomicrons transported through lacteals into the thoracic duct and then into lymph circulation.

23. Hemoglobin S.

- **Sickle cell disease—it is also called as HbS disease**
- Prevalence—1 in 1 lakh birth
- Molecular basis of disease—the genes for alpha chain and beta chains of Hb reside on chromosome numbers 16 and 11, respectively. Mutation in these genes gives different forms of Hb. In HbS case, due to mutations in gene in 11th chromosome,

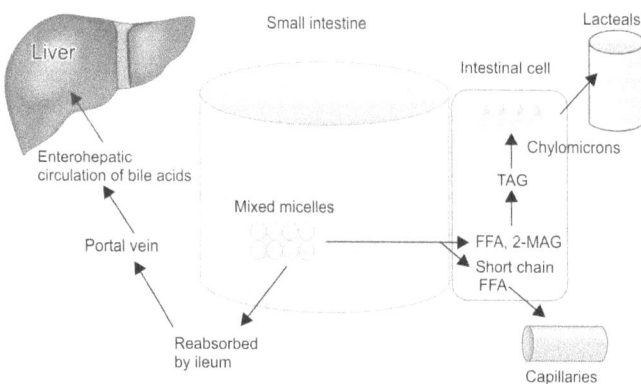

Fig. 20: Absorption of TAG.

there is displacement of glutamate with valine at 6th position of beta chain. The substitution of hydrophilic glutamic acid by hydrophobic valine causes a localized stickiness on the surface of the molecule. The deoxygenated HbS may be with protrusion on one side and cavity on the other side, so that many molecules can adhere and polymerise. This leads to the structural changes in RBC into sickle shape
- **Symptoms**—sickled cells form small plugs in capillaries. Occlusion of major vessels can lead to infarction of affected organs. Death will occur in second decade of life. HbS gives protection against malaria

Laboratory Diagnostic Procedures

- **Electrophoresis**—electrophoresis at alkaline pH shows a slower moving band than HbA. At this pH carboxyl group of glutamic acid is negatively charged. But lack of this charge on HbS makes it less negatively charged, and decreases the mobility towards positive pole. In acidic pH HbS moves faster than HbA
- **Sickling test**—blood smear is prepared and reducing agent, such as sodium dithinite is added and RBCs are observed for sickling under light microscope.

Management

Blood transfusion (overload the iron), antisickling agents like urea, cyanate and aspirin which interfere with polymerization.

24. Isoenzymes.
Refer 2003 Short Note 5.

25. Structure of cell membrane.
Refer 2008 Short Note 5.

26. Define BMR. What are the factors that can affect BMR?
Refer 2005 Short Note 26.

27. Define oxidative phosphorylation. Explain chemiosmotic theory.
Refer 2006 Short Note 5.

28. Galactosemia.
Refer 2005 Short Note 7.

29. Ketogenesis.
Refer 2005 Essay Question 2.

30. Glucose tolerance test.

This is a well standardized test which is highly useful to diagnose diabetes mellitus in doubtful cases. The ability of a person to metabolize a given load of glucose is referred to as glucose tolerance. Usually an oral glucose tolerance test is performed in the clinical laboratory.

Indications

- Patient has suggestive symptoms of diabetes mellitus but has inconclusive values of fasting blood sugar
- During pregnancy—excessive weight gaining, past history of big baby or miscarriage
- To rule out benign renal glycosuria.

Preparation of patient:

The patient is instructed to do following ways:
- To take normal carbohydrate diet for three days prior to the test
- To avoid drugs which influence the blood glucose level at least for 2 days prior to the test
- Not to do strenuous exercise on the previous day
- Not to take food after 8 PM the previous night to ensure 12 hours fasting
- Not to smoke during the test
- To report at the laboratory at 8 AM sharp in empty stomach.

Procedure

A sample of blood (2 mL) and urine sample are collected in the fasting state. Then the patient is given a glucose load of 75 g dissolved in a glass of water which the patient should drink slowly. The glucose water may be flavored to reduce the tendency to vomit. The blood and urine samples are collected at half an hour intervals for the next two and a half hours. Glucose is estimated in all blood samples and urine samples are tested for glucose by Benedict's qualitative test. A graph is plotted with blood glucose concentration on the Y-axis and the time in hours in the X-axis.

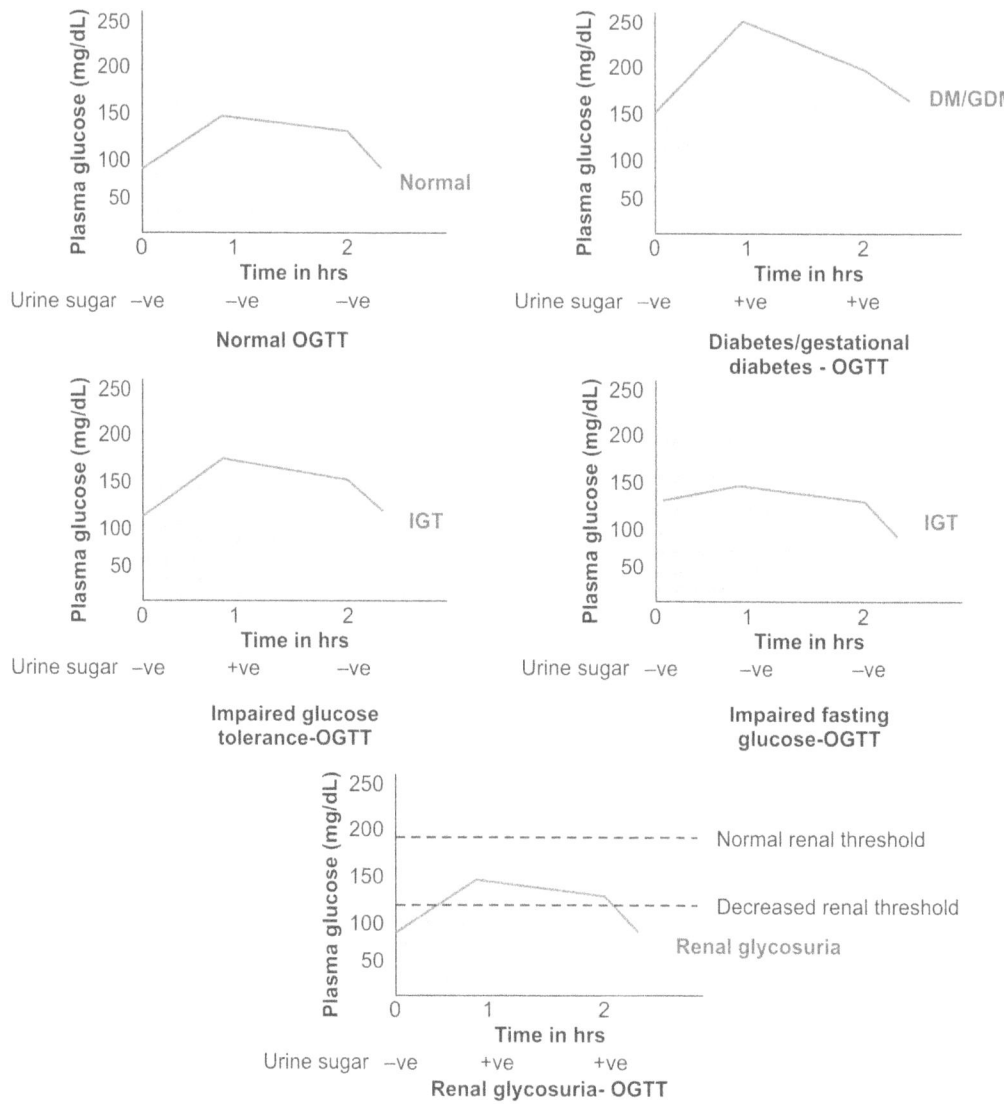

Fig. 21: Various types of glucose tolerance tests.

Types of GTT
- Oral
- Intravenous (for suspected cases of malabsorption)
- Corticosteroid stressed GTT to detect any latent diabetes.

Interpretation of GTT

Normal GTT (Fig. 21)
- Fasting blood sugar value is between 80–100 mg%
- The glucose level rises sharply and a peak is reached at 1 hour
- The blood glucose level comes to normal in 2 hours
- All the urine samples are negative for glucose.

31. Transamination reactions.
Refer 2008 Short Note 14.

32. Renal regulation of pH.
Refer 2005 Essay Question 4.

33. Gout.
Refer 2005 Short Note 17.

34. Mutation.
An alteration in genetic material results in mutation. Change in nucleotide sequence of DNA. Out of every 10^6 cell divisions, one mutation occurs.

Types
- Point mutation
- Silent mutation
- Mis-sense mutation—acceptable, partially acceptable and unacceptable
- Nonsense terminator codon mutation
- Frame shift mutation.

Point Mutation

Single base change/single nucleotide change.
- Transition—pyrimidine is changed to pyrimidine and purine is changed to purine **(Fig. 22)**
- Transversion: Change from purine to any one of pyrimidine and change of pyrimidine to any one of purines **(Fig. 22)**.

Silent Mutation

Type of point mutation where there will be no detectable effect.

Missense Mutation

Point mutation leading to the formation of another defective amino acid to get a defective protein. It has three types:
1. Acceptable – Hb (hikari) – Beta chain 61 Lys – asparagines—no functional consequences
2. Partially acceptable – HbS – partial abnormal function – Beta 6 Glu to valine
3. Unacceptable missense- Nonfunctioning protein – HbM – a 58 His – tyrosine.

Nonsense Terminator Codon Mutation

For examples, beta thalassemia—the codon for tyrosine UAC is mutated to a terminator codon–UAA/UAG—result in premature termination.

Frame shift Mutation

Due to deletion or insertion of nucleotides in mRNA to generate altered mRNAs which produce garbled proteins.

35. Differences between DNA and RNA.

S.No.	Characteristics	DNA	RNA
1.	Monomeric units	A,G,C, and thymidylate	A,G,C, and uridylate
2.	Sugar	Deoxyribose	Ribose
3.	Nature of strand/s	Double stranded helix	Single stranded
4.	Base pairs	A=T; G≡C	A= U; G≡C
5.	Types	A-DNA; B-DNA; Z- DNA	mRNA, tRNA, rRNA, snRNA
6.	Function	Carry genetic information. Synthesis of RNA transcription	Involved in the synthesis of proteins translation
7.	Alkali hydrolysis	Not possible	Possible due to presence of OH group in 2' position

36. Oncogenes.
Refer 2005 Short Note 20.

37. Post-translational modification.
Refer 2006 Short Note 27.

38. Formation of creatine.
Creatine and creatinine are the nonprotein nitrogenous substances present in normal urine. They are synthesized from three amino acids namely—arginine, glycine and methionine. The synthesis occurs in kidney, liver and muscles **(Fig. 23)**.

Synthesis of Creatine from Glycine
- **At the mitochondria of kidney**—glycine combines with arginine and the methyl group is transferred from arginine to glycine to form guanidoacetic acid and ornithine by an amido transferase.
- **At liver**—guanidoacetic acid receives a methyl group from S-adenosyl methionine (SAM) to form creatine

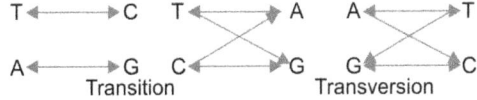

Fig. 22: Types of point mutation.

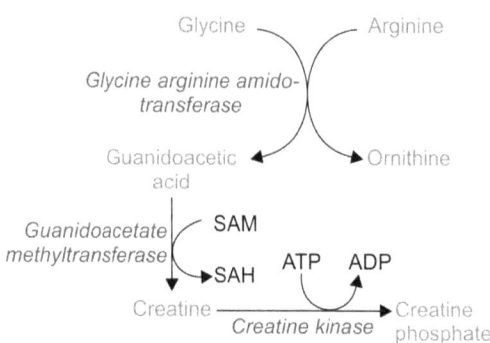

Fig. 23: Synthesis of creatine.

- **In the muscles**—creatine kinase (CK) in muscles converts creatine to creatine phosphate which acts as a high energy molecule involved in resynthesis of ATP from ADP during muscle contraction. (Lohmann's reaction). It is the storage form of energy in muscles
- Creatine loses water to form creatinine which is excreted by the kidneys by a nonenzymatic spontaneous reaction.

Clinical Application

- Normal serum level of creatinine is 0.7–1.4 mg/dL; serum creatine is 0.2–0.4 mg/dL
- Serum creatinine is a marker of renal failure. Creatinine clearance test is used to measure GFR.

39. Alkaptonuria.
Refer 2004 Short Note 11.

40. Southern blotting.
Refer 2005 Short Note 38.

III. SHORT ANSWER QUESTIONS

1. Name the essential fatty acids.
Essential fatty acids are those which cannot be synthesized by the body but have to be supplemented in the diet. They are polyunsaturated fatty acids. They are:
1. Linoleic acid (18°C) - ω6
2. Linolenic acid (18°C) - ω3
3. Arachidonic acid (20°C) - ω6—it can be formed if the dietary supply of linolenic acid is sufficient. So it cannot be strictly categorized under essential fatty acid.

2. Significance of HMP shunt pathway.
Refer 2005 Short Note 2.

3. Benedict's test.
- This reaction is commonly used to find out the presence of glucose in urine to diagnose a case of diabetes mellitus
- In alkaline medium sugars form enediols which reduce the cupric ions (Cu^{2+}) present in copper sulfate to cuprous ion (Cu^+) to form yellow precipitate of cuprous hydroxide or red precipitate of cuprous oxide
- 0.5 mL of glucose solution is boiled with 5 mL of Benedict's reagent for 2 minutes and then allowed to cool. Copper is reduced to produce green, yellow, orange or red precipitate depending upon the concentration of sugar. It is a semi-quantitative test **(Fig. 24)**.

Components of Benedict's reagent and their role

Benedict's reagent contains:
- Sodium carbonate to provide alkaline medium
- Copper sulfate for the reduction of copper ions
- Sodium citrate—Stabilising agent.

4. Inhibitors of citric acid cycle.
- Aconitase:
  - Inhibited by fluroacetate
  - It is a noncompetitive inhibition

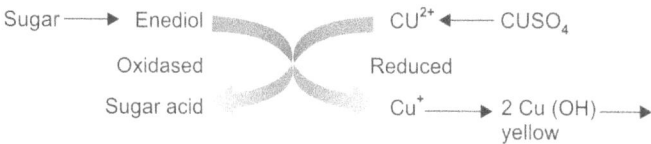

Fig. 24: Principle of Benedict's test.

- α-ketoglutarate dehydrogenase:
  - Inhibited by arsenite
  - It is a noncompetitive inhibition
- Succinate dehydrogenase:
  - By malonate
  - It is a competitive inhibitor.

5. Chloride shift.

- Hb is the major blood buffer in RBCs and it acts along with bicarbonate system
- It has 38 histidine residues
- **In the tissue level:** The oxyHb releases O_2 to the tissues which is facilitated by low pO_2, low pH and high pCO_2 and CO_2 produced is returned to the lungs carried by Hb where CO_2 is eliminated in expired air
- **In the RBC:** CO_2 is converted to carbonic acid by carbonic anhydrase resulting in decrease in pH and Hb becomes deoxy-Hb
- DeoxyHb neutralizes carbonic acid to increase the pH and there will be increase in bicarbonate and decrease in pCO_2
- To maintain electroneutrality, chloride ions enter into RBC for each bicarbonate ion leaves. This is called **Chloride shift (Fig. 25)**.

6. Functions of calcium.

Refer 2007 Essay Question 6.

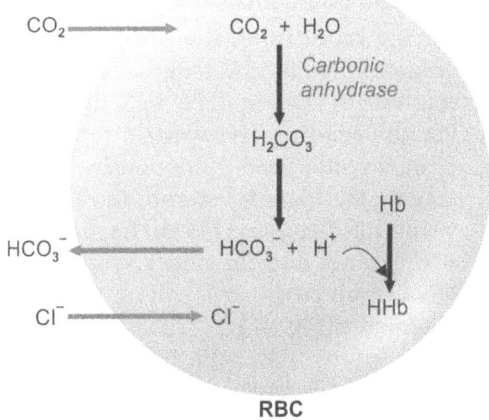

Fig. 25: Chloride shift.

7. Lipotropic factors.

Fatty liver can be prevented by taking lipotropic factors, such as choline, lecithin, methionine, vitamin E, selenium and omega-3 fatty acids.

Lipotropic Factors

They are choline, lecithin, methionine, vitamin E, selenium and omega-3 fatty acids. They are required for the normal mobilization of fat from liver. When they are deficient fat gets deposited in liver causing fatty liver.

Mode of Actions

- Choline—it reverses fatty changes in liver
- Lecithin and methionine—they help to synthesize apoproteins and choline
- Selenium and vitamin E-antioxidants
- Omega-3 fatty acids—present in marine oils and also has a protective action.

8. Normal blood levels of: 1. Cholesterol, 2. Bilirubin, 3. Sodium, 4. Potassium.

Total cholesterol	140-200 mg/dL
Bilirubin (unconjugated)	*0.2-0.6 mg/dL*
Bilirubin (conjugated)	0-0.2 mg/dL
Sodium	136-145 mmol/L
Potassium	3.5-5 mmol/L

9. Phospholipids.

Refer 2004 Short Notes 1.

10. Fluorosis.

- Excessive intake of fluoride (more than 2 ppm) is toxic to the body
- The manifestations include mottling of enamel, stratification and discoloration of teeth (more than 5 ppm)—dental fluorosis
- In the advanced stages (more than 20 ppm), hypercalcification of limb bones and ligaments of spine get calcified leading to crippling of the individual—skeletal fluorosis
- These manifestations are collectively referred to as fluorosis
- A level more than 20 ppm is toxic leading to fluorosis, which causes osteoporosis, osteosclerosis and brittle bones. Genu

valgum is the characteristic feature. Fluorosis leads to blood concentration of fluoride of 50 µg/dL.

Prevention of Fluorosis

- To drink fluoride free water
- To avoid intake of jowar rich in fluoride.
- To restrict in using fluoride containing toothpaste
- Vitamin C supplementation.

11. Name the buffer systems of blood.

Buffers resist changes in pH when small quantities of an acid or an alkali are added. Various buffers in blood are:
- Bicarbonate buffer system
- Phosphate buffer system
- Protein buffer system.

Bicarbonate Buffer System

(Bicarbonate carbonic acid system) ($NaHCO_3$/H_2CO_3)—it is the most important buffer in plasma and it accounts for 65% of buffering capacity in plasma.

12. Sources of carbon and nitrogen in purine ring.

Sources of Carbon and Nitrogen in Purine ring (Fig. 26)

- **N1**—aspartate
- **C2**—formyltetrahydrofolic acid
- **N3, N9**—glutamine
- **C 4, C5, N7**—glycine
- **C6**—respiratory CO_2
- **C8**—methenyltetrahydrofolic acid.

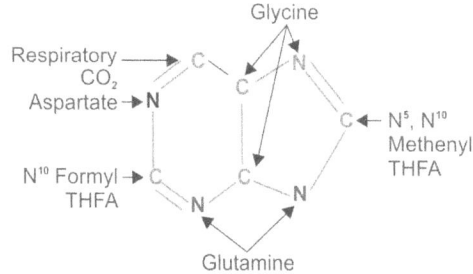

Fig. 26: Sources of carbon and nitrogen in purine ring.

13. Wobble hypothesis.

- 61 codons code for 20 amino acids. Thus, there must be "degeneracy" in the genetic code—multiple codons must decode the same amino acid
- The degeneracy of the genetic code resides mostly in the last nucleotide of the codon. 1 triplet suggesting that the base pairing between this last nucleotide and the corresponding nucleotide of the anticodon is not strictly by the Watson-Crick rule. This is called wobble hypothesis
- For example, the two codons for arginine, AGA and AGG, can bind to the same anticodon having a uracil at its 5'end (UCU). Similarly, three codons for glycine—GGU, GGC, and GGA—can form a base pair from one anticodon, CCI.

14. Write the enzyme defect in: (1) Lesch-Nyhan Syndrome (2) Orotic aciduria.

1. **Lesch-Nyhan syndrome**—it is a X-linked inborn error of purine metabolism complete deficiency of (hypoxanthine-guanine phosphoribosyltransferase) (HGPRTase) which acts in purine salvage pathway
2. **Orotic aciduria**—autosomal recessive condition
   - This condition results from absence of either or both the enzymes orotate phosphoribosyl transferase (ORPTase) and OMP decarboxylase of pyrimidine synthetic pathway.

15. Okazaki fragments.

- During replication, the polymerase III holoenzyme binds to template DNA and synthesizes DNA in the 5' to 3' direction. On the leading (forward) strand, the DNA is synthesized continuously. On the lagging (retrograde) strand, the DNA is synthesized in short (1–5 kb) fragments
- RNA primer and the newly synthesized DNA molecules are called **Okazaki fragments (Fig. 27)**
- After many Okazaki fragments are generated, the replication complex begins to remove the RNA primers and the gaps are filled with the proper base paired

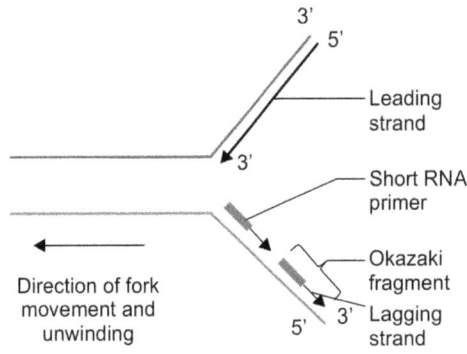

Fig. 27: Okazaki fragments.

deoxynucleotides, the fragments of newly synthesized DNA are joined by the enzyme DNA ligases.

16. What are xenobiotics?

Xenobiotics are strange or foreign compounds which are antigens which may be accidentally ingested or taken as drugs or compounds produced in the body by bacterial metabolism.

Various Xenobiotics
- Compounds accidentally ingested like preservatives, food additives and adulterants
- Drugs taken for therapeutic purposes
- Endogenous compounds which has to be eliminated by the body like bilirubin, steroids
- Compounds produced by bacterial metabolism, e.g. amines produced by decarboxylation of amino acids like histamine from histidine; cadaverine from lysine; putrescine from ornithine; tyramine from tyrosine and trytamine from tryptophan.

Detoxification
It is the process by which these xenobiotics are detoxified in the body which occurs in 2 phases.

17. Causes of metabolic acidosis.

Refer 2004 Short Note 16.

Causes of High anion gap metabolic acidosis—accumulation of acid
- Renal failure—H⁺ excretion is less.
- DKA—keto acid production is more
- Lactic acidosis—hypoxia, circulatory failure, many drugs, and bacterial metabolism increases lactic acid
- Methanol, ethanol also causes lactic acidosis.

Causes of Normal anion gap metabolic acidosis both anions and cations lost but acidosis present
- Diarrhea—loss of bicarbonate from intestinal secretions
- Hyperchloremic metabolic acidosis in renal tubular acidosis which may be due to either failure to secrete acid or conserve bicarbonate; acetazolamide treatment.

18. Name the important compounds formed from glycine.

Metabolic Products
- Methylenetetrahydrofolate by glycine cleavage system to join one-carbon pool
- Glucose—it is a glucogenic amino acid.

Special Products
- Creatine, creatine phosphate and creatinine
- Heme
- Purine nucleotides
- Glutathione
- Conjugating agent
- Constituent of most of the proteins are more in collagen.

19. Inhibitors of protein biosynthesis.

Reversible Inhibitors in Prokaryotes

a. **Antibiotics—bacteriostatic**
- Tetracyclins—bind to 30S, prevents attachment of aminoacyl tRNA—to the ribosomal acceptor site
- Chloromycetin—inhibits peptidyl transferase
- Erythromycin and clindamycin—prevents translocation.

b. **Bactericidal antibiotics**
- Aminoglycosides
  - Streptomycin is irreversible inhibitor of 30S ribosomes
  - Low concentration—misreading mRNA

- Pharmacological concentration—prevents initiation complex; total inhibition of translation.

Inhibitors—Eukaryotes

- Cycloheximide—inhibits both human and bacterial peptidyl transferase (60S)
- Diphtheria toxin—Inactivates → eEF2 by attaching ADP to eEF2; prevents translocation
- Ricin toxin (Castor bean seed)—inhibts translation.

Inhibitors—Prokaryotes and Eukaryotes

- Puromycin—structural analog of tyrosinyl tRNA incorporated into the peptide chain causing inhibition of elongation in both prokaryotes and eukaryotes
- It acts as a research tool.

20. Apoptosis.

- For growth and differentiation, old cells need to be destroyed. Removal of aged or damaged cells is done by the process of apoptosis. It is also called programed cell death
- The term literally means 'dropping off'
- Stress and other stimuli like apoptotic gene products can activate apoptosis
- *Caspases, p53, c-fos, Rb* are genes responsible for apoptosis
- Antiapoptotic gene is *bcl-2*
- Free radical damage causes increased permeability of mitochondria
- This leads to mitochondrial swelling and leads to release of cytochrome C. This acts as a trigger for apoptosis
- Nuclear shrinkage, chromatin condensation, membrane blebbing occurs during apoptosis.

MBBS Examination 2009

ANSWER ALL QUESTIONS

I. **Essay questions** (10/15 Marks each)
1. a. Sources and fate of acetyl-CoA, explain the de novo synthesis of cholesterol and its regulation.
   b. De novo synthesis of cholesterol and its regulation.
2. Explain a) How pyruvate enters the Kreb's citric acid cycle for oxidation? b) How many ATPs are produced in this pathway?
3. Name the compounds derived from glycine. Explain any two in detail.
4. Describe in detail the mechanism of regulation of blood pH.
5. What are porphyrias? Classify different types of porphyrias and give the enzyme defect and biochemical findings.
6. What is oxidative phosphorylation? Discuss the steps of the same and mention its significance.
7. Name liver function tests with diagnostic significance of each. Write in detail the biochemical tests of any three done in your laboratory.
8. Describe the pathway for synthesis of urea from ammonia. What is normal blood urea level? Name the conditions in which blood urea level is increased and give the biochemical basis.

II. **Short notes** (5 Marks each)
1. Write a note on chemiosmotic theory. (hypothesis).
2. Active transport.
3. Uronic acid pathway.
4. Insulin.
5. Wald's visual cycle.
6. Collagen.
7. Glycosaminoglycans.
8. Chromatography.
9. Levels of organization of proteins.
10. Calcium homeostasis.
11. Phenylketonuria.
12. Formation of uric acid.
13. Porphyria.
14. Urea cycle.
15. ELISA.
16. Active methionine.
17. Flame photometer.
18. Bilirubin formation and excretion.
19. Plasma proteins.
20. Replication.
21. Classify RNA and explain the functions.
22. Hyperuricemia.
23. Renal glycosuria.
24. Cardiac troponin (CTI/CTT).
25. Structure of cholesterol and its importance in the body.
26. Beriberi.
27. Enzyme poisons.
28. Flurosis.
29. What is protein-energy malnutrition (PEM)? What are the types of PEM? Write the importance features.
30. Functions of vitamin C.
31. Denaturation.
32. Reverse transcription.
33. Sphingolipidoses.
34. Gout.
35. Metabolic acidosis.
36. Tumor markers.
37. Colorimeter.
38. Functions of adrenal cortical hormones.
39. Plasmid.
40. Functions of albumin.

III. Short answer questions
(2/3 Marks each)
1. Key enzymes of glycolysis.
2. Fatty liver.
3. Lipid peroxidation.
4. Zymogens.
5. BMR.
6. Normal levels of: i) BUN ii) Fasting serum glucose iii) LDH iv) ALT.
7. tRNA.
8. Vitamin K.
9. Limiting amino acid.
10. Isoenzymes.
11. Detoxification by conjugation.
12. Glutathione.
13. Metabolic acidosis.
14. Codons.
15. Renal function test.
16. Orotic aciduria.
17. Wobble hypothesis.
18. Van den Bergh's test.
19. Rickets.
20. γ-Globulins.
21. Effect of temperature on enzyme activity.
22. Define epimer. Name two epimers.
23. Phosphatidylinositol importance.
24. Biochemical functions of selenium.
25. Benedict's test.
26. Ribose and deoxyribose.
27. Lysosomes.
28. Bence Jones protein.
29. Bile salts.
30. Cori cycle.
31. Maple syrup urine disease.
32. Alkali reserve.
33. Biological value of proteins.
34. Carcinogenic virus.
35. Electrophoretic technique and its importance.
36. Methemoglobin.
37. Importance of glucose-6-phosphate dehydrogenase deficiency.
38. G proteins.
39. Renal threshold substances.
40. Carbon monoxide.

I. ESSAY QUESTIONS

1. a. Sources and fate of acetyl-CoA, explain the de novo synthesis of cholesterol and its regulation.

Sources of Acetyl-CoA (Fig. 1)
- Pyruvate derived from aerobic glycolysis is oxidatively decarboxylated to acetyl-CoA by pyruvate dehydrogenase in mitochondria
- Beta-oxidation of even chain fatty acids like palmitic acid (16°C) and stearic acid (18°C) will produce acetyl-CoA occurs in mitochondria
- Carbon skeleton of ketogenic amino acids like phenylalanine, tyrosine, leucine are catabolized to produce acetyl-CoA.

Fate of Acetyl-CoA
- **TCA cycle**—two carboned acetyl-CoA enter into the citric acid cycle in the mitochondria and condenses with 4C oxaloacetate and completely oxidized to produce energy in the form of ATP and CO_2 and water. It is the final common oxidative pathway of all the foodstuffs
- **Synthesis of fatty acids**—acetyl-CoA enters into the cytoplasm through the inner membrane of mitochondria as citrate by ATP citrate lyase to synthesize fatty acids (de novo synthesis) with the help of NADPH.

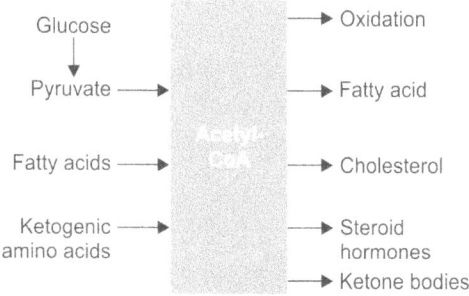

Fig. 1: Sources of acetyl-CoA.

- **Ketone body synthesis**—during starvation and other conditions like uncontrolled diabetes mellitus: Three molecules of acetyl-CoA condense to form ketone bodies are: Acetone, acetoacetate, beta-hydroxybutyrate occurs in cytoplasm
- **Cholesterol synthesis**—three molecules of acetyl-CoA are condensed to form cholesterol by reductive synthesis with the help of NADPH. In adrenal cortex and in reproductive organs like testes, ovaries cholesterol is converted to steroid and sex hormones, respectively
- **Acetylcholine formation**—acetyl-CoA combines with choline to form acetylcholine which is a neurotransmitter in brain and in nerve synapses
- **Detoxication**—acetyl-CoA acts as a detoxifying agent to detoxify sulfonamide drugs by acetylation
- **Acetylation** of amino sugars for **glycoprotein synthesis**
- **Acetylation** of neuramnic acid to synthesise gangliosides
- **N-acetylglutamate** (NAG) acts as an activator of the rate-limiting enzyme of urea cycle—carbamoyl phosphate synthetase I.

b. **Explain the De novo synthesis of cholesterol and Its regulation.**

Refer 2004 Essay Question 2.

2. **Explain a) How pyruvate enters the Kreb's citric acid cycle for oxidation? b) How many ATPs are produced in this pathway?**

ENTRY OF PYRUVATE INTO KREB'S CYCLE

Pyruvate the end product of aerobic glycolysis in the cytosol is converted to acetyl-CoA by the action of the multi-enzyme pyruvate dehydrogenase (PDH) complex.

Conversion of Pyruvate to Acetyl-CoA by PDH (Fig. 2)

The 3 enzymes present in pyruvate dehydrogenase complex are:
1. **Pyruvate Decarboxylase (enzyme I)**—it catalyses oxidative decarboxylation with the help of TPP as its coenzyme. Hydroxyethyl TPP is formed
2. **Dihydrolipoyl transacetylase (enzyme 2)**—the hydroxyethyl group of TPP is oxidized to acetyl group by this enzyme and then acetyl group is transferred from TPP to lipoamide to form acetyl-lipoamide
3. **Dihydrolipoyl dehydrogenase (enzyme 3)**—this enzyme oxidizes lipoamide and at the end all the cofactors are reformed
- The coenzymes of pyruvate dehydrogenase are 5 in number—NAD$^+$, FAD, CoA, lipoic acid and TPP

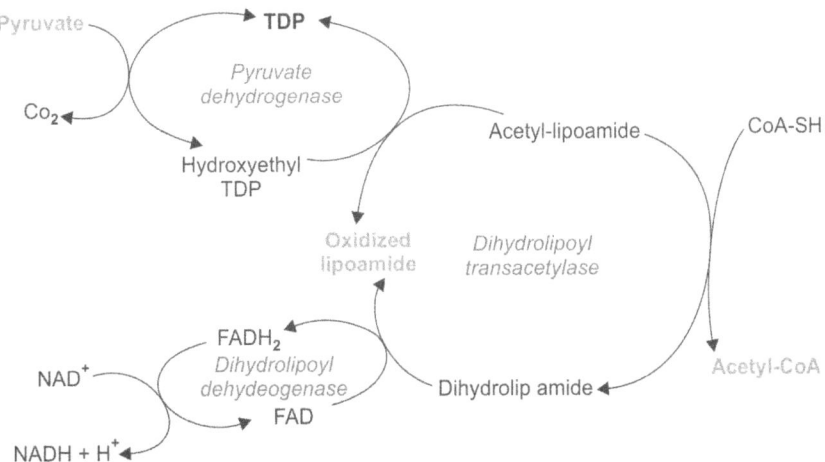

Fig. 2: Pyruvate dehydrogenase complex.

- Thus pyruvate is converted to acetyl-CoA and enters into TCA cycle.

TCA Cycle

Refer 2004 Essay Question 1
- The TCA cycle is a series of reactions in mitochondria that oxidize acetyl residues and reduce coenzymes which on re-oxidation are linked to the formation of ATP
- **Other name**—*citric acid cycle or Kreb's cycle or tricarboxylic acid cycle*
- **Intracellular location**—mitochondria.

Steps of TCA Cycle (Fig. 3)

Preparatory phase:
Acetyl-CoA enters into the TCA cycle in the mitochondria and joins with 4C oxaloacetate which is considered as a catalyst

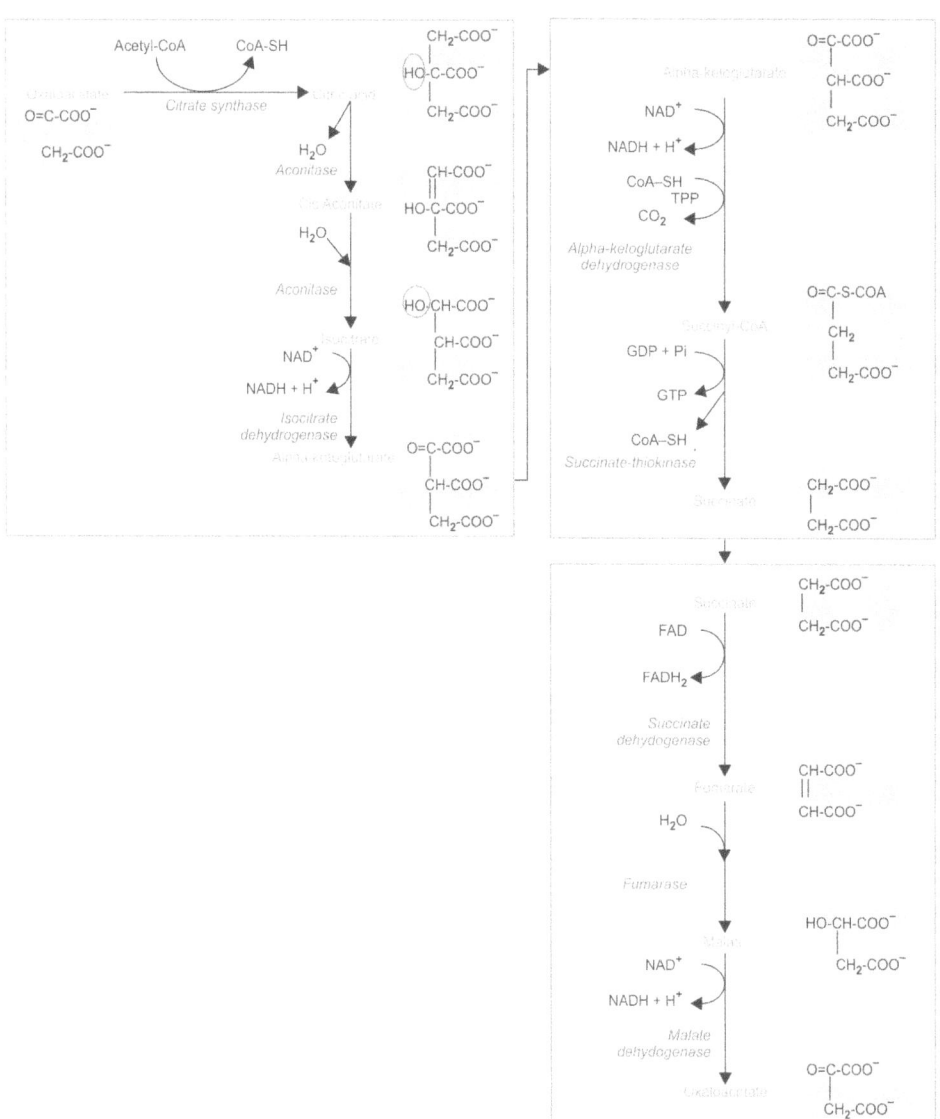

Fig. 3: Steps of TCA cycle.

Sources of acetyl-CoA:
- Glycolysis (aerobic) ends in pyruvate. Then pyruvate → acetyl-CoA
- Beta oxidation of fatty acid → acetyl-CoA
- Ketogenic amino acids → acetyl-CoA.

Step 1: Formation of citric acid
- Oxaloacetate condenses with acetyl-CoA to form citrate
- It is catalyzed by citrate synthase
- It is an irreversible step.

Step 2: Formation of isocitrate
- Citrate is isomerized to isocitrate by aconitase
- Here the intermediate is cis-aconitate
- It is a reversible step.

Step 3: Formation of α-ketoglutarate
- Isocitrate is dehydrogenated to form oxalosuccinate
- It is unstable and undergoes spontaneous decarboxylation to form α-Ketoglutarate (α-KG). It is catalyzed by isocitrate dehydrogenase. NADH generated enters into ETC to generate ATP (2-5).

Step 4: Formation of succinyl-CoA
- α-KG is oxidatively decarboxylated to form succinyl-CoA by α-Ketoglutarate dehydrogenase
- It is a multienzyme complex with 3 subunits. It is an irreversible step. NADH enters into ETC. Five coenzymes are needed—NAD$^+$, FAD, TPP, CoA, lipoate.

Step 5: Generation of succinate (substrate level phosphorylation)
- This reaction is an example for substrate level phosphorylation
- Succinyl-CoA → succinate
- It is catalyzed by succinate thiokinase.

Step 6: Formation of fumarate
- Succinate is dehydrogenated to fumarate by succinate dehydrogenase
- Oxidative phosphorylation is through FAD to produce 1.5 ATP.

Step 7: Formation of malate
- Fumarate to malate conversion is done by fumarase.

Step 8: Regeneration of oxaloacetate
- Finally malate is oxidized to oxaloacetate by malate dehydrogenase
- Malate → oxaloacetate → acetyl-CoA
- Oxaloacetate acts as a catalyst which again joins with another molecule of acetyl-CoA to continue another cycle.

Significance
- Complete oxidation of acetyl-CoA
- ATP generation
- Final common oxidative pathway
- Anaplerotic role.

Energetics

Step No.	Reactions	Coenzyme	ATP (old calculation)	ATP (new calculation)
3	Isocitrate to α-KG	NADH	3	2.5
4	α-KG to succinyl-CoA	NADH	3	2.5
5	Succinyl-CoA to succinate	GTP	1	1
6	Succinate to fumarate	FADH$_2$	2	1.5
8	Malate to oxaloacetate	NADH	3	2.5
Total ATP			12	10

Regulation
- Citrate synthase—inhibited by ATP (allosteric inhibitor)
- Isocitrate dehydrogenase—activated by ADP; inhibited by ATP and NADH
- α-KG dehydrogenase—inhibited by succinyl-CoA and NADH
- Availability of ADP—cellular need of ATP and availability of ADP inside the cells to regulate the TCA cycle.

3. **Name the compounds derived from glycine. Explain any two in detail.**

Refer 2004 Essay Question 3.
Glycine is the simplest, nonessential and glucogenic amino acid.

Synthesis of Glycine:
Glycine is derived from serine, threonine and from CO_2 and NH_3 by glycine synthase.

Compounds Formed from Glycine (Fig. 4)

- Creatine, creatine phosphate and creatinine (glycine + arginine + S-adenosyl methionine)
- Heme (glycine + succinyl-CoA)
- Purine bases and nucleotides—C4, C5 and N7
- Glutathione (Gamma-glutamylcysteinyl-glycine)
- Conjugation for xenobiotics
- Constituent of proteins like collagen (glycine + proline + hydroxyproline)
- Methylene tetrahydrofolate by glycine cleavage system
- Glucose—it is glucogenic.

Creatine Production from Glycine

- Creatine and creatinine are the non-protein nitrogenous substances present in normal urine. They are synthesized by 3 amino acids—arginine, glycine and methionine. The synthesis occurs in kidney, liver and muscles (Fig. 5)
- Normal serum level of creatinine is 0.7–1.4 mg/dL; serum creatine is 0.2–0.4 mg/dL
- Serum creatinine is a marker of renal failure. Creatinine clearance test is used to measure GFR.

Production of Heme

Succinyl-CoA combines with glycine catalyzed by the enzyme ALA synthase in the presence of the coenzyme pyridoxal phosphate in the mitochondria to form alpha-amino-beta-keto-adipic acid which is converted by the same enzyme to delta aminolevulinic acid. It is the rate-limiting step in heme synthesis (Fig. 6).

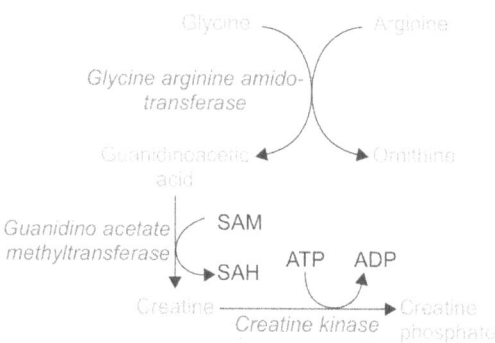

Fig. 5: Synthesis of creatine.

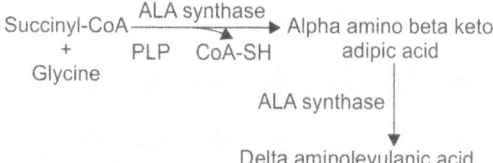

Fig. 6: Role of glycine in heme synthesis.

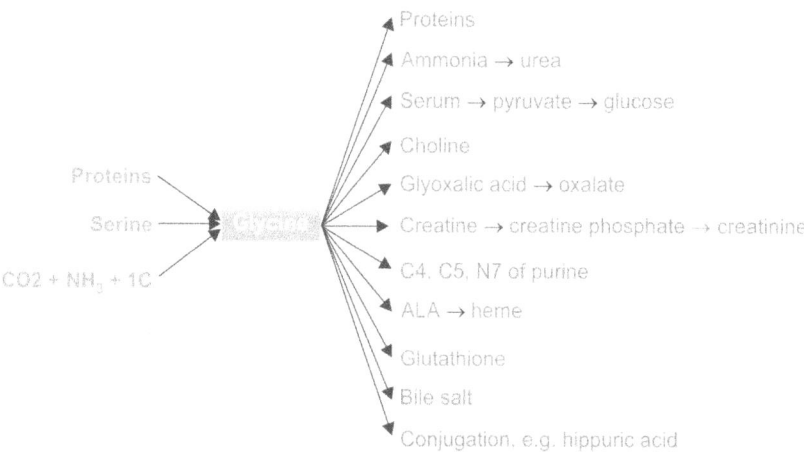

Fig. 4: Products derived from glycine.

4. **Describe in detail the mechanism of regulation of blood pH.**

Refer 2005 Essay Question 4.

5. **What are porphyrias? Classify different types of porphyrias and give the enzyme defect and biochemical findings.**

Refer 2008 Essay Question 2.
- Porphyrias are a group of inborn errors of metabolism associated with biosynthesis of heme. These are characterized by increased production and excretion of porphyrins and/or their precursors
- Congenital porphyrias are classified into: a. Hepatic b. Erythropoietic c. Hepato-erythropoietic **(Fig. 7)**.
    - **Hepatic porphyria:**
        - *Acute intermittent porphyria—uroporphyrinogen-I synthase*

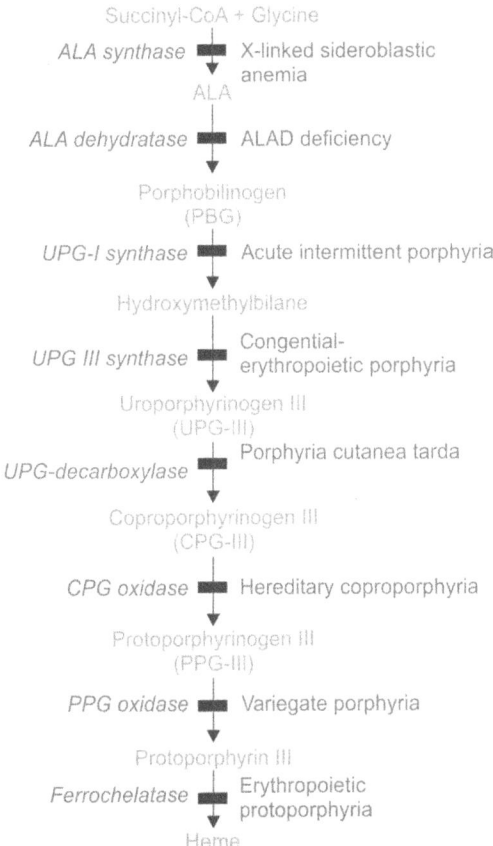

Fig. 7: Enzyme deficiencies in porphyrias.

deficiency **(AD):** This leads to secondary increase in activity of ALA. The levels of ALA and PBG are elevated in blood and urine. Urine is dark on voiding due to photo-oxidation of PBG to porphobilin. Symptoms appear intermittently. Patients will have acute abdominal pain. An attack is precipitated by starvation and symptoms are relieved by glucose infusion. Patients may have neurological abnormality like sensory and motor disturbances, agitation and confusion. Patients may have neuropsychiatric problems
- *Variegate porphyria*—protoporphyrinogen oxidase deficiency (AD):
    * Acute hepatic—1/100,000
    * Deficiency—protoporphyrinogen oxidase
    * Accumulation—urinary ALA, protoporphyrinogen IX, coproporphyrin-III
    * Scarring following photosensitive eruption
    * Photosensitivity, abdominal pain, neuropsychiatric **symptoms**.
- *Hereditary coproporphyria*—due to coproporphyrinogen-III oxidase deficiency (AD):
    * It is an autosomal dominant (AD) condition
    * Uroporphyrin and coproporphyrin are excreted in urine and in feces. Urine is colored
    * Symptoms are similar to acute intermittent porphyria but milder
    * Photosensitivity, abdominal pain, neuropsychiatric symptoms are present.
- *ALA dehydratase deficiency*:
    * Abdominal pain, neuropsychiatric symptoms present
    * Increased excretion of urinary ALA, coproporphyrin-III
- *Porphyria cutanea tarda (AD):*
    * Uroporphyrinogen decarboxylase deficiency

- Here patients are more prone for photosensitivity. The urobilinogens get accumulated and when patients come under light they spontaneously form urobilin which is a potent oxidant and destroys skin cells and causes scarring
- Patients have gross skin malformations leading to monster like appearance, and they prefer night. Sunscreens are mildly effective
- Uroporphyrins excreted in urine. It is colored urine.
  - **Erythropoietic:**
    - *Erythropoietic protoporphyria (AD) hereditary protoporphyria:*
      * Due to ferrochelatase deficiency or heme synthase
      * Autosomal dominant condition
      * Photosensitivity++
      * Porphyrins or their precursors are not excreted in urine
      * Protoporphyrin level—increased in plasma, RBCs and feces. RBCs show fluorescence.
    - *Congenital erythropoietic porphyria - AR*
      * Uroporphyrinogen-III synthase deficiency
      * Autosomal recessive disorder
      * Photosensitivity++
      * Dark urine—uroporphyrinogen I and coproporphyrinogen I—Urine—portwine appearance
      * Dermatitis and scarring—monkey faces, mutilation of nose, ear and cartilage
      * Erythrodontia
    - *ALA synthase deficiency*
      * Erythroid form
      * X-linked sideroblastic anemia
      * RBC count and Hb—decreased
    - *Protoporphyria*
- **Acquired porphyria:**
  - Due to lead poisoning
  - Drug induced—barbiturates, antifungal—grisofulvin
  - Due to inhibition of ferrochelatase
  - Associated anemia.

6. What is oxidative phosphorylation? Discuss the steps of the same and mention its significance.

Refer 2006 Short Note 5.

7. Name liver function tests with diagnostic significance of each. Write in detail the biochemical tests of any three done in your laboratory.

The tests used to diagnose liver disease are called liver function tests. They are:

1. Tests based on hepatic excretory function:
   a. Serum bilirubin
   b. Urine Bile pigments—bilirubin, bile salts, urobilinogen
   c. Fecal urobilinogen
   d. Dye excretion test—bromsulphophthalein (BSP) test.
2. Markers of liver injury—estimation of liver enzymes:
   a. Serum alanine aminotransferase (ALT)
   b. Serum aspartate aminotransferase (AST)
   c. Serum alkaline phosphatase (ALP)
   d. Serum gamma-glutamyl transferase (GGT).
3. Tests based on synthetic function: Synthesis of plasma proteins—estimation of:
   a. Total plasma proteins
   b. Serum albumin, globulin, A/G ratio
   c. Prothrombin time.
4. Special tests—estimation of:
   a. Ceruloplasmin
   b. Ferritin
   c. Alpha-1 antitrypsin (AAT)
   d. Alpha-fetoprotein (AFP).
5. Tests based on detoxification function—estimation of:
   a. Blood ammonia and bilirubin
   b. Hippuric acid test.

Explanation of three Tests in Detail

1. Synthetic function—total plasma proteins, serum albumin, globulins
   - Almost all plasma proteins with exception of immunoglobulins are

synthesized by liver. Normal total serum proteins level is 6 – 8 g/dL
- Albumin is quantitatively the most important protein synthesized by the liver, and reflects the extent of functioning liver cell mass. Normal albumin level is 2.5-3.5 g/dL
- In hepatocellular diseases hypoalbuminemia occurs
- Normal serum globulin level is 2-3.5 g/dL. In chronic inflammatory disorders, such as hepatitis and in cirrhosis of liver hyperglobulinemia will be present
- A/G ratio—since albumin has a half life of 20 days in all chronic diseases of liver, the albumin level is decreased. A reversal of A/G ratio is seen in cirrhosis of liver. Normal A/G ratio is 1.2: 1–2.5: 1
- Estimation of total proteins is done by Biuret method and serum albumin is estimated by bromocresol green method. Globulin is calculated by subtracting albumin values from total protein
- It is also estimated by doing electrophoresis of proteins and calculated by densitometry.

2. **Prothrombin time (synthetic function)**
   - Since prothrombin is synthesized by the liver, it is a useful indicator of liver function
   - The half life of prothrombin is 6 hours only. Therefore prothrombin time (PT) indicates the recent function of liver
   - PT is prolonged only when more than 80% of liver function is lost
   - In vitamin K deficiency PT is prolonged. To differentiate liver dysfunction from that of vitamin K deficiency, vitamin K is given to the patient and PT is measured. Elevated PT even after administration of vitamin K indicates liver dysfunction.

3. **van den Bergh test (hepatic excretory function)**
   - Estimation of Bilirubin
   - The serum bilirubin estimation is based on van den Bergh reaction in which diazotised sulfanilic acid reacts with bilirubin to form a purple colored complex, azobilirubin. Normal serum does not give a positive Van den Bergh test
   - When bilirubin is conjugated, the purple color is produced immediately on mixing with the reagent, the response is said to be van den Bergh direct positive
   - When the bilirubin is unconjugated, the color appears only after addition of alcohol, so it is said to be van den Bergh indirect positive
   - When both conjugated and unconjugated bilirubin are present, it produces an immediate color which intensifies on adding alcohol. It is then said to be biphasic
   - In hemolytic jaundice, unconjugated bilirubin is elevated so indirect positive
   - In obstructive jaundice, conjugated bilirubin is elevated, so direct positive
   - In hepatic jaundice, both conjugated and unconjugated bilirubin are elevated so it is biphasic.

8. **Describe the pathway for synthesis of urea from ammonia. What is normal blood urea level? Name the conditions in which blood urea level is increased and give the biochemical basis.**

Refer 2006 Essay Question 9.
- Urea is the end product of protein catabolism. It is synthesized in the liver mitochondria and cytoplasm. Ammonia and the alpha amino group of aspartic acid are the sources of the two nitrogen atoms of urea.
- The cycle is also called as Kreb's Henseleit urea cycle or Ornithine cycle
- First line of defence against ammonia is done by trapping of NH_3 by glutamic acid to form glutamine in the brain cells
- Second line of defence is by the formation of urea which is the end product of protein metabolism in liver.

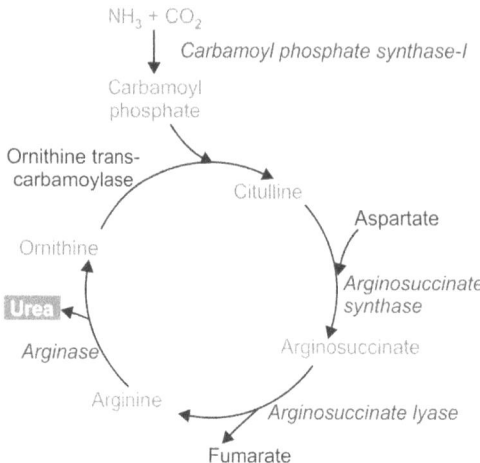

Fig. 8: Urea cycle.

Steps of Urea Formation (Fig. 8)

Site: In liver, first two steps of urea cycle are taken place in liver mitochondria and other steps are taken place in cytosol.

- **Step 1: Formation of carbamoyl phosphate**
  - One molecule of ammonia condenses with CO_2 in the presence of two molecules of ATP to form carbamoyl phosphate by the enzyme carbamoyl phosphate synthetase-I. (CPS-1). This occurs in liver mitochondria
  - This is the **rate-limiting step**. It is an irreversible step and regulated allostearically by N-acetylglutamate (NAG).
- **Step 2: Formation of citrulline:** Mitochondria
  - The carbamoyl group is transferred to the NH_2 group of ornithine by ornithine transcarbamoylase (OTC)
  - Citrulline enters into the cytoplasm to continue further reactions.
- **Step 3: Formation of argininosuccinate**
  - One molecule of aspartic acid adds to citrulline forming a carbon to nitrogen bond which provides second nitrogen of urea by argininosuccinate synthetase
  - Two high energy phosphate bonds are utilized.
- **Step 4: Formation of arginine**
  - Argininosuccinate is cleaved by argininosuccinate lyase (argininosuccinase) to arginine and fumarate. Fumarate inhibits this step
  - Fumarate enters into TCA cycle to be converted to malate which is then converted to oxaloacetate
  - Oxaloacetate is transaminated to aspartate. This is a link between TCA cycle and urea cycle.
- **Step 5: Formation of urea**
  - Hydrolysis of arginine gives rise to urea and ornithine by the enzyme arginase
  - Ornithine returns to the mitochondria to react with another molecule of carbamoyl phosphate to proceed the next cycle.

Urea Level in Blood

Normal blood urea level is 20-40 mg/dl. Urinary excretion of urea is 15-30 g/day

Urea level may be increased due to high protein intake and inborn errors of urea cycle. Increased blood urea level leads to uremia.

Causes for elevation in urea level

- Prerenal:
  - Increased protein breakdown after surgery, fever
  - Diabetic coma, thyrotoxicosis
  - Dehydration—vomiting, diarrhea
  - Intestinal obstruction
- Renal—acute glomerular nephritis, nephrosis, pyelonephritis, hypertension, polycystic kidney
- Postrenal—obstruction: Stones, stricture, enlarged prostate, tumor—growth in bladder.

II. SHORT NOTES

1. **Write a note on chemiosmotic theory. (hypothesis).**

Refer 2006 Short Note 5.

2. Active transport.

Plasma membrane regulates the passage of various biomolecules into the interior and to the exterior of cells. This is mediated by two types of transport mechanisms—active and passive transport (passive diffusion)

Active transport—movement of molecules across the membrane against concentration gradient with the help of energy is known as active transport.

Salient Features

- It requires energy in the form of ATP
- Transport is unidirectional
- It requires transporters which are integral proteins
- Saturated at higher concentration of solutes, e.g. sodium pump, calcium pump.

Two types of active transport

1. Primary active transport—sodium pump, calcium pump
2. Secondary active transport—cotransport (symport) and counter transport (antiport).

Primary Active Transport (Fig. 9)

Sodium Pump

- Cell has low sodium and high potassium. This is maintained by Na^+K^+ activated ATP are called as sodium pump. It pumps sodium ions out of the cell and potassium ions from outside to inside generating an electrochemical gradient.

Physiological importance of sodium/potassium pump:

- Cell volume is controlled by this pump
- Excitability of neurons and muscles is rendered by this process
- Sugars and amino acids are transported by this pump.

Clinical significance: Cardiac glycosides like digitonin and ouabain inhibit ATPase enzyme by inhibiting dephosphorylation. Digitalis is hence used in the treatment of congestive failure by enhancing the contractility of cardiac muscle.

Calcium pump

ATP dependent calcium pump functions to regulate muscle contraction through the sarcoplasmic reticulum found in skeletal muscles. Ca^{++} concentration is low in muscle fibers during resting condition. Sudden release of large amounts of Ca^{++} results by nervous stimulation causing muscle contraction. Two calcium ions are transported for each ATP hydrolysis.

Secondary Active Transport (Fig. 10)

- Here energy is provided by ATP indirectly for active transport of ions or molecules against concentration gradient
- Two types of secondary active transport are:
  1. Symport or cotransport
  2. Antiport or counter-transport
     1. Symport or cotransport system—transfer of one molecule depends on the simultaneous transfer of another molecule in the same direction, e.g. glucose and many amino acids are transported against concentration gradient by this mechanism
     2. Antiport or counter-transport system—transport of two solutes or ions in opposite direction, e.g. sodium-calcium counter-transport, sodium-hydrogen counter-transport,

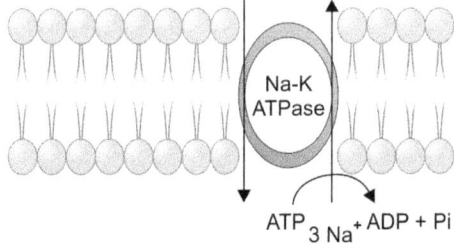

Fig. 9: Primary active transport.

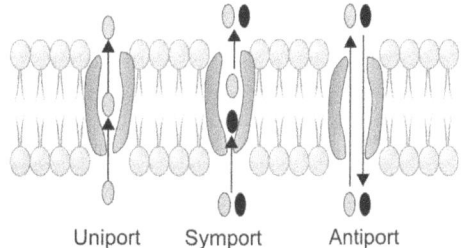

Fig. 10: Secondary active transport.

chloride—bicarbonate exchange in RBC.
- Uniport system—transport of single solute across the membrane, e.g. glucose transporters, calcium pump.

3. Uronic acid pathway.

It is an alternate pathway of glucose metabolism.

Uronic Acid Pathway (Fig. 11)

- In this pathway glucose is converted to active UDP glucose which is then dehydrogenated to form UDP-glucuronic acid
- UDP-glucuronidase removes UDP to convert it into D-glucuronic acid which is reduced to L-gulonic acid
- Removal of one water molecule from gulonic acid gives rise to L-gulonolactone
- Gulonolactone oxidase converts it into ascorbic acid in lower animals. As this enzyme is absent in human beings, vitamin C cannot be synthesized in man
- L-gulonic acid is oxidized to L-xylulose which is then converted to xylitol and D-xylulose. These pentoses enter into pentose phosphate pathway.

Importance of this Pathway

- It provides UDP-glucuronic acid (active form of glucuronic acid). UDP-glucuronic acid is used for:
  - Conjugation of bilirubin
  - Conjugation of steroids
  - Conjugation of various drugs which will make them more soluble and hence easily excretable
  - Glycosaminoglycan synthesis.
- It provides pentoses to HMP pathway.

4. Insulin.

Refer 2006 Short Note 20.

5. Wald's visual cycle.

Refer 2008 Short Note 8.

6. Collagen.

- The major structural protein found in connective tissue is collagen
- It is a Greek word means the substance to produce glue
- About 25-30% of the total weight of protein in the body is collagen.

Structure of Collagen

- Tropocollagen (molecular weight—285 kDa) is made up of three polypeptides chains

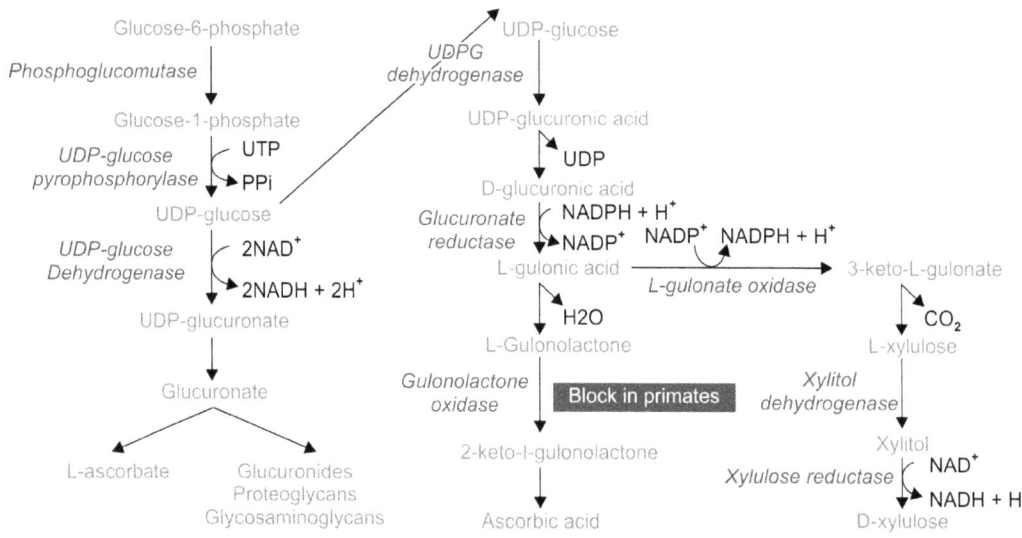

Fig. 11: Uronic acid pathway.

- Each polypeptide chain of collagen has about 1,000 amino acids. About 33% of these amino acids is glycine which occupies every third residue. The repetitive amino acid sequence is Gly-X-Y series in which X and Y are commonly proline and hydroxyproline or lysine and hydroxylysine.

Synthesis
- It is synthesized by fibroblasts as a large precursor procollagen (molecular weight—360 KD)
- Then it is cleaved by specific peptidases to form tropocollagen
- Hydroxylation of proline and lysine residues of collagen (post-translational modification) is done intracellularly and finally forms collagen. This process needs ascorbic acid
- Glycosylation of hydroxylated polypeptides are done by galactosyl and glucosyl-transferases
- Outside the fibroblast cells, procollagen is cleaved by specific peptidases to remove about 150 amino acids from N-terminal area and 300 amino acids from C-terminal end to form mature tropocollagen
- Tropocollagen molecules are then assembled into rodlike collagen by forming covalent crosslinks. Tropocollagen molecules are arranged in quarter staggered array to form collagen fibres with triple stranded, quarter staggered arrangement (Fig. 12).

Functions
- Serves to hold together the cells in tissues
- Major fibrous element of tissues like bone, teeth, tendons, cartilage and blood vessels are formed by collagen
- To give support to organs
- To provide alignment of cells so that anchoring is possible. This helps in proliferation and differentiation of cells

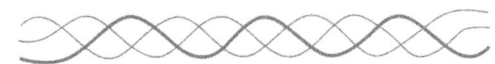

Fig. 12: Triple helical collagen fiber.

- In blood vessels, if collagen is exposed, platelets adhere and thrombus formation is initiated.

Abnormalities in Collagen
- **Osteogenesis imperfecta**—it is due to a mutation in type I collagen where glycine residue is replaced by cysteine. This disrupts the triple helix near carboxy-terminus causing brittle bones and skeletal deformities
- **Ehlers-Danlos syndrome (EDS)**—it is due to defective type III collagen formation due to defective lysyl oxidase or lysyl hydroxylase. This causes weakening of collagen, loose skin, hypermobile and lax joints. There will be hyperextensibility of skin and joints. There are around 10 types of EDS
- **Alport syndrome**—due to abnormal type IV collagen, basement membrane of kidney, glomerular apparatus is abnormal. Hematuria progresses to renal failure in these cases
- **Menke's disease**—deficiency of copper results in defective function of lysyl oxidase enzyme. This results in reduced crosslinkage of collagen
- **Other disorders**—homocystinuria, deficiency of vitamin C, lathyrism.

7. Glycosaminoglycans.
- Glycosaminoglycans (GAGs) or mucopolysaccharides are heteropolysaccharides containing the repeating units of disaccharides made up of uronic acid and amino sugars
- They are the essential components of connective tissue structure.

Common Glycosaminoglycans
- Hyaluronic acid
- Chondroitin sulfate
- Dermatan sulfate
- Heparin
- Heparan sulfate
- Keratan sulfate.

Structure of Glycosaminoglycans

- They are made up of repeating units of disaccharides made up of uronic acid and amino sugars—polymer of both
- This polymer is attached covalently to extracellular core proteins to form proteoglycans except hyaluronic acid. It looks like a bottle brush
- Proteoglycans join with one molecule of hyaluronic acid to form aggregates which is stabilized by link proteins
- Uronic acid present in GAGs are either glucuronic acid or its epimer iduronic acid. Keratan sulfate does not contain uronic acid
- The amino sugars are glucosamine or galactosamine
- Except hyaluronic acid all GAGs contain sulfates donated by the active sulfate PAPS
- They are usually unbranched.

Common GAGs in Details

Site of Occurrence

Extracellular connective tissues of arterial wall, bones, cartilages, synovial fluid, vitreous humor of eye.

1. **Hyaluronic acid (Fig. 13)**
   - Anionic, nonsulfated glycosaminoglycan
   - **Site of occurrence**—present in loose connective tissues, tendons
   - **Repeating units**—composed of D-glucuronic acid and N-acetylglucosamine, linked by β-1, 4 and β-1, 3 glycosidic bonds
   - **Functions**—acts as lubricant and shock absorber. It helps in migration of cells in reproduction in embryogenesis and in wound healing.

Chondroitin sulfate (Fig. 14)

- **Site of occurrence**—it is present in ground substance of connective tissues present in cartilage, bone, tendons, cornea and skin
- **Repeating units**—it is made up of repeating units of glucuronic acid and N-acetylgalactosamine to which sulfate group is attached
- **Functions**—it provides an endoskeletal structure to maintain the structure and shape of the tissues like cartilage

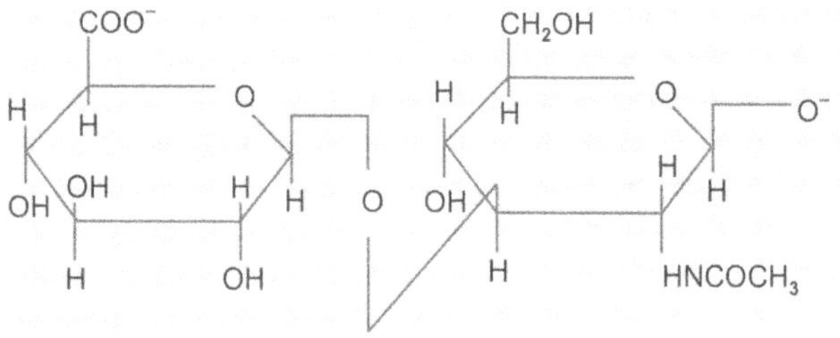

Fig. 13: Hyaluronic acid.

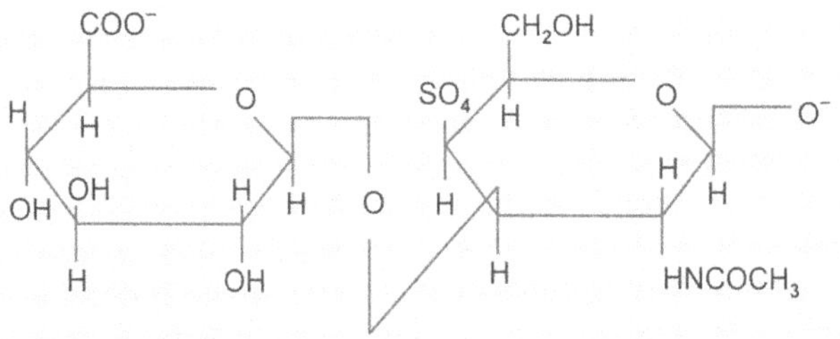

Fig. 14: Chondroitin sulfate.

- **Therapeutic uses**—it is used to treat osteoarthritis as anti-inflammatory agent, stimulating the synthesis of proteoglycans.

Dermatan sulfate
- **Site of occurrence**—it is present in connective tissues present in skin, blood vessels and heart valves
- **Repeating units**—it is made up of repeating units of L-iduronic acid and N-acetylgalactosamine to which sulfate group is attached
- **Functions**—it provides transparency to the cornea and maintains the shape of eye.

Heparin (Fig. 15)
Produced mainly by mast cells of liver.
- **Site of occurrence**—intracellular component of mast cells which line the arteries of liver, lung and skin
- **Repeating units**—highly sulfated glycosaminoglycan made up of glucosamine and glucuronic or iduronic acid
- **Functions**—it acts as an anticoagulant, causing release of lipoprotein lipase enzyme to act on the triglycerol.

Heparan sulfate (Fig. 15)
- **Site of occurrence**—skin, aortic walls, fibroblast
- **Repeating units**—made up of glucosamine and glucuronic or iduronic acid like heparin. Glucosamine may be acetylated
- **Functions**—it acts as receptors in plasma membrane and mediates cell communications and cell growth. Responsible for charge selectiveness in glomerular filtration.

Keratan sulfate
- **Site of occurrence**—loose connective tissue, cartilage, cornea
- **Repeating units**—made up of N-acetylglucosamine and galactose. **No uronic acid**
- **Functions**—it provides transparency of the cornea.

8. Chromatography.

Definition: It is a separative procedure for separating components of a solution by differences in migration rate as the solution (mobile phase) is passed through a stationary phase. The term is derived from the Greek word chroma, means color. This is used to separate almost all biological substances including proteins, carbohydrates, lipids and nucleic acids.

Types of Chromatography
- Adsorption chromatography
- Partition chromatography
- Gel infiltration (size exclusion) chromatography
- High pressure liquid chromatography
- Ion exchange chromatography
- Affinity chromatography.

Adsorption Chromatography
- In this technique the separation is based on differences in adsorption at the surface of a solid stationary medium
- The common adsorbing substances are alumina, silicates or silica gel
- These are packed into columns and the mixture of proteins to be separated is

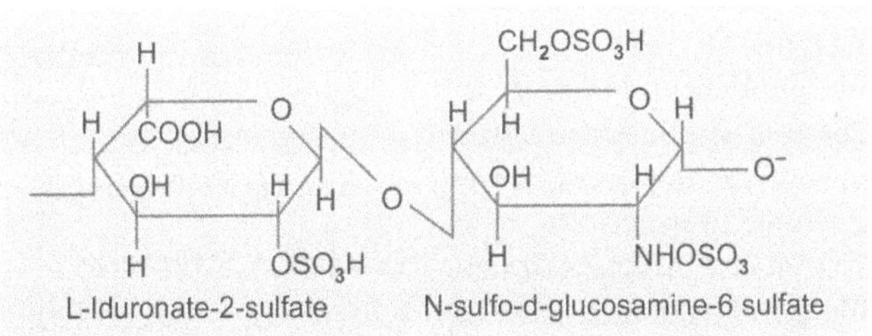

Fig. 15: Heparin and heparan sulphate.

applied in a solvent on the top of the column
- The components get adsorbed on the column of adsorbent. The eluent from the column is collected as equal fractions and the concentrations of each measured.

Partition Chromatography

- This is a technique of chromatography which includes different types depending on the phases between which the components are partitioned, e.g. solid-liquid, liquid –liquid, gas-liquid, etc.
- This is used for the separation of mixtures of amino acids and peptides
- There is a stationary phase which may be either solid or liquid and a mobile phase which may be a liquid or gas
- The components of mixture to be separated are partitioned between the two phases depending on the partition coefficient (solubility) of the particular substances
- The types of partition chromatography are: i) Paper chromatography ii) Thin layer chromatography.
  i. **Paper chromatography:**
     - In this type the stationary phase is water held on a solid support of filter paper (cellulose)
     - The mobile phase is a mixture of immiscible solvents like water, a nonpolar solvent and an acid or base, e.g. butanol-acetic acid- water, phenol- water - ammonia
     - Chromatography can be done with the mobile phase applied from top is called descending type or bottom ascending type.
     - A few microliters of the mixture to be separated is applied as a small spot at one end of the paper 1" away from the edges. In ascending type the paper is placed in a glass trough containing the solvent and allowed to move in the paper
     - It takes 14 to 16 hours
     - The distance to which each component moves depends on its partition coefficient.
  ii. **Thin layer chromatography:**
     - This is liquid-liquid chromatography
     - Thin layer of silica gel is spread on a glass plate
     - Sample is applied as small spots
     - The plates placed in a trough containing the solvent. It takes 3-4 hours.

Visualization of Chromatography

- After the run is over, the paper or the plate is dried
- Location reagents, such as ninhydrin will be sprayed for amino acids and proteins; sulfuric acid sprayed for phospholipids and diphenylamine for sugars
- Spots are identified and the distance traveled by the solute and solvent are marked and Rf value calculated.

Importance of Rf Value

Rf value is the ratio of distance traveled by substance to the distance traveled by the solvent. It is constant for a particular solvent system.

9. Levels of organization of proteins.

Refer 2003 Essay Question 3
Proteins have different levels of structural organization. They are **(Figs. 16 and 17)**:
- Primary structure
- Secondary structure
- Tertiary structure
- Quaternary structure

Primary Structure

- It denotes the number and sequence of amino acids in the protein
- Primary structure is maintained by **peptide bond (CO -NH bond)**, e.g. **insulin**.

Secondary Structures

- It denotes the configurational relationship between residues which are about 3-4 amino acids apart in linear structure

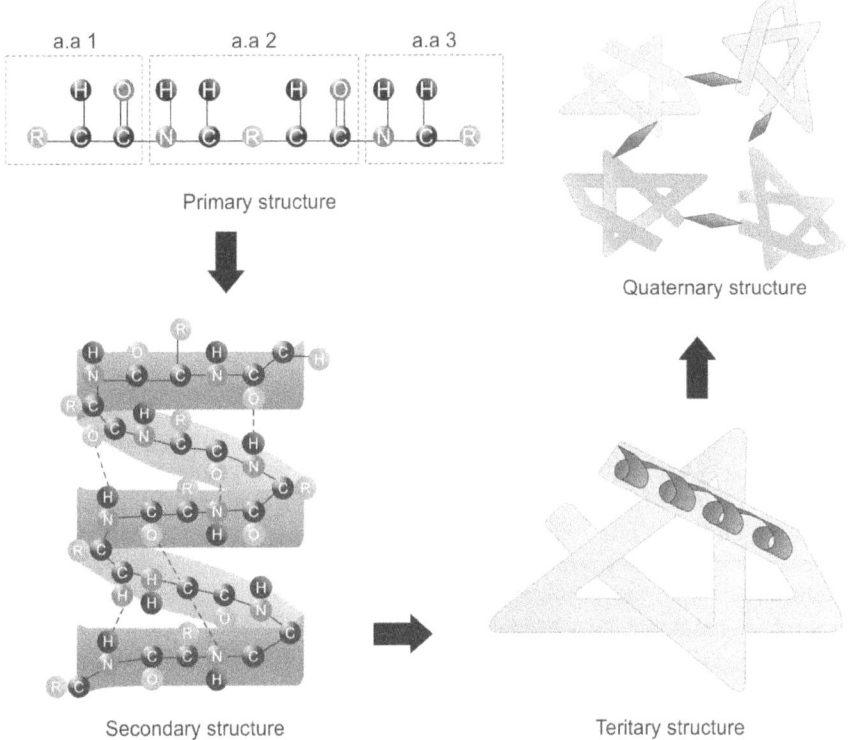

Fig. 16: Level of organization of proteins.

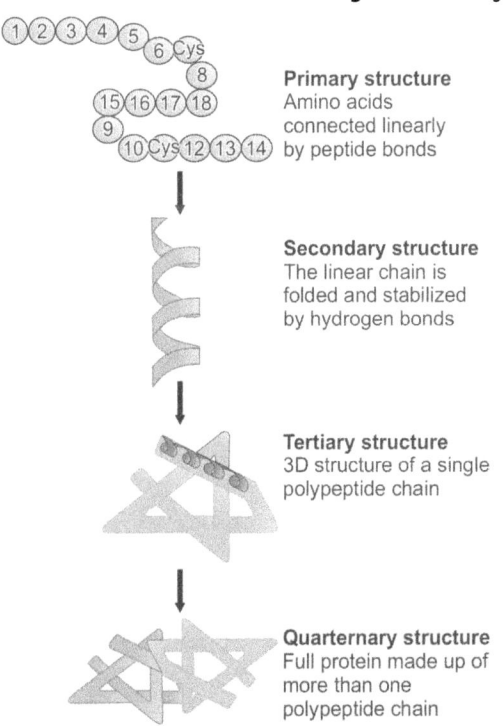

Primary structure
Amino acids connected linearly by peptide bonds

Secondary structure
The linear chain is folded and stabilized by hydrogen bonds

Tertiary structure
3D structure of a single polypeptide chain

Quaternary structure
Full protein made up of more than one polypeptide chain

Fig. 17: Structures of protein.

- This structure is maintained by non-covalent forces or bonds like hydrogen bonds, electrostatic (ionic) bonds, hydrophobic bonds and van der Waals forces
- The types of secondary structure are- i) Alpha helix, e.g. alpha keratin, ii) Beta pleated sheet, beta bends (reverse turns, beta turns), nonrepetitive secondary structure and supersecondary motifs.

Tertiary Structure

- It denotes the 3 dimensional structure of whole protein by further folding, e.g. myoglobin
- It defines the stearic relationship of amino acids which are far apart from each other in linear structure, but are close in the 3 dimensional aspects
- Secondary, tertiary and quaternary structures are maintained by hydrogen bonds, electrostatic bonds, hydrophobic bonds and weak van der Waals forces
- Domains are the fundamental, functional and 3 dimensional structural units of

polypeptides. The domains are connected with flexible areas of protein.

Quaternary Structure

- This occurs only in proteins which have more than one polypeptide chain—polymeric proteins
- These polypeptides aggregate to form quaternary structure to get one functional protein
- Each polypeptide chain (**Fig. 18**) is termed as subunit or monomer. Depending on the number of polypeptide chains, the proteins are dimer (2 chains), trimer (3 chains), and tetramer (4 chains) and so on
- If the protein has two copies of the same polypeptide chains they are termed as homodimer and if it has two different polypeptide chains they are called as heterodimer
- For example, hemoglobin is a heterotetramer having 2 alpha chains and 2 beta chains
- Quaternary structures are maintained by hydrogen bonds, electrostatic bonds, hydrophobic bonds and weak van der Waals forces.

10. Calcium homeostasis.

Refer 2004 Essay Question 4.

11. Phenylketonuria.

Refer 2005 Essay Question 3.

- Phenylketonuria is the inborn error of metabolism in phenylalanine metabolism
- It is an autosomal recessive disease with an incidence of 1: 10,000 births

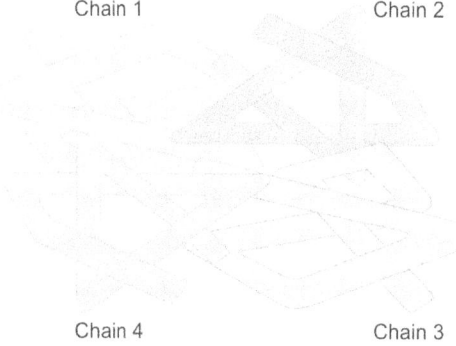

Fig.18: Quaternary structure of proteins.

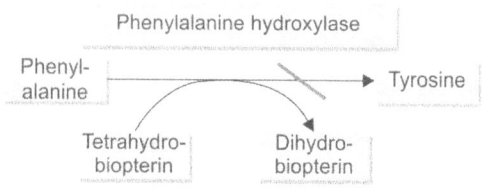

Fig. 19: Phenylketonuria.

- It is due to deficiency of phenylalanine hydroxylase
- So phenylalanine is not converted into tyrosine and it accumulates hyperphenylalaninemia
- The excess of phenylalanine is converted to phenylpyruvate, phenyllactate, and phenylacetate and phenylacetylglutamine. Phenylpyruvate, phenyllactate, phenylacetate are excreted in urine (**Fig. 19**).

Clinical Manifestations

- The child is mentally retarded
- Convulsions, tremors, agitation, hyperactivity may be present
- The child often has hypopigmentation due to reduced availability of tyrosine for melanin production
- Phenyllactate in sweat causes mousy body odor.

Laboratory Diagnosis

- Blood level of phenylalanine is elevated—Normal level is 1mg/dL which is elevated to >20 mg/dL
- This is confirmed by Tandem mass spectroscopy
- Guthrie's test is confirmative
- Urine ferric chloride test is positive
- DNA probes—to diagnose the defects in phenylalanine hydroxylase and dihydrobiopterin reductase.

Treatment

- Early detection
- Low phenylalanine diet—tapioca based diet which has low phenylalanine is the treatment of choice
- Gene therapy is under trial.

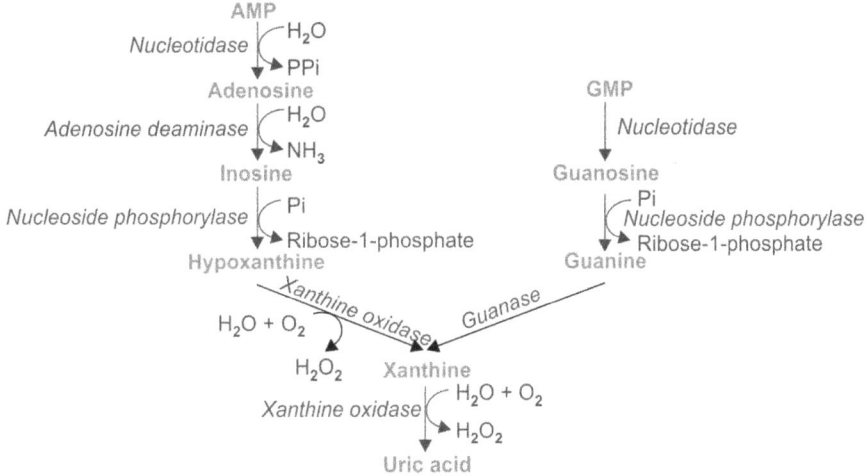

Fig. 20: Synthesis of uric acid.

12. Formation of uric acid.

Purines are adenine, guanine, xanthine and hypoxanthine.

Purine catabolism leads to the production of uric acid.

Steps for formation of uric acid (Fig. 20)

- **Step 1:** Adenosine monophosphate (AMP) is converted to adenosine by **nucleotidase** by the removal of phosphate. GMP is also converted to guanosine by nucleotidase
- **Step 2: Adenosine deaminase** converts adenosine to inosine by the removal of ammonia
- **Step 3:** By the addition of one phosphate, **nucleoside phosphorylase** enzyme removes ribose-1-phosphate from inosine and guanosine to form hypoxanthine and guanine, respectively
- **Step 4:** Guanine is converted to xanthine by guanase enzyme. Hypoxanthine is acted by xanthine oxidase to form xanthine. Hydrogen peroxide is released
- **Step 5:** Xanthine is converted to uric acid by the enzyme xanthine oxidase. Hydrogen peroxide is released which is decomposed to water and oxygen by catalase enzyme.
  - Xanthine oxidase is a metalloenzymes containing molybdenum (Mo) and iron. It is competitively inhibited by allopurinol
  - Uric acid is excreted in urine
  - Normal urinary excretion of uric acid is 500–700 mg/day
  - Normal blood level of uric acid is 2-5 mg/dL for females and 3-7 mg/dL for males.

13. Porphyria.

Refer 2008 Essay Question 2; 2nd part

14. Urea cycle.

Refer 2006 Essay Question 9.

15. ELISA.

- Enzyme-linked immunosorbent assay (ELISA) is a nonisotope immunoassay
- ELISA is used widely to measure hormone, growth factors, tumor markers, bacterial and viral antigens, etc.
- Here the antigen is labeled with a stable enzyme, whereas in radioimmunoassay a radioisotope is used.

Principle (Figs. 21 A and B)

- Enzymes used as labels catalyse color change in the substrate which is then detected
- The amount of enzyme-labeled antigen bound is inversely proportional to the

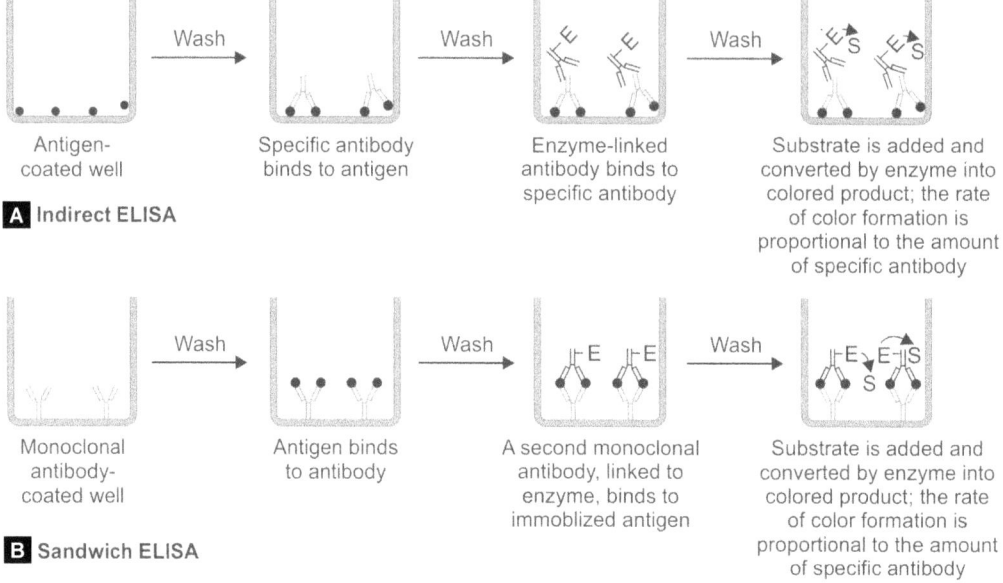

Figs. 21A and B: ELISA.

amount of antigen in the serum being analysed
- Commonly used enzyme substrate combinations are: Alkaline phosphatase with substrate p-nitrophenyl and horseradish peroxidase with tetramethylbenzidine
- Two types of ELISA are:
  1. Antibody detection—indirect ELISA (single antibody)
  2. Antigen detection—sandwich ELISA (double antibody).

Antibody Detection: Indirect ELISA

- This is used to detect small quantities of antibodies
- HIV antibodies—are detected by the following methods:
  - Specific antigen to the antibody coated well is taken
  - Then the sample (serum) is added and incubated. The antibody in patient's sample binds to the antigen and fixed
  - Next a second antibody conjugated with the enzyme peroxidase is added to the antigen-antibody already formed. Remaining is washed
  - Now the Ag-Ab-Ab-enzyme complex is obtained
  - Now a substrate for the enzyme which will form a colored product is added. The color developed is directly proportional to the concentration of the analyte antibody.

Antigen Detection: Sandwich ELISA

- Assay of thyroid hormone is done by the following methods:
  - Specific antibody is fixed to the antigen coated well of a microtiter plate
  - Sample is added to the well and incubated at 37°C. The antigen in patient's sample is fixed to the antibody. Excess antigen are washed out
  - Next a specific antibody tagged with an enzyme like horseradish peroxidase is added which will bind to the antigen (secondary Ag). Remaining is washed
  - The Ab-Ag-Ab-enzyme complex is now obtained
  - Then a substrate for the enzyme which will form a colored product is added. The color developed is directly

proportional to the concentration of the analyte antigen.

16. Active methionine.
Refer 2007 Essay Question 4.

17. Flame photometer.
This is an analytical instrument used for quantitative analysis of sodium, potassium, calcium and lithium in biological fluids like blood, serum, urine, etc.

Principle

- The solution containing the substance to be measured is passed as a very fine spray into the air supply of a burner
- In the flame, the solution evaporates and the substance is converted to the atomic state
- As the temperature rises, the thermal energy of the flame excites these electrons so that they are able to absorb one more quanta of thermal energy and move into higher energy orbit farther from the nucleus
- The electron in the higher energy orbits are prone to return to lower energy orbits
- In doing so, the energy previously absorbed is released as quanta of light, the wavelength of which are characteristic of the substance thus giving rise to emission spectrum
- Part of the light which is emitted in all directions is collected by a reflector and falls on a detector
- The light intensity and hence the detector output is directly proportional to the concentration of the substance in the flame.

Parts (Fig. 22)

- **Nebulizer**—it produces a fine spray of droplets of uniform size necessary for constant emission of light
- **Burner and flame**—when supplied with fuel and air at constant pressure produced with the help of a compressor the burner will produce a steady flame. If the sample is in the distilled water, the flame will be blue in color
- **Diaphragm**—functions as a slit
- **Capillary tube**—the free lower end is used to insert into the sample and the other end is focussed over the flame
- **Filter**—monochromatic filter. The principal wavelengths used are—589 nm for sodium, 766 nm for potassium, 554 nm for calcium, 671 nm for lithium
- **Detector**—a photosensor which converts light energy to electrical energy. The intensity of light compared with that of standard and the result is calculated
- **Output devices**—digital display or an eternal recorder. The amplified signal from the photomultiplier operates this device
- **Output tube**—to release the waste solution
- **Compressor**—it pumps air at high pressure and mixes it with fuel and is fed into the flame.

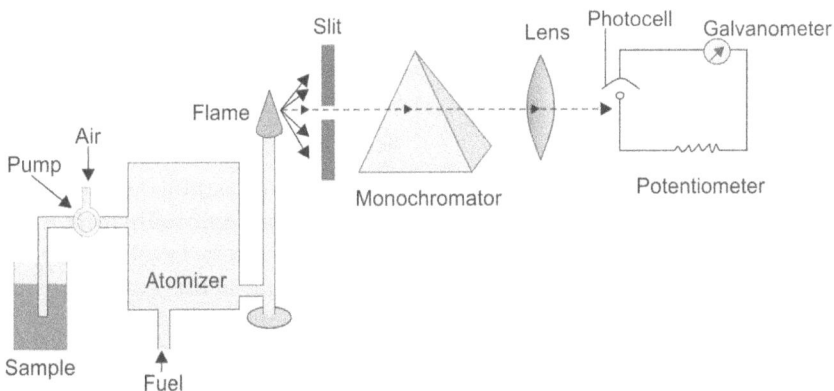

Fig. 22: Flame photometer.

18. Bilirubin formation and excretion.
Refer 2005 Short Note 3.

19. Plasma proteins.
- The total protein content of plasma is 6-8 g/dL
- Plasma proteins consist of albumin, globulins (α_1, α_2, β and γ) and fibrinogen
- Albumin—3.5-5 g/dL; Globulins—2.5-3.5 g/dL and fibrinogen—200-400 mg/dL
- Normal albumin: Globulin ratio is 1.2:1-1.5:1.

Albumin
It is produced by the liver and of 69,000 D molecular weight. It is a globular protein elliptical in shape and it has 585 amino acids arranged in one polypeptide chain

Functions of Albumin
- Transport protein—it transports various substances like bilirubin, free fatty acid, drugs like aspirin, hormones like thyroxine, steroid hormones, minerals like calcium, copper, etc.
- Colloid osmotic pressure—it maintains colloid osmotic pressure in vascular and extravascular compartments. It contributes to plasma oncotic pressure. It cannot pass between intracellular and extracellular compartment. So exerts a net osmotic pressure. The osmotic pressure of plasma is about 278-305 mOsm/kg which is necessary for the movement of water from ECF to ICF in arteriolar end and reverse in venular end of capillaries
- Buffer—albumin has the maximum buffering capacity. 16 histidine residues are present in albumin which can bind to H$^+$ and can function as a buffer
- Nutrition—liver takes up amino acids from diet and converts it into albumin. It is then released in blood and taken up by other tissues by pinocytosis. So albumin is a source of amino acids for the cells. PEM is characterized by hypoalbuminemia which results in growth retardation and edema. Human albumin is used in the treatment of liver diseases, hemorrhage, shock and burns.

Globulin
Globulins are globular proteins bigger in size than albumin.
There are different fractions present with globulins. They are: α_1-globulins, α_2-globulins, β-globulins and γ-globulin.
- α_1-globulins—they include retinol binding protein (RBP), α_1-feto protein, α_1-antitrypsin, α_1-acid glycoprotein (AAG), HDL and prothrombin
- α_2-globulins—they include ceruloplasmin, transcortin, haptoglobin, thyroxine binding protein (TBP), α_2-macroglobuliin (AMG)
- β-globulin—they include hemopexin, transferrin, β_2-microglobulin (BMG), C-reactive protein (CRP), low density lipoprotein (LDL)
- γ-globulins – IgG, IgM, IgA, IgD, IgE. They act as antibodies.
  - Most of them are transport proteins, e.g. thyroxine binding globulin (TBG), RBP, transcortin and transferrin
  - Haptoglobin binds with free Hb and prevents the loss of iron and hemopexin binds with free heme and prevents loss of iron.

Clotting Factors
There are 12 Clotting factors—I, II, IV to XIII present along with plasma proteins. Except calcium (factor IV) all others are proteins produced by the liver. They are in the inactive zymogen form and activated when the coagulation process is initiated.

Acute Phase Reactants
CRP, ceruloplasmin, alpha-1 antitrypsin, alpha-2 macroglobulin are acute phase reactants. Their levels increase in the blood during acute conditions like fever, inflammations, etc.

20. Replication.
Refer 2007 Essay Question 9.

21. Classify RNA and explain the functions.

- Nucleic acids are classified into deoxyribonucleic acid (DNA) and ribonucleic acid (RNA)
- RNA can be classified into messenger RNA (mRNA), ribosomal RNA (rRNA), transfer RNA (tRNA), small nuclear RNA (snRNA)
- **Components**—it is a polymer of purine and pyrimidine ribonucleotides of adenine, guanine, cytosine, and uracil linked by 3'5'- phosphodiester bonds.

Functions

- **Messenger RNA (mRNA):**
  - It is synthesized from DNA by transcription. Its precursor is the heterogenous nuclear RNA (hnRNA) from which it is synthesized by post-transcriptional modification
  - It has a poly A tail at its 3' end and a cap at 5' end consisting of 7-methyl-GTP
  - It contains the codons for protein synthesis which serve as a template for protein synthesis. It is attached to ribosome on which protein synthesis occurs.
- **Transfer RNA (tRNA) or soluble RNA:**
  - It shows extensive internal base pairing
  - It has clover leaf like structure
  - It contains unusual bases. They are dihydrouracil (DHU), pseudouridine (Y) and hypoxanthine. Many bases are methylated
  - It acts as an adapter molecule in carrying a specific amino acid for a particular codon in mRNA and helps in protein synthesis—translation
  - It has an acceptor arm, anticodon arm, DHU arm and pseudouridine arm.
    - **Acceptor arm is at 3' end**—it carries the amino acids. It has seven base pairs. The end sequence is CCA-3'. The 3' end hydroxyl group is bonded with carboxyl end of amino acids.
    - **Anticodon arm of tRNA**—it is present at the opposite side of acceptor arm. It recognizes the triplet nucleotide codon present in mRNA
    - **DHU Arm of tRNA**—it contains dihydrouridine. DHU arm serves as the recognition site for enzymes
    - **Pseudouridine arm of tRNA**—it contains pseudouridine and it is involved in binding tRNA to ribosomes
- **Ribosomal RNA (rRNA)**—it is a component of ribosomes. Ribosomes are made up of many polypeptides and rRNA
- **Small nuclear RNA (snRNA)**—these are small nuclear RNAs. They are involved in the process of removal of introns and splicing of exons of mRNA precursors.

Ribozymes—some RNA are capable of enzymatic functions like peptidyl transferase.

22. Hyperuricemia.
Refer 2008 Short Note 18.

23. Renal glycosuria.
Refer 2007 Short Note 22.

24. Cardiac troponin (CTI/CTT).
- Troponins are markers of MI.
- The troponin complex consists of 3 components which are as follows:
  1. **Troponin C**—C for calcium binding subunit
  2. **Troponin I (actomyosin ATPase inhibitory subunit)**—it is increased in blood within 4 hours after onset of symptoms, peaks at 14-24 hours and remains elevated for 3-5 days
  3. **Troponin T (TnT) (tropomyosin binding subunit)**—it increases after 6 hours of MI, peaks at 72 hours and then remains elevated up to 7-10 days. It is not increased in muscle injury, whereas CK2 may be elevated
- **High sensitive TnT (hnTnT):** Elevated level of this reveals the early diagnosis of AMI.

25. Structure of cholesterol and its importance in the body.

- It is an animal sterol and it means '*solid bile alcohol*'

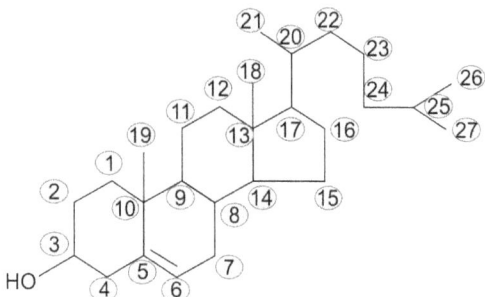

Fig. 23: Structure of cholesterol.

- It derives its name from Greek word 'cholesterine' means bile solid
- It has 27 carbon atoms totally
- It has a steroid nucleus with cyclopentanoperhydrophenanthrene ring system made up of 3 cyclohexane rings A, B and C and a cyclopentane ring D containing 19 carbon atoms and 8 carbon side chain attached to D ring at C17. OH group attached to C3 of A ring. One double bond between C5 and 6 in ring B
- Two methyl groups are attached to C10 and C13
- It is amphipathic in nature with polar head at C3-OH group and a nonpolar steroid nucleus and hydrocarbon chain at C17
- In the body it exists as cholesterol ester with a fatty acid attached to the OH at C3 (Fig. 23).

Functions of Cholesterol

- Major structural constituent of cell membranes and lipoproteins
- Precursor of steroid hormones, sex hormones, vitamin D and bile acids
- It has an insulating effect on nerve fibres.

26. Beriberi.
Refer 2006 Short Note 7.

27. Enzyme poisons.
- Certain poisons act as irreversible non-competitive inhibitors
- There is no competition between substrate and these inhibitors
- They usually bind to different domains than the substrate binding site
- K_m value is not changed; V_{max} is reduced
- Increase in substrate concentration will not abolish noncompetitive inhibition
- For example, cyanide inhibits cytochrome oxidase, iodoacetate inhibits enzymes with SH group in their active site.

28. Flurosis.
Refer 2008 Short Question 10.

29. What is protein-energy malnutrition (PEM)? What are the types of PEM? Write the importance features.
Refer 2006 Short Note 23.

30. Functions of vitamin C.
Refer 2005 Essay Question 5.

31. Denaturation.
- Denaturation is the disruption or disorganization of native or biologically active protein structure
- The loss of secondary, tertiary and quaternary structure of proteins without alteration of the primary structure (amino acids connected by peptide bonds) is called denaturation (Fig. 24).

Agents of Denaturation
- Physical agents—mild heating, X-rays, UV radiation, high pressure, vigorous shaking may lead to denaturation
- Chemical agents—acids, alkali, organic solvents, heavy metals (Pb, Hg), treating with urea, salicylates, detergents.

Characteristics of Denaturation
- The biological activity of the protein is lost due to loss of higher structures

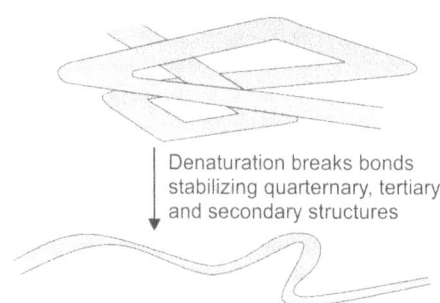

Fig. 24: Denaturation.

- Physical, chemical and biological properties of proteins are lost
- **Physical alterations**—native helical structure is lost; primary structure intact
- **Chemical alterations**—protein becomes insoluble, viscosity increased, maximum precipitation, decreased surface tension and diffusion; unfolding of proteins
- These proteins are vulnerable to proteolytic enzymes, so cooked food is easily digestible than uncooked food
- Denaturation is usually irreversible
- It is sometimes reversible if the agent causing the denaturation is removed. This is called renaturation, e.g. salicylates denature Hb and when it is removed, Hb is renatured
- **Renaturation**—denaturation is many times reversible if the agent causing the denaturation is removed, e.g. salicylates denature Hb and when it is removed, Hb is renatured, immunoglobulins treated with urea.

32. Reverse transcription.

- Synthesis of DNA from RNA by reverse transcriptase enzyme is known as reverse transcription
- Genetic material for many living organisms is in DNA. DNA-dependent RNA polymerase is involved in transcription (production of mRNA from DNA)
- But some viruses and other organisms have only RNA as their genetic material. Retro viruses are RNA viruses, e.g. HIV
- Reverse transcriptase is RNA-dependent DNA polymerase
- The enzyme reverse transcriptase will make DNA strand from RNA. Usually transcription is the production of mRNA from DNA. So this process of making DNA from RNA is named as reverse transcription
- Once the virus infects human cells, the viral RNA is converted into DNA by reverse transcription and this DNA is known as cDNA—complementary DNA
- The single-stranded DNA acts as template to produce double-stranded (ds) DNA. This DNA is incorporated into human genome and it leads to the production of viral proteins and RNA.

33. Sphingolipidoses.

It is the inherited lipid storage disease. Sphingolipidoses are lysosomal storage disorders arising in degradation of sphingolipids. They are due to accumulation of certain lipids in lysosomes due to defect in the following enzymes:

Disease	Enzyme deficiency	Symptoms
Tay-Sachs disease	Hexosaminidase A	Mental retardation, blindness, weakness
Fabry's disease	α-galactosidase	X-lined recessive kidney failure only in males
Krabbe's disease	β-galactosidase	Mental retardation, demyelination
Gaucher's disease	β-glucosidase	Enlarged liver and spleen, erosion of long bones
Niemann-Pick disease	Sphinomyelinase	Enlarged liver and spleen, mental retardation
Farber's disease	Ceramidase	Hoarseness, dermatitis, skeletal deformation

- **Tay-Sachs disease**—hexosaminidase A deficiency. Accumulation of GM2 Ganglioside. It is characterized by mental (retardation), blindness, muscular weakness
- **Fabry's disease**—α-galactosidase deficiency. Accumulation of globotriaosylceramide. It is characterized by skin rash, (kidney) failure (full symptoms only in males; X-linked recessive)
- **Krabbe's disease**—β-galactosidase deficiency. Accumulation of galactosylceramide. It is characterized by (mental retardation) and demyelination
- **Niemann-Pick disease**—(sphingomyelinase deficiency). Accumulation of sphingomyelin. It is characterized by enlarged liver and spleen, mental retardation; fatal in early life

- **Farber's disease**—(Ceramidase deficiency). Accumulation of sphingosine. It is characterized by hoarseness, dermatitis, skeletal deformation, and mental retardation; fatal in early life
- **Metachromatic leukodystrophy**—(Arylsulfatase deficiency). Accumulation of 3-sulfo-galactosylceramide. It is characterized by mental retardation and psychologic disturbances in adults; demyelination.

34. GOUT.
Refer 2005 Short Note 17.

35. Metabolic acidosis.
Refer 2004 Short Note 16.

36. Tumor markers.
Refer 2003 Short Note 20.

37. Colorimeter.
- Colorimetry is the measurement of colors
- So the substance to be estimated colorimetrically should be either colored or capable of forming chromogens by the addition of reagents
- The instrument used is called colorimeter.
- It acts as an absorptiometer by measuring the amount of light absorbed by the colored substance
- Colorimeter is used to quantitate biological substances.

Principle—colored solutions have the property of absorbing certain wavelengths of light and transmitting others. This property is based on Beer-Lambert's law

Beer's law

When monochromatic light passes through a colored solution, the amount of light transmitted decreases exponentially with the increase in concentration of the colored substance. In other words the intensity of the color is directly proportionate to the concentration of the colored particle in solution.

Lambert's law
- Amount of light absorbed by a colored solution depends on the length of the column or the depth of the liquid through which light passes
- Colorimeter is based on the above said principles.

Instrument (Fig. 25)
Colorimeter consists of a light source usually a tungsten filament lamp, a monochromator to allow a particular wavelength of light, slit cuvette containing the sample solution and a photoelectric cell which converts light energy to electrical energy.

The monochromatic light after passing the filter is allowed to fall on the colored solution kept in the cuvette. The solution absorbs part of the light and the remaining light is allowed to fall on the photocells which convert light into an electrical signal. The electrical signal generated is directly proportional to the intensity of the light falling on the detector. These signals are measured by a galvanometer and read as absorbance or optical density (OD) values.

38. Functions of adrenal cortical hormones.
- Adrenal cortex has 3 different zones and each secretes hormones under the influence of adrenocorticotropic hormones of anterior pituitary
- The outer zone of adrenal cortex—zona glomerulosa produces C21 steroids and mineralocorticoids

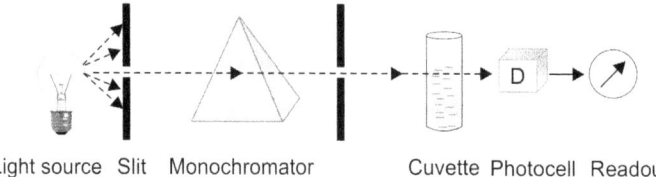

Light source   Slit   Monochromator   Cuvette   Photocell   Readout

Fig. 25: Colorimeter.

- Middle zone—zona fasciculris produces glucocorticoids
- The innermost zona reticularis produces androgens and estrogens.

Functions of Glucocorticoids

- Carbohydrates metabolism—gluconeogenetic enzymes stimulated, glycolytic enzymes suppressed leading to hyperglycemia
- Lipids—increased lipolysis leading to mobilization of fats and depositing in unusual sites like neck
- Proteins—catabolism increased → amino acids go for gluconeogenesis
- Bones—it inhibits osteoblast function causing osteoporosis
- Immune system—suppresses immune system by lysis of lymphocytes. Anti-inflammatory and antiallergic.

Mineralocorticoids

Aldosterone causes increased reabsorption of sodium and water from the distal tubules leading to:
- Reduced urine formation
- Increasing the BP
- Increased K excretion.

Sex Hormones

- **Estrogens**
  - Maturation and functioning of secondary sex organs in females
  - Maintenance of pregnancy
  - Progestins—implantation of ovum and maintenance of pregnancy
- **Androgens**—maturation and functioning of secondary sex organs in males.

39. Plasmid.

Plasmids are commonly used cloning vectors in recombinant DNA technology. Chimeric or hybrid DNA molecules can be constructed in **cloning vectors** typically bacterial plasmids, bacterial phages, or cosmids which then continue to replicate in a host cell under their own control systems. In this way, the chimeric DNA is amplified **(Fig. 26)**.

- **Bacterial plasmids**
  - They are cloning vectors which are small, circular, duplex DNA molecules
  - Their natural function is to confer antibiotic resistance to the host cell
  - They are present as single or multiple copies in the bacterium
  - They can replicate independently from their parent DNA as episomes
  - The DNA sequence of the plasmids are well known and so the restriction sites are easily identified
  - Plasmids are used in cloning of small pieces of DNA which are less than 10 kilobases. As the plasmids are smaller they can be separated from the host chromosome easily after the recombination
- Bacteriophage vectors—viral DNA
  - They can be propagated to high copy numbers—several hundred per cell
  - They can accept large pieces of DNA upto 20 kilobase (kb).
- Cosmid vectors—they are recombinant plasmids and bacteriophage constructed from plasmid and viral DNA
  - They can accept larger pieces of DNA of 35 to 50 kb.
- Other vectors—Bacterial artificial chromosome (BAC), P1vectors which can accept DNA of 50 to 250 kb and yeast artificial chromosome (YAC) which can accept 0.5 to 3 M.

40. Functions of albumin.

- The total protein content of plasma is 6-8 g/dL
- Plasma proteins consist of albumin, globulins—($\alpha 1, \alpha 2, \beta$ and γ) and fibrinogen
- Albumin—3.5-5 g/dL; Globulins—2.5-3.5 g/dL and fibrinogen - 200-400 mg/dL
- Normal albumin: Globulin ratio is 1.2:1-1.5:1

Albumin

- It is produced by the liver and of 69,000 D molecular weight. It is a globular protein

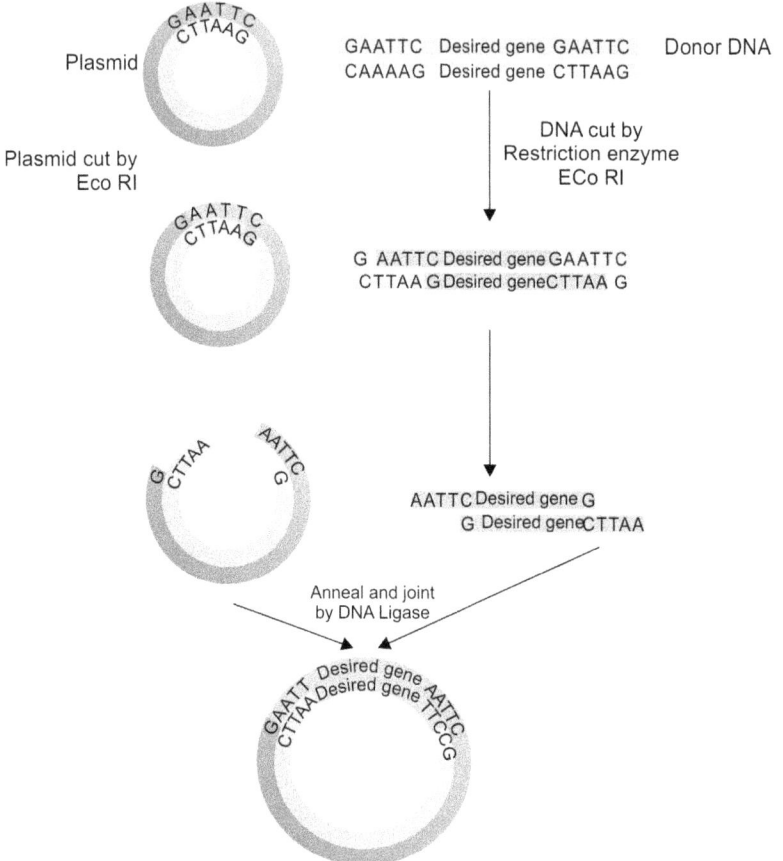

Fig. 26: Use of plasmids in making chimeric DNA in recombinant DNA technology.

elliptical in shape and it has 585 amino acids arranged in one polypeptide chain.

Functions of Albumin

- Transport protein—it transports various substances like bilirubin, free fatty acid, drugs like aspirin, hormones like thyroxine, steroid hormones, minerals like calcium, copper, etc.
- Colloid osmotic pressure—it maintains colloid osmotic pressure in vascular and extravascular compartments. It contributes to plasma oncotic pressure. It cannot pass between intracellular and extracellular compartment. So exerts a net osmotic pressure. The osmotic pressure of plasma is about 278-305 mOsm/kg which is necessary for the movement of water from ECF to ICF in arteriolar end and reverse in venular end of capillaries
- Buffer—albumin has the maximum buffering capacity. 16 histidine residues are present in albumin which can bind to H^+ and can function as a buffer
- Nutrition—liver takes up amino acids from diet and converts it into albumin. It is then released in blood and taken up by the other tissues by pinocytosis. So albumin is a source of amino acids for the cells. PEM is characterized by hypoalbuminemia which results in growth retardation and edema. Human albumin is used in the treatment of liver diseases, hemorrhage, shock and burns.

III. SHORT ANSWER QUESTIONS

1. Key enzymes of glycolysis.
- All catalyse irreversible reactions.
  1. Glucokinase—it phosphorylates glucose to glucose-6-phosphate. It has a higher km for glucose than hexokinase
  2. Phosphofructokinase (PFK)—It converts fructose-6-phosphate to fructose 1, 6-bisphosphate
  3. Pyruvate kinase—it converts PEP to pyruvate.

2. Fatty liver.
Fatty liver refers to the deposition of excess fat—triacylglyceride in the liver cells. Progression of fatty liver ends in cirrhosis of liver (**Fig. 27**).

Causes of Fatty Liver
- Increased mobilization of nonesterified fatty acids from adipose tissue
- Increased lipolysis in adipose tissue in diabetes and in starvation
- More synthesis of fatty acid from glucose
- Decreased oxidation of fat by hepatic cells
- Toxic injury to liver is due to poisoning by carbon tetrachloride, arsenic, lead compounds
- Hepatitis B infection
- Obesity due to excessive calorie intake
- Protein-energy malnutrition causes reduced apoprotein synthesis and hence fatty liver
- Alcoholism—most common cause in India.

Prevention
It can be prevented by taking lipotropic factors, such as choline, lecithin, methionine, vitamin E, selenium and omega-3 fatty acids.

Lipotropic Factors
They are choline, lecithin, methionine, vitamin E, selenium and omega-3 fatty acids. They are required for the normal mobilization of fat from liver. When they are deficient fat gets deposited in the liver causing fatty liver.

Mode of Actions
- Choline—it reverses fatty changes in liver
- Lecithin and methionine—they help to synthesize apoproteins and choline
- Selenium and vitamin E—antioxidants
- Omega-3 fatty acids—present in marine oils and also has a protective action.

3. Lipid peroxidation.
- It is auto-oxidation of lipids exposed to toxic oxygen radicals to cause damage to tissues in vivo
- It is a chain reaction to get continuous supply of free radicals to initiate and elongate peroxidation
- Antioxidants are the substances which can prevent lipid peroxidation, e.g. vitamin E, selenium
- PUFA present in the cell membrane are easily destroyed by peroxidation.

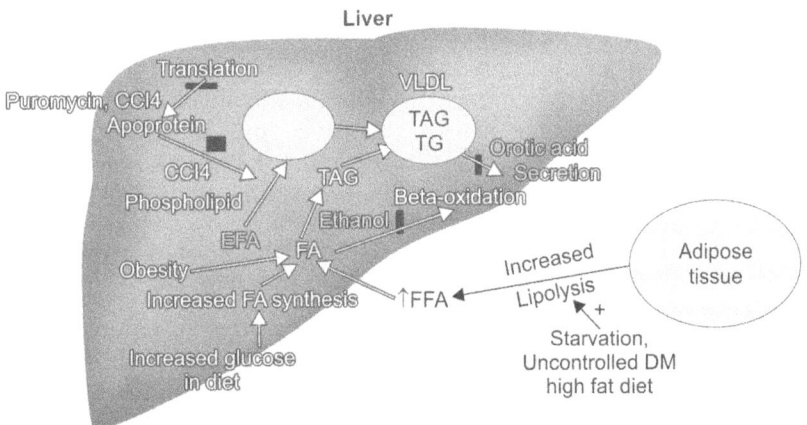

Fig. 27: Fatty liver.

- There are 3 phases of lipid peroxidation:
  1. **Initiation phase**
     - Primary event is the production of R' (carbon centered radical) or ROO' (lipid peroxide radical) by the interaction of PUFA with free radicals
       - Reaction 1A: $RH + OH' \rightarrow R' + H_2O$
       - Reaction 1B: $ROOH \rightarrow ROO' + H^+$
     The R' and ROO' are degraded to malondialdehyde which can be estimated to measure the lipid peroxidation.
  2. **Propagation phase**
     - R' reacts with molecular oxygen forming peroxyl radical which can attack another PUFA
       - Reaction 2: $R' + O_2 \rightarrow ROO'$
       - Reaction 3: $ROO' + RH \rightarrow ROOH + R'$
     - The net result is the formation of ROOH—hydroperoxide
     - This occurs as a chain reaction or propagation
     - Accumulation of this lipid damages lead to the destruction of membranes.
  3. **Termination phase**
     - The above reaction proceeds until one peroxyl radical combines with another peroxyl radical to form inactive products.
       - Reaction 4A: $ROO' + ROO' \rightarrow ROOR + O_2$
       - Reaction 4B: $R' + R' \rightarrow R - R$
       - Reaction 4C: $ROO' + R' \rightarrow RO - RO$

4. **Zymogens.**

- Zymogen or proenzyme is the inactive precursor form of the enzyme
- They undergo irreversible covalent activation by breakdown of one or more peptide bonds and get activated, e.g. trypsinogen → trypsin, chymotrypsinogen → chymotrypsin.

5. **BMR.**

Refer 2005 Short Note 26.

6. **Normal levels of: i) BUN; ii) Fasting serum glucose; iii) LDH; iv) ALT.**

Parameter	Normal value
BUN	8-20 mg/dL
Fasting serum glucose	70-110 mg/dL
LDH	100-200 U/L
ALT	13-35 U/L

7. **tRNA.**

Refer 2006 Short Note 18.

8. **Vitamin K.**

- **Common name:** Antihemorrhagic vitamin, coagulation vitamin
- **Structure:** The vitamin K is a derivative of naphthoquinone attached to isoprenoid units
- **Vitamin K3 types**—vitamin K1—phylloquinone vitamin. It has found in plants; Vitamin K2—menaquinone—found in microorganisms and animals; Vitamin K3—menadione (no isoprenoid units)—alkylated form.

Sources—green leafy vegetables, cabbage, cauliflower, tomato.

Metabolism of Vitamin K

- The vitamin is synthesized by intestinal bacteria and so need not to be taken through diet. Its absorption depends on chylomicrons and bile salts, and it is finally stored in liver.

Functions

Vitamin K is involved in post-translational modifications of clotting factors, such as factor II, VII, IX and X which undergo gamma carboxylation to get active forms.

Carboxylation of Clotting Factors and Significance (Fig. 28)

- All the pre-translational clotting factors contain glutamic acids at their ends of polypeptide chains which are converted to gamma carboxyglutamic acid in the

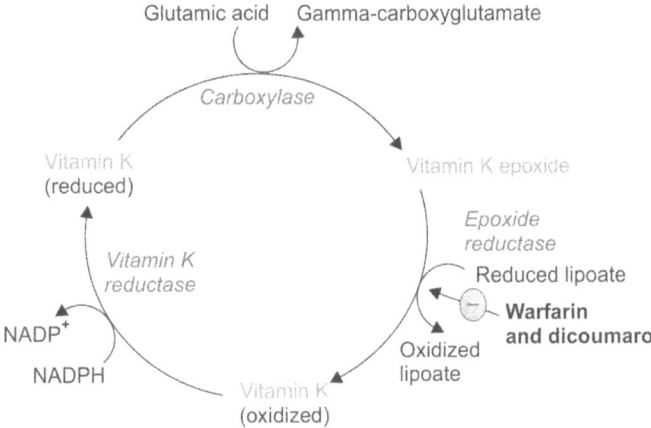

Fig. 28: Vitamin K cycle.

presence of carboxylase, O_2, CO_2, vitamin K (quinone form), $NADP^+$ and H^+
- These carboxylated clotting factors now possess two negative charges on their γ-carboxyglutamate which in turn chelate with two positive charges of Ca^{++}; This complex converts prothrombin to thrombin
- Bone protein osteocalcin also gets activated by gamma-carboxylation and also other structural proteins of kidney, lung and spleen
- This gamma-carboxylation is inhibited by warfarin and dicoumarol by competitive inhibition of epoxide reductase enzyme.

Deficiency of Vitamin K

The deficiency is uncommon because its adequate supply is made by intestinal bacteria, and also through diet. However, the deficiency may occur due to malabsorption syndrome, diarrhea, and antibiotic therapy. Symptoms are:
- Bleeding, ecchymotic patches
- The major feature of deficiency is increased both bleeding time and clotting times.

9. Limiting amino acid.

- Some of the proteins do not contain one or more essential amino acids. These limit the weight gain or growth of the animals when those proteins are fed to the animals. They are known as limiting amino acids for that particular protein
- Limiting amino acids in:
  a. Rice and wheat—(lysine and threonine) rectified by feeding pulse proteins
  b. Zein—(tryptophan and lysine) meat proteins rectify this
  c. Bengal gram—(cysteine and methionine) rectified by cereals proteins.

Protein	Limiting amino acids	Has to be supplemented
Rice	Lysine, threonine	Pulse proteins
Zein	Tyrtryptophen, lysine	Meat proteins
Tapioca	Phenylalanine, tyrosine	Fish protein
Bengal gram	Cyseine, metionine	Cereals

10. Isoenzymes.

- Multiple molecular forms of an enzyme catalyzing the same reaction are isoenzymes or isozymes, e.g. lactate dehydrogenase—5 isoenzymes (LDH1, 2, 3, 4 and 5), creatine kinase—3 isoenzymes (CK 1, 2, 3) and alkaline phosphatase
- They are physically distinct forms of the same enzyme activity
- They are synthesized from various tissues and hence useful to study the disorders of those organs.

Examples

A. Lactate Dehydrogenase:
- There are 5 isoenzymes. They are LDH1, LDH2, LDH3, LDH4, and LDH5
- LDH is a tetramer with 4 subunits
- Isoenzymes of LDH help in the diagnosis of heart and liver diseases.
- Flipped pattern is observed in myocardial infarction (LDH 1 > LDH 2)
- Increased activity of LDH 5 is an indicator of liver diseases.

11. Detoxification by conjugation.

Refer 2004 Short Note 14.

12. Glutathione.

- Glutathione is gamma-glutamylcysteinyl-glycine. It is a tripeptide of biochemical importance. Glutamate combines with cysteine to form gamma-glutamylcysteine, which combines with glycine to form glutathione. Each step needs one ATP.

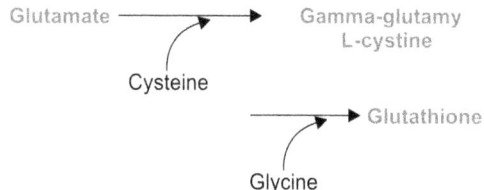

Functions of Glutathione

- **Role in absorption of amino acids in intestines, kidney tubules and in brain**—glutathione is involved in Meister cycle which is needed for absorption and transport of neutral amino acids in intestines, kidney tubules and brain
- **Coenzyme role**—glutathione is needed as a cofactor for:
  - Maleylacetoacetate isomerase, converting maleylacetoacetate to fumaryl acetoacetate
  - Cysteic acid → Taurine
- **To maintain the integrity of RBC membrane**—glutathione present in the RBC is needed for inactivation of free radicals formed inside. Glutathione peroxidase and glutathione reductase enzymes play important role in keeping glutathione in reduced state
- **Conversion of metHb**—metHb cannot transfer oxygen. Glutathione helps in the reduction of metHb to normal Hb
- **Conjugation reactions**—glutathione (GSH) acts as a conjugation agent in detoxification reactions
- **Activation of enzymes**—glutathione keeps certain enzymes with -SH groups in their active site in reduced form.

13. Metabolic acidosis.

Refer 2004 Short Note 16.

14. Codons.

- The letters A, G, T, and C correspond to the nucleotides—adenine, guanine, thymine, and cytosine are found in DNA
- They are organized into three-letter code words called codons, and the collection of these codons makes up the genetic code
- Twenty different amino acids are required for the synthesis of the cellular complement of proteins; thus, there must be at least 20 distinct codons that make up the genetic code
- Codons consisting of two nucleotides each could provide for only 16 (4^2) specific codons, whereas codons of three nucleotides could provide 64 (4^3) specific codons. It is now known that each codon consists of a sequence of three nucleotides, i.e. it is a triplet code
- Three of the 64 possible codons do not code for specific amino acids; these have been termed **nonsense codons**. These nonsense codons are utilized in the cell as termination signals.

15. Renal function test.

Classification of RFT
- **To screen for kidney diseases**
  - Urine analysis—physical, chemical and microscopic examination which are follows:
    a. Physical examination:
      * Volume (24-hours urinary output)
      * Appearance—color
      * pH
      * Specific gravity
      * Osmolality
      * Smell.

b. **Chemical examination:**
  * Qualitative analysis for abnormal constituents of urine mainly glucose, protein and blood
c. Microscopic examination of the centrifuged sediment of urine:
  * For RBC, WBC, pus cells, crystals—to rule out urinary stones and casts
- Plasma urea, creatinine and electrolytes.

2. **To assess Glomerular function**
   - **Glomerular filtration rate (GFR)**—normal GFR is 120-125 mL/min. This is reduced in renal failure
   - **Clearance tests**—done to assess the glomerular filtration and renal blood flow
   - **Renal clearance of a substance is the volume of plasma from which the substance is completely cleared by the kidney in 1 minute**
   - **Clearance** = mg of substance excreted per min/mg of substance per mL of plasma;
   $C = UxV/P$ where C = Clearance of the substance; U = Concentration of the substance in urine; P = Concentration of the substance in plasma; V= Volume of urine passed per minute.
   - Clearance tests—this test is done by using either endogenous markers, such as urea or creatinine or exogenous markers like Inulin, [51]cr-labelled EDTA, [99]Tec-labelled EDTA.

3. **To assess tubular functions**
   - **Renal** tubules reabsorb or secrete certain substances, concentrate the urine and acidify the urine. So it is important for maintaining specific gravity and osmolality of urine
   - **The following are the tubular function tests:**
     a. **SG—specific gravity of urine-**
     b. Urine **concentration test (fluid deprivation test)**
     c. **Measurement of osmolality**
     d. **Dilution tests**
     e. **Urinary acidification test** (acid load test—ammonium chloride loading test)
     f. **Fractional excretion of bicarbonate, sodium and phosphate in urine**—also help in assessing renal tubular functions.

16. Orotic aciduria.

- It is an autosomal recessive disease
- This occurs due to the error in pyrimidine metabolism
- There are 2 types—type I and II
  1. **Type I orotic aciduria**—the condition results from absence of either or both of the enzymes Orotate phosphoribosyl transferase (ORPTase) and OMP decarboxylase—the enzymes of pyrimidine synthesis
  2. **Type II orotic aciduria**—the condition results from the absence of the enzyme OMP decarboxylase—the enzyme of pyrimidine synthesis **(Fig. 29)**.

Clinical Features

- Growth is retarded and megaloblastic anemia present. Bone marrow cells are

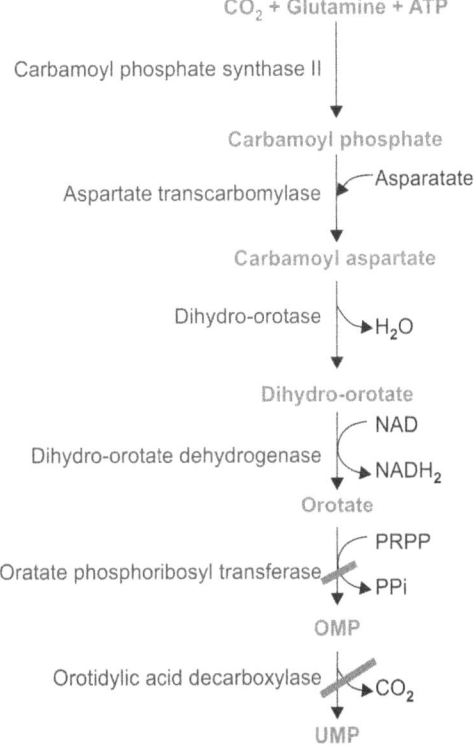

Fig. 29: Orotic aciduria.

rapidly dividing cells which are affected leading to anemia.
- Orotic acid crystalluria—orotate crystals are excreted in urine which may cause urinary tract obstruction in type I. Type II will have orotidinuria also in addition
- Treatment is by feeding cytidine or uridine. They are converted into UTP which can act as feedback inhibitor. Remission with oral uridine
- Orotic aciduria also occurs in urea cycle defect like ornithine transcarbamylase deficiency, since carbamoyl phosphate accumulates and gets diverted to pyrimidine.

17. Wobble hypothesis.
Refer 2008 Short Question 13.

18. Van den Bergh test.
Refer 2008 Short Note 16.

19. Rickets.
Deficiency of vitamin D causes: a) Rickets in children and b) Osteomalacia in adults.

Rickets in Children
- Because of the poor mineralization of bones, they become soft and pliable
- Main features are—bossing of frontal bones, pigeon chest, knock knees, bow legs and rickety rosary—enlargement of epiphysis at the lower end of ribs and costochondral junction causing beading of ribs
- Harrison's sulcus—a transverse depression from the costal cartilage to axilla due to indentation of lower ribs to diaphragm.

20. γ-globulins.
- Immunoglobulins are γ-globulins which act as antibodies. The antibody has a high specificity for a particular antigen only. The antibody's structure is complementary to that specific antigen
- The different classes of Ig are IgG, IgM, IgA, IgD and IgE, IgG depending on the type of heavy chains. Gamma (γ), IgM – Mu (μ), IgA – Alpha (α), IgD-Delta (δ), IgE – Epsilon (ε). The light chains of immunoglobulins are either kappa (κ) or lambda (λ).

IgG
- IgG consists of two heavy chains and two light chains. Heavy chains are of gamma type
- Variable and constant regions are seen in both light and heavy chains. VL and VH are variable and constant regions in light chains and VH and CH are in heavy chains
- The variable regions are important for antigen binding and recognition
- IgG is the major antibody is 75 to 80%
- They are produced by B cells and are involved in secondary immune response
- It crosses placenta and is a reason for Rh isoimmunization (**Fig. 30**).

21. Effect of temperature on enzyme activity.
- The velocity of enzyme catalyzed reaction increases with increase in temperature upto a maximum and then declines
- When we draw a graph for velocity against temperature, a bell shaped curve is obtained
- The temperature at which maximum amount of the substrate is converted to the product per unit is called the optimal temperature. Most of the enzymes work at optimal temperature ranges between 37-50°C, except some, e.g. thermobacillus (Taq pol II)
- Temperature coefficient or Q_{10} is the factor by which the rate of catalysis is increased by a rise of 10°C. it is usually between 0°C and 40°C (**Fig. 31**).

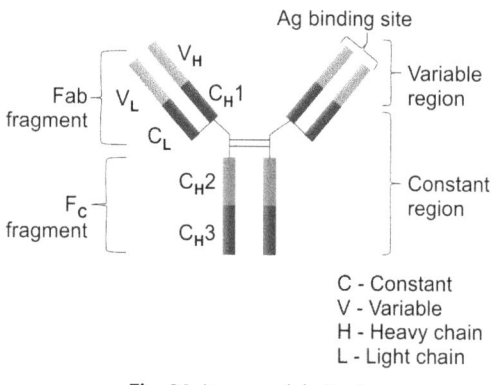

C - Constant
V - Variable
H - Heavy chain
L - Light chain

Fig. 30: Immunoglobulin-G.

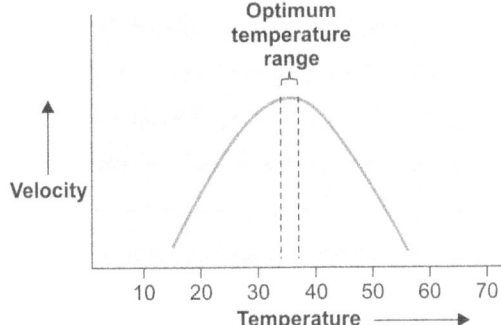

Fig. 31: Effects of temperature on enzyme velocity.

22. Define epimer. Name two epimers.

Isomers differing as a result of variations in configuration of the OH and H with regard to a single carbon atom other than the reference carbon atom—on carbon atoms 2, 3, and 4 of glucose are known as epimers.
- Biologically, the most important epimers of glucose are mannose and galactose formed by epimerization at carbons 2 and 4, respectively.

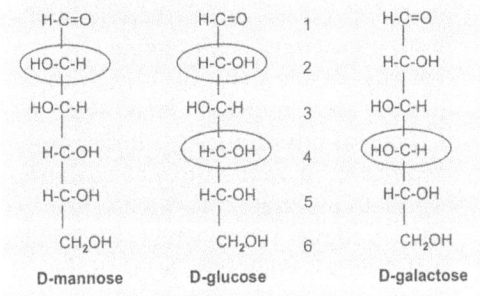

Fig. 32: Epimers.

23. Importance of phosphatidylinositol 4,5-bisphosphate.

Phosphatidylinositol (PIP2)
- It is one of the glycerophospholipid—compound lipid
- Its functional group is inositol which esterifies phosphatidic acid
- Phosphatidylinositol 4,5-bisphosphate (PIP2) acts as second messenger in mediating hormone action on biological membrane, e.g. TRH, catecholamines, oxytocin.

24. Biochemical functions of selenium.

- Selenium is an important trace elements
- Normal serum level—50 to 100 mg/dL
- RDA—50 to 100 mg/day

Function
- Antioxidant function—the requirement of vitamin E reduces with increase in selenium intake. Both spare the action of one another
- Selenium-containing enzymes—glutathione peroxidase antioxidant enzyme which protects RBC from free radicals contains selenium
- 5'-deiodinase (thyroid metabolism)—in selenium deficiency it leads to hypothyroidism
- It is necessary for spermatogenesis
- Selenium is a constituent of selenocysteine which is the 21st amino acid
- Deficiency of selenium—leads to Keshan disease characterized by multifocal myocardial necrosis, cardiac arrhythmias and cardiac enlargement
- Selenium toxicity is called selenosis which produces symptoms of hair loss, falling of nails, diarrhea and loss of weight.

25. Benedict's test.

Refer 2008 Short Question 3.

26. Ribose and deoxyribose.

- They are aldopentoses having 5 carbon atoms
- Deoxygenation occurs at 2nd carbon in deoxyribose
- D-ribose is a structural element of ribonucleic acid, and coenzymes like ATP, NAD, NADP and flavoproteins
- Ribose is an intermediate products of pentose phosphate pathway
- Deoxyribose is a structural element of DNA.

27. Lysosomes.

- They are tiny cellular organelles. They are bags of enzymes which are hydrolases
- These enzymes hydrolyze polysaccharides, proteins, lipids and nucleic acids having pH around 5. They catalyze degradative reactions

- The marker enzyme of lysosomes is acid phosphatase
- When the lysosomal membrane is disrupted the released enzymes can hydrolyze other substrates leading to tissue damage
- Example for lysosomal damage results in inflammation and arthritis is gout.

28. Bence Jones protein.

- Monoclonal light chains are excreted in urine in conditions like multiple myeloma. They are called Bence Jones protein. This is due to asynchronous production of H and L chains or due to deletion of portions of L chains
- This is seen in the electrophoresis as myeloma band or monoclonal bands
- The Bence Jones protein precipitate when heated between 45-60°C and redissolve above 80° or below 45°C. Bradshaw test is also positive
- These proteins will block renal tubules leading to renal failure.

Bradshaw's test

- This is a positive test for multiple myeloma to show the presence of Bence Jones protein. Few mL of concentrated hydrochloric acid is taken in a test tube and few mL of urine is layered over it. A white ring of precipitate is formed to give positive result for Bradshaw's test.

29. Bile salts.

Refer 2004 Short Note 9.
- Bile salts are sodium or potassium salts of taurocholic or glycocholic acids
- They are produced from cholesterol by 7-alpha-hydroxylase and present in bile
- They are water insoluble, toxic and conjugated by glycine or taurine
- They emulsify the lipids into droplets to form mixed micelles and thereby increase the surface area of the particles and lower the surface tension
- Micellar formation helps in absorption of lipids.

30. Cori cycle.

Cori cycle (lactic acid cycle) (Fig. 33)

Definition: Transferring lactate from muscle tissues to liver and resynthesis of glucose in liver is known as Cori's cycle.

Effects
- In contracting muscle, pyruvate is reduced to lactate which gets accumulated in muscle and may lead to muscular cramps in strenuous muscular exercise
- It rescues lactate for further use (gluconeogenesis) and counteracts lactic acidosis.
- It is of less importance in starvation but important in more normal situations especially in certain cells, such as matured RBC, medulla, retina which are lacking mitochondria and virtually anaerobic

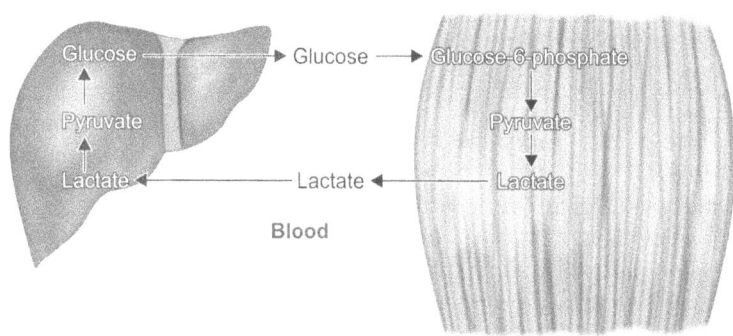

Fig. 33: Cori cycle.

- Lactate is carried from skeletal muscle to liver through blood. In the liver lactate is converted to pyruvate and by gluconeogenesis it is converted to glucose which is then transported to muscles for energy supply.

31. Maple syrup urine disease.
Refer 2007 Essay Question 10.

32. Alkali reserve.
- Bicarbonate represents the reserve of alkali available for the neutralization of strong acids
- The alkali reserve has to be sufficiently high to meet the acid load
- If it is too low to give a ratio of 1, all the HCO_3^- would have been exhausted within a very short time; and buffering will not be effective
- Under physiological circumstances, the ratio of 20 (a high alkali reserve) ensures high buffering efficiency against acids
- The normal bicarbonate level in serum 24 mmol/L.

33. Biological value of proteins.
- It is one of the parameters for the assessment of nutritive value of proteins
- It is the ratio between the amount of nitrogen retained and nitrogen absorbed during a specific interval.

34. Carcinogenic virus.
- Viruses cause cancers in humans and animals by activating oncogenes or damaging tumor suppressor genes or by other mechanisms
- Two types of oncogenic viruses are:
  1. DNA viruses, e.g. herpes virus; adenovirus, papova viruses
  2. RNA viruses, e.g. rous sarcoma virus contains reverse transcriptase
- DNA virus infects the host cell and binds tightly to host cell DNA and causes alteration in gene expression and transforms into altered protein synthesis
- RNA viruses use RNA as genome. RNA gets copied by reverse transcriptase to produce single-stranded DNA which will be copied to form double-stranded viral DNA or provirus. Provirus then gets integrated into host cell genome and transform into neoplastic cell. Example are:
  - Epstein-barr virus (EBV):
    - Burkitt's lymphoma is caused by EBV
    - It infects the B lymphocytes
    - The B cells are immortalized. But they are dependent on B cell growth factor for proliferation
    - Next it causes transposition of oncogenes, so that they get BCGF independence
    - But the cells divide slowly. Then the virus activates the c-myc oncogene which causes cancer
    - EBV is linked with nasopharyngeal carcinoma.
  - Human papilloma virus—it has circular double-stranded DNA. There are more than 100 HPV types. Types 16 and 18 cause cervical cancer
  - Hepatitis B virus hepatoma.

35. Electrophoretic technique and its importance.
Refer 2006 Short Note 30.

36. Methemoglobin.
- Methemoglobin (MetHb) is a type of Hb variant. The iron in the heme is in ferrous form normally. When it is oxidized to ferric form then it is called methemoglobin
- Normally the metHb level in blood is less than 1%. It has decreased capacity of transporting oxygen
- Small quantities of metHb formed are reduced by metHb reductase systems using NADH and cytochrome b5. Remaining is reduced using NADPH dependent enzyme. Glutathione dependent metHb reductase system is also present
- **Methemoglobinemia**—increase in metHb level in blood is known as methemoglobinemia. It is manifested as cyanosis
- Two types – Congenital and acquired
  1. Congenital methemoglobinemia—cytochrome b5 reductase deficiency is the cause for this. Oral administration of methylene blue reduces the symptoms.

2. Acquired methemoglobinemia—may be due to intake of: a) Water containing nitrates; b) Absorption of aniline dyes; c) Drugs like acetaminophen, sulfanilamides, amyl nitrate ingestion.

G6PD deficiency causes reduced availability of NADPH for the RBCs. At that time the NADPH-dependent methemoglobin reductase will be inactive leading to methemoglobinemia.

37. Importance of glucose-6-phosphate dehydrogenase deficiency.

- Hexose monophosphate pathway is an alternate pathway in carbohydrate pathway
- It has two phases of reactions which as follows:
  1. Phase I oxidative phase—irreversible phase
  2. Phase II (nonoxidative phase)—reversible

Oxidative Phase

- **Step 1:** Rate-limiting step catalyzed by glucose-6-phosphate dehydrogenase enzyme which is NADP dependent. One NADPH is produced

$$\text{Glucose-6-phosphate} \xrightarrow[\text{NADP} \quad \text{NADPH} + H^+]{\text{Glucose-6 phosphate dehydrogenase}} \text{6-phosphogluconolactone}$$

Glucose-6-phosphate dehydrogenase deficiency—congenital

- It is the most common inborn error of metabolism. It is X-linked recessive trait
- This will lead to drug induced hemolytic anemia
- The deficiency is manifested only when exposed to certain oxidant drugs or toxins like primaquine for malaria or ingestion of toxic glycosides in Fava beans (favism)
- Sulfa drugs may also precipitate hemolysis. This leads to jaundice and severe anemia.

This disease offers resistance to plasmodium infection and protects the individual from malaria since the parasite requires reduced glutathione which is not available in the G6PD deficiency.

38. G proteins.

Refer 2006 Short Note 32.

39. Renal threshold substances.

- Compounds whose excretion in urine is dependent on blood level are known as threshold substances
- At normal or low plasma levels they are completely reabsorbed and are not excreted in urine
- But when the blood level is elevated the tubular reabsorptive capacity (tubular maximum or Tm) is saturated and the excess will be excreted in urine
- Normal renal threshold:
  - For glucose is 180 mg/dL;
  - Lactate—60 mg/dL;
  - Bicarbonate—28 mEq/L;
  - Calcium—10 mg/dL
- For glucose the renal threshold is 175-180 mg/dL above which glucose will be seen in urine. The tubular reabsorptive capacity (tubular maximum or Tm) for glucose is 375 mg/min (T_{max})
- In renal glycosuria the renal threshold for glucose is reduced and so glucose is excreted in urine even though the blood glucose level is normal.

40. Carbon monoxide.

Carbon monoxide is a colorless, odorless gas that is produced in large quantities by vehicles and exhaust from industries. It is one of the air pollutants.

- It has 200 times more affinity than oxygen towards hemoglobin
- When one molecule of CO binds with Hb, it forms carboxyhemoglobin
- It increases affinity of oxygen toward Hb, so the Hb will not release oxygen. This carboxyhemoglobin is unsuitable for oxygen transport
- Automobile exhaust in closed space is the cause of CO poisoning most common
- Cigarette smoker has 4% CO-Hb
- When the CO-Hb level in blood exceeds 20%—breathlessness, headache, nausea, vomiting ensues. At 40-60% death can occur
- Oxygen administration is the effective treatment.

MBBS Examination 2010

ANSWER ALL QUESTIONS

I. Essay questions (10/15 Marks each)

1. Define enzymes. Classify enzymes with suitable examples. Explain the concept of active site of enzymes.
2. Describe the steps of HMP shunt pathway. What is its significance? How is it regulated?
3. Discuss about nucleic acids under following headings: a) Types, b) Functions, c) Components, d) Chargaff's rule of DNA composition, e) Different forms of DNA double helix and f) Differences between DNA and RNA.
4. Describe the steps of s-adenosyl-methionine cycle. Explain the term transmethylation with five suitable examples.
5. Describe the citric acid cycle. How is it regulated? What is its amphibolic role?
6. Describe the chemistry, absorption, functions and deficiency manifestations of vitamin A.
7. Describe the separation of serum proteins by paper electrophoresis. Draw the pattern of electrophoresis in: i) Multiple myeloma, ii) Nephrotic syndrome.
8. How is blood pH regulated?

II. Short notes (5 Marks each)

1. Nutritional importance of proteins.
2. Describe the requirement, sources, metabolic functions and deficiency manifestations of folic acid.
3. Explain with a neat labeled diagram of fluid mosaic model of biological membrane.
4. Total parenteral nutrition and its importance.
5. Transfer RNA (tRNA).
6. Explain the metabolism and functions of HDL.
7. What are glycoproteins? Give three examples and its importance.
8. Chemiosmotic theory.
9. Rapoport-Luebering shunt pathway and its significance.
10. What are nucleotides? Name any three biologically important nucleotides and their importance.
11. Give an account of the formation of specialized products from glycine.
12. Explain the term transamination and its salient features.
13. Polymerase chain reaction and its applications.
14. Blotting techniques.
15. Gene therapy.
16. Write an account of salvage pathway in purine nucleotide synthesis. Add a note on Lesch–Nyhan syndrome.
17. Post-translational modification.
18. What are porphyrias? Describe any three porphyrias in detail.
19. Give an account of water distribution and its balance in the body.
20. What are isotopes? What are its applications in biochemistry?
21. Inhibitors of electron transport chain.
22. Transport of bilirubin.
23. Vitamin E.
24. Substrate level phosphorylation.
25. Gluconeogenesis.
26. Regulation of enzyme activity.
27. Abnormal hemoglobins/hemoglobinopathies.

28. Digestion and absorption of triacylglycerol.
29. Biomedical importance of derivatives of cholesterol.
30. Significance and disorders of pentose phosphate pathway.
31. Genetic code.
32. Formation of epinephrine.
33. Cytochrome P450.
34. Purine salvage pathway.
35. Dehydration.
36. LAC operon.
37. Orotic acidurias.
38. Phenylketonuria.
39. Water toxicity.

III. Short answer questions

(2/3 Marks each)

1. Why sucrose is called a nonreducing disaccharide?
2. Name the essential fatty acids.
3. Name any four biologically important compounds derived from cholesterol.
4. What are phospholipids? Give two examples.
5. Name the essential amino acids.
6. Mention any two biological functions of albumin.
7. Name the amino acids required for purine biosynthesis.
8. Sickle cell hemoglobin.
9. Specific dynamic action.
10. Write the principle and significance of Biuret test.
11. Okazaki pieces.
12. Differences between CPS I and CPS II
13. Metabolic role of magnesium.
14. Anion gap.
15. Rothera's test.
16. Gout.
17. Fluorosis.
18. van den Berg test.
19. Mutarotation.
20. Subcellular organelles.
21. Free radicals.
22. Basal metabolic rate.
23. Causes of fatty liver.
24. Renal glycosuria.
25. Role of HDL as scavenger of cholesterol.
26. FIGLU.
27. Dietary fibers.
28. Xeroderma pigmentosum.
29. Functions of parathyroid hormone.
30. Mention two second messengers.
31. Symport.
32. Oxytocin.
33. Addison's disease.
34. Functions of glucagon.
35. Gamma-aminobutyric acid.
36. Hartnup's disease.

I. ESSAY QUESTIONS

1. **Define enzymes. Classify enzymes with suitable examples. Explain the concept of active site of enzymes.**

DEFINITION

Enzymes are biocatalysts which are proteins in nature (except ribozymes). They are specific in their reaction. They are heat labile and colloidal and are required in small quantities for their action.

Classification

A. **As per the site of location:**
   a. Intracellular enzymes within the cellular organelles, e.g. cytosol—enzymes of glycolysis, mitochondria-enzymes of TCA cycle
   b. Extracellular enzymes—secreted from the cells but function outside the cells, e.g. digestive enzymes—pepsin, trypsin.

B. **As per the diagnostic use—plasma enzymes**
   a. Plasma specific or plasma functional enzymes—they have definite functions in plasma found in high concentration than in tissues mostly synthesized in liver, e.g. lipoprotein lipase, pseudocholinesterase
   b. Plasma nonspecific or plasma nonfunctional enzymes—they have no definite function in plasma; they may be absent or present in low amounts in

plasma. During the damage of tissues of its origin, its level is elevated in plasma, e.g. amylase, acid phosphatase.

C. **As per the types of reaction catalyzed**: For example, dehydrogenases—removes hydrogen atom. Proteases—hydrolase proteins

D. **IUB systems of classification—6 classes**: As per this system enzymes are represented as EC number with 4 digits (IUB system) First digit represent the class, second for the subclass, third for the sub-subclass, and fourth represents specific enzyme in list.

CLASSES: (OTHLIL) (6 CLASSES)

- **O**xidoreductases—these class of enzymes catalyze oxidations and reductions.
  $$AH_2 + B \rightarrow A + BH_2$$
  For example, alcohol dehydrogenase, oxidases, reductases
- **T**ransferases—these classes of enzymes catalyze transfer of moieties between substrate, such as amino acids, glycosyl, methyl, or phosphoryl group.
  $$A\text{-}R + B \rightarrow A + B\text{-}R$$
  For example hexokinase, transaminase
- **H**ydrolases—these classes of enzymes catalyze hydrolytic cleavage of C-C, C-O, C-N, and other bonds by adding of water.
  $$A\text{-}B + H_2O \rightarrow A\text{-}OH + B\text{-}H$$
  For example, acetylcholine + $H_2O \rightarrow$ choline + acetate catalyzed by acetylcholine esterase
- **L**yases—these classes of enzymes catalyze cleavage of C-C, C-O, C-N, and other bonds by elimination, leaving double bonds without adding water.
  For example, fructose-1, 6-bisphosphate $\xrightarrow{\text{Aldolase}}$ glyceraldehyde-3-phosphate + DHAP
- **I**somerases—these classes of enzymes catalyze geometric or structural changes within a molecule.
  For example, Racemases, epimerase, cis-trans isomerases
- **L**igases—these classes of enzymes catalyze the joining together of two molecules coupled to the hydrolysis of ATP.

For example, acetyl-CoA + ATP $\rightarrow$ malonyl CoA + ADP + Pi.

CONCEPT OF ACTIVE SITE OF ENZYME

- This is the region of the enzyme where the substrate binding and catalysis occurs
- Active site occupies a smaller portion of the enzyme
- It contains specific amino acid residues and possesses three dimensional structure
- Situated in a cleft or crevice of the enzyme molecule
- It is not rigid but flexible in structure and shape to promote proper substrate binding by conformational changes
- Substrate binds to the enzymes at the active site by noncovalent bonds[s]
- Substrate binds to the enzymes[E] at the active site to form enzyme-substrate complex[ES] which is the first step in enzyme catalysis
  $$E + S \leftrightarrow ES \rightarrow E + P$$
- After the catalysis the product [P] is released and the enzyme becomes free for further use
- Depending upon the substrate binding to the active site of the enzymes, two models have been proposed to explain the mechanism of enzyme action.

1. **Lock and key model**—rigid template model, Fischer's template theory: The active site is rigid and complementary to the substrate. The substrate fits into active site like lock and key. This could not explain the flexibility shown by enzymes
2. **Koshland's induced fit model**—this model explains that the enzymes are not rigid and preshaped. When the substrate interacts with the enzyme it induces a conformational change to produce the substrate binding site.

2. **Describe the steps of HMP shunt pathway. What is its significance? How is it regulated?**

- **HMP shunt:** Hexose monophosphate shunt—alternate pathway for oxidation of glucose

- **Other names**: Pentose phosphate shunt or Warburg-Dickens-Horecker pathway, phospogluconate oxidative pathway
- **Occurrence**: Liver, adipose tissue, RBC, mammary glands, testes, adrenal gland.

Steps of HMP Shunt Pathway (Reactions) (Fig. 1)

- There are two phases:
  1. Phase I: Oxidative phase—irreversible phase
  2. Phase II: Nonoxidative phase—reversible phase.

Oxidative Phase

- Rate-limiting step catalyzed by glucose-6-phosphate dehydrogenase enzyme which is NADP dependent. One NADPH is produced

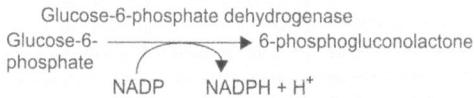

- Hydrolysis of 6-phosphogluconolactone to 6-phosphogluconate by hydrolase enzymes

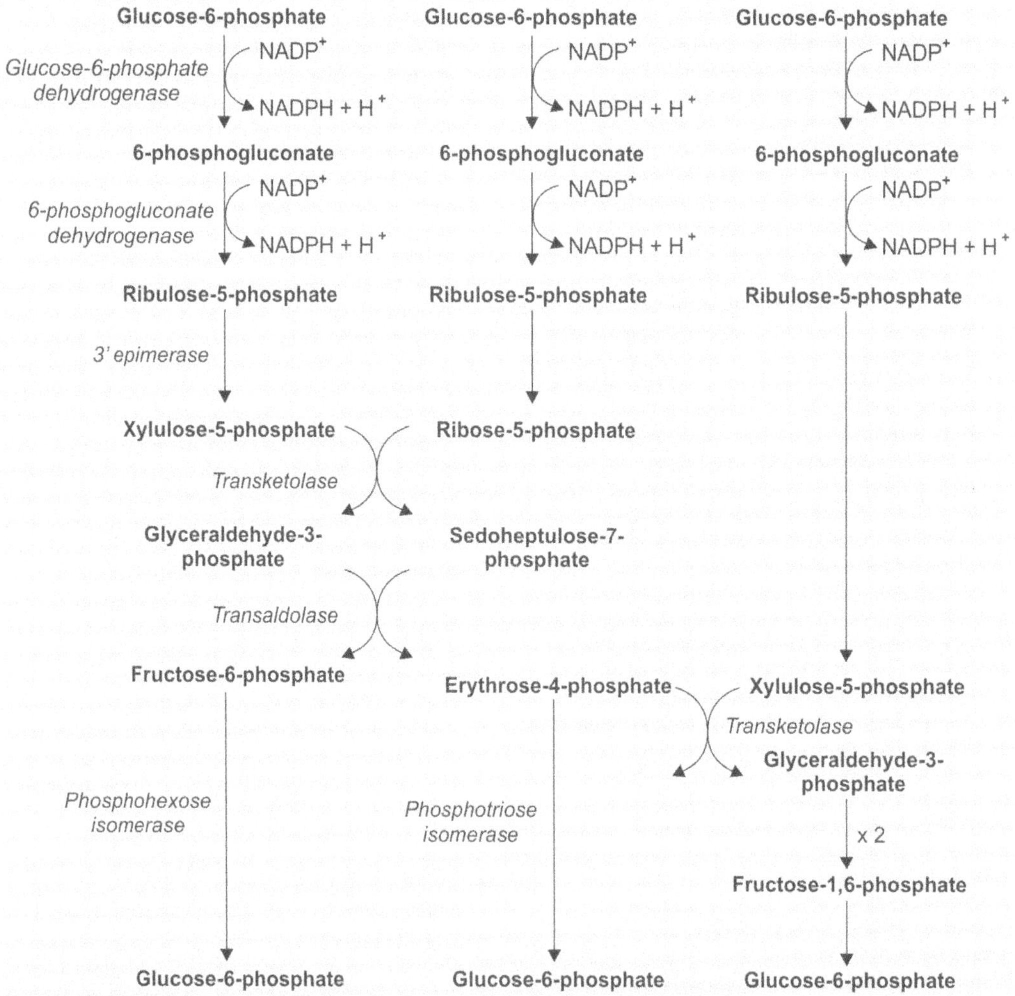

Fig. 1: HMP shunt.

- Oxidation and decarboxylation of 6-phosphogluconate to form ribulose-5-phosphate by phosphogluconate dehydrogenase.

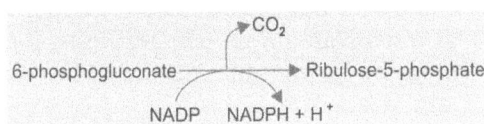

Nonoxidative Phase

- Isomerization—ribulose-5-phosphate is isomerized to ribose-5-phosphate by keto isomerase or epimerised to xylulose 5-phosphate by epimerase

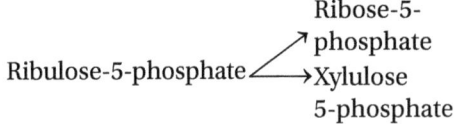

- **Transketolase reaction**: TPP dependent reaction

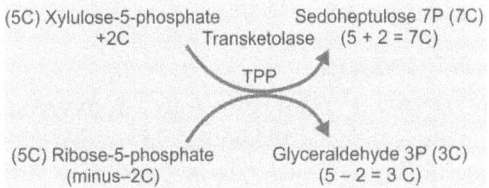

7C-ketose sedoheptulose and 3C–aldose glyceraldehyde 3-phosphate are generated.
- **Transaldolase reaction**: 3C from Sedoheptulose 7-phosphate are removed and joined with glyceraldehyde 3-phosphate to form 6C ketose fructose 6-phosphate

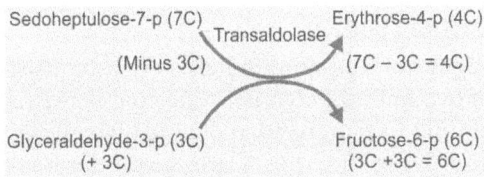

- Second transketolase reaction-TPP dependent

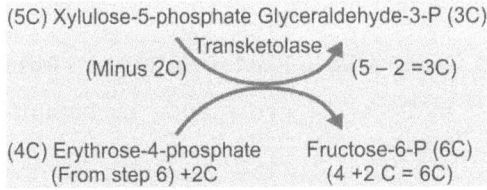

- Regeneration of glucose-6-phosphate.
  - two molecules of glyceraldehyde-3-phosphate from above point are condensed to form fructose-6-phosphate (3 × 2 = 6 C). This is then converted to glucose-6-phosphate by reversal of glycolysis by fructose 1, 6-bisphosphatase.

Significance of Hmp Pathway

Biochemical Significance (Oxidative Phase)

- Biosynthesis of pentoses-ribose-5-phosphate for the synthesis of nucleotides and nucleic acids like DNA, RNA, ATP, NAD, FAD
- Provides way for interconversion of pentoses and hexoses (both phases)
- Generation of NADPH which acts as reducing equivalents for:
  - Reductive synthesis of fatty acids, bile acids, cholesterol
  - NADPH is needed for the integrity of RBC membrane
  - Antioxidant—free radical scavenger
  - Helps to prevent met, Hb formation
  - Detoxifies drugs by liver microsomes P450 enzymes.

Clinical Significance

- **Glucose-6-phosphate dehydrogenase deficiency:**
  - X linked recessive trait
  - Cells having the deficient enzyme have lower rate of NADPH production and deficiency of reduced glutathione leading to hemolysis
  - This deficiency is manifested only when exposed to certain drugs, such as primaquine (antimalarial)
  - Fava beans consumption and sulfa drugs also precipitate hemolysis
  - Methemoglobinemia will be seen in circulation in glucose-6-phosphate deficiency. There is no cyanosis
  - This disease offers resistance to plasmodium infection and protects the individual from malaria since the parasite requires reduced glutathione which is not available in G6PD deficiency

- Transketolase activity of RBC is used to measure the deficiency level of thiamine
- Genetic defect in transketolase enzyme will lead to Wernick Korsakoff syndrome (encephalopathy) seen in alcoholics.

Regulation of HMP Shunt
- Rate-limiting enzyme—glucose-6-phosphate dehydrogenase is regulated by NADPH by competitive inhibition. Oxidative phase is controlled by NADPH
- Insulin induces G6PD enzyme and increase the overall pathway
- Nonoxidative phase is controlled by the requirement of pentoses.

3. Discuss about nucleic acids under following headings: a. Types, b. Functions, c. Components, d. Chargaff's rule of DNA composition, e. Different forms of DNA double helix and f. Differences between DNA and RNA.

A. TYPES OF NUCLEIC ACIDS

- Nucleic acids are classified into deoxyribonucleic acid (DNA) and ribonucleic acid (RNA)
- DNA is further classified into B-DNA, A-DNA, and Z-DNA
- RNA can be classified into messenger RNA (mRNA), ribosomal RNA (rRNA), transfer RNA (tRNA), small nuclear RNA (snRNA).

B. FUNCTIONS OF NUCLEIC ACIDS

DNA
- DNA is the genetic material in the cell. It is the chemical basis of hereditary and it is organized into genes which are the fundamental units of genetic information
- The genes in DNA encode proteins which are necessary for cellular function
- It is involved in the synthesis of RNA—by transcription. Proteins are then synthesized by translation
- It provides template for replication of the information into daughter DNA.

RNA
- Messenger RNA (mRNA)—it is synthesized from DNA by transcription. It contains the codons for protein synthesis which serve as a template for protein synthesis. It is attached to ribosome on which protein synthesis occurs
- Transfer RNA (tRNA)—it acts as an adapter molecule in carrying a specific amino acid for a particular codon in mRNA and helps in protein synthesis—translation
- Ribosomal RNA (rRNA)—it is component of ribosomes. Ribosomes are made up of many polypeptides and rRNA
- Small nuclear RNA (snRNA)—these are small nuclear RNAs. They are involved in the process of removal of introns and splicing of exons of mRNA precursors
- Ribozymes—some RNA are capable of enzymatic functions like peptidyl transferases.

COMPONENTS

- **DNA**—it contains four deoxyribonucleotides as backbone—deoxyadenylate, deoxyguanylate, deoxycytidylate and thymidylate units which are held by 3'5'-phosphodiester bonds
- **RNA**—it is a polymer of purine and pyrimidine ribonucleotides of adenine, guanine, cytosine and uracil linked by 3'5'-phosphodiester bonds.

C. STRUCTURE OF DNA (WATSON–CRICK MODEL) (FIG. 2)

Right handed double helix—DNA consists of two helical polynucleotide chains twisted around in right handed double helix. Purine and pyrimidine bases are inside the helix. Phosphate and deoxyribose units are on the outside. The planes of bases are perpendicular to the helical axis. Sugars are kept at right angles to the bases.

D. BASE PAIRING RULE–CHARGAFF'S RULE

- In DNA, the two strands are complementary to each other

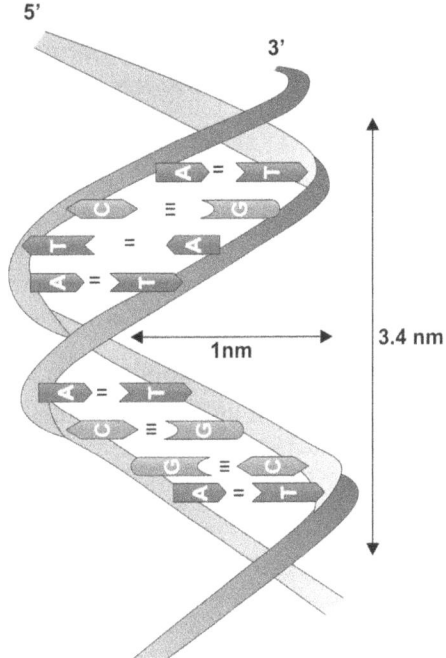

Fig. 2: Structure of DNA.

- The number of adenine molecules are equal to thymine molecules (A=T) and number of cytosine molecules are equal to guanine molecules (C=G)
- Adenine pairs with thymine by 2 hydrogen bonds (A=T); guanine pairs with cytosine by 3-hydrogen bonds (G≡C). This is called Chargaff's rule.

Hydrogen bonding—adenine pairs with thymine by 2 hydrogen bonds (A=T); Guanine pairs with cytosine by 3-hydrogen bonds (G≡C). GC bond is stronger than AT bond.

Antiparallel—the two strands of DNA run antiparallel to each other. One strand runs in 5' to 3' direction, while the opposite strand runs in 3' to 5' direction.

Structure of helix:
- Diameter or width of the helix is 20Å (1.9 to 2.0 nm)
- It has a pitch of 3.4 nm per turn
- Within a single turn 10 base pairs are seen.
- Adjacent pairs are separated by 0.34 nm
- It has a major groove (1.2 nm) and a minor groove (0.6 nm) which wind along the molecule, parallel to the phosphodiester backbone
- Proteins interact with the bases in these grooves.

E. DIFFERENT FORMS OF DNA DOUBLE HELIX

DNA exists in six structural forms. They are—A-DNA, B-DNA, C-DNA, D-DNA, E-DNA and Z-DNA. Out of these A, B, and Z forms are important.

- **B-DNA**—it has the classic Watson–Crick model. It is the commonest form. The DNA is a right handed helix. It has two polydeoxyribonucleotide strands twisted around each other. The two strands are antiparallel. One strand runs from 5' to 3' direction and other on 3' to 5' direction. The width of double helix is 2 nm. Each turn of helix is 3.4 nm with 10 pairs of nucleotides. The sugar forms as backbone in which base is attached. The bases in two strands form hydrogen bonds and they are arranged according to Chargaff's rule
- **A-DNA**: It is right handed helix having 11 base pairs per turn
- **Z-DNA**: It is a left handed helix containing 12 base pairs per turn. The polynucleotide strands of DNA move in a zigzag fashion.

S. No.	Property	A-DNA	B-DNA	Z-DNA
1.	Shape	Broadest	Medium	Narrow
2.	Type of helix	Right handed	Right handed	Left handed
3.	Base pairs per turn	11	10	12
4	Helix diameter	25.5Å	23.7Å	18.4Å
5.	Pitch per turn of helix	25.3Å	35.4Å	45.6Å
6.	Major groove	Narrow	Wide	Flat
7.	Minor groove	Very broad	Narrow	Very narrow

F. DIFFERENCES BETWEEN DNA AND RNA

S. No.	Characteristics	DNA	RNA
1.	Monomeric units	A, G, C, and thymidylate	A, G, C, and uridylate
2.	Sugar	Deoxyribose	Ribose
3.	Nature of strand/s	Double stranded helix	Single stranded
4.	Base pairs	A=T; G≡C	A=U; G≡C
5.	Types	A-DNA; B-DNA; Z-DNA	mRNA, tRNA, rRNA, snRNA
6.	Function	Carry genetic information. Synthesis of RNA—transcription	Involved in the synthesis of proteins—translation

4. Describe the steps of S-adenosyl-methionine cycle. Explain the term trans-methylation with five suitable examples.

METHIONINE METABOLISM

- Methionine is a sulfur containing amino acid; it is an essential, glucogenic amino acid
- From methionine the other sulfur containing amino acid—cysteine is produced.

Steps of Methionine Metabolism (Fig. 3)

- Activation of Methionine to S-Adenosyl Methionine (SAM)
  S-adenosylmethionine cycle (Fig. 4):

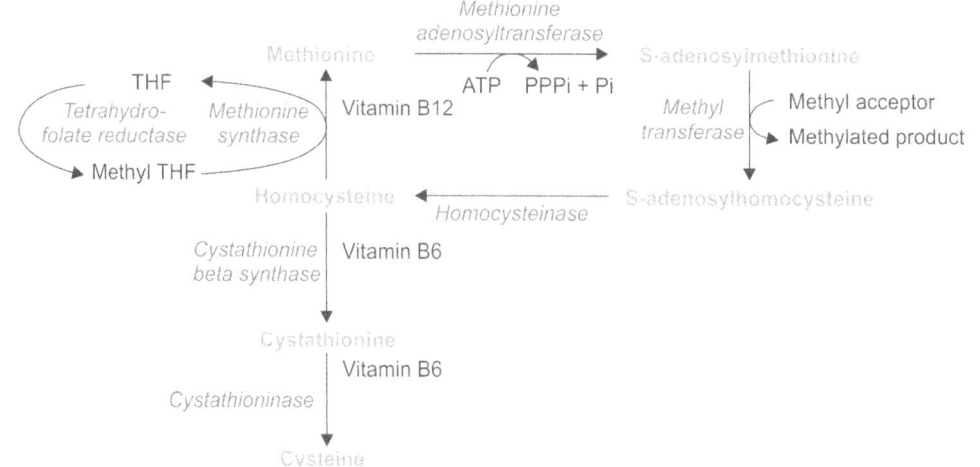

Fig. 3: Methionine metabolism.

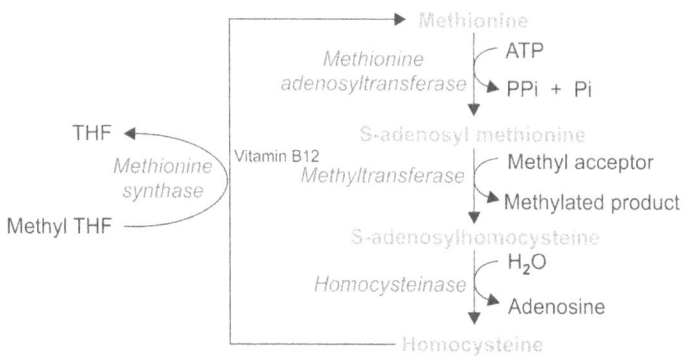

Fig. 4: S-adenosyl methionine cycle.

- Methionine adenosyltransferase enzyme transfers the adenosyl group to the sulfur atom of methionine to form the active methionine S-adenosyl methionine.
- **Transfer of methyl group to other acceptors (transmethylation)**—SAM donates methyl group to methyl acceptors by methyl transferases to form S-adenosyl-homocysteine (SAH)
- **Formation of homocysteine**—from S-adenosylhomocysteine adenosine group is removed by adenosine homocysteinase to form homocysteine
- **Resynthesis of methionine**—homocysteine forms methionine by homocysteine methyltransferase. This step uses methyltetrahydrofolate which becomes THFA in the presence of B12
- **Formation of cysteine**—homocysteine combines with serine to form cystathionine using cystathionine synthase in the presence of PLP. Cystathionine is hydrolyzed to cysteine and homoserine by cystathioninase. PLP acts as a coenzyme for this step also. This is trans-sulfuration reaction
- **Final oxidation of homoserine**—homoserine is deaminated and decarboxylated to propionyl-CoA which is converted to methylmalonyl-CoA and then to succinyl-CoA with the help of deoxyadenosyl-cobalamin. Succinyl-CoA enters into TCA cycle and hence methionine is a glucogenic amino acid.

TRANSMETHYLATION REACTION

It is acceptance of a methyl group from a donor like S-adenosyl methionine by an acceptor resulting in the formation of a methylated compound.
- Transmethylation reaction requires SAM which is obtained by accepting adenosyl group from ATP by methionine by methionine adenosyltransferase.

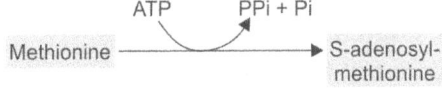

The examples for transmethylation reactions are:

Methyl acceptor	Methylated product
Guanidoacetic acid + SAM	Creatine
Serine + SAM	Choline
Epinephrine + SAM	Metanephrine
Norepinephrine + SAM	Epinephrine
tRNA + SAM	Methylated tRNA

5. **Describe the citric acid cycle. How is it regulated? What is its amphibolic role?**

Refer 2004 Essay Question 1.

6. **Describe the chemistry, absorption, functions and deficiency manifestations of Vitamin A.**

Refer 2006 Essay Question 7.

7. **Describe the separation of serum proteins by paper electrophoresis. Draw the pattern of electrophoresis in: i. Multiple myeloma, ii. Nephrotic syndrome.**

SEPARATION OF SERUM PROTEINS BY PAPER ELECTROPHORESIS

Principle
- The term electrophoresis refers to the movement of charged particles through an electrolyte when subjected to an electric field
- Cations (positively charged ions) move towards cathod and anions (negative) to anode
- When a biological mixture is subjected to electrophoresis, the compounds in the mixture move in relation to their net charge, size, molecular weight and mass and gets separated according to these characteristics, so that the desired compound can be identified and isolated.

Applications
It is used for the separation of serum proteins, serum lipoproteins, isoenzymes, immunoglobulins, abnormal hemoglobin and many other compounds.

Technique (Horizontal) (Fig. 5)
- The apparatus consists of two troughs filled with barbitone buffer solution (pH 8.6) through which electric current is passed

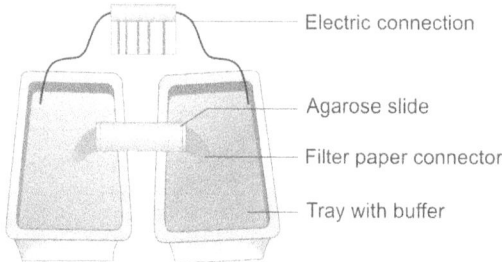

Fig. 5: Electrophoresis apparatus.

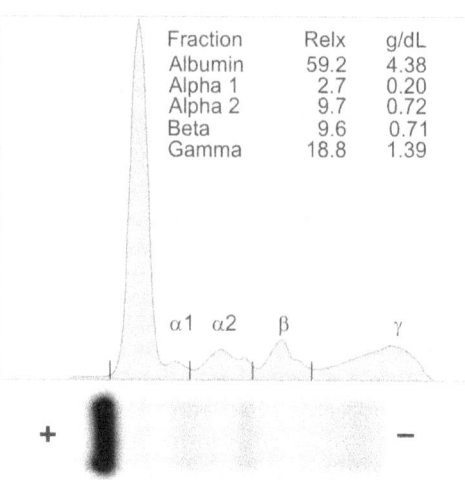

Fig. 6: Normal electrophoretic pattern.

Fraction	Rel%	g/dL
Albumin	59.2	4.38
Alpha 1	2.7	0.20
Alpha 2	9.7	0.72
Beta	9.6	0.71
Gamma	18.8	1.39

- Whatman No. 3 filter paper is cut into strips of 2 cm width and soaked in buffer solution
- Filter paper is suspended over the glass rod fixed in the apparatus. The two ends of the strip should dip in the buffer solution in the inner compartments of the two troughs
- The outer compartments of the two troughs contain electrode through which current is passed
- A drop of serum is mixed with a drop of bromophenol blue dye. Using a 0.1 mL pipette, 0.05 mL of the mixed serum is applied as a fine streak on the center of the paper supported by glass rod
- The chamber is closed with the lid and the current is switched on adjusting it to 180-200 volts
- The moving boundary of the migrating proteins, stained blue can be seen moving towards anode
- At the end of 5 hours run, the current is switched off and the strips are removed, and dried in the hot air oven with temperature $110°C$ for ½ an hour
- Then the dried strips are put in the dish containing bromophenol blue staining solution overnight
- Next day morning, the stained strips are washed in 2% acetic acid solution twice or thrice to remove the excess stain
- Then they are kept in a fixative solution of 2% sodium acetate in 10% acetic acid for 6 minutes
- Then, the papers are dried in the hot air oven for 15 minutes. If necessary blue color can be developed further by exposing to ammonia vapor and the various bands are observed.

Clinical Significance

Electrophoretogram of serum proteins is helpful in detecting changes in the individual protein fractions in serum and in detecting abnormal bands in certain diseased conditions.

In a normal electrophoretogram the proportions of the various protein bands are as follows (**Fig. 6**. Normal electrophoretic Pattern):

- Albumin – about 60%
- α_1 globulin – about 4%
- α_2 globulin – about 8%
- β-globulin – about 12%
- γ-globulin – about 16%

PATTERN OF ELECTROPHORESIS IN CERTAIN DISEASES (FIGS. 7A TO D)

- **Multiple myeloma**—abnormal paraprotein M band/myeloma band seen between β- and γ regions
- **Nephrotic syndrome**
  - Albumin—reduced
  - α_2 globulin—markedly increased.
- Chronic liver disease (cirrhosis liver)
  - Albumin—reduced
  - γ-globulin—increased
- Agammaglobulinemia (congenital disorder)
  - γ band faint, other bands—unaltered.

8. **How is blood pH regulated?**

Refer 2005 Essay Question 4.

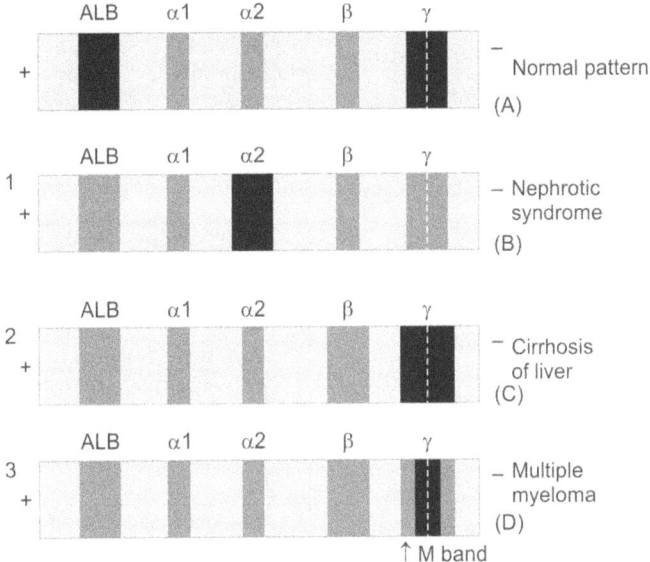

Figs. 7A to D: Electrophoretic pattern in diseases.

II. SHORT NOTES

1. Nutritional importance of proteins.

- Proteins are the major building block of our body, 10–15% of energy is provided by proteins in diet
- Proteins are the sources of essential amino acids, such as isoleucine, leucine, threonine, lysine, methionine, phenylalanine, tryptophan and valine
- Histidine and arginine are the semi-essential amino acids
- Growing children requires lot of essential amino acids in food
- Safe level of protein intake is 0.75 g/day
- **Nitrogen balance:**
  - A normal healthy adult is said to be in nitrogen balance that means the dietary intake of N_2 equals the daily loss through urine, feces and skin. When excretion exceeds intake, it is negative nitrogen balance, when intake exceeds excretion, it is positive nitrogen balance.
- **Factors affecting nitrogen balance:**
  - Growth: Positive nitrogen balance during growing period
  - Hormones: Growth hormones insulin, androgen, +ve nitrogen balance
  - Pregnancy: Positive nitrogen balance
  - Convalescence: Positive nitrogen balance
  - Acute illness: After trauma, surgery, burns, negative nitrogen balance
  - Protein deficiency: Negative nitrogen balance.
- **Nutritional indices:**
  - **Assessment of nutritional value**—the protein is given to an animal and the weight gain is assessed
  - **Biological value**—it is the ratio between the nitrogen retained and nitrogen absorbed during a specific interval.

$$\frac{\text{Retained nitrogen}}{\text{Absorbed nitrogen}} \times 100$$

2. Describe the requirement, sources, metabolic functions and deficiency manifestations of folic acid.

FOLIC ACID

The Latin word folium means **leafy vegetables**.

Chemistry

It is composed of pteridine, para-aminobenzoic acid (PABA) and glutamic acid.

Pteridine + PABA + glutamic acid → Pteroylglutaminc acid or folic acid.

Source

- Rich: Yeast, green leafy vegetables (folium)
- Moderate: Cereals, pulses, oil seeds and eggs.

Recommended Dietary Allowance

- Adult: 200 µg/day
- Pregnancy: 400 µg/day.

BIOCHEMICAL FUNCTIONS (FIG. 8)

Coenzyme form of folic acid—tetrahydrofolate

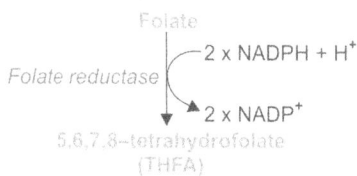

- Folic acid is first reduced to 7, 8 dihydrofolic acid and further reduced to 5, 6, 7, 8 tetrahydrofolic acid (THFA) by folate reductase enzyme
- THFA is a carrier of one carbon groups. One-carbon groups play a vital role in donating carbon atoms for the synthesis of different types of compounds

Different one-Carbon Compounds

Group	Structure
Formimino	HN=CH-
Formyl	HCO
Methyl	$-CH_3$
Methylene	$-CH_2-$
Methenyl	=CH

[N^5 and N^{10} atoms of THFA carry the one-carbon groups]

S. No.	Folic acid derivative	One-carbon group transferred	Compounds produced
1.	N^5, N^{10} methylene THFA	Methylene (CH_2)	Serine-glycine interconversion-dTMP Glycine cleavage system
2.	N^5, N^{10} methenyl THFA	Methenyl (=CH)	C_8 of purine ring
3.	Formyl THFA	Formyl	C_2 of purine ring
4.	N^5, N^{10} methylene THFA	Methylene (CH_2)	dTMP in DNA
5.	N^5-methyl-THFA	Methyl (CH_3)	N_5-methyl $-H_4F$-methylcobalamin and homocysteine to produce methionine
6.	N^5-formimino THFA	Formimino (-CH=NH)	Histidine –FIGLU

Causes of Folate Deficiency

- Pregnancy
- Dietary deficiency
- Defective absorption
- Hemolytic anemia
- **Folate trap (Fig. 8):** When vitamin B_{12} is deficient, methyl-THFA cannot be converted to THFA. B_{12} takes up this methyl group to form methylcobalamine to supply the methyl group to homocysteine to form methionine. So methyl-THFA gets trapped inside the cell in B_{12} deficiency the following reaction (reaction given in **Fig. 9**)cannot take place, leads to folate deficiency.

Deficiency Manifestations

- Reduced DNA synthesis
- Macrocytic anemia
- Hyper-homocysteinemia
- Birth defects—neural tube defects in fetus
- Cancer.

Assessment of Folate Deficiency

FIGLU excretion test or Histidine load test
Histidine is metabolized to formiminoglutamic acid from which formiminogroup is removed by THFA. Therefore in folate deficiency, FIGLU is excreted in urine.

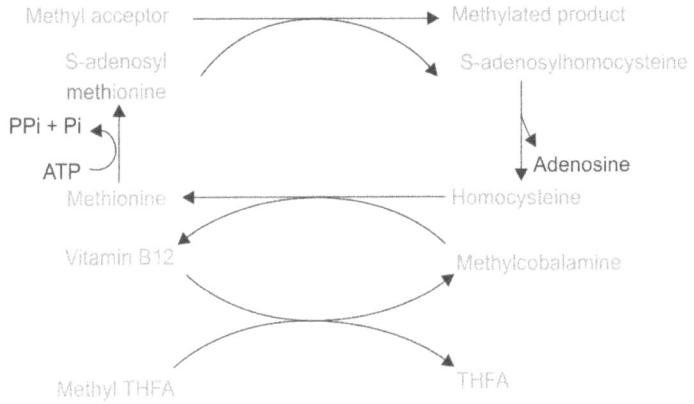

Fig. 8: Folate trap.

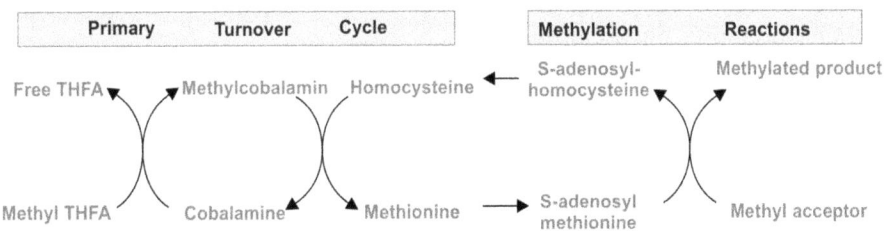

Fig. 9: Transmethylation reaction of folic acid.

Folate antagonists:
- Sulfonamides
- Aminopterine
- Primethamine.

3. **Explain with a neat labeled diagram of fluid mosaic model of biological membrane.**

- Cell membrane is also called as plasma membrane
- It protects the intracellular organelles from outer environment and provides selective permeability for cell function
- The structure of cell membrane was described by **Singer and Nicolson as fluid mosaic model**.

STRUCTURE OF CELL MEMBRANE (FIG. 10)

- Cell membrane has selective permeability
- Outer cell membrane has ectoenzymes, such as 5'nucleotidase and alkaline phosphatase
- Plasma membranes are made up of lipids, proteins and small amount of carbohydrates—present as glycoproteins and glycolipids
- The **matrix** of a membrane is a polar bilipid layer
- **Fluid mosaic model**—the lipid bilayer shows free lateral movement and so it is said to be fluid in nature (flip flop movement is restricted)
- **The fluidity of the membrane depends upon:**
  a. The cholesterol content of the membrane alters fluidity. Fluidity is less when cholesterol level is high
  b. This also depends upon the temperature (Tm) which is inversely proportional
  c. The nature of fatty acids—fluidity increases when there is more unsaturated fatty acids.
- **Phospholipids:**—these are arranged in bilayers with polar head oriented towards

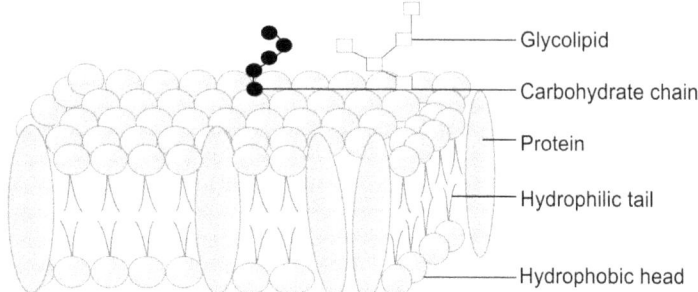

Fig. 10: Structure of cell membrane.

extracellular side and a hydrophobic nonpolar tail towards cytoplasmic side. Choline containing phospholipids are found in the external layer. Ethanolamine and serine containing phospholipids are in the inner layer
- **Thickness**: Single layer thickness of 25Å thick. Head portion—10Å and tail 15Å thick. Total thickness 50–80Å
- **Membrane proteins:**
  a. Peripheral proteins—present on the surfaces of the bilayer. They are attached by ionic and polar bonds to polar heads of lipids. They anchor proteins to lipid bilayer
  b. Integral membrane proteins deeply embedded in the bilayer and attached by hydrophobic bonds or vander waals forces
  c. Transmembrane proteins—they span the whole bilayer. They serve as receptors or hormones, ion channels, etc.

4. Total parenteral nutrition and its importance.

Other name: Intravenous hyperalimentation or total parenteral feeding.
- In patients who cannot or should not use their GI tract (unconscious, major surgery), total parenteral feeding has to be resorted
- It contains glucose and amino acids
- About 10–30% glucose, 1–1.5 g/kg protein, a fat emulsion containing 1–4 g fat/kg body weight, along with multivitamins and trace element solution are commonly used
- The solution should also contain adequate amounts of Na, K, Ca, Mg
- The solution may be infused through one of the large vessels like sub-clavian vein to superior vena cava, where the blood flow is sufficient to dilute the hypertonic solution
- Common problems related to parenteral nutrition are—fluid overload, sodium retention, and hypoglycemia.

5. Transfer RNA (tRNA).

Refer 2004 Short Note 12.

6. Explain the metabolism and functions of HDL.

- Main transport form of cholesterol from peripheral tissues to liver
- Anti-atherogenic known as good cholesterol
- Involved in reverse cholesterol transport.
- High density lipoprotein (HDL) sub-fractions—HDL-I (Bad and contains only Apo E), HDL-2
- Good and anti atherogenic, HDL-3 contains Apo A-II and its role is controversial.

METABOLISM OF HDL (FIG. 11)
- Intestinal cells synthesize HDL which is discoidal in shape

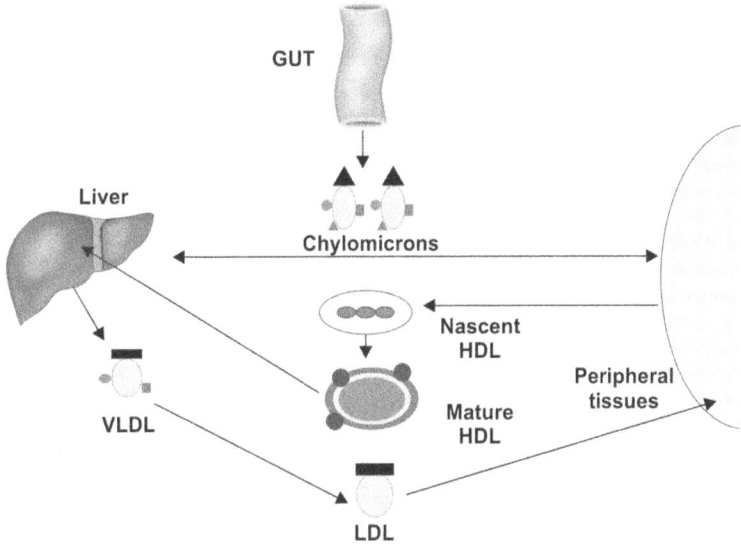

Fig. 11: Metabolism of lipoproteins.

- Free cholesterol derived from peripheral tissue is taken up by HDL. It is mediated by ABC protein which is a cholesterol efflux regulator protein (CETP)
- The esterified cholesterol moves into the interior of HDL disc
- Mature HDL is sphere in shape and loaded with cholesterol esters–HDL-3
- These spheres are taken up by liver cells by apo A-I mediated receptor mechanism
- Hepatic lipase hydrolyses HDL phospholipid and TAG, and CE is released into liver cells
- CETP transfers cholesterol from HDL to VLDL and LDL in exchange for TAG to form HDL-2.

FUNCTIONS OF HDL

- Anti-atherogenic known as good cholesterol
- Involved in reverse cholesterol transport
- HDL subfractions—HDL 1 (bad and contains only Apo E), HDL–2
- Good and anti-atherogenic, HDL-3 contains Apo A-II and its role is controversial
- Acts as a reservoir for apoproteins which can be donated to or received from other lipoproteins
- As an anti-oxidant it prevents the oxidation of LDL.

7. What are glycoproteins? Give three examples and its importance.

GLYCOPROTEINS

- They are conjugated proteins
- When the carbohydrate chains are attached to a polypeptide chain it is caked proteoglycans. If the carbohydrate content is less than 10% it is named as glycoprotein. If the carbohydrate content is more than 10% it is named as mucoprotein
- Glycoproteins are present in all tissues and in cell membranes as glycocalyx
- They play important role as enzymes, hormones, transport proteins, structural proteins and receptors
- Glycophorin is the major membrane glycoprotein of erythrocytes. It is a transmembrane protein
- The oligosaccharide chains of glycoproteins are composed of many carbohydrate residues. They are—glucose, mannose, galactose, N-acetylgalactosamine, arabinose, L-fucose, N-acetylneuramnic acid (NANA)

- Glycosylation occurs in the Golgi complex
- Other carbohydrates usually present in glycoproteins are—pentoses like arabinose and xylose, hexoses like mannose and galactose and l-fructose (methyl pentose)
- The oligosaccharide chains are mostly branched without repeating units
- Glycoproteins differ from mucoproteins in their carbohydrate content—glycoprotein has less than 4% carbohydrate whereas it may be more than 4% in mucoproteins
- Oligosaccharides are attached by O-glycosidic linkage to the oxygen of serine and threonine or by N-glycosidic linkage to side chain nitrogen of asparagines residues.

FUNCTIONS OF GLYCOPROTEINS

- Structural substance—collagen, bacterial cell wall
- Enzymes—ribonuclease—B, prothrombin
- Transport proteins—ceruloplasmin (carries Cu), transferrin (Fe)
- Hormones—TSH, thyroglobulin
- Immunity—immunoglobulin, blood group antigens
- Lubricant—mucin
- Message transfer—receptor proteins on cell surfaces
- Cell adhesion—selectins, integrins.

8. Chemiosmotic theory.
Refer 2006 Short Note 5.

9. Rapoport-Luebering shunt pathway and its significance.
Refer 2007 Short Note 18.

10. What are nucleotides? Name any three biologically important nucleotides and their importance.

- Nucleotides are nitrogenous base + pentose sugar + phosphate group
- They are the phosphorylated nucleosides
- The phosphate group is attached to the hydroxyl group of pentoses by an ester linkage
- Depending on the nature of the pentoses, the nucleotides are of 2 types—(1) Ribonucleotides; (2) Deoxyribonucleotides
- Depending upon the number of phosphate groups added they are known as—1 P-Monophosphates (MP), 2P-Diphosphates (DP) and 3P-Triphosphates (TP)
- **Ribonucleotides**
  a. Adenosine ribonucleotides:
   - AMP—cyclic AMP: Major metabolic regulator and second messenger in hormonal action
   - ATP: Energy currency of cell; high energy phosphate. It helps in the formation of active methionine (SAM) involved in transmethylation; it is also needed for the synthesis of certain coenzymes like NAD, FAD, etc.
  b. Guanosine ribonucleotides: GMP, GDP and GTP
   - Cyclic GMP: Major metabolic regulator and second messenger in hormonal action
   - GTP: Involved in protein synthesis as energy source.
  c. Uridine ribonucleotides: UMP, UDP and UTP
   - UDP sugars act as donors of sugar for the synthesis of glycogen (UDP-glucose)
   - UDP-galactose—for the synthesis of glycoproteins and proteoglycans
   - UDP-glucuronate is a conjugating agent for conjugation of bilirubin, drugs, etc.
  d. Cytosine ribonucleotides—CDP, CDP and CTP
   - CDP choline is needed for the synthesis of sphingomyelin.
  e. Hypoxanthine nucleotide:
   - Ionosine MP—IMP: Precursor or parent nucleotide of purine ribonucleotides.

Deoxyribonucleotides

- d-AMP, d-GMP, d-CMP, d-thymidine – dTMP: They are present in DNA.

11. Give an account of the formation of specialized products from glycine.
Glycine is the simplest amino acid.

METABOLIC PRODUCTS (FIG. 12)

- Methylene tetrahydrofolate by glycine cleavage system to join one carbon pool
- Glucose—It is glucogenic
- Creatine, creatine phosphate and creatinine
- Heme
- Purine nucleotides
- Glutathione
- Conjugating agent
- Constituent of most of the proteins—more in collagen.

SPECIAL PRODUCTS FORMED FROM GLYCINE

- **Creatine production from glycine (Fig. 13):**
  - Creatine and creatinine are the non-protein nitrogenous substances present in normal urine. They are synthesized by 3 amino acids—arginine, glycine and methionine. The synthesis occurs in kidney, liver and muscles
  - Normal serum level of creatinine is 0.7–1.4 mg/dL; serum creatine is 0.2–0.4 mg/dL
  - Serum creatinine is a marker of renal failure. Creatinine clearance test is used to measure GFR.
- **Production of heme (Fig. 14):**
  - Succinyl-CoA combines with glycine catalysed by the enzyme ALA synthase in the presence of the coenzyme pyridoxal phosphate in the mitochondria to form alpha-amino-beta-ketoadipic acid which is converted by the same enzyme to delta-aminolevulinic acid. It is the rate-limiting step in heme synthesis
- **Synthesis of purine (Fig. 15):**
  - Whole molecules of glycine are contributed for the formation of C_4, C_5 and N_7 of purine ring.

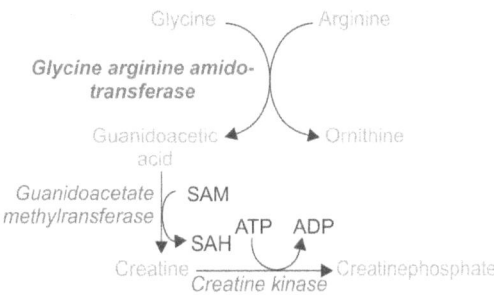

Fig. 13: Synthesis of creatine.

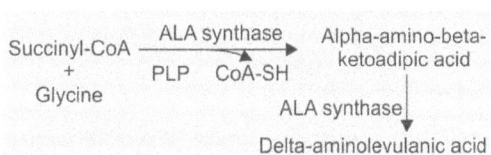

Fig. 14: Role of glycine in heme synthesis.

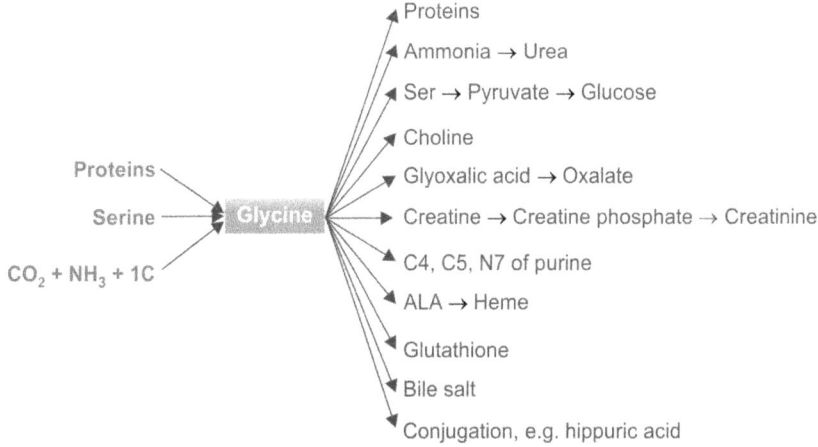

Fig. 12: Metabolic fate of glycine.

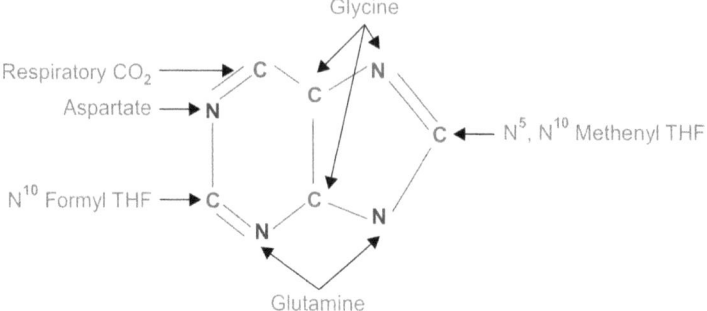

Fig. 15: Contribution of glycine to form purine ring.

- **Conjugating agent:** Glycine acts as a conjugating agent
  - It conjugates bile acids to produce conjugated bile acids which are less toxic. Glycocholic acid and glycolchenodeoxycholic acid are the conjugated primary bile acids
  - In the liver glycine conjugates benzoic acid and detoxifies it to form hippuric acid which is easily excreted from urine.

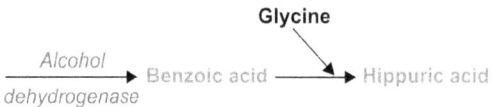

- **Neurotransmitter:** Glycine acts as an inhibitory neurotransmitter by opening chloride specific channels. It causes over-excitation in high concentration
- **Glutathione formation:** Glutathione is gamma-glutamylcysteinylglycine. It is a tripeptide of biochemical importance. Glutamate combines with cysteine to form gamma-glutamylcysteine which combines with glycine to form glutathione. Each step needs one ATP

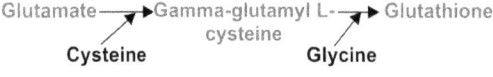

12. Explain the term transamination and its salient features.

Refer 2008 Short Note 14.

13. Polymerase chain reaction and its applications.

POLYMERASE CHAIN REACTION (FIG. 16)

It is an in vitro DNA amplification procedure in which millions of a particular sequence of DNA can be produced within few hours.

- Two primers of about 20-30 nucleotides with complementary sequence of the flanking region are needed
- Step 1—Separation: DNA strands are separated by heating at 95°C for 15-2 minutes
- Step 2—Annealing: The primers are annealed by cooling to 50°C for 0.5-2 minutes. Then they hybridize with their complementary single-stranded DNA separated already
- Step 3—Polymerization: New DNA strands are synthesized by Taq polymerase. This enzyme is derived from bacteria that found in hot springs. The polymerase reaction is allowed to take place at 72°C for 30 seconds in presence of dNTPs of adenine, guanine, cytosine and thymine to duplicate both strands of DNA
- Step 4: Steps 1, 2 and 3 are repeated to double up the DNA strands. After 20 cycles one million times amplifications will occur
- These cycles are repeated by automated instrument called tempcycler.

Clinical Applications

- Detection of infectious diseases: Tuberculosis and viral diseases like HIV and hepatitis. PCR detects even one bacillus present in the specimen and PCR is used in the diagnosis of viral infections like hepatitis C and HIV
- Medicolegal cases: PCR allows the DNA in a single cell or in a hair follicle to be analyzed. This is highly useful in forensic medicine to identify the criminal
- PCR is especially useful for prenatal diagnosis
- Diagnosis of genetic disorders: By using PCR technique, mutant genes are amplified to diagnose certain inborn errors of metabolism by amplifying the particular genes, e.g. sickle cell anemia, cystic fibrosis, etc.

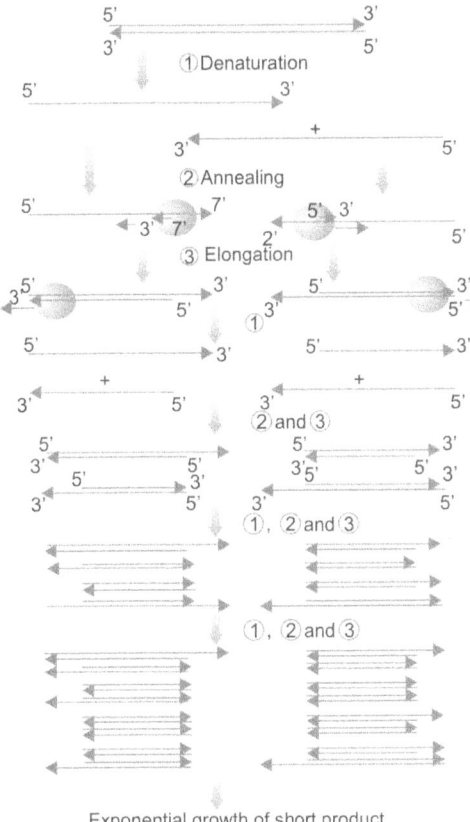

Fig. 16: Polymerase chain reaction.

14. Blotting techniques (Fig. 17).

Blotting is a technique for transferring DNA, RNA and proteins on to a carrier so they can be separated, and often follows the use of a gel electrophoresis. The southern blot is used for transferring DNA, the northern blot for RNA and the western blot for protein.

- **Northern Blot (Fig. 18)**
  - Northen blot technique is used for detection of specific RNA sequences. It was developed by James Alwine and George stark at Stanford university.
  - RNA is isolated from several biological samples, e.g. tissues—then electrophoresed and blotted on to a membrane. This is then probed with radioactive cDNA. There will be RNA-

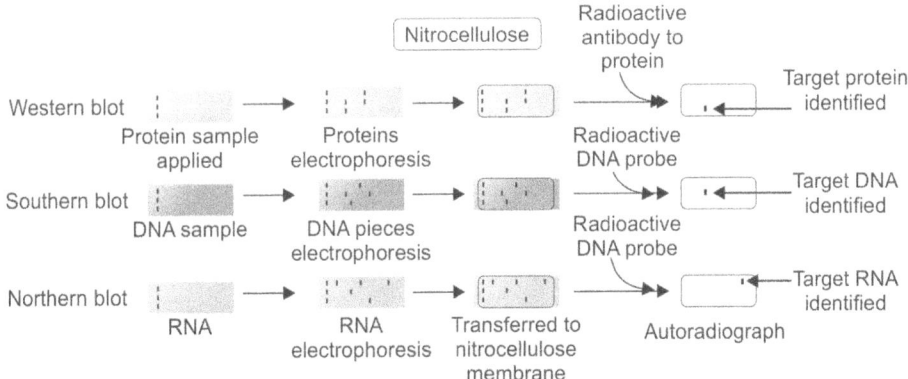

Fig. 17: Blotting techniques.

DNA hybridization. This is used to detect gene expression in a tissue.

- **Western Blot (Fig. 19)**
  - The proteins are isolated from the tissue and electrophoresis is done
  - The separated proteins are then transferred on to a nitrocellulose membrane
  - After fixation, it is probed with radioactive antibody and autoradiographed
  - Alternately the specific antibody is poured over, washed and a second antibody carrying horseradish peroxidase is added. Hydrogen peroxide and a chromogen are layered. This technique is useful to identify the specific protein.

- **Southern Blot**
  - This technique was found out by EM Southern
  - This technique is based on DNA hybridization technique
  - Used to detect specific DNA segment
  - **Steps:**
    - DNA is extracted from the tissues
    - It is fragmented using restriction endonucleases
    - The cut fragments are electrophoresed in agarose gel

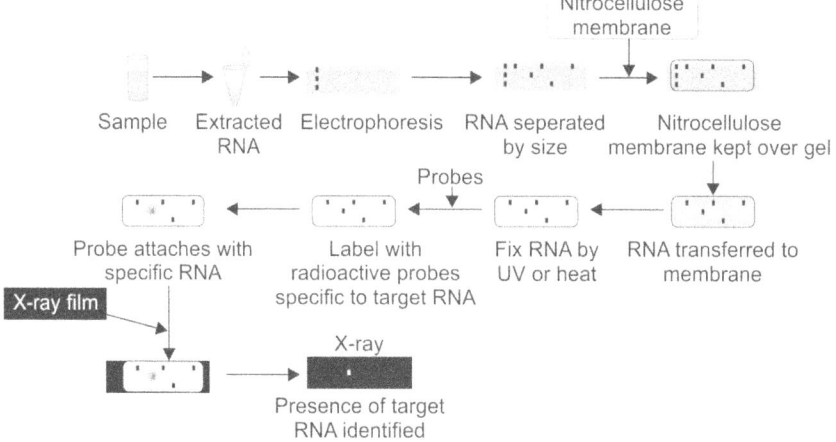

Fig. 18: Northern blot.

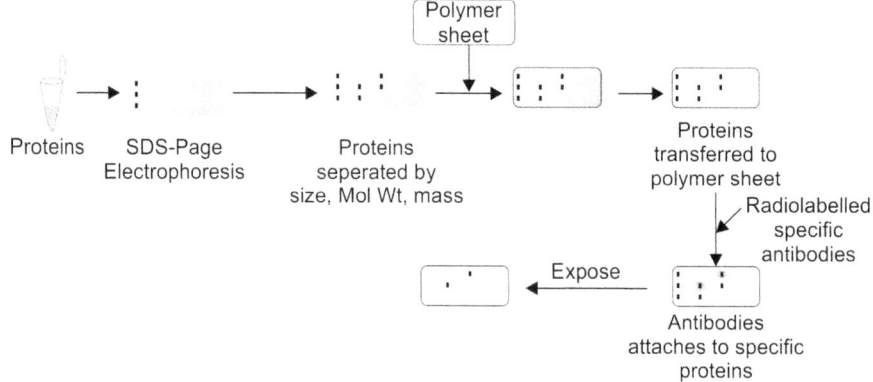

Fig. 19: Western blot.

- It is then treated with NaOH to convert DNA to single stranded DNA
- The gel is then blotted over a nitrocellulose membrane
- An exact replica of the pattern in the gel is reproduced in the membrane. The DNA gets attached to the membrane
- The DNA is fixed to the membrane at 80°C
- A radioactive DNA probe which is complementary to the desired DNA fragment is applied
- This probe gets attached to the desired DNA (DNA hybridization)
- The membrane is washed and a radiographic film is exposed on the membrane
- The X-ray is developed to identify the DNA.

15. Gene therapy.

GENE THERAPY (FIG. 20)

It is an intracellular delivery of genes to generate a therapeutic effect by correcting an existing abnormality. Somatic gene therapy is the insertion of new gene into somatic cell of the patient. Germ cell gene therapy is considered as unethical.

Procedure

- The healthy gene should be isolated
- This gene is incorporated into a vector or carrier like viruses as expression cassette
- The vector is then delivered to the target cells
- There are 3 ways of applying gene carrying vectors:
  1. Exvivo strategy: Patients cells are cultured in the laboratory, the new genes are infused into the cells and the modified cells are administered back to the patient
  2. In situ strategy: When the vector containing the gene is injected intravenously or directly into the tissue
  3. In vivo strategy: The vector is injected directly to the target cell itself. For example, cystic fibrosis gene to the respiratory tract cells.
- The vectors used for gene delivery are:
  a. Retroviruses:
     - They are RNA viruses that replicate through DNA intermediate. Moloney Murine leukemia virus is commonly used. The *gag, pol, env* genes are deleted from the virus rendering it incapable of replication inside human body
     - In human cells the reverse transcriptase carried by the vector converts RNA to DNA, which is integrated to target cell DNA.
  b. Adenoviruses
  c. Plasmid liposome complex
  d. Gene gun method.

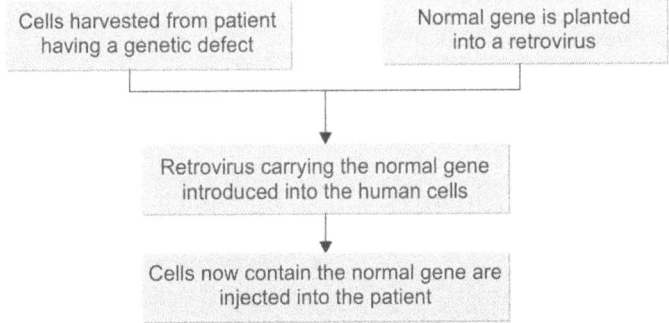

Fig. 20: Gene therapy.

Applications: Gene therapy is effective in inherited disorders caused by single genes. Various diseases like severe combined immunodeficiency (SCID), Duchenne muscular dystrophy, cystic fibrosis, familial hypercholesterolemia are treated by gene therapy.

16. Write an account of salvage pathway in purine nucleotide synthesis. Add a note on Lesch–Nyhan syndrome.

Refer 2004 Short Note 15.

17. Post-translational modification.

Refer 2007 Short Note 31.

18. What are porphyrias? Describe any three porphyrias in detail.

Refer 2008 Essay Question 2.

Porphyrias are a group of inborn errors of metabolism associated with biosynthesis of heme. These are characterized by increased production and excretion of porphyrins and/or their precursors.

Porphyrias are (**Fig. 21**):

- **Acute intermittent porphyria**—uroporphyrinogen I synthase deficiency
  - This leads to secondary increase in activity of ALAs
  - The levels of ALA and PBG are elevated in blood and urine
  - Urine is dark on voiding due to photo oxidation of PBG to phorphobilin. Symptoms appear intermittently
  - Patients will have acute abdominal pain. An attack is precipitated by starvation and symptoms are relieved by glucose infusion
  - Patients may have neurological abnormalities like sensory and motor disturbances, agitation and confusion. Patients may have neuropsychiatric problems.
- **Congenital erythropoietic porphyria**:
  - Uroporphyrinogen-III synthase deficiency
  - Autosomal recessive disorder
  - Photosensitivity present and dark urine are the symptoms.

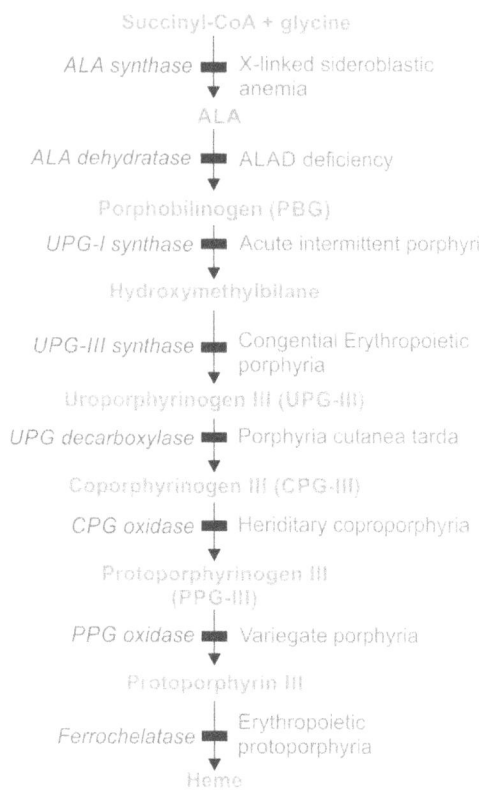

Fig. 21: Enzyme deficiencies in porphyrias.

- **Porphyria cutanea tarda**:
  - Uroporphyrinogrn decarboxylase deficiency
  - Here patients are more prone for photosensitivity
  - The urobilinogens accumulate and when patients come under light they spontaneously form urobilin which is a potent oxidant and destroys skin cells and causes scarring
  - Patients have gross skin malformations leading to monster like appearance, and they prefer night. Sunscreens are mildly effective.
- **Hereditary coproporphyria**: Due to coproporphyrinogen-III oxidase deficiency
- **Variegate porphyria**: Protoporphyrinogen oxidase deficiency
- **Erythropoietic protoporphyria**: Ferrochelatase deficiency.

19. Give an account of water distribution and its balance in the body.

Body is composed of 60–70% of water. The water distribution is given in the following diagram.

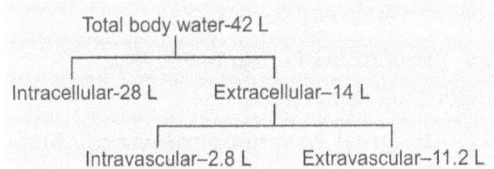

Intake and Output of Water
- Source of water intake:
  - Drinking water—stimulated by thirst
  - Water from food
  - Carbohydrate, proteins, fats generate water on catabolism.
- Output of water: Water is excreted through kidneys—urine, through lungs, skin and stools.

Water Balance
- Due to osmolality when sodium moves from one compartment to another, water also moves to maintain isotonicity. So the regulation of sodium and water are considered together
- **Regulation of water and Electrolyte balance:**
- **Renin-angiotensin system**: When there is fall in ECF volume, the renal blood flow decreases and this is sensed by the juxtaglomerular apparatus leading to secretion of Renin. Renin stimulates production of angiotensin which gets converted to angiotensin II. angiotensin II stimulates production of aldosterone
- **Aldosterone**: It acts on DCT and causes increased reabsorption of sodium and water
- **Antidiuretic hormone (ADH):** Antidiuretic hormone is produced in response to hypovolemia. It stimulates water reabsorption in the tubules and stimulates thirst
- **Atrial natriuretic peptide (ANP):** In hypervolemia atrial natriuretic peptide is produced which inhibits renin and aldosterone secretion.

20. What are isotopes? What are its applications in biochemistry?

ISOTOPES
- Isotopes are elements having same atomic number (protons) but different mass number (neutrons + protons). For example, ^{131}I and ^{125}I are isotopes of iodine
- Isotopes are stable or unstable. Unstable isotopes emit alpha, beta or gamma rays to become stable isotopes. This emission of radiation is called radioactivity. These isotopes are called radioactive isotopes
- This radioactivity can be measured and used for quantification or identification of the target analyte.

Uses of Isotopes
- **To study the metabolic pathways**: For example, when 14C labeled acetoacetate is given, its incorporation into Palmitic acid can be studied (fatty acid synthesis)
- **Half life**: When a radioactive compound is administered in the body, the half life of the particular compound can be estimated. For example, radiolabeled albumin has a half life of 20 days. ^{51}Cr labeled RBCs have a life span of 120 days
- **Thyroid function**: ^{131}I when given intravenously goes into thyroid gland and is incorporated into thyroxine. Using this the functions of thyroid gland like uptake, coupling and other functions can be studied
- **To diagnose thyroid diseases**: In hyperthyroidism the radiation from thyroid will be high and low in hypothyroidism
- **Bone scanning**: ^{90}Sr labeled dye is used to detect osteoblastoma since this element enters osteoblasts
- **Radioimmunoassays (RIA):** Instead of enzymes and color forming substrates in ELISA, RIA uses radiolabeled substrates which emit radiation which is proportional to the concentration of the analyte (direct method)

- **Therapeutic applications**: Gamma rays are used as ionizing radiations. It causes death of malignant cells attacking the DNA
  - Gamma rays of cobalt ^{60}Co is used to treat cancer cervix
  - ^{32}P is used for the treatment of polycythemia and chronic leukemia
  - ^{131}I is used to treat thyroid cancer and thyrotoxicosis.

21. Inhibitors of electron transport chain.
Refer 2005 Short Note 24.

22. Transport of bilirubin.
Refer 2005 Short Note 3.

23. Vitamin E.
Refer 2004 Short Note 10.

24. Substrate level phosphorylation.
- Production of ATP at the substrate level of certain metabolic pathways without the involvement of ETC
- Energy is trapped directly from the substrate without the help of the ETC.

Example:

1. Glycolysis

- A) Energy of 1, 3-BPG is trapped to synthesize 1 ATP with the help of bisphosphoglycerate kinase

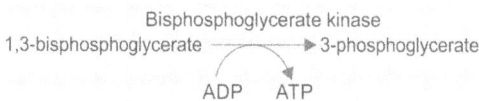

- B) Energy of PEP trapped to synthesize 1 ATP with the help of pyruvate kinase.

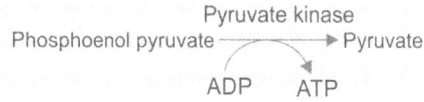

2. TCA cycle:

- Energy of succinyl-CoA is trapped to synthesize 1 ATP with the help of succinate thiokinase.

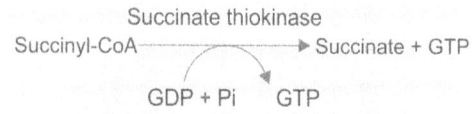

25. Gluconeogenesis.
Refer 2008 Essay Question 6.

26. Regulation of enzyme activity.
Refer 2006 Short Note 2.

27. Abnormal hemoglobins/hemoglobinopathies.
Hemoglobin is a conjugated protein made up of a prosthetic group called heme and protein part globin. Globin is a complex tertiary structure composed of two alpha and two beta chains. **The genes for these proteins are located in chromosomes 16 and 11, respectively.** Any mutation in these genes gives rise to abnormal structure of hemoglobin which shows altered haemoglobin function.

The following lists the major types of hemoglobinopathies

A. Qualitative or structural hemoglobinopathies

1. **HbS: Sickle Cell Hb**:
   - The glutamic acid in the 6th position of beta chain of Hb is changed to valine. This change of amino acid causes sickling of RBC
   - The sickled RBC plugs in capillaries and may cause occlusion of major vessels and lead to infarction of organs.

2. **HbE:**
   - It is the second most variant occurring after HbS
   - The glutamic acid at 26th position replace by lysine in beta chain. This variant is most prevalent in West Bengal.

3. **HbC (Cooley's hemoglobin):** Glutamate at 6th position of beta chain is replaced by lysine
   - It is mostly seen in blacks. Homozygous have a mild to moderate hemolytic anemia.

4. **HbD:**
   - It does not produce sickling
   - It is found in Punjab. Beta 21 glutamic acid is replaced by glutamine.
5. **HbM:**
   - Group of variants where substitution occurs in the proximal or distal histidine residues of α and β chains
     A 58 His $\to$ Tyrosine (Hb M Boston)
     B 92 His $\to$ Tyrosine (Hb M Hyde park)
   - Tendency of heme to get oxidized to hemin is more to form methemoglobin. O_2 binding is decreased causing cyanosis.

B. **Quantitative hemoglobinopathies:**
   It is due to lack or decreased synthesis of either α or β globin chain
   For example, thalassemia
   1. **α-thalassemia:** α-globin chain synthesis is reduced. Excess of β chain and δ chain formation
   2. **β-thalassemia:** β-globin chain synthesis is reduced.

28. Digestion and absorption of triacylglycerol.

Refer 2008 Short Note 22.

29. Biomedical importance of derivatives of cholesterol.

Cholesterol is catabolized to bile acids (BA) and salts, vitamin D and sex and steroid hormones.

Bile Acids and Bile Salts

Primary BA: Cholic acid and chenodeoxycholic acids
Secondary bile acids: Lithocholic acid and deoxycholic acid and their conjugated sodium and potassium salts.

Steps

- Cholesterol is hydroxylated at 7th position by 7 α-hydroxylase enzyme which is the **rate-limiting enzyme** which needs NADPH and vitamin C and converted into 7α-hydroxycholesterol
- This in turn is acted by 12-α-hydroxylase with the addition of CoA-SH in the presence of NADPH to form cholyl-CoA and chenodeoxycholyl-CoA with the removal of 3C propionate. This forms 24 carbon cholic acid or chenodeoxycholic acid
  - The so formed 24C bile acids conjugated with glycine/taurine to produce glycocholic acid or taurocholic acid
  - They are the sodium or potassium salts of primary and secondary bile acids.

Functions of Bile Salts

- They facilitate the lipid digestion
- They act as detergent in the formation of lipid micelle.

Vitamin D and calcitriol

- Cholecalciferol is 7-dehydrocholesterol (7-DHC) which is an intermediate of cholesterol metabolism
- 7-DHC is rich in malphigian layer of epidermis. The bond between 9 and 10 of 7-DHC is cleaved and converted into cholecalciferol by the action of UV light

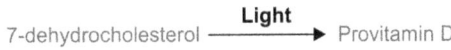

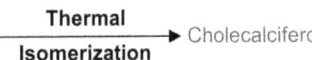

Activation of provitamin D (colecalciferol) into active vitamin D (calcitriol) takes place in two different sites—liver and kidney

Biochemical Functions of Calcitriol

- Vitamin D acts as steroid hormone. It binds to specific cytoplasmic receptors which interacts with DNA and induces the synthesis of mRNA for specific proteins calbindin which is a calcium-binding protein will lead to biological action
- **Effect on intestine**—calcitriol induces the synthesis of calbindin and helps in the absorption of calcium and phosphorus from the intestines
- **Effects on bone**—calcitriol stimulates the activity of osteoblasts which help in mineralization of bones. They secrete alkaline phosphatase enzyme which in

turn increases the ionic concentration of phosphate and calcium
- **Effects on kidney**—calcitriol increases the reabsorption of calcium and phosphorous from the renal tubules thereby conserving both minerals.

Steroid and Sex Hormones (Fig. 22)

- Steroid hormones—glucocorticoids and mineralocorticoids from adrenal cortex. Glucocorticoids mainly affect glucose metabolism
- Mineralocorticoids—mainly aldosterone increases sodium reabsorption from renal tubules leading to sodium retention.
  Sex hormones—from gonads and sex organs
    i. Ovarian hormones—from pregnenolone—estrogens, progesterone—maintains pregnancy and they help in maturation and function of female secondary sex organs
    ii. Testicular hormones—androgens—testosterone and estrogens maturation of male secondary sexual characters.

30. Significance and disorders of pentose phosphate pathway.

Refer 2005 Short Note 2 and 2010 Essay Question 2

31. Genetic code.

Refer 2005 Short Note 19.

32. Formation of epinephrine (Fig. 23).

- **Catecholamines:** Catecholamines are derived from tyrosine. They include—epinephrine, norepinephrine, DOPA and dopamine
- These hormones are secreted by adrenal glands
- Tyrosine is first hydroxylated to DOPA by tyrosine hydroxylase. It requires tetra-hydrobiopterin and NADPH
- DOPA is decarboxylated to form dopamine by DOPA decarboxylase, a PLP dependent enzyme. Dopamine is a catecholamine

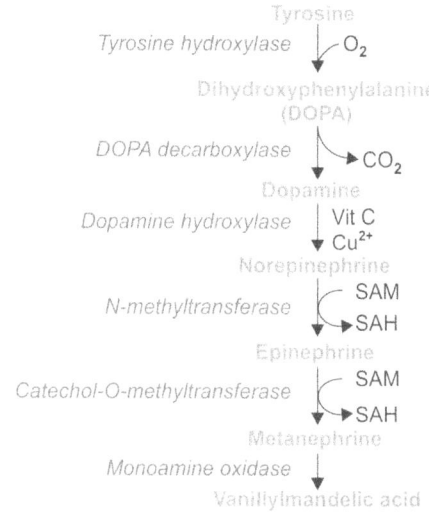

Fig. 23: Formation of epinephrine.

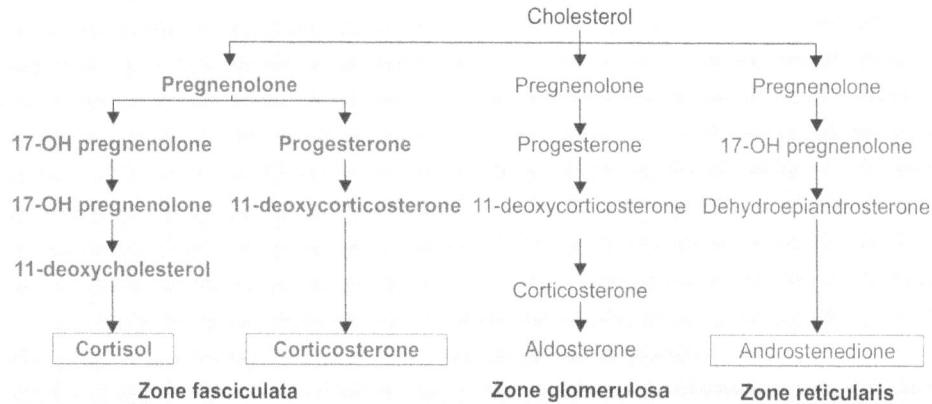

Fig. 22: Formation of steroid and sex hormones.

which is a neurotransmitter. In Parkinsonism dopamine level is reduced. L-DOPA is used as a drug in Parkinsonism
- Dopamine is hydroxylated to norepinephrine by dopamine hydroxylase
- Norepinephrine is methylated to epinephrine by methyltransferase which needs SAM which is the methyl donor
- Epinephrine is methylated to metanephrine and oxidized to vanillylmandelic acid (VMA) and excreted in urine. Level of VMA is elevated in pheochromocytoma and in neuroblastoma.

33. Cytochrome 450.

Refer 2004 Short Note 20.

34. Purine salvage pathways.

Refer 2004 Short Note 15.

35. Dehydration.

It is a disorder of water balance.
- Dehydration is a condition characterized by water depletion in the body. It may be due to insufficient intake or excessive loss of water
- The loss of water exceeds the intake of water.

TYPES

1. Simple dehydration: Loss of water without the loss of electrolytes
2. Combined deficiency of water and electrolytes.

CAUSES OF DEHYDRATION

- Deficient water intake: Starvation, dysphagia, weakness, coma
- Excessive loss of water: Diarrhea, vomiting, excessive sweating, fluid loss in burns, adrenocortical dysfunction, kidney diseases, diabetes insipidus, etc.

FEATURES

- The volume of ECF is decreased with rise in electrolyte concentration and osmotic pressure
- Water moves from ICF to ECF, resulting in cell shrinkage and increased protein breakdown
- ADH secretion increased leading to water retention and low urine volume
- Plasma proteins and blood urea concentrations are increased
- Water depletion may be either depletion of water alone or along with electrolytes
- The clinical features are increased pulse rate, low blood pressure, sunken eyeballs, decreased skin turgor, lethargy, fever, confusion and coma
- **Treatment:** Plenty of water should be taken. Intravenous administration of 5% glucose solution should be given, if the patient cannot drink orally. If electrolytes are also lost, sufficient electrolytes must also be given. The cause for dehydration must be identified and treated.

36. LAC operon.

Refer 2004 Short Note 19.

37. Orotic acidurias.

OROTIC ACIDURIAS (FIG. 24)

- It is an inborn error of metabolism found in pyrimidine metabolism
- It is an autosomal recessive disease
- There are 2 types—type I and II
    1. **Type I orotic aciduria**: The condition results from absence of either or both of the enzymes Orotate phosphoribosyl transferase (ORPTase) and OMP decarboxylase—the enzymes of pyrimidine synthesis
    2. **Type II orotic aciduria**: The condition results from absence of the enzyme OMP decarboxylase—the enzyme of pyrimidine synthesis.

Clinical Features

- Growth is retarded and megaloblastic anemia present. Bone marrow cells are rapidly dividing cells which are affected leading to anemia
- Orotic acid crystalluria: Orotate crystals are excreted in urine which may cause

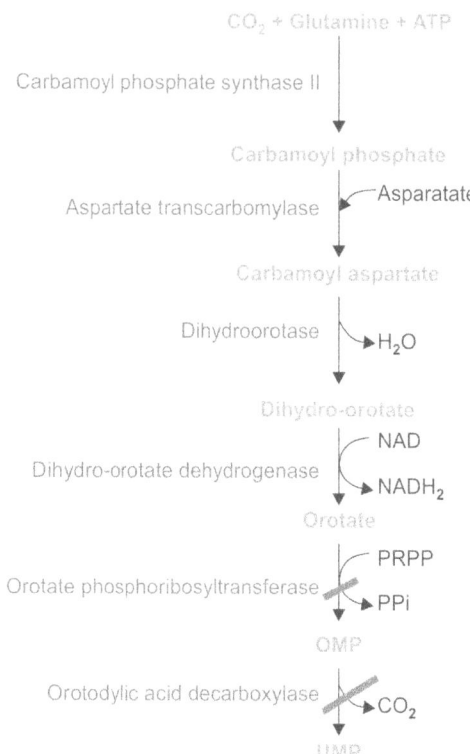

Fig. 24: Synthesis of pyrimidine nucleotides and disorders.

urinary tract obstruction in type I. Type II will have orotidinuria also in addition
- Treatment is by feeding cytidine or uridine. They are converted into UTP which can act as feedback inhibitor. Remission with oral uridine
- Orotic aciduria also occurs in urea cycle defect like ornithine transcarbamoylase deficiency, since carbamoyl phosphate accumulates and gets diverted to pyrimidine.

38. Phenylketonuria.

- **It is an** inborn error of metabolism in phenylalanine metabolism

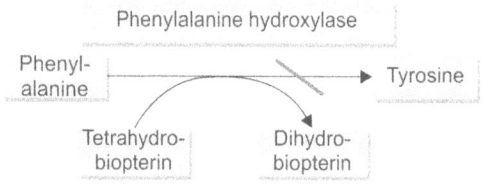

- It is an autosomal recessive disease with an incidence of 1: 10,000 births
- It is due to deficiency of phenylalanine hydroxylase
- So phenylalanine is not converted into tyrosine and it accumulates hyperphenylalaninemia
- The excess of phenylalanine is converted to phenylpyruvate, phenyllactate, and phenylacetate and phenylacetyl glutamine. Phenylpyruvate phenyllactate, phenylacetate are excreted in urine.

Clinical Manifestations

- The child is mentally retarded
- Convulsions, tremors, agitation, hyperactivity may be present
- The child often has hypopigmentation due to reduced availability of tyrosine for melanin production
- Phenyllactate in sweat causes mousy body odor.

Laboratory Diagnosis

- Blood level of phenylalanine is elevated—normal level is 1 mg/dL which is elevated to >20 mg/dL
- This is confirmed by Tandem mass spectroscopy
- Guthrie's test is confirmative
- Urine ferric chloride test is positive
- DNA probes—to diagnose the defects in phenylalanine hydroxylase and dihydrobiopterin reductase.

Treatment

- Early detection
- Low phenylalanine diet—tapioca based diet which has low phenylalanine is the treatment of choice
- Gene therapy is under trial.

39. Water toxicity.

Overhydration or water intoxication is caused by excessive water retention in the body.

Causes

- Excessive intake of large volumes of salt free fluids
- Renal failure

- Psychogenic polydipsia
- True polydypsia
- In ADH secreting tumors
- Syndrome of inappropriate antidiuretic hormone secretion (SIADH)
- Excessive intravenous administration in cases of trauma and postsurgery.

Clinical Features

- There will be dilution of ECF and ICF with decrease in osmolality
- Headache, lethargy and convulsions may occur

To differentiate psychogenic from true polydypsia, water deprivation test may be used.
Treatment: To stop water intake, diuretics and administration of hypertonic saline.

III. SHORT ANSWER QUESTIONS

1. Why sucrose is called a nonreducing disaccharide?

- Sucrose is a disaccharide made up of an aldohexose-glucose and a ketohexose-fructose and there is no free aldehyde or keto group
- The functional group of sucrose is used in the formation of 1–4 linkage. Hence there is no free functional group and no free anomeric carbon.
- The anomeric carbon of both monosaccharide units is involved in glycosidic bond. Hence it is a nonreducing sugar.

2. Name the essential fatty acids.

Essential fatty acids cannot be synthesized by the body but have to be supplemented in diet. They are polyunsaturated fatty acids. They are:
- Linoleic acid (18 C)-ω6
- Linolenic acid (18 C)-ω3
- Arachidonic acid (20C)-ω6—can be formed, if the dietary supply of linolenic acid is sufficient. So it cannot be strictly categorised under essential fatty acid.

3. Name any four biologically important compounds derived from cholesterol.

- Bile acids and bile salts
  - Primary BA: Cholic acid and chenodeoxycholic acids
  - Secondary bile acids
  - Lithocholic acid and deoxycholic acid and their conjugated Na and potassium salts.
- Steroid hormones: Glucocorticoids and mineralocorticoids
- Sex hormones - Progestrone, testosterone and estrogens
- Vitamin D and calcitriol.

4. What are phospholipids? Give two examples.

Refer 2004 Short Note 1.
They are compound lipids which contain esters of fatty acids with glycerol or sphingosine, nitrogenous base, and phosphate group.

Types of Phospholipids

I. **Glycerophospholipids:** Made up of fatty acid ester with glycerol two types. There are of:
  A. **Nitrogenous-glycerophospholipids:** They are made up of fatty acid ester with glycerol, phosphate, and nitrogenous group as functional group. Alcohol is glycerol, e.g. lecithin (Phosphatidylcholine), cephalin
  B. **Non-nitrogenous glycerophospholipids,** e.g. phosphatidylinositol.
II. **Sphingophospholipids:** They are made up of esters of fatty acids with sphingosine as the alcohol (FA + sphingosine = Ceramide), e.g. sphingomyelin.

5. Name the essential amino acids.

Refer 2005 Short Note 40.
Essential amino acids are indispensable amino acids which cannot be synthesized in the body but have to be supplemented by diet. They are:
- Arginine, histidine, isoleucine, leucine. Threonine, lysine, methionine, phenylalanine, tryptophan and valine
- Arginine and histidine are semi-essential amino acids which can be synthesized in adults but not by growing children.

6. Mention any two biological functions of albumin.

Refer 2009 Short Note 40.

- **Transport protein**: It transports various substances like bilirubin, free fatty acid, drugs like aspirin, hormones like thyroxine, steroid hormones, minerals like calcium, copper, etc.
- **Colloid osmotic pressure**: It maintains colloid osmotic pressure in vascular and extravascular compartments. It contributes to plasma oncotic pressure. It cannot pass between intracellular and extracellular compartment. So exerts a net osmotic pressure. The osmotic pressure of plasma is about 278–305 mOsm/kg, which is necessary for movement of water from ECF to ICF in arteriolar end and reverse in venular end of capillaries.

7. Name the amino acids required for purine biosynthesis.

- N1—aspartate
- N3, N9—glutamine
- C4, C5 and N7—glycine.

8. Sickle cell hemoglobin.

Refer 2008 Short Note 23.

SICKLE CELL HEMOGLOBIN

- In the 6th position of β chain of hemoglobin, when glutamate is replaced by Valine, HbS results
- The hemoglobin can carry oxygen, but when deoxygenated, the Hb sticks with other Hb molecules leading to the formation of sickle shaped plugs which can obstruct vasculature
- This also leads to reduced life span of RBC leading to hemolytic anemia.

Types

- Sickle cell disease—homozygous—severe manifestations
- Sickle cell trait—heterozygous—symptoms only in precipitating conditions.

Diagnosis

Hemoglobin electrophoresis reveals S band which is diagnostic.

9. Specific dynamic action.

- It is represented as thermogenic effect of food. The heat is produced after intake of food which is due to energy expenditure for digestion and absorption of food form reserved energy (diet induced thermogenesis)
- Specific dynamic action can be considered as the activation of energy needed for various chemical reactions. This activation energy is to be supplied initially. This activation energy is varied to different food
- For example, for carbohydrate—5%, for proteins—30% and for fat—15%, etc.
- Hence an extra calorie should be provided to account for the loss of energy as SDA
  - Energy requirement of an individual depends upon—occupation, physical activity and lifestyle which can be divided into 3 groups—sedentary, moderate and heavy. Heavy workers need high BMR
  - Energy requirement is calculated by the energy required for: 1. BMR—basal metabolic rate; 2. SDA—specific dynamic action; 3. Physical activity.

10. Write the principle and significance of Biuret test.

- **Principle**: This is a general test for proteins. Compounds which contain two or more peptide bonds will answer this. Dipeptides and free amino acids do not give Biuret positive. The violet or purple color is due to the formation of the co-ordination complex between cupric ions and nitrogen atoms of the peptide bonds
- **Reagents**: 5% sodium hydroxide and 1% copper sulfate (Biuret reagent)
- **Procedure**: 2 mL of protein solution, 2 mL of 5% NaOH is added and mixed well. Then 2–3 drops of 1% copper sulfate solution is added. Protein gives a violet or purple colored complex.

11. Okazaki pieces.

Refer 2008 Short Answer Question 15.

12. Differences between CPS-I and CPS-II.

Carbamoyl phosphate synthetase I (CPS-I) is the rate-limiting enzyme of urea cycle. Carbamoyl phosphate synthetase II (CPS-II) is the enzyme of pyrimidine synthesis.

Differences Between CPS-I and CPS-II

S. No	Features	CPS-I	CPS-II
1	Site	Mitochondria	Cytosol
2	Pathway	Urea cycle	Pyrimidine synthesis
3	Positive effector	N-acetyl-glutamate	Nil
4	Source of nitrogen	Ammonia	Glutamine
5	Inhibitor	Nil	CTP

13. Metabolic role of magnesium.

- Magnesium is an important intracellular cation
- Total body Mg is 25 g, out of which 60% is complexed with calcium in bone
- RDA: 400 mg/day for men; 300 mg/day for women
- Normal serum level is 1.8 to 2.2 mg/dL
- Functions:
  a. Activator of many enzymes like alkaline phosphatase, hexokinase, fructokinase, phosphofructokinase, adenylyl cyclase. ATP is also needed for these reactions
  b. It prevents neuromuscular irritability
  c. It helps in insulin dependent uptake of glucose and Mg improves glucose tolerance.
- Deficiency of Mg leads to neuromuscular irritability
- Hypomagnesemia may be due to vomiting, diarrhea, PEM, cirrhosis and diuretic therapy
- Hypermagnesemia may be due to excessive intake, renal failure, rickets, hyperparathyroidism, etc.

14. Anion gap.
Refer 2005 Short Note 33.

15. Rothera's test.

- Ketone bodies appear in urine under pathological conditions, such as diabetes mellitus with ketosis, starvation ketosis, persistent vomiting, Von Gierke's disease and alkalosis
- The major ketone bodies are three—acetone, acetoacetic acid and beta-hydroxybutyric acid
- Ketone bodies in urine are identified by Rothera's test, rapid tests, such as ketostix strips and acetest tablets.
- **Rothera's test:**
  - **Principle:** Freshly prepared sodium nitroprusside reacts with ketone bodies and form a purple colored ferropentacyanide complex. This test is specific for acetoacetate and beta-hydroxybutyrate
  - **Procedure:** 5 mL of urine is saturated with solid ammonium sulfate and few drops of sodium nitroprusside added, followed by addition of ammonia. A purple ring develops in presence of ketone bodies in urine.

16. Gout.
Refer 2005 Short Note 17.

17. Fluorosis.
Refer 2008 Short Answer Question 10.

18. van den Berg test.
Refer 2008 Short Note 16.
- The serum bilirubin estimation is based on van den Bergh reaction, in which diazotised sulfanilic acid reacts with bilirubin to form a purple colored complex, azobilirubin. Normal serum does not give a positive van den Bergh test
- When bilirubin is conjugated, the purple color is produced immediately on mixing with the reagent, the response is said to be van den Bergh direct positive
- When the bilirubin is unconjugated, the color appears only after addition of alcohol, so it is said to be van den Bergh indirect positive
- When both conjugated and unconjugated bilirubin are present, it produces an immediate color which intensifies on adding alcohol. It is then said to be biphasic
- In hemolytic jaundice—unconjugated bilirubin is elevated so indirect positive
- In obstructive jaundice—conjugated bilirubin is elevated so direct positive
- In hepatic jaundice—both conjugated and unconjugated bilirubin are elevated so biphasic.

19. Mutarotation.

It is defined as the change in optic rotation by the interconversion of α and β forms of D-glucose to an equilibrium mixture with respect to time.

α –D-glucose ⇌ Equilibrium mixture
+112°   of α and β-D –Glucose
               +52.7°

               ⇌ β-D –glucose
                 +18.7°

The specific optic rotation of α and β-D-glucose are +112° and + 18.7°, respectively. Freshly prepared a D-Glucose solution dissolved in water gradually changes its optic rotation from + 112° to + 52.7° with respect to time to form an equilibrium mixture containing 1/3 of alpha anomers and 2/3 of beta anomers.

Similarly α and β forms of both pyranose and furanose forms of fructose interconvert through open chain form and at equilibrium, fructose has a specific rotation of -92°.

20. Subcellular organelles.

- An organelle is a subcellular entity which is limited by membranes, e.g. nucleus, mitochondria. They can be isolated by high speed ultracentrifugation
- They can be identified by the presence of markers. For example, DNA—marker for nucleus, ATP synthase—mitochondria.

21. Free radicals.

- Free radicals are molecules or molecular species that contain one or more unpaired electrons which are capable of independent existence
- It is a molecule or molecular fragment that contains one or more unpaired electrons in its outer orbital. It is generally represented by a superscript dot, (R). They are constantly produced during the oxidation of foodstuffs, due to leaks in ETC. About 1-4% of oxygen is converted to free radicals in our body, e.g. superoxide anion radical (O_2^-)
- Lipid peroxide radical (ROO)
- **Characteristics:** Extreme reactivity, short life span, damage to various tissues, generation of new free radical by chain reaction.

22. Basal metabolic rate.

Refer 2005 Short Note 26.

23. Causes of fatty liver.

Refer 2009 Short Answer Question 2.

24. Renal glycosuria.

Refer 2007 Short Note 22.

25. Role of HDL as scavenger of cholesterol.

HDL cycle is the main transport form of cholesterol from peripheral tissues to liver for excretion through the bile or for utilization.

Metabolism

- Intestinal cell synthesize HDL which is discoidal in shape
- Lecithin cholesterol acyltransferase (LCAT) binds to the nascent HDL and converts free cholesterol to cholesterol ester. Thus HDL becomes spherical in shape (HDL 3)
- Free cholesterol derived from peripheral tissue is taken up by HDL 3. It is mediated by ATP binding cassette protein 1 (ABC protein)
- The esterified cholesterol moves into the interior of HDL disc
- Mature HDL spheres are taken up by liver cells by apo AI mediated receptor mechanism
- Hepatic lipase hydrolyses HDL phospholipid and TG, and CE are released into liver cells
- Cholesterol ester transfer protein (CETP) transfers cholesterol from HDL to VLDL and LDL in exchange for TG.

Significance

- By this cycle, cellular and lipoprotein cholesterol is delivered back to the liver where excess cholesterol is excreted into bile for excretion in the feces
- This prevents deposition of cholesterol in the tissues and this cycle is thought to be anti-atherogenic and high level of HDL

cholesterol confers a decreased risk of coronary heart disease.

26. FIGLU (Fig. 25).

- Histidine is metabolized to formimino-glutamic acid from which formimino group is removed by THFA. Therefore in folate deficiency, FIGLU is not converted to glutamate and FIGLU is excreted in urine in excess (more than 30 mg/day)
- Histidine → Urocanic acid → FIGLU → glutamate; THFA → formimino THFA
- Normal FIGLU excretion in urine is <30 mg/day
- **FIGLU** excretion test is a sensitive indicator for folic acid deficiency.

27. Dietary fibers.

Refer 2008 Short Note 10.

28. Xeroderma pigmentosum.

- It is an autosomal recessive condition in which there is defect in nucleotide excision repair mechanism
- Pyrimidine dimers are formed in the skin cells which are exposed to UV light. The patient becomes highly sensitive to UV rays. Sunlight causes blisters in the skin
- Because of the defective repair system, the cells cannot repair the damaged DNA resulting in skin cancer. Death occurs in second decade due to skin cancer
- This is also caused by defects in the genes coding for any of the XP proteins required for the repair.

29. Functions of parathyroid hormone.

PTH is secreted by four parathyroid glands embedded in the thyroid tissue by the chief cells. Decreased serum calcium leads to release of PTH from parathyroids. PTH activates adenylyl cyclase in target cells and increases intracellular calcium concentration. A protein kinase is activated which activates enzyme systems. PTH acts on:

- **PTH and bones**—PTH causes demineralization in bones. It activates pyrophosphatase in osteoclasts leading to bone resorption and solubilising calcium. Calcium is released into the bloodstream and increases blood calcium level. This leads to loss of bone matrix
- **PTH and kidneys**—PTH causes decreased renal excretion of calcium and increased excretion of phosphates and increased reabsorption of calcium leading to increased blood calcium level
- **PTH and intestines**—PTH stimulates increased production of Vitamin D_3 which acts on intestine to absorb more calcium leading to increased calcium level in blood.

30. Mention two second messengers.

- Group I hormones having cell surface receptors which act through second messengers.
- Examples for second messengers are
  - Calcium
  - Cyclic AMP and GMP
  - Phosphatidyl inositol.

31. Symport (Fig. 26).

- Symport is a type of active transport requiring energy
- It is a co-transport system
- One molecule of ATP is utilized for this reaction. The substances are moved against concentration gradient.
- The opposite of symport is antiport

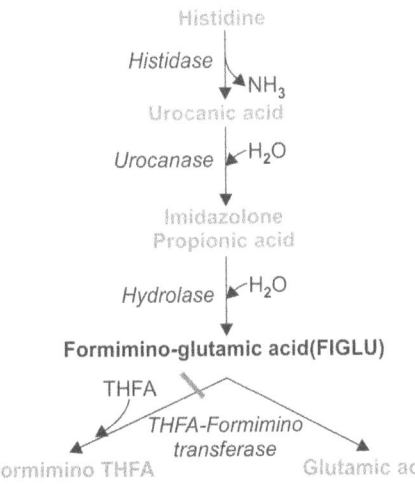

Fig. 25: Metabolism of histidine.

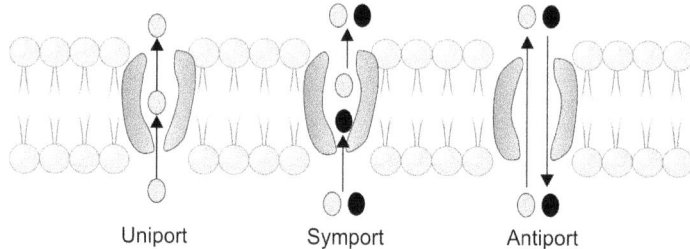

Fig. 26: Symport.

- Transfer of one molecule depends on the simultaneous transfer of another molecule in the **same direction**
- For example, glucose and many amino acids are transported against concentration gradient by this mechanism, sodium glucose transporter (SGLT).

32. Oxytocin.

- Oxytocin is a hormone synthesized by posterior pituitary
- It is a nanapeptide molecule with 9 amino acids
- The stimulant for oxytocin secretion from the pituitary is suckling of the nipple of the mother by the newborn baby
- It causes the pregnant uterus to contract and induce labor. It causes contraction of myoepithelial cells of the breast leading to ejection of milk from breast. Oxytocin inhibits synthesis of steroids by the ovary.

33. Addison's disease.

Reduced production of cortisol from the adrenal cortex leads to Addison's disease. It may be primary due to adrenal dysfunction or secondary due to pituitary or hypothalamic dysfunction.

There will be hypoglycemia, loss of weight, anorexia, muscle wasting, impaired cardiac function, low blood pressure, decreased Na^+ and increased K^+ level in serum. Patients are more prone for stress.

34. Functions of glucagon.

- Glucagon is a hyperglycaemic hormone synthesized by alpha cells of islets of Langerhans 1 of pancreas
- Its action is opposite to that of insulin
- Glucagon increases blood glucose by the following mechanisms:
  - Inhibiting glycolysis—inhibits glucokinase, phosphofructokinase, pyruvate kinase
  - Stimulating gluconeogenesis—by stimulating PEPCK, pyruvate carboxylase, fructose 1, 6-bisphosphatase, glucose-6-phosphatase
  - Stimulates glycogenolysis—by activating phosphorylase
  - Inhibits glycogenesis—by inactivating glycogen synthase.

35. Gamma-aminobutyric acid (Fig. 27).

- Glutamate on decarboxylation produces gamma-aminobutyric acid (GABA)
- It is produced in brain. GABA is an inhibitory neurotransmitter because it

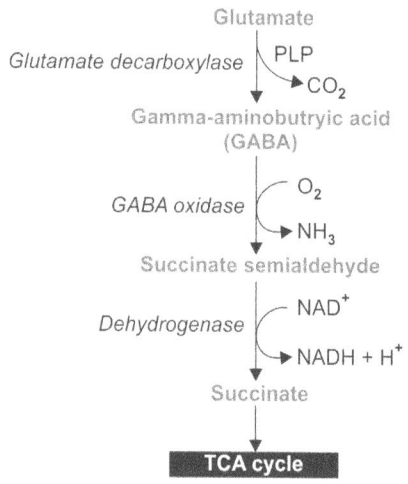

Fig. 27: Synthesis of GABA.

opens chloride channels in postsynaptic membranes in CNS
- It inhibits nerve transmission in the brain, calming nervous activity by opening the chloride channel
- Glutamate and GABA are the most abundant neurotransmitters in the central nervous system, and especially in the cerebral cortex.

36. Hartnup's disease.

- It is an autosomal recessive disorder connected to tryptophan transport
- It is named after the family of Hartnup in whom the disorder was described first
- It is due to defective amino acid transport during absorption of amino acids from the intestines and also during reabsorption of amino acids from renal tubules
- This leads to the deficiency of tryptophan and nicotinic acid and NAD
- Neurological and pellagra like symptoms are present
- Aminoaciduria will be present due to failure of amino acid-especially-tryptophan transport in renal tubules
- Increased excretion of indole compounds will be detected by Obermeyer test
- Treatment: Supplementation of niacin and high protein diet.

MBBS Examination 2011

ANSWER ALL QUESTIONS

I. **Essay questions** (10/15 Marks each)
1. Describe the chemistry, sources, daily requirement, biochemical functions and deficiency manifestations of vitamin B12.
2. Describe how cholesterol is synthesized in our body. What are the products formed from cholesterol?
3. Write in details about the initiation, elongation and termination of transcription. Give an account of post-transcriptional processing.
4. Write in detail about the absorption, transport, daily requirement and deficiency manifestation of iron.
5. Describe in detail TCA cycle and the energetics of the same. Justify why TCA cycle is called an amphibolic cycle.
6. Describe in detail the components and chemiosmotic theory of electron transport chain.
7. a. What is cloning? Mention the various types of cloning. b. Describe in detail the steps involved in recombinant DNA technology.
8. Describe the role of: (i) plasma and (ii) renal buffers in maintaining acid base homeostasis.

II. **Short notes** (5 Marks each)
1. Active form of vitamin D and its biochemical role.
2. Catabolism of hemoglobin.
3. Protein-energy malnutrition.
4. Ketogenesis.
5. Fatty acid synthase complex.
6. Glycogen metabolism.
7. Enzyme inhibition.
8. Glycosylated hemoglobin.
9. Oxidative phosphorylation (chemiosmotic theory).
10. Regulation of blood glucose.
11. Synthesis and mechanism of action of nitric oxide.
12. Homocystinurias.
13. Hyperuricemias.
14. Metabolic acidosis.
15. Phase two detoxification (conjugation)
16. Cyclic AMP.
17. Assessment of hypothyroidism.
18. Mutations.
19. Electrophoresis.
20. Antioxidants.
21. Role of niacin as coenzyme.
22. Classification of hyperlipidemias and their clinical importance.
23. Sphingolipidoses.
24. Biochemical role of vitamin C.
25. Cori cycle and glucose-alanine cycle.
26. High density lipoprotein cycle.
27. Glycogenolysis.
28. Isomerism in carbohydrates.
29. Balanced diet.
30. Fructose intolerance (hereditary fructose intolerance)
31. Purine salvage pathway.
32. Explain the types and functions of immunoglobulins.
33. Phenylketonuria
34. Fluorosis.
35. Serum protein electrophoresis.
36. Cell cycle.

37. Role of parathormone in calcium, phosphate homeostasis.
38. Define xenobiotics and add a note on the various detoxification reactions.
39. Mutation.
40. Secondary structure of protein.

III. Short answer questions
(2/3/4 Marks each)

1. Zymogen.
2. Name two zinc containing enzymes.
3. Ferritin.
4. Define Km.
5. Functions of selenium.
6. What are cytochromes?
7. Brown adipose tissue.
8. Lactose intolerance.
9. Define respiratory quotient.
10. Functions of vitamin K.
11. Name the major intracellular and extracellular anion.
12. Principle of flame photometer.
13. Metabolic roles of zinc and selenium.
14. Orotic aciduria
15. Chimeric DNA.
16. Osmolality.
17. Anti-HIV drugs.
18. Compounds formed from glycine.
19. Write the normal serum sodium and potassium level.
20. What are monoclonal and polyclonal antibodies?
21. Markers for lysosomes and mitochondria.
22. Fluorosis.
23. Role of Apo-CII.
24. Define metalloenzymes with two examples.
25. Pulmonary surfactant—structure and clinical importance.
26. Iodine number and its importance.
27. What is the function of lipoprotein lipase?
28. Structure of lecithin.
29. Net protein utilization.
30. Chondroitin sulfate—structure.
31. Double reciprocal plot (Lineweaver-Burk plot).
32. Alkaline phosphatase as a diagnostic tool.
33. What are the different forms of calcium in blood?
34. RDA and functions of iodine.
35. Why arachidonic acid is not considered 'purely' an essential fatty acid?
36. Urea cycle disorders cause orotic aciduria. Explain.
37. Acidosis causes hyperkalemia. Why?
38. Define frameshift mutation with an example.
39. We need two primers for polymerase chain reaction. Justify.
40. Mechanism of action of chloromphenicol.
41. Mention the amino acids which take part in one-carbon pool.
42. Mention the enzymes which require selenium as cofactor.
43. Lesch-Nyhan syndrome presents with hyperuricemia. Explain.
44. Hypothyroidism presents with hypercholesterolemia. Why?
45. Histidine load test.
46. Mention two tumor markers and specify the diagnostic application.
47. M band.
48. Beer Lambert's law.
49. Mention two transmethylation reactions.
50. Enzyme deficiency in albinism. Mention two clinical features.

I. ESSAY QUESTIONS

1. Describe the chemistry, sources, daily requirement, biochemical functions and deficiency manifestations of vitamin B12.

Refer 2006 Short Note 8.

2. Describe how cholesterol is synthesized in our body. What are the products formed from cholesterol?

Refer 2004 Essay Question 2.

3. Write in details about the initiation, elongation and termination of transcription. Give an account of post-transcriptional processing.

TRANSCRIPTION

It is the process of formation of mRNA from DNA. Message from DNA is copied in the language of nucleotides (A, G, C, U) (Anti-template strand)

Coding strand ←5' G-T-C-A-A-C-G-3'
Template strand 3' C-A -G-T-T-G-C-5' →
↓
mRNA TRANSCRIPT 5' G -U-C-A-A-C-G-3'
∧∧∧∧∧∧∧∧∧∧∧∧∧∧

- Each DNA strand has a template strand which is transcribed to mRNA. It has the complementary sequence of mRNA
- The opposite strand of DNA is known as coding strand or anti-template strand. It has the same sequence as that of mRNA but all the U are changed to T.

Transcription Unit

It is the region of DNA which includes the gene for mRNA synthesis and also the regions of initiator, promoter and terminator regions.

Promoters

Starting signals at promoter site–10^5 initiation sites in human beings.
- TATA Box—prokaryotes; Goldberg-Hogness box in eukaryotes
- Transcription frequency signals–upstream
- Enhancers and silencers
- **TATA Box-pribnow box**: 6 nucleotides-5'-TATAAT-3' 10 bp upstream to the left of transcription start site
- 35 sequence second consensus nucleotide sequence (5'-TTGACA-3')–35 bp left of transcription start site
- The TATA box is bound by 34 kDa TATA-binding protein (TBP) which in turn binds several other proteins called TBP-associated factors (TAFs). This complex of TBP and TAFs is referred to as TFIID.
- **Eukaryotic promoter region: Goldberg-hognness box** (TATA box):
- 25 bp upstream of start site
- II consensus sequence—CAAT box
- Additional—GC box-(GGGCGG)
- CIS acting genetic elements
- Binding sites for general transcription factors-protein
- The process of transcription differs in prokaryotes and eukaryotes mainly in the RNA polymerase enzymes involved.
(Students can write any one–Prokaryotes or Eukaryotes).

TRANSCRIPTION IN BACTERIA (PROKARYOTES)

- **Bacterial RNA polymerase**—it is the prime enzyme for transcription
- It is a multisubunit enzyme of 350 kDa
- The core enzyme has 2 Identical α subunits, 2 unidentical β, β' subunits, one (Ω) omega subunit, one sigma (σ) factor and two Zn molecules
- Beta subunit fixes initiation site. Sigma factor recognizes promoter site and increases the affinity of holoenzyme to the promoter site **(Fig. 1)**.

Transcription–Steps: Prokaryotes

1. Initiation:
- Unwinding of DNA helix and the sigma factor recognizes two base sequences on the coding strand and initiates the transcription by RNA polymerase.
- RNA polymerase binds to the promoter site and moves forward to form preinitiation complex
- I nucleotide on mRNA gets attached to initiation site-β subunit and it becomes the 5' end of mRNA usually a purine nucleotide is the first unit. This is the initiation of transcription
- Attachment of next nucleotide (complementary) (formation of phosphodiester bond) enzyme moves on and on
- Release of σ factor after 10-20 nucleotides are polymerized **(Fig. 2)**.

2. Elongation

The RNAP moves along the DNA template. New nucleotides are attached to mRNA complementary to the template DNA according to the base pair rule. The synthesis is from 5' to 3' end. As the RNAP moves on DNA template, the DNA helix unwinds downstream

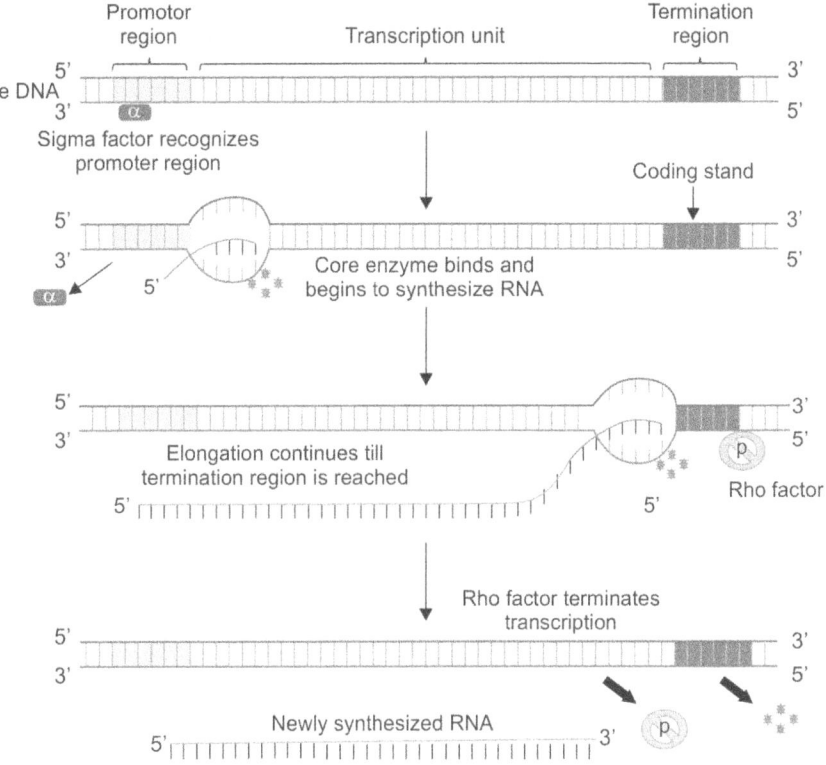

Fig. 1: Process of transcription in prokaryotes.

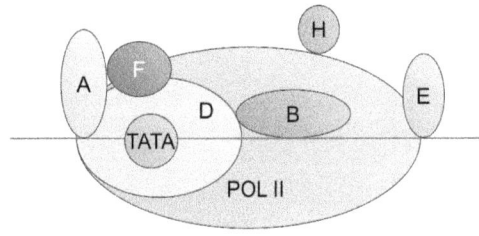

Fig. 2: Transcription—initiation.

and winds upstream forming a transcription bubble **(Fig. 3)**.

3. Termination

They are of 2 types:
1. **Rho-independent termination (Fig. 4):**
   - Termination signal in the DNA is given as a complementary palindromic sequence in DNA, i.e. ATT CGG GGG AAA followed by TTT CCC CCG AAT, so that a U turn is formed in mRNA

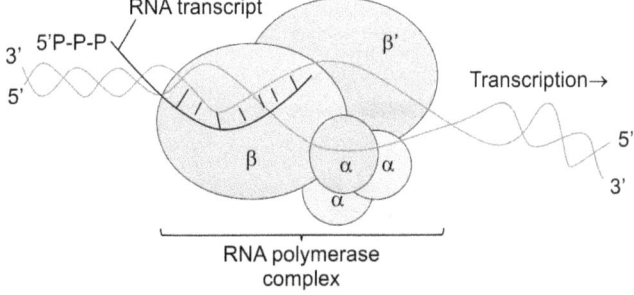

Fig. 3: Elongation—transcription.

- RNA transcript forms stable hairpin turn process slows down
- Two-fold symmetry due to palindromes-in hairpin turn of RNA
- Base of stem of the hairpin is rich in G and C
- Beyond hairpin turn-string of 'U's; U =A-weak-separation of new RNA.

2. **Rho-dependent termination (Fig. 5):**
   - Rho-dependent—addition of r (Rho) factor—binds to C-rich region near 3' end and migrates along behind RNAP in 5'-3'
   - At termination site—Rho factor displaces DNA and dissociates RNA molecule.

Inhibitors–Prokaryotes

1. **Rifampicin**—inhibits initiation by binding to b subunit of RNAP
2. **Actinomycin D–chemotherapy**—binds to DNA template and interferes the movement of RNAP.

TRANSCRIPTION IN EUKARYOTES

Mammalian RNA Polymerase

- Three major classes of RNAP –I (A), II (B), III (C)
- Type I (A)—is responsible for synthesis of rRNA (28S, 18S and 5.8S). It is not sensitive to α amanitin toxin—(Amanita phalloides- potsonous mushroom)
- Type II (B)—is the main enzyme which synthesize hnRNA (mRNA) and snRNA. It is highly sensitive to even low concentration of a amanitin
- Type III (C)—synthesize tRNA and 5S RNA. Moderately sensitive to high concentration of α amanitin.

Steps

Similar to prokaryotes—initiation, elongation and termination.
Promoters are different in eukaryotes.

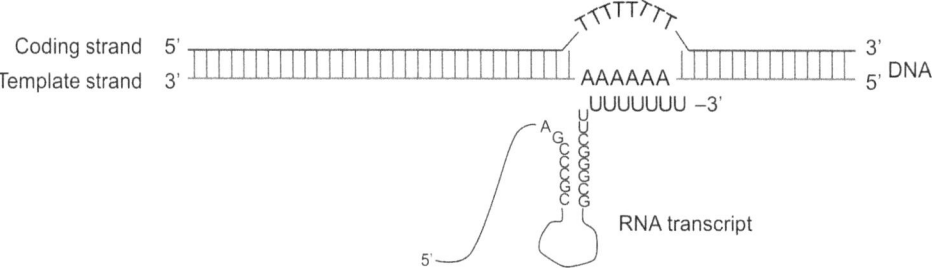

Fig. 4: Termination (Rho-independent).

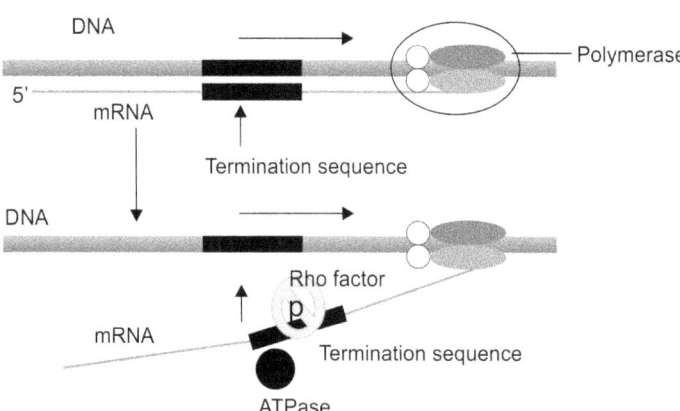

Fig. 5: Rho-dependent termination.

Eukaryotic Promoter Region

- Goldberg-hognness box (tata box):-25 bp upstream of start site
- Second consensus sequence—CAAT box
- Additional—GC Box (GGGCGG)
- CIS acting genetic elements
- Binding sites for general transcription factors—protein
- **Eukaryotic promoters**—decide where transcription is to commence and how frequently this event is to occur
- **Tata binding protein (TBP)** 30kDa, bind to TATA box—in turn bind to **TAFs–TBP Associated Factors**
- TBP + TAFs = TFIID
- Binding of TFIID to TATA sequence—first step in the formation of transcription complex.

Transcription Factors

- 4 factors + RNAP II—initiation of TATA box promoter
- TF—transacting elements—cytosol
- TFIIA—binds to TATA box along with TFIID
- TFIIB—binds to RNAP II and facilitates binding of TFIID and A on TATA box ATPase activity
- TFIIE—binds preinitiation complex—starts transcription in the presence of RNAP
- TFIID—recognizes and binds to TATA box, independent of RNAP II-TBP + TAFs—in minor grooves
- RNAP I and RNAP III—need specific TF
- Other factors—F, H, J.

Enhancers (Fig. 6)

- Increase rate of transcription
- Upstream to 5' side
- Downstream 3'
- Activators—enhancers with DNA sequences response elements that bind specific transcription factors
- Silencers—decrease the rate of transcription.

POST-TRANSCRIPTIONAL PROCESSING

A. Modification in mRNA:

- **Splicing (Fig. 7)**
  - The long primary transcripts have coding regions called exons and uncoding regions called introns
  - The introns should be removed and the exons should be spliced together. This is done by using snRNA
  - They attach with the terminal portions of introns and cleave at one end forming a lariat
  - This lariat is removed and the exons reattached by nucleophilic attack of terminal base of 1st exon to terminal base of 2nd exon.
- **Formation of Poly A tail:** The 3' end of mRNA is attached with 20-250 adenine nucleotides. This is to protect the 3'end from the attack of 3' exonuclease present in the cytoplasm
- **5' capping:** The 5' end is capped by 7 methyl-guanosine triphosphate. This will prevent the attack of cytoplasmic 5' exonuclease attack on mRNA
- **Methylation:** N_6 of adenine molecules and 2' hydroxy group of ribose are methylated.

B. Modification in tRNA:

- Trimming, converting the existing bases into unusual bases
- Addition of CCA nucleotides to 3' terminal end of tRNAs.

C. Ribosomal RNA:

Preribosomal RNA is synthesized originally are converted to ribosomal RNAs by post-transcriptional modifications.

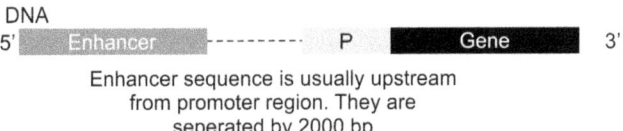

Enhancer sequence is usually upstream from promoter region. They are seperated by 2000 bp

Fig. 6: Enhancer.

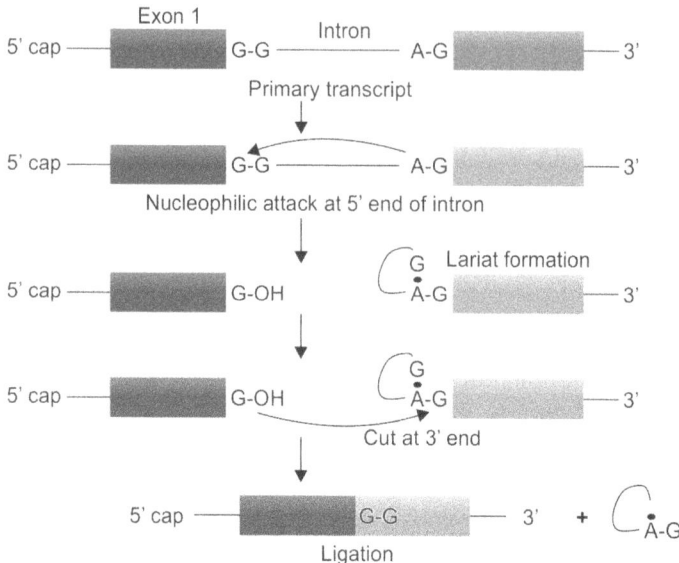

Fig. 7: Post-transcriptional processing of mRNA—splicing.

4. **Write in detail about the absorption, transport, daily requirement and deficiency manifestation of Iron.**

Refer 2006 Essay Question 8.

5. **Describe in detail TCA cycle and the energetics of the same. Justify why TCA cycle is called an amphibolic cycle.**

Refer 2004 Essay Question 1.

6. **Describe in detail the components and chemiosmotic theory of electron transport chain.**

Refer 2007 Essay Question 7.

7. a. **What is cloning? Mention the various types of cloning. b. Describe in detail the steps involved in recombinant DNA technology.**

A. CLONING

A clone is a large population of identical molecules, bacteria, or cells that arise from a common ancestor.

Types

- **Molecular cloning**—cloning of gene— when a gene of interest is introduced into a bacterial DNA to produce chimeric or recombinant DNA which is then amplified
- **Animal cloning**—when a cell from an animal is grown to an exact duplicate of that animal it is known as "cloning of an animal"
- **Molecular cloning** allows for the production of a large number of identical DNA molecules which can then be characterized or used for other purposes.
- This technique is based on the fact that chimeric or hybrid DNA molecules can be constructed in cloning vectors typically bacterial plasmids, bacterial phages, or cosmids which then continue to replicate in a host cell under their own control systems
- In this way, the chimeric DNA is amplified.

B. RECOMBINANT DNA TECHNOLOGY: (MOLECULAR CLONING)

When a gene of one species is transferred to another gene of different species, it is called recombinant DNA technology or genetic engineering. Usually there will be a combination of human DNA and bacterial DNA. The DNA thus formed is called as recombinant DNA or chimeric DNA or hybrid DNA

Preparation of DNA recombination **(Fig. 8)**:
1. **Preparation of specific human gene:** The mRNA of the desired gene is extracted and by using reverse transcriptase enzyme is complementary copy of that mRNA called complementary DNA (cDNA) is produced
2. **Preparation of chimeric DNA molecules:** Vectors are hosts like bacteria in which the desired gene is inserted into their genome. Restriction endonuclease is the enzyme which cuts DNA at specific sites. Using a restriction enzyme like EcoRI both the human DNA and plasmid DNA of the vectors are cut. They are cut in such a way that the ends of both the DNA are sticky and anneal with each other. DNA ligase forms phosphodiester linkages between both ends and joins them. The resulting hybrid DNA with the desired gene is called chimeric DNA
3. **Cloning of chimeric DNA (Fig. 9):**
   A. Transfection—the plasmid is introduced into the host cell by a process called transfection. Host *E. coli* cells are incubated with plasmid vectors in a hypertonic medium containing calcium. The calcium ion channels are opened through which the plasmid is imbibed into the host cell.
   B. Cloning—clone is a large population of identical cells arising from a common ancestor molecule. The cells are allowed to divide so that a large population of cells with the chimeric DNA is obtained.
4. **Checking the viability of the process:** Plasmid pBR-325 *contains chloram-*

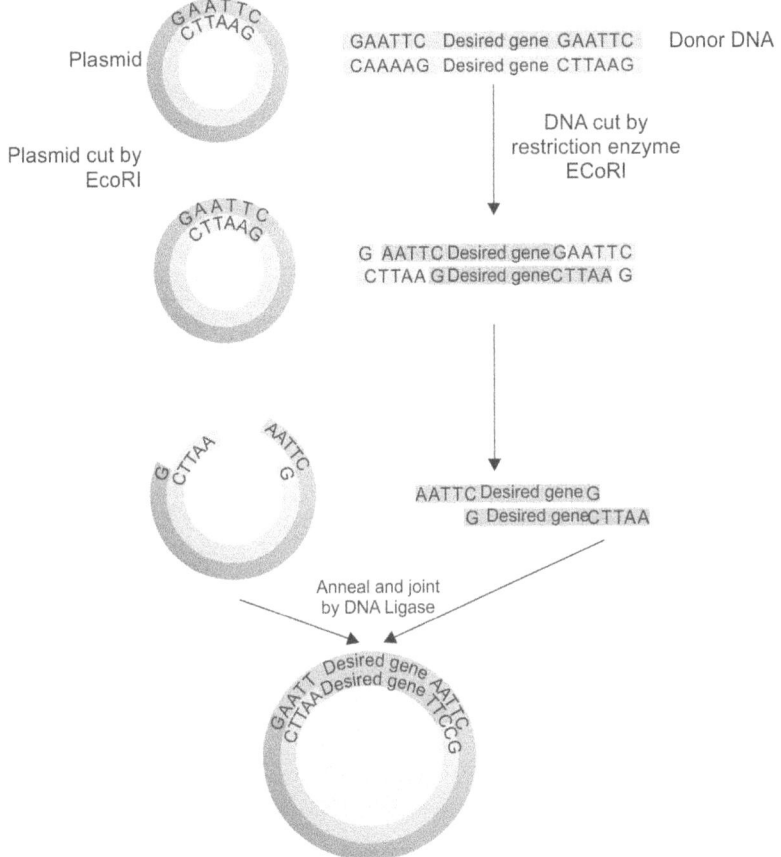

Fig. 8: Procedure of DNA recombination.

phenicol resistance gene (Cmr), *ampicillin resistance* (Apr) and *tetracycline resistance* (Tcr) genes. When this plasmid is cut by the EcoRI enzyme it will cut in the middle of *Cmr* gene. When the foreign DNA is inserted, the chloramphenicol resistance will be lost. This process functions as a marker for hybrid DNA

5. **Selection of colony with the desired gene:** After the transfection, the bacteria are cultured in a medium containing ampicillin and tetracycline. Wild bacteria are killed in that medium and the bacteria containing the cloned plasmid will grow. To check whether the colony contains the desired plasmid, a part of the colony is subjected to chloromphenicol media. If the bacterium dies, then it is the colony that contains the hybrid DNA plasmid

6. **Expression vectors:** Vector carrying a foreign gene which can produce the desired protein is called expression vector. Thus the human proteins like insulin can be harvested from such cultures.

Applications

- Large scale production of therapeutic human proteins can be obtained, e.g. human recombinant insulin for diabetic patients
- Vaccines with genetic material of bacteria and viruses can be produced
- Genetic probes can be produced to:
  - Identify genetic diseases during antenatal period

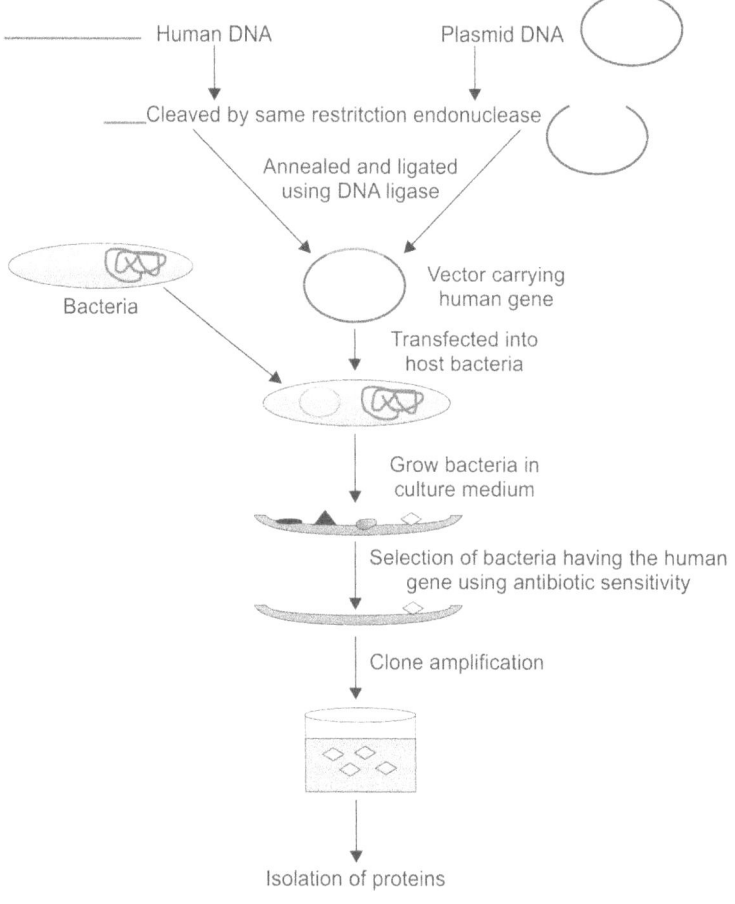

Fig. 9: Cloning.

- Diagnosis of virus and bacteria in blood using their DNA
- To pinpoint location of a gene in chromosome
- To identify mutations in genes
- To detect activation of oncogenes.
• Gene therapy—normal genes could be inserted into the patient's cells where it is defective, e.g. adenosine deaminase deficiency. Prenatal diagnosis by amniocentesis.

8. **Describe the role of: (i) plasma and (ii) renal buffers in maintaining acid base homeostasis.**

Refer 2003 Essay question 4.

II. SHORT NOTES

1. **Active form of vitamin D and its biochemical role.**

BIOSYNTHESIS OF ACTIVE VITAMIN D

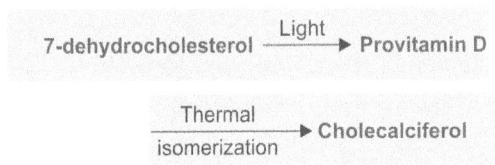

- 7-DHC is rich in malphigian layer of epidermis. The bond between 9 and 10 of 7-DHC is cleaved and converted into cholecalciferol by the action of UV light. That is why this is called as sunshine vitamin
- Vitamin D is a prohormone. Activation of provitamin D (cholecalciferol) into active vitamin D (calcitriol) takes place in two different sites:

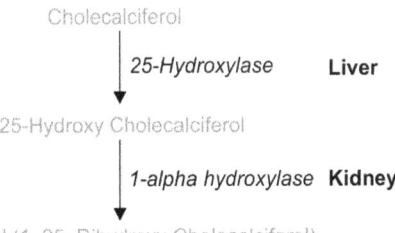

1. **25 hydroxylation of Cholecalciferol in liver**—cholecalciferol through blood reaches the liver cells and undergoes hydroxylation at 25th carbon. This reaction is catalyzed by 25-hydroxylase to form 25-hydroxycholecalciferol
2. **In plasma**—25-HCC is bound to vitamin D binding protein
• **1 hydroxylation in kidney**—the active form of vitamin D is synthesized at kidney. 25-hydroxycholecalciferol is hydroxylated at 1st position and converted into 1, 25-dihydroxycholecalciferol/calcitriol. It is the **active form of vitamin D.**

BIOCHEMICAL FUNCTIONS OF CALCITRIOL

The active form of vitamin D is calcitriol which is 1, 25-dihydroxycholecalciferol

Calcitriol acts as steroid hormone. It binds to specific cytoplasmic receptors which interacts with DNA and induces the synthesis of mRNA for specific proteins called calbindin which is a calcium-binding protein which will lead to biological actions **(Fig. 10)**.
• **Effect on intestine**—calcitriol induces the synthesis of calbindin and helps in the absorption of calcium and phosphorus from the intestines
• **Effects on kidney**—calcitriol increases the reabsorption of calcium and phosphorous from the renal tubules thereby conserving both the minerals
• **Action on bones**—calcitriol increases the activity of osteoblasts and hence mineralization of bones is increased. It remodels the activity of osteoclasts and osteoblasts. It prevents rickets and osteomalacia.

2. **Catabolism of hemoglobin.**

Refer 2005 Short Note 3.

3. **Protein-energy malnutrition.**

Refer 2004 Short Note 4.

4. **Ketogenesis.**

Refer 2005 Essay Question 2.

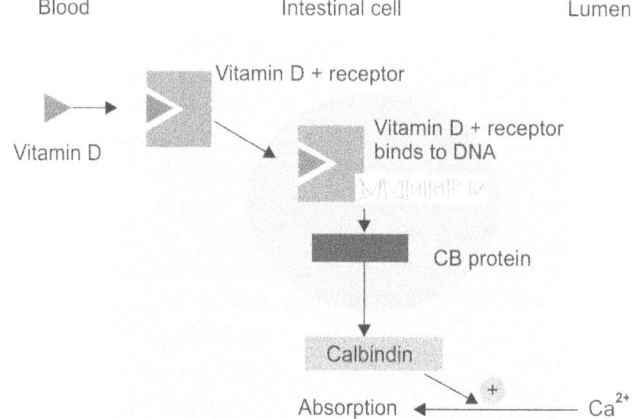

Fig. 10: Absorption of calcium by calcitriol.

5. Fatty acid synthase complex.

- It is the multienzyme complex. It catalyzes the synthesis of fatty acid from acetyl-CoA
- It is a dimer with identical subunits. Each subunit is organized into 3 domains with 7 enzymes **(Fig. 11)**.

Domain 1: Other name: Condensing unit

It is the initial substrate binding site. Enzymes are: i) Beta-ketoacyl synthase; ii) acetyl transferase; iii) malonyl transacylase.

Domain 2: Other name: Reduction unit

It contains dehydratase, enoyl reductase, beta-ketoacyl reductase and acyl carrier protein (ACP).

Domain 3: Other name: Releasing unit

It contains thioesterase or deacylase

Advantage of multienzyme complex

- Intermediates of the reaction can easily interact with the active site of enzyme

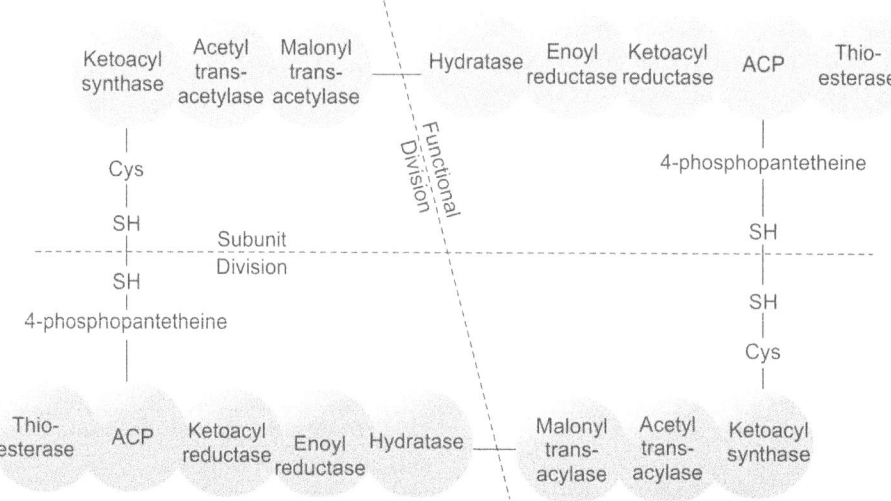

Fig. 11: Domains of fatty acid synthase complex.

- One gene codes for all the enzymes, so they are equimolecular in concentration
- Efficiency of the synthetic process is enhanced.

6. Glycogen metabolism.
Refer 2006 Essay Question 1.

7. Enzyme inhibition.
Refer 2005 Essay Question 1.

8. Glycosylated hemoglobin.
Refer 2007 Short Note 15.

9. Oxidative phosphorylation (chemiosmotic theory).
Refer 2006 Short Note 5.

10. Regulation of blood glucose.
Refer 2005 Essay Question 6.

11. Synthesis and mechanism of action of nitric oxide.

Nitric oxide (NO) is an uncharged molecule having an unpaired electron, so it is a highly reactive free radical.

SYNTHESIS

- Nitric oxide is formed from arginine using molecular oxygen by **the enzyme nitric oxide synthase (NOS)** which is a heme containing enzyme. Cofactors are FAD, FMN, NADPH and tetrahydrobiopterine. Calmodulin activates this enzyme
- The product formed are NO + citrulline. The enzyme is a dioxygenase as both atoms of O_2 are utilized to form two products **(Fig. 12)**.

Isoenzymes of NOS

There are 3 isoenzymes of NOS produced from three different genes which are as follows:

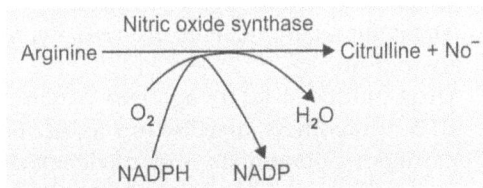

Fig. 12: Synthesis of nitric oxide.

1. **Neuronal NOS**—NOS-1 or nNOS present in central and peripheral neurons
2. **Macrophage NOS**—NOS-2 or inducible NOS (iNOS) mainly seen in macrophages and neutrophils. It is induced by inflammation
3. **Endothelial NOS**: NOS-3 or eNOS seen in endothelial cells, platelets, endocardium and myocardium. It produces arterial relaxation.

Mechanism of action of Nitric Oxide

- NOS is activated by acetylcholine
- NO diffuses into adjacent smooth muscle and activates guanylate cyclase leading to formation of cyclic GMP (cGMP). cGMP activates protein kinase in smooth muscles which dephosphorylates myosin light chain leading to the relaxation of muscles. Hence NO is a vasodilator.

Physiological actions

- **Blood vessels**—NO is a potent vasodilator produced by endothelial cells. NO maintains normal blood pressure. It dilates coronary, cerebral, renal and muscle arteries. Excess production of NO leads to refractory hypotension
- **Central nervous system (CNS)**—glutamate acts on N-methyl-D-aspartate (NMDA) receptors to cause calcium influx which activates NOSn. NO causes release of CRH, GHRH and LHRH hormones
- **Macrophages**—NOSi enzymes of macrophages produce NO. NO being a free radical kills the bacteria in the phagosome
- **Platelets**—NO inhibits the platelet adhesion and its function
- **Intestinal system**—it reduces motility and relaxation of sphincters.

12. Homocystinurias.
Refer 2014, Short Note 24
- These are the inborn errors of metabolism in methionine metabolism **(Fig. 13)**. These are autosomal recessive disorders of about 1:200,000 child births

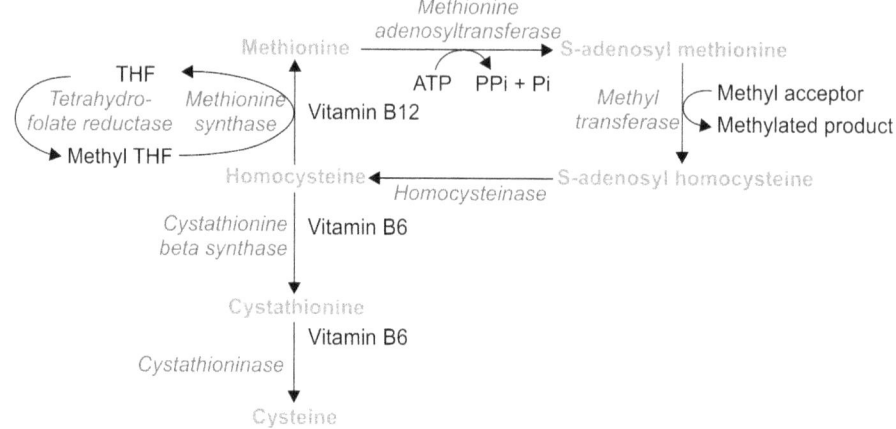

Fig. 13: Methionine metabolism.

- Normal homocysteine level in blood is 5-15 μmol/L. It is highly increased in disease conditions. In elderly people in vitamin B6 or B12 deficiency, smokers, alcoholics and in hypothyroidism also the level is increased. Large amounts of homocystine are excreted in urine in these conditions
- Hyperhomocysteinemia is a risk factor for coronary heart disease. It is seen in smokers, alcoholics, and hypothyroidism
- Other disorders associated with homocystinuria are neurological disorders, pre-eclampsia of pregnancy, chronic pancreatitis.

Congenital homocystinurias are due to the following causes:
- Cystathionine beta synthase deficiency—type I
- Deficient N^5, N^{10} methylene THFA reductase—type II
- Cobalamine deficiency—type III
- Defective intestinal absorption of vitamin B12—Type IV.

Cystathionine beta synthase deficiency:
- Methionine and homocysteine levels are increased in blood and in urine
- Marked decrease in plasma cysteine level
- Clinical features: Mental retardation, Charlie Chaplin gait, skeletal deformities and ectopia lentis in eyes are seen

- Homocysteine activates Hageman's factor causing platelet aggregation leading to intravascular thrombosis
  - Cyanide-nitroprusside test will be positive in urine. Urinary homocysteine levels are elevated
  - Treatment is a diet low in methionine and rich in cysteine.

Cobalamin deficiency: N5 methyl-THFA-homocysteine-methyl-transferase is dependent on B12. So in B12 deficiency, homocysteine cannot be converted to methionine. Hence, hyperhomocysteinemia occurs

Deficient N^5, N^{10} Methylene THFA reductase:
- This leads to reduced methionine synthesis with increase in homocysteine level in urine
- There will be behavioral changes and vascular abnormalities.

Acquired Hyperhomocysteinemia
- Nutritional deficiency of vitamins like cobalamin, folic acid and pyridoxine
- Metabolic—chronic renal diseases, hypothyroidism
- Drug induced—folate agonists, vitamin B12 antagonists, pyridoxine agonists, estrogen antagonists and nitric oxide antagonists.

13. Hyperuricemias.
Refer 2008 Short Note 18.

14. Metabolic acidosis.
Refer 2004 Short Note 16.

15. Phase two detoxification (conjugation).
Refer 2004 Short Note 14.

16. Cyclic AMP.
Refer 2005 Short Note 8.

17. Assessment of hypothyroidism.
- **Free T3 and T4**—ELISA techniques to quantitate this free fraction. The values of free hormones are not affected by the amount of carrier proteins in blood
- **Binding proteins:**
  - The abnormalities in the level of binding proteins may be reflected as abnormal hormone levels
  - Radioactive iodine labeled T_3 is added to the patient's serum and and it will occupy the free binding sites on TBG.
- **Plasma TSH**—in primary hyperthyroidism, TSH level is elevated due to lack of feedback but in secondary hyperthyroidism, TSH level as well as T_3 and T_4 levels are low
- **TRH response test**—TRH will stimulate TSH. If the hypothalamic pituitary-thyroid axis is normal, the T_3 and T_4 secretion is increased. An abnormal response is observed in hyperthyroidism and hypopituitrism
  - **Interpretation:**
    - In primary hypothyroidism, T3, T4 values are low and the most sensitive test is TSH. TSH levels will be elevated in clinical hypothyroidism
    - In secondary hypothyroidism, which is due to pituitary dysfunction, T3, T4 and TSH will be low. In these patients, TRH will be low. To check the hypothalamo-pituitary-thyroid axis, TRH stimulation test can be done.

18. Mutations.
Refer 2008 Short Note 34.

19. Electrophoresis.
Refer 2006 Short Note 30.

20. Antioxidants.
Antioxidants are compounds which prevent lipid peroxidation or rancidity by free radicals or control the oxidation process.

Types

I. **As per the nature**
   - **Naturally occurring antioxidants**—for examples, vitamin E and C, selenium, β-carotene
   - **Chemicals**—butylated hydroxyanisole (BHA), butylated hydroxytoluene (BHT).

II. **As per their action:** Two types: a) Preventive and b) Chain breaking antioxidants
   a. **Preventive antioxidants**
      - They will inhibit the initial production of free radicals. They are: Catalase, glutathione peroxidase and EDTA
      - Catalase: $2H_2O_2 \rightarrow O_2 + H_2O$
      - Glutathione peroxidase: $2H_2O_2 \rightarrow 2H_2O$
      - EDTA.
   b. **Chain breaking antioxidants**
      - They inhibit the propagative phase.

      $$O_2 + O_2 + 2H^+ \rightarrow H_2O_2 + O_2$$

      - They include superoxide dismutase, uric acid and vitamin E
      - Vitamin E would intercept the peroxyl free radical and inactivate it before a PUFA can be attacked

      $$T\text{-}OH + ROO' \rightarrow TO' + ROOH$$

      - The phenolic hydrogen of alpha tocopherol reacts with the peroxyl radical converting it to a hydroperoxide product

- The tocoperoxyl radical thus formed is stable and will not propagate the cycle any further
- This oxidative form of vitamin E is converted to vitamin E by ascorbic acid. Ascorbic acid becomes dehydroascorbate by reacting with Vitamin E radical. Two molecules of dehydroascorbate combine together to form ascorbate
- Other antioxidants are ceruloplasmin, caffeine and beta carotene.

Some antioxidants used in therapy are vitamin C, vitamin E, dimethylthiourea, dimethylsulfoxide, allopurinol.

21. Role of niacin as coenzyme.

- Niacin is one of the water-soluble vitamins
- It can be synthesised from tryptophan. 60 mg of tryptophan will give rise to I mg of niacin.

CoEnzymes

Nicotinamide adenine dinucleotide (NAD$^+$, NADH$^+$)

Nicotinamide adenine dinucleotide phosphate (NADP$^+$)

- NAD$^+$/NADH take part in oxidation reduction reactions
- NADPH mostly takes part in reductive biosynthesis.

NAD$^+$ Dependent Enzymes

I. **Carbohydrate metabolism:**
   a. Glycolysis:
      1. Glyceraldehyde-3-phosphate dehydrogenase: Glyceraldehyde-3-phosphate → 1, 3-BPG
      2. Lactate dehydrogenase (lactate → pyruvate).
   b. Pyruvate dehydrogenase:
      $$\text{Pyruvate} \xrightarrow{\text{NAD, FAD, CoA, TPP, lipoic acid}} \text{acetyl-CoA}$$
   c. TCA cycle:
      1. Isocitrate $\xrightarrow{\text{Isocitrate dehydrogenase/NAD}}$ oxalosuccinate
      2. α-ketoglutarate $\xrightarrow{\text{α-KG dehydrogenase/5 coenzymes}}$ succinyl-CoA
      3. Malate $\xrightarrow{\text{Malate dehydrogenase/NAD}}$ fumarate

II. **Lipid metabolism:-beta oxidation**
   1. Beta hydroxy acyl-CoA dehydrogenase
      Beta hydroxy acyl-CoA $\xrightarrow{\text{NAD}}$ beta-keto acyl-CoA

III. **Amino acid metabolism:**
   1. Glutamate dehydrogenase
      Glutamte $\xrightarrow{\text{NAD}}$ α-ketoglutarate

NADPH Generating Reactions

HMP pathway
1. Glucose-6-phosphate dehydrogenase:
   Glucose-6-phosphate $\xrightarrow{\text{NADP}}$ 6 phosphogulonolactone + NADPH
2. 6-phosphogluconate dehydrogenase:
   6-phosphogulonolactone → 3-keto-6-phosphogluconate + NADPH
3. Cytoplasmic isocitrate dehydrogenase
4. Malic enzyme—malate → pyruvate.

NADPH Utilizing Reactions (Reductive Synthesis)

- Fatty acid synthesis: Fatty acid synthase complex
- Cholesterol synthesis: HMG-CoA → mevolanate. HMG-CoA reductase (rate-limiting step in cholesterol synthesis)
- Bile acid synthesis
- Methemoglobin → hemoglobin
- Phenylalanine → tyrosine; phenylalanine hydroxylase
- Folate → dihydrofolate → tetrahydrofolate; folate reductase
- Bile acid synthesis—7 α-hydroxylase
- Steroid synthesis—hydroxylation steps.

22. Classification of hyperlipidemias and their clinical importance.

- Frederickson's classification of hyperlipoproteinemias are also called as dyslipoproteinemias
- They are 5 types which are explained here

Type	Name	Defect	Clinical features
Type I	Familial LP lipase deficiency Apo C II deficiency	LP lipase deficiency	Chylomicrons, TAG increased Eruptive xanthomas, hepatomegaly Creamy layer over clear plasma
Type II a	Familial hypercholesterolemia	LDL receptor defect, apo B increased	LDL, cholesterol increased TAG normal, clear plasma Atherosclerosis, tuberous xanthoma
Type II b	_____	Apo B, apo C II increased	LDL, VLDL, cholesterol increased Corneal arcus Slightly cloudy plasma
Type III	Familial dyslipoproteinemia/broad beta disease or remnant removal disease	Apo E, apo C II increased	VLDL, chylomicron Cholesterol increased. Palmar xanthoma, cloudy plasma, risk of vascular disease
Type IV	Familial hypertriacylglycerolemia	Overproduction of VLDL, apo C II	VLDL, TAG, cholesterol increased Associated with diabetes, obesity, cloudy or milky plasma
Type V	Familial lipoprotein excess	Secondary to other causes	VLDL, chylomicron, TAG increased, cholesterol level normal, risk of heart diseases, creamy layer over milky plasma

Importance of Hyperlipoproteinemias

- Elevation of lipids in plasma leads to the deposition of cholesterol on the arterial walls leading to atherosclerosis affecting commonly the coronary and cerebral vessels. This will lead to ischemic heart disease and cerebrovascular accidents
- Deposition of lipids in subcutaneous tissues leads to xanthomas of various types
- Eruptive xanthomas—small yellow nodules with deposition of TG
- Tuberous xanthomas—yellow plaques containing cholesterol and TG found over the elbows and knees
- Xanthelesma—lipid deposits under the periorbital skin made up of cholesterol
- Tendinous xanthomata found over tendons
- Deposition of lipids around the cornea leads to corneal arcus indicating hypercholesterolemia.

Management

- Restriction of fat intake
- Supplementation of diet with PUFA and lipid lowering drugs
- For example, statin group of drugs to decrease cholesterol
- Restriction of body weight
- Regular exercise.

23. Sphingolipidoses.

Refer 2009 Short Note 33.

24. Biochemical role of vitamin C.

Refer 2005 Essay Question 5.

25. Cori cycle and glucose alanine cycle.

CORI CYCLE (lactic acid cycle) (FIG. 14)

Definition: Transferring lactate from muscle tissues to liver and resynthesis of glucose in liver is known as Cori cycle.

Effects

- In contracting muscle, pyruvate is reduced to lactate which gets accumulated in muscle and may lead to muscular cramps in strenuous muscular exercise
- It rescues lactate for further use (gluconeogenesis) and counteracts lactic acidosis
- It is of less importance in starvation but important in more normal situations especially in certain cells, such as matured RBC, medulla, retina which are lacking mitochondria and virtually anaerobic
- Lactate is carried from skeletal muscle to liver through blood. In the liver lactate is converted to pyruvate and by gluconeogenesis it is converted to glucose which is then transported to muscles for energy supply.

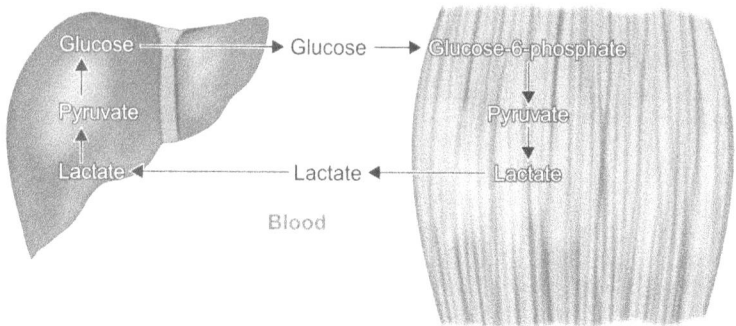

Fig. 14: Cori cycle.

GLUCOSE-ALANINE CYCLE: (CAHILL CYCLE)

- Alanine synthesized in muscle is transported to liver where it is converted to glucose **(Fig. 15)**
- Muscle protein → alanine $\xrightarrow{Transamination}$ pyruvate $\xrightarrow{Gluconeogenesis}$ glucose.

Significance

- Liver maintains glucose output by gluconeogenesis of alanine
- It also maintains nitrogen balance.

26. High density lipoprotein cycle.

Refer 2010 Short Note 6.
Other name: Reverse cholesterol transport

HDL CYCLE:

- HDL cycle is the main transport form of cholesterol from peripheral tissues to liver for excretion through the bile or for utilization.

Metabolism

- Intestinal cell synthesize HDL which is discoidal in shape
- Lecithin cholesterol acyltransferase (LCAT) binds to the nascent HDL and converts free cholesterol to cholesterol ester. Thus HDL becomes spherical in shape (HDL 3)

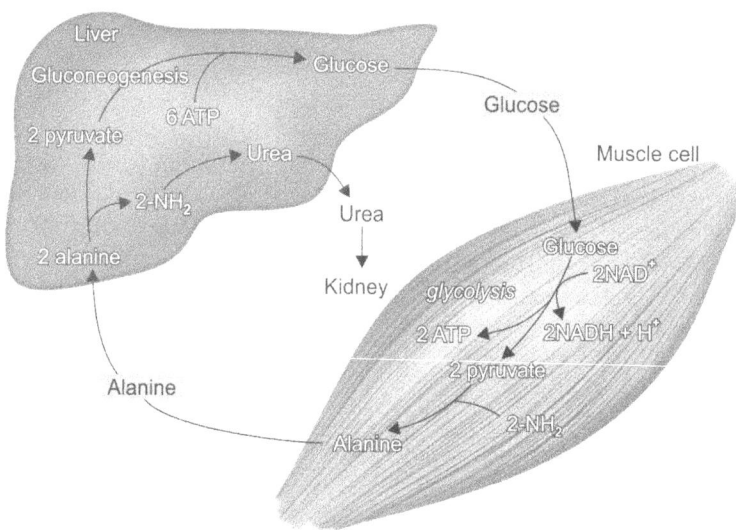

Fig. 15: Glucose alanine cycle.

- Free cholesterol derived from peripheral tissue is taken up by HDL 3. It is mediated by ABC protein (ATP binding cassette protein 1)
- The esterified cholesterol moves into the interior of HDL disc
- Mature HDL spheres are taken up by liver cells by ApoA1 mediated receptor mechanism
- Hepatic lipase hydrolyses HDL phospholipid and TAG
- The released cholesterol esters are taken into liver cells to be converted to bile acids and excreted through bile
- Cholesterol ester transfer protein (CETP) transfers cholesterol from HDL to VLDL and LDL in exchange for TG.

Significance

- By this cycle, cellular and lipoprotein cholesterol is delivered back to the liver where excess cholesterol is excreted into bile. **This is known as reverse cholesterol transport**
- Excretion of cholesterol needs esterification with PUFA. Thus PUFA helps in lowering cholesterol in the body and so cholesterol is an antiatherogenic
- This prevents deposition of cholesterol in the tissues and this cycle is thought to be antiatherogenic and high level of HDL cholesterol confers a decreased risk of coronary heart disease.

Functions

- **Antiatherogenic known as good cholesterol**
- **Involved in reverse cholesterol transport.**
- HDL subfractions—HDL 1 (bad and contains only ApoE), HDL 2
- Good and antiatherogenic HDL 3 contains apoA2 and its role is controversial
- Act as a reservoir for apoproteins which can be donated or received from other lipoproteins
- As antioxidant it prevents the oxidation of LDL.

27. Glycogenolysis.

Refer 2006 Essay Question 1.

28. Isomerism in carbohydrates.

- Sugars exhibit various forms of isomerism. Glucose with four asymmetric carbon atoms can form 16 isomers as per Vant Hoff's formula (2^n) where 'n' is the number of asymmetric carbon ($2^4 = 16$)
- **D-and-L isomerism**—the designation of a sugar isomer as the D form or of its mirror image as the L form. It depends on the orientation of H and OH groups on the penultimate carbon (carbon adjacent to primary alcohol) **(Fig. 16)**.
  Enantiomers—in D and L isomerism, the groups attached to carbon atoms of glucose 2, 3, 4, and 5 are totally reversed to produce mirror images. These 2 forms—D and L isomers are known as **Enantiomers.**
  Diastereoisomerism—configurational changes with regard to C2, C3 and C4 will produce eight different aldohexoses and this is known as **diastereoisomerism.** Out of these 8 differ aldohexoses, only 3 are seen in human beings. They are glucose, galactose and mannose.
- **Optic isomerism**—when a beam of plane polarized light is passed through a freshly prepared solution of carbohydrates, it will rotate either to the right or left. Dextrorotatory are compounds that rotate the plane of polarized light to the right D (+) and levorotatory are compounds that rotate the light to the left L (-).

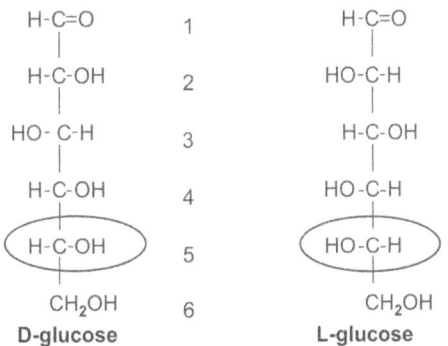

Fig. 16: D-and-L isomerism.

- **Pyranose and furanose ring structures (Fig. 17):** The stable ring structures of monosaccharides are similar to the ring structures of either pyran (a six-membered ring) or furan (a five-membered ring). For glucose in solution, more than 99% is in the pyranose form
- **Alpha and beta anomers:** C1 of aldoses and C2 of ketoses are known as anomeric carbon atom. Sugar can exist in 2 forms represented by α and β anomers. In alpha form the hydroxyl group is attached to C1 below the plane of the ring and in beta form OH group is above the plane of the ring. These α and β forms are called as anomers **(Fig. 18)**
- **Epimers:** Isomers differing as a result of variations in configuration of the OH and H with regard to a single carbon atom other than the reference carbon atoms, e.g. carbon atoms 2, 3, and 4 of glucose are known as epimers. The important epimers of glucose are mannose with respect to 2nd carbon and galactose with respect to carbon 4 **(Fig. 19)**
- **Aldose-ketose isomerism:** Fructose has the same molecular formula as glucose but differs in its structural formula, since there is a potential keto group in position 2 of fructose, whereas there is a potential aldehyde group in position 1 of glucose **(Fig. 20)**.

29. Balanced diet.

Refer 2007 Short Note 14.

30. Fructose intolerance (hereditary fructose intolerance).

FRUCTOSE INTOLERANCE

It is an inborn error of fructose metabolism.

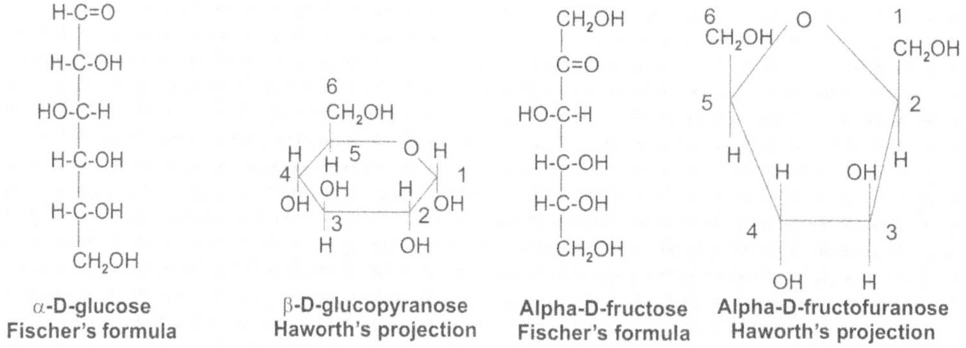

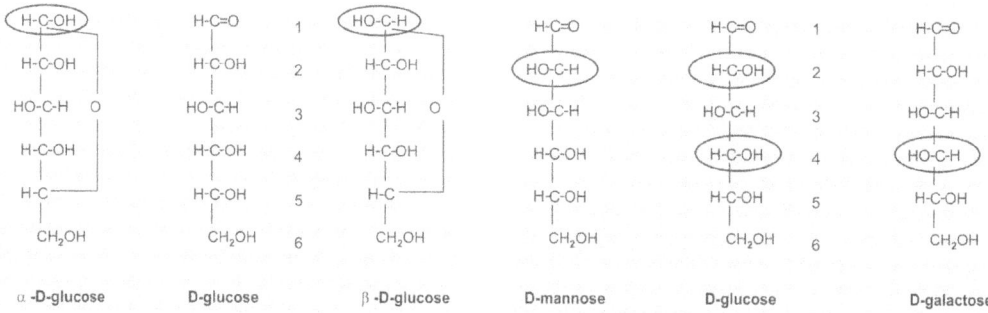

Fig. 17: Glucopyranose and fructopyranose—alpha and beta.

Fig. 18: Alpha and beta anomers.

Fig. 19: Epimers.

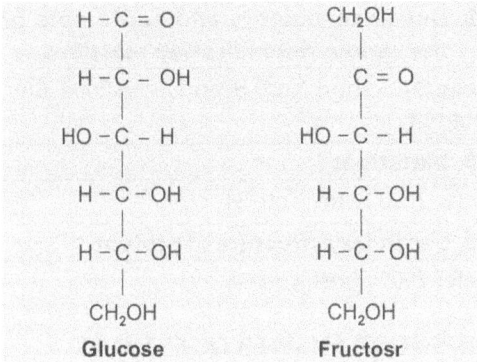

Fig. 20: Aldose-ketose isomerism.

Cause

Due to the absence of hepatic **aldolase B**, this cleaves fructose-1-phosphate

Fructose → fructose-1-phosphate $\xrightarrow{\text{aldolase B}}$ glyceraldehyde + DHAP

So there will be accumulation of fructose-1-phosphate which inhibits fructokinase causing impaired clearance of fructose from blood **(Fig. 21)**.

Clinical Features

- Accumulation of fructose-1-phosphate (F-1-p) leads to liver and kidney damage
- Fructose-induced **hypoglycemia** despite the presence of high glycogen reserve due to inhibition of glycogenolysis and gluconeogenesis.

Treatment

Diet low in fructose and sucrose.

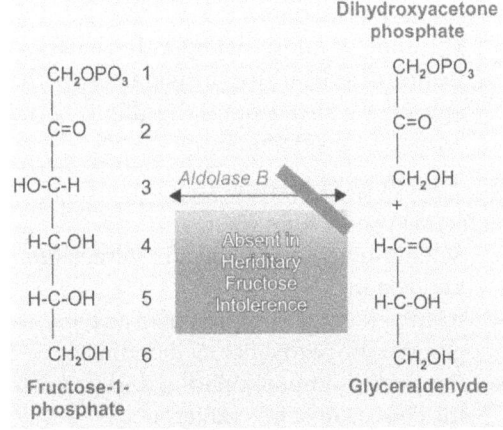

Fig. 21: Hereditary fructose intolerance.

31. Purine salvage pathway.
Refer 2004 Short Note 15.

32. Explain the types and functions of immunoglobulins.
Refer 2008 Short Note 11.

33. Phenylketonuria.
Refer 2003 Short Note 12.

34. Fluorosis.
Refer 2008 Short Answer Question 10.

35. Serum protein electrophoresis.
Refer 2006 Short Note 30.

36. Cell cycle.

- The term cell cycle refers to the events occurring during the period between two mitotic divisions. It is divided into G1 (gap 1), S (synthesis), G2 (gap 2) and M (mitosis) phase
- The cell division is taking place in M phase. The daughter cells then enter either to G_0 (dormant/resting) phase or re-enter the cell cycle when there is necessity for growth or repair
- In normal cell population most of cells are in G_0 phase
- Interphase is the period between the end of M phase and beginning of next mitosis
- In G1 phase, proteins and RNA content increase
- In S phase, DNA is synthesized, only once becoming tetraploid
- In G2 phase, cytoplasmic enlargement takes place **(Fig. 22)**

Cell Cycle and Cyclins (Fig. 23)

- CDK2—cyclin E directs the cells in G1 phase to enter into S phase
- CDK2—cyclin A pushes the cells to complete S phase and cyclin A, B make cells complete the G2 phase and enter into M phase.

37. Role of parathormone in calcium, phosphate homeostasis.
Refer 2010 Short Answer Question 32.

- Parathormone (PTH) is secreted by the chief cells of parathyroid glands

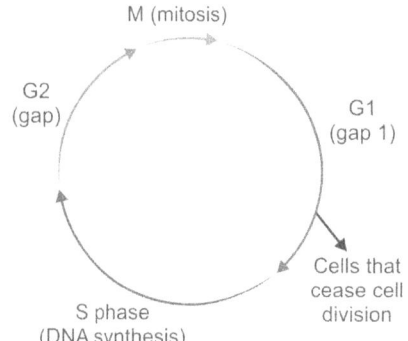

Fig. 22: Cell cycle.

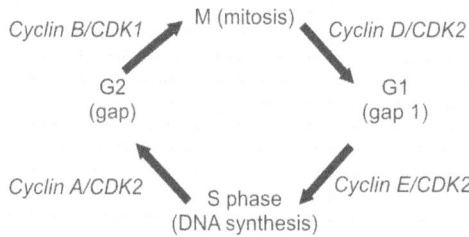

Fig. 23: Role of cyclin dependent kinases.

- It binds with a receptor protein on the surface of the target cells. This activates adenylyl cyclase
- PTH has 3 major sites of action—intestine, bone and kidney. All these 3 actions of PTH increase the serum calcium level
    1. **In intestines**—stimulates production of 1 alpha-hydroxylation of 25 hydroxycalciferol to produce the biologically active form of vitamin D (calcitriol) in the kidney which increases the absorption of calcium from the intestine
    2. **In bone**—facilitates mobilization of calcium from bone by increasing the number of osteoclasts and activating pyrophosphatase in osteoclasts. It stimulates secretion of collagenase from osteoclasts causing loss of matrix and bone resorption
    3. **In kidney**—maximizes tubular reabsorption of calcium within the kidney, thus resulting in minimal losses of calcium and increased excretion of phosphate.

38. Define xenobiotics and add a note on the various detoxification reactions.

Refer 2005 Short Note 16 and Refer 2004 Short Note 14.

39. Mutation.

Refer 2008 Short Note 34.

40. Secondary structure of protein.

Refer 2007 Short Note 25.

III. SHORT ANSWER QUESTIONS

1. Zymogen.

Refer 2009 Short Answer Question 4.

2. Name two zinc containing enzymes.

Zinc containing enzymes—carbonic anhydrase, alcohol dehydrogenase.

3. Ferritin.

- The storage form of iron is ferritin normal level 20-250 ng/mL
- Iron (Fe^{2+}) entering the mucosal cells is oxidized to ferric form (Fe^{3+}) by the enzyme ferroxidase
- Fe^{3+} combines with apoferririn to form ferritin (storage form of iron)
- From the mucosal cells it enters into the bloodstream if there is anemia.

4. Define K_m.

Refer 2003 Short Note 8.

- K_m value or Michaelis-Menten constant is defined as the substrate concentration at half maximal velocity in an enzyme-catalyzed reaction
- K_m value is a constant and a characteristic feature of a given enzyme (signature of the enzyme). It also denotes the affinity of the enzymes for substrates.

5. Functions of selenium.

Refer 2008 Short Note 12.

- Selenium acts a nonspecific intracellular antioxidant
- It is an essential component of enzymes—glutathione peroxidise, 5' deiodinase
- Prevents lipid peroxidation and protects the cells against free radicals

- It binds with certain heavy metals and protects the body from their toxic effects
- It is necessary for the normal development of spermatozoa.

6. What are cytochromes?

Refer 2006 Short Note 25.
- They are copper containing hemoproteins present in METC. They are cytochrome b, c, c1 and aa3
- Complex III of METC is known as cytochrome oxidase. It is a cluster of iron sulfur hemoproteins—cytochrome b and c1
- Cytochrome c is a heme containing peripheral protein. It collects electrons from complex III and delivers it to complex IV
- Cytochrome aa3 are called cytochrome oxidase which is complex IV. It includes 4 redox centers—cytochrome a, a3, and 2 copper ions.

7. Brown adipose tissue.

- Brown adipose tissue is active in hibernating animals and in newborn babies which is essential for maintaining body temperature
- They have good blood supply, rich content of mitochondria (which gives brown color) but low activity of ATP synthase
- Thermogenin is an uncoupling protein (UCP) present in inner mitochondrial membrane of brown adipocytes and it acts as a natural uncoupler of oxidative phosphorylation
- Hence, the energy of oxidation is not conserved for ATP synthesis but dissipated as heat to maintain the body temperature
- Thus, the tissue is extremely active in some species in arousal from hibernation, in animals exposed to cold (nonshivering thermogenesis), and in heat production in the newborn animal
- Though not a prominent tissue in humans, it is present in normal individuals where it could be responsible for **"diet-induced thermogenesis."**

8. Lactose intolerance.

- It is due to the absence or deficiency of lactase or beta galactosidase enzyme
- In lactose intolerance due to the absence of lactase enzyme, lactose remains accumulated and it becomes a substrate for bacterial fermentation. This causes production of H_2 and CO_2 gases. These accumulated gases and osmotically active products draw water from the intestinal lumen causing abdominal discomfort, diarrhea and dehydration
- Cause may be congenital or acquired
- Acquired lactose intolerance occurs due to sudden change in milk containing diets.

Treatment

Lactobacillus in curd, yeast. Patient should not be given milk in this condition.

9. Define respiratory quotient.

- Respiratory quotient (RQ) is the measurement of the ratio of the volume of carbon dioxide produced in L/g to volume of oxygen consumed in L/g
- RQ of fats, carbohydrates and proteins are 0.7, 1.0 and 0.8, respectively.

10. Functions of vitamin K.

Refer 2009 Short Answer Question 8.
Vitamin K is involved in post-translational modifications of clotting factors, such as factor II, VII, IX and X which undergo gamma carboxylation to get active form, e.g. prothrombin is activated to thrombin by carboxylation helped by vitamin K.

11. Name the major intracellular and extracellular anion.

- Intracellular anions—sulfate and phosphate
- Extracellular anions—chloride, bicarbonate.

12. Principle of flame photometer.

- When introduced to flame the analyte elements like Na, K, Ca and Li emit a light at characteristic wavelength

- The intensity of the light is measured at the particular wavelength of the material and it is directly proportional to the concentration of the element.

13. Metabolic roles of zinc and selenium.
Refer 2008 Short Note 12.

14. Orotic aciduria.
Refer 2010 Short Note 37.

15. Chimeric DNA.
When a gene of one species is transferred to another gene of different species it is called recombinant DNA technology or Chimeric DNA. The process by which it is produced is known as genetic engineering. Usually there will be a combinations of human DNA and bacterial DNA. The DNA thus formed is called as recombinant DNA or chimeric DNA or hybrid DNA.

16. Osmolality.
- It is the osmotic pressure exerted by the number of moles per kilogram of solvent
- Osmolality of plasma varies from 285 to 295 mOsm/kg
- It is a measure of solute particles present in the fluid medium
- Sodium and its associated anions make the largest contribution 90% to plasma osmolality
- It is measured by osmometer
- Plasma osmolality can be measured from the concentration of sodium, potassium, urea and glucose which is as follows: 2 (Na) + 2 (K) + urea + glucose
- This calculation is simplified—osmolality = 2 × plasma Na (when plasma glucose and urea are normal).

17. Anti-HIV drugs.
Reverse transcriptase inhibitors—they inhibit reverse transcriptase (RT) of HIV virus.
- Nonnucleoside analogues, e.g. nevirapine
- Nucleoside analogues, e.g. azidothymidine, zidovudine
- Nucleotide analogues, e.g. adefovir
- Protease inhibitors—inhibit HIV protease, e.g. nelfinavir
- Combination of drugs—combination like highly active antiretroviral therapy (HAART).

18. Compounds formed from glycine.
Refer 2004 Essay Question 3.
1. Creatine, creatine phosphate and creatinine. (glycine + arginine + S-adenosylmethionine)
2. Heme (glycine + succinyl-CoA)
3. Purine bases and nucleotides –C4, C5 and N7
4. Glutathione (gamma-glutamylcysteinyl-glycine)
5. Conjugation for xenobiotics
6. Constituent of proteins like collagen. (glycine + proline + hydroxyproline)
7. Methylene tetrahydrofolate by glycine cleavage system
8. Glucose—it is glucogenic.

19. Write the normal serum sodium and potassium level.
- **Sodium (Na)**—135-145 mmol/L
- **Potassium (K)**—3.5-5 mmol/L

20. What are monoclonal and polyclonal antibodies?
- **Monoclonal antibodies**—they are antibodies produced from a single clone of B cells from a single ancestor. They express same affinity towards a particular part of the antigen (epitope). They produce one type of antibody specific for one epitope and they are homogenous
- **Polyclonal antibodies**—they are antibodies against a single antigen but produced by different B cells. Each type of antibody is specific for a single epitope. They are heterogeneous mixture of antibodies each one specific for various epitopes on the antigen.

21. Markers for lysosomes and mitochondria.

Organelles	Marker enzyme
Lysosomes	Cathepsin
Mitochondria	ATP synthase

22. Fluorosis.
Refer 2008 Short Answer Questions 10.

23. Role of Apo CII.
- The protein part of lipoprotein is called apolipoprotein
- Apolipoproteins are synthesized in liver
- APO CII—it activates lipoprotein lipase.

Apoproteins	Blood level (mg/dL)	Site of production	Components	Functions
APO CII	5	Liver	Chylomicron, VLDL	Clearance of TAG, activates lipoprotein lipase

24. Define metalloenzymes with two examples.
- Metalloenzymes are enzymes which require metals ions for their activity. These enzymes hold the metals tightly and are not readily exchanged
- For example, carbonic anhydrase—zinc, phenol oxidase, copper.

25. Pulmonary surfactant—structure and clinical importance.
- Dipalmitoyl lecithin, phosphatidyl-glycerol, cholesterol and surfactant proteins A, B and C are the constituents of lung surfactant produced from the lung epithelium
- This is needed for the normal functioning of lungs. It decreases the surface tension of the aqueous layer of lung and prevents collapse of lung alveoli
- Low levels of lung surfactant in newborn children leads to respiratory distress syndrome (RDS) which is the most common cause for neonatal mortality
- Administration of natural or artificial surfactants is of therapeutic benefit.

26. Iodine number and its importance.
- It is defined as the number of grams of iodine taken up by 100 g of fat
- It is an index of the degree of unsaturation and is directly proportional to the content of unsaturated fatty acids
- Higher the iodine number, higher is the degree of unsaturation
- It also helps to identify adulteration.

Food substances	Iodine No.
Butter	28
Sunflower oil	30

27. What is the function of lipoprotein lipase?
- It is one of the enzymes acting on lipids.
- Its function is to hydrolyse TGL present in chylomicron and VLDL into fatty acids and glycerol
- It is located in the endothelial layer of capillaries of adipose tissue, muscles and heart
- It is not present in liver
- Lack of APO CII leads to decreased activity of LPL and consequent accumulation of chylomicrons and VLDL in blood
- Insulin increases LPL activity.

28. Structure of lecithin.
- Lecithin is phosphatidylcholine
- It is a glycerophospholipid containing choline
- It is a nitrogen containing phospholipid
- The alpha and beta positions are esterified with fatty acids (PUFA) which is present in beta carbon
- Phosphoric acid attached to the third position to which choline is attached.

$$CH_2-O-CO-R_1$$
$$R_2-COO-CH$$
$$CH_2-O-\overset{O}{\underset{O}{\overset{\|}{P}}}-O-CH_2-CH_2-N^+(CH_3)_3$$

29. Net protein utilization.
- It is one of the nutritional indices of proteins
- It denotes nutritional quality and availability of a protein
- Net protein utilization (NPU) = retained nitrogen/intake of nitrogen × 100

- NPU is a better index than biological value of proteins.

30. Chondroitin sulfate—structure.

Refer 2007 Short Notes 16.

[Structure of chondroitin sulfate showing COO⁻, CH₂OH, SO₄, OH, H, HNCOCH₃ groups]

It is one of the mucopolysaccharides or glycosaminoglycans which are under the classification of heteropolysaccharides. Usually attached to proteins as part of proteoglycan.

Site of occurrence—it is present in ground substance of connective tissues present in cartilage, bone, tendons, cornea and skin.

Repeating units—it is made up of repeating units of glucuronic acid and n-acetylgalactosamine to which sulfate group is attached.

Functions—it provides an endoskeletal structure to maintain the structure and shape of the tissues like cartilage.

Therapeutic uses—it is used to treat osteoarthritis as anti-inflammatory agent.

31. Double reciprocal plot (Lineweaver-Burk plot) (Fig. 24).

- It is also called as Lineweaver-Burk plot
- Sometimes the determination of enzyme activity needs very high substrate concentration which is impractical
- A linear form of the Michaelis-Menten equation circumvents this difficulty and permits V_{max} and K_m to be extrapolated from initial velocity data obtained at lower concentrations of substrate

$$V_i = \frac{V_{max}[S]}{K_m + [S]}$$

Invert,

$$\frac{1}{V_i} = \frac{K_m + [S]}{V_{max}[S]}$$

Factor:

$$\frac{1}{V_i} = \frac{K_m}{V_{max}[S]} + \frac{[S]}{V_{max}[S]}$$

And simplify:

$$\frac{1}{V_i} = \left[\frac{K_m}{V_{max}}\right]\frac{1}{[S]} + \frac{1}{V_{max}}$$

- This equation is got by taking the reciprocal of the Michaelis–Menten equation
- When $1/v_i$ is plotted against $1/[S]$ a straight line is obtained with the slope equal to K_m/V_{max}
- Such a plot is called a **double reciprocal** or **Lineweaver-Burk plot (Fig. 24)**.

Significance

- Double reciprocal or Lineweaver-Burk plot of $1/v_i$ versus $1/[S]$ is used to evaluate K_m and V_{max} values
- It can be used to determine the kinetic mechanisms of enzyme inhibitors.

32. Alkaline phosphatase as a diagnostic tool.

- It is a marker of obstructive jaundice
- It is also increased in bone disorders
- Six isoenzymes of alkaline phosphatase (ALP)
- Alpha-1 ALP; alpha-2 heat labile ALP; Alpha-2 heat stable ALP; pre-beta ALP; gamma-ALP, leukocyte ALP (LAP)

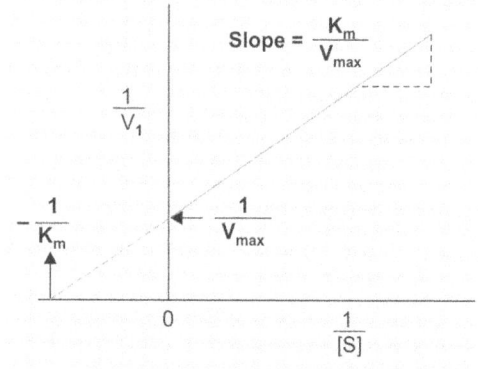

Fig. 24: Double reciprocal plot.

- They are due to the difference in the carbohydrate content
- Increase in alpha-1 ALP—obstructive jaundice; alpha-2 ALP—indicates hepatitis; and pre-beta ALP—indicates bone diseases; gamma-ALP—indicates ulcerative colitis; LAP—increased in lymphomas.

33. What are the different forms of calcium in blood?

- Total calcium level—9-11 mg/dL
- Three forms of calcium in blood:
  1. Ionized calcium (active form)—5 mg/dL.
  2. Protein bound Ca—4 mg/dL
  3. Protein complexed with phosphate, HCO_3^-, citrate—1 mg/dL.

34. RDA and functions of Iodine.

- RDA—150 –200 mg/day
- Iodine deficiency is common in India and iodized salt can prevent this.

Functions

- Only biological role of iodine helps in the formation of thyroxine and triiodothyronine
- About 80% of body iodine is stored in thyroglobulin as iodothyroglobulin in thyroid glands
- Radioactive iodine is useful in thyroid scanning I^{131}.

35. Why arachidonic acid is not considered 'purely' an essential fatty acid?

- Arachidonic acid (20C)-ω6—can be synthesized in the body, if the dietary supply of linolenic acid is sufficient. So it cannot be strictly categorized under essential fatty acid
- Arachidonic acid is semiessential because it can be produced form linoleic acid.

36. Urea cycle disorders cause orotic aciduria. Explain.

- In condition like hyperammoninemia type II (ornithine transcarbamylase deficiency) carbamoyl phosphate is not converted to citrulline and other metabolites of urea cycle. So carbamoyl phosphate gets accumulated
- Carbamoyl phosphate is also a precursor of pyrimidine synthesis. So it is channeled to pyrimidine synthesis
- Orotic acid is an intermediate in pyrimidine synthesis
- Orotic aciduria results from absence of either or both the enzymes—ORPTase, OMP decarboxylase of pyrimidine synthetic pathway.

37. Acidosis causes hyperkalemia. Why?

- In acidosis, to reduce serum H^+ levels, K^+ inside the cells gets exchanged for H^+ using H^+K^+ antiporter
- So extracellular K^+ increases leading to hyperkalemia
- The reverse occurs in metabolic alkalosis (hypokalemia) occurs.

38. Define frameshift mutation with an example.

- When a base is added or deleted in a nucleotide, the reading frameshifts to produce a 'garbled' protein
- For example, addition of A in this strand changes the reading frame and thereby the amino acid composition is also changed from the region of addition or deletion

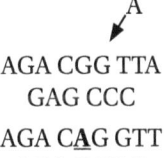

AGA CGG TTA
GAG CCC
AGA CAG GTT
AGA GCC C

- Frameshift mutation leads to premature chain termination of polypeptide to produce nonfunctional polypeptides as in thalassemia.

39. We need two primers for polymerase chain reaction. Justify.

- DNA polymerase is the enzyme needed for synthesis of new strand of DNA using the template single strand. It synthesizes the strand from 5' to 3' direction
- A primer is needed for DNA polymerase to start DNA synthesis (RNAP does not need a primer)

- A primer is a small strand of nucleotide which is complementary to the template strand
- Since two strands of DNA are complementary to each other we need a forward primer for one strand and reverse primer for other strand. So two primers are needed for polymerase chain reaction.

40. Mechanism of action of chlorophenicol.

- Chloramphenicol (chloromycetin) inhibits peptidyl transferase which is important in elongation of translation process of protein synthesis in bacteria. So it kills bacteria
- It does not inhibit human peptidyl transferase. So it can be given to humans as antibiotic in bacterial infections.

41. Mention the amino acids which take part in one-carbon pool.

- Glycine, serine, tryptophan and histidine
- Beta carbon of serine
- 1 carbon in ring of tryptophan
- Alpha carbon of glycine
- 1 carbon in ring of histidine via formiminoglutamate (Fig. 25).

42. Mention the enzymes which require selenium as cofactor.

- Glutathione peroxidase (antioxidant)
- 5'-deiodinase (thyroid metabolism).

43. Lesch-Nyhan syndrome presents with hyperuricemia. Explain.

- It is an X-linked inborn error of purine metabolism. Incidence 1: 10,000 due to complete deficiency of HGPRTase which is a purine salvage pathway enzyme
- So the salvage pathway is stopped and PRPP gets accumulated which will go for increased purine synthesis and catabolism of purines leads to the formation of more uric acid
- Hyperuricemia leads to nephrolithiasis and gout develops in later life

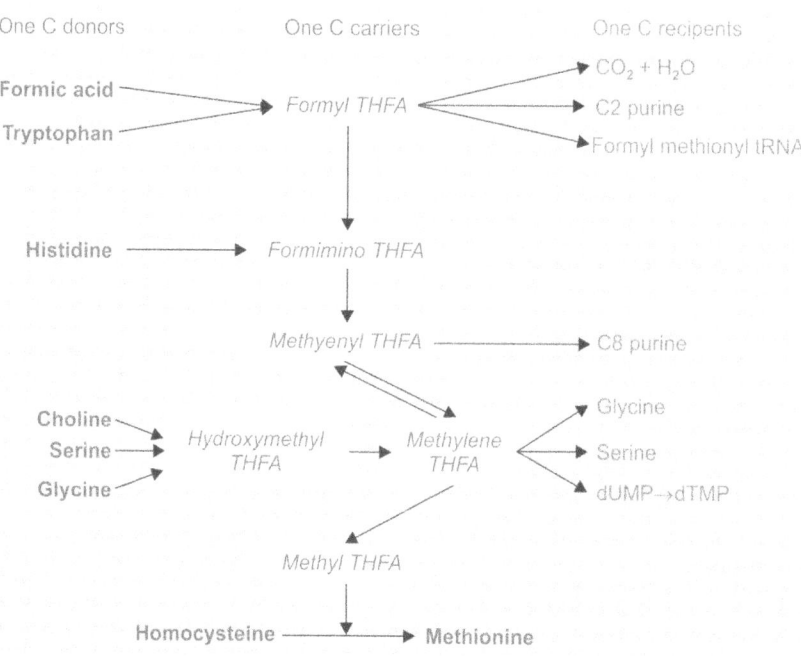

Fig. 25: Amino acids in one-carbon pool.

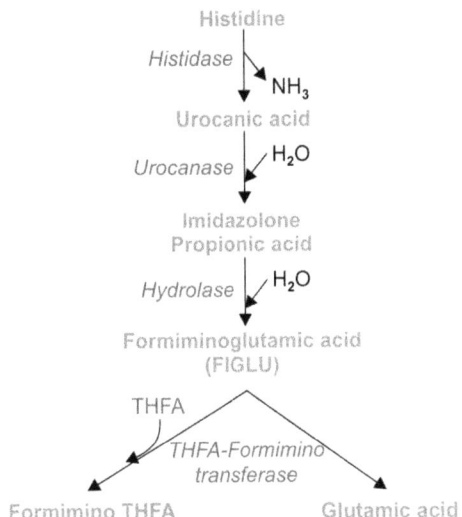

Fig. 26: Histidine metabolism.

- It is also characterized by self-mutilation and mental retardation.

44. Hypothyroidism presents with hypercholesterolemia. Why?

- Thyroid hormone increases catabolism of lipoproteins which are carriers of cholesterol
- So in hypothyroidism, lipoprotein catabolism is reduced leading to hypercholesterolemia.

45. Histidine load test (Fig. 26).

It is also known as formiminoglutamic acid (FIGLU) excretion test.
- Histidine is normally metabolized to formiminoglutamic acid, from which formimino group is removed by tetrahydrofolate. So in folate deficiency, FIGLU is excreted in urine. So this test is used for diagnosis of folate deficiency
- About 5 g of histidine is given orally 3 times at 4 hours intervals. 24-hours urine is collected and FIGLU assay—normal less than 30 mg of FIGLU excreted in per day urine. This level is increased in folic acid deficiency.

46. Mention two tumor markers and specify the diagnostic application.

- Tumor markers are the biological substances synthesized and released by cancer cells
- They are found in an increased level in blood and other body fluids and tissues
- Tumor markers are substances whose presence or elevation in body is used to identify or confirm the presence or to monitor the prognosis of the cancer
- Carbohydrate antigens, e.g. carcinoembryogenic antigen (CA125) ovarian and endometrial cancer
- Enzymes, e.g. prostate specific antigen—prostate cancer.

47. M band.

- In multiple myeloma, light chain immunoglobulins are produced more so there will be a prominence in gamma globulin region in electrophoresis
- It is of monoclonal origin of immunoglobulins. This is called as the myeloma band or monoclonal band (M band). It is diagnostic of multiple myeloma.

48. Beer-Lambert law.

Principle—colored solutions have the property of absorbing certain wavelengths of light and transmitting others. This property is based on Beer-Lambert law

Beer's law—when monochromatic light passes through a colored solution, the amount of light transmitted decreases exponentially with the increase in concentration of the colored substance. In other words the intensity of the color is directly proportionate to the concentration of the colored particle insolution

Lambert law—amount of light absorbed by a colored solution depends on the length of the column or depth of the liquid through which light passes.

Colorimeter is based on the above said principles.

49. Mention two transmethylation reactions.

Transmethylation reaction is acceptance of a methyl group from a donor like s-adenosyl methionine (SAM) by an acceptor resulting in the formation of a methylated compound.
- Transmethylation reaction requires SAM which is obtained by accepting adenosyl group from ATP by methionine by methionine adenosyltransferase.

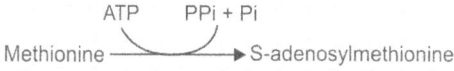

The examples for transmethylation reactions are:

Methyl acceptor	Methylated product
Guanidoacetic acid	Creatine
Serine	Choline

50. Enzyme deficiency in albinism. Mention two clinical features.

- It is an autosomal recessive disorder with incidence of 1 in 20,000
- It is due to deficiency of tyrosinase leading to melanin deficiency
- Ocular fundus—hypopigmented and color of iris may be red or gray. Patient will have nystagmus, photophobia and decreased visual acuity
- Skin is hypopigmented and sensitive to UV rays. Skin contains nevi and melanomas. Hair is also white.

MBBS Examination 2012

ANSWER ALL QUESTIONS

I. Essay questions (10/15 Marks each)

1. Describe the components and reactions of electron transport chain. Add a note on its inhibitors.
2. Describe the dietary sources, daily requirement, biochemical function and symptoms of vitamin C deficiency.
3. a. Describe the metabolism of tyrosine.
   b. Inborn errors associated with tyrosine metabolism.
4. a. Enumerate the liver function tests and how van den Bergh test distinguishes different types of jaundice.
   b. Importance of van den Bergh test in differentiating types of jaundice.
5. What are the components of mitochondrial electron transport chain? Describe the events and inhibitors of oxidative phosphorylation.
6. Explain the significance and reactions of hexose monophosphate shunt and disorders associated to it.
7. With the help of a figure, describe the process by which DNA replication takes place in a cell.
8. a. What are the functions of sodium in the body?
   b. What is the reference range for levels of serum sodium?
   c. Describe the working of the renin-angiotensin-aldosterone system to maintain optimal amounts of sodium in the body.
   d. Briefly discuss disorders associated with derangements in sodium homeostasis.

II. Short notes (5 Marks each)

1. Balanced diet.
2. Causes of hypoglycemia.
3. Allosteric inhibition.
4. Obesity.
5. Alkaptonuria.
6. Functions of mitochondria.
7. Glycosylated hemoglobin (HbA1C).
8. Neoglucogenesis (gluconeogenesis).
9. Thalassemias.
10. Purine salvage pathway.
11. Post-translational modifications.
12. Electrophoresis.
13. Repair mechanism of DNA.
14. Salvage pathway of purine synthesis.
15. Functions of glucocorticoids.
16. Functions of albumin.
17. Precipitation reactions of proteins.
18. Renal tubular function tests.
19. Role of kidney in regulating the pH of blood.
20. Immunoglobulins.
21. Isoenzymes of lactate dehydrogenase and their significance.
22. Functions, deficiency symptoms of vitamin thiamine.
23. Calcium homeostasis and its disorder. Disorders of calcium homeostasis.
24. Metabolic adaptation in Fed state.
25. What are the various mucopolysaccharides? Add a note on hyaluronic acid.
26. Lineweaver-Burk plot and its significance.
27. Enzymes, coenzymes, inhibitors of pyruvate dehydrogenase reaction.
28. Alcohol metabolism.

29. Fredrickson classification of hyperlipoproteinemias.
30. Mention the types of heteropolysaccharides and their functions.
31. Secondary structure of proteins/alpha helix.
32. Structure of an immunoglobulin with the help of a figure.
33. Causes and manifestations of gout.
34. Transamination reactions.
35. Role of lungs in maintenance of pH of blood.
36. Conjugation reactions involved in metabolism of xenobiotics.
37. Principle and applications of electrophoresis.
39. Tumor markers.
40. Salvage pathway for purines and its importance in the body.
38. Functions of tyrosine in the body.

III. Short answer questions
(2/3/4 Marks each)

1. Markers of nucleus and mitochondria.
2. Name 2 tumor markers.
3. Functions of phospholipids.
4. Name the essential fatty acids.
5. Active forms of thiamine and riboflavin.
6. Name the ketone bodies.
7. Significance of Rapaport–Leubering cycle.
8. Name two glycogen storage diseases.
9. Significance of HMP shunt.
10. Name the derivatives of cholesterol.
11. Name the urea cycle disorders.
12. Causes of increased blood urea level.
13. Name the derivatives of tryptophan.
14. Fluorosis.
15. Parameter for the assessment of nutritive value of proteins.
16. Restriction endonucleases.
17. Mutagens.
18. Lesch-Nyhan syndrome.
19. Denaturation of proteins.
20. Differences between DNA and RNA.
21. What are the enzymes required for DNA replication?
22. What is the principle of affinity chromatography?
23. What are the causes of respiratory acidosis?
24. Maple syrup urine disease.
25. Urea clearance.
26. Bence Jones protein.
27. What are oncogenes?
28. Beer–Lambert law.
29. What are the forces that stabilize secondary structure of proteins?
30. Name the basic amino acids.
31. Cardiolipin.
32. Mention the types of fatty acid oxidation.
33. What are the products of arachidonic acid?
34. Carnitine.
35. Anomerism.
36. How hemoglobin binds to oxygen?
37. K_m value and its significance.
38. Bronze diabetes.
39. WHO criteria for diagnosis of diabetes mellitus.
40. Zellweger's syndrome.
41. Outline the distribution of water in the various compartments of the body.
42. What is the mechanism of action of steroid hormones?
43. List four features of the genetic code.
44. Explain the clinical relevance of serum creatinine levels.
45. What is meant by the polymerase chain reaction? List two of its applications.
46. What are the reference levels of glucose and protein in cerebrospinal fluid? How are they affected in bacterial meningitis?
47. What is meant by quaternary structure of a protein? Name a protein, abundantly found in blood that has a quaternary structure.
48. Name the bases found in nucleic acids.
49. List four causes of respiratory acidosis.
50. What are the functions of glutathione?

I. ESSAY QUESTIONS

1. **Describe the components and reactions of electron transport chain. Add a note on its inhibitors.**
Refer 2007 Essay Question 7.

2. **Describe the dietary sources, daily requirement, biochemical function and symptoms of vitamin C deficiency.**
Refer 2005 Essay Question 5.

3. a. **Describe the metabolism of tyrosine.**
Refer 2015 Essay Question 6.
Synthesis of tyrosine—tyrosine is an aromatic amino acid. It is hydroxylated phenylalanine.

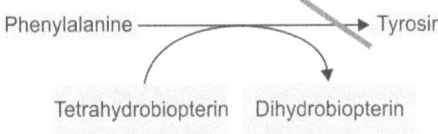

Conversion of Phenylalanine to Tyrosine by hydroxylation

Phenylalanine hydroxylase enzyme hydroxylates phenylalanine to tyrosine in the presence of the cofactor tetrahydrobiopterin, and coenzymes—NADPH and NADH. It is an irreversible reaction. Further tyrosine is catabolized by various steps to form fumarate (glucogenic pathway) and acetoacetate (ketogenic pathway).

- Tyrosine is an aromatic amino acid. It is synthesized from phenylalanine. It is both glucogenic and ketogenic.

Catabolism of Tyrosine (Fig. 1)

- **Transamination**—tyrosine is transaminated by tyrosine transaminase using PLP and alpha-ketoglutarate to form p-hydroxyphenylpyruvate and glutamic acid. This step is induced by glucocorticoids
- **Synthesis of homogentisic acid (dihydroxyphenyl acetate)**—p-hydroxyphenylpyruvate is converted to homogentisate by hydroxylase enzyme. It is a copper containing enzyme. Ascorbic acid is required for this reaction
- **Formation of maleylacetoacetate**—by the cleavage of aromatic ring homogentisate is converted to maleyl-acetoacetate by a dioxygenase called homogentisate oxidase which contains an iron atom at its active site
- **Isomerisation of maleyl to fumarylacetoacetate**—maleylacetoacetate is converted to its isomer fumarylacetoacetate by isomerase using glutathione (GSH) as its cofactor
- **Hydrolysis of fumarylacetoacetate**—fumarylacetoacetate is cleaved into fumarate (glucogenic) and acetoacetate (ketogenic) by a hydrolase enzyme.

Other products formed from Tyrosine

- Melanin pigments
- Catecholamines
- Thyroxine
- Tyramine

Synthesis of Melanin (Fig. 2)

- Tyrosine is hydroxylated by tyrosinase to dihydroxyphenylalanine (DOPA). It is a mono-oxygenase containing copper
- Tyrosinase acts again on DOPA to form DOPA quinone
- Decarboxylation and oxidation of DOPA quinone converts it to indolequinone, which is polymerized to melanin.

Catecholamines (Fig. 3)

- Tyrosine is first hydroxylated to DOPA by tyrosine hydroxylase. It requires tetrahydrobiopterin and NADPH
- DOPA is decarboxylated to form dopamine by DOPA decarboxylase, a PLP dependent enzyme. Dopamine is a catecholamine which is a neurotransmitter. In Parkinsonism dopamine level is reduced. L-DOPA is used as a drug in Parkinsonism
- Dopamine is hydroxylated to norepinephrine by dopamine hydroxylase
- Norepinephrine is methylated to epinephrine by methyl transferase which needs SAM which is a methyl donor.

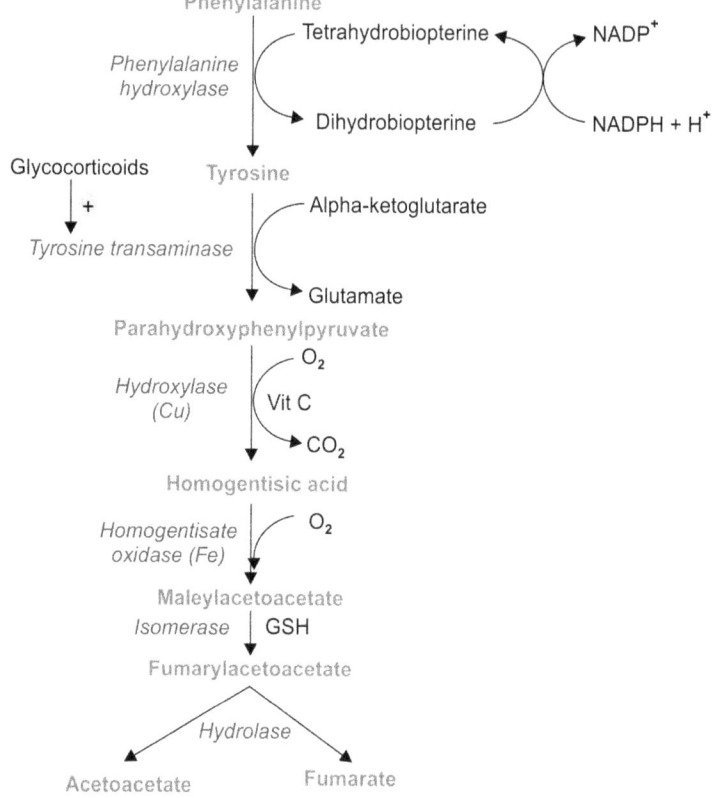

Fig. 1: Catabolism of tyrosine.

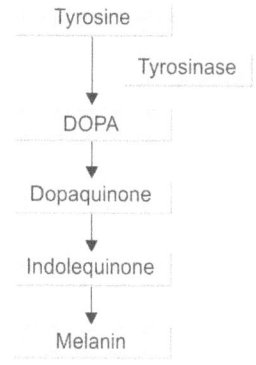

Fig. 2: Formation of melanin.

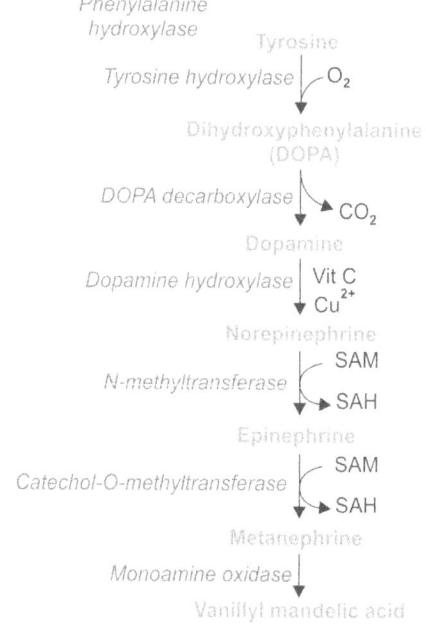

Fig. 3: Catechloamine.

- Epinephrine is methylated to metanephrine and oxidized to vanillyl mandelic acid (VMA) and excreted in urine
- Normal level of excretion of VMA is 2-6 mg/day urine. This is elevated in pheochromocytoma and in neuroblastoma.

Thyroid Hormones

Specific tyrosine molecules are iodinated to form mono- and Di-triiodothyronine and thyroxine (T4).

Tyramine

- Tyrosine is decarboxylated to tyramine by intestinal bacteria which is one of the reasons for food allergy.

b. Inborn errors associated with tyrosine metabolism.

Refer 2016 Short Note 7 for elaborate answer.

Phenylketonuria (PKU)

It is an autosomal recessive disease with an incidence of 1:10,000 births. It is due to deficiency of phenylalanine hydroxylase.

Alkaptonuria

- It is an autosomal recessive condition affecting 1:250,000 births
- It is due to the defect in homogentisate oxidase enzyme
- Urine turns black on standing. FeCl3 test is positive. Benedict's test is strongly positive since homogentisate is a reducing agent. Generally it is a harmless condition.

Albinism

- It is an autosomal recessive disorder with incidence of 1 in 20,000
- It is due to deficiency of tyrosinase leading to melanin deficiency.

Hypertyrosinemias

a. Tyrosinemia type I (hepatorenal tyrosinemia):
   - It is an autosomal recessive condition affecting 1.5/1,000 births
   - It is due to fumarylacetoacetate hydrolase deficiency.
b. Tyrosinemia type II (oculocutaneous tyrosinemia—Richner Hanhart syndrome):
   - It is due to deficiency of tyrosine transaminase.
c. Tyrosinemia type III (neonatal tyrosinemia):
   - Due to absence of para-hydroxyphenyl-pyruvate hydroxylase.
d. Hawkinsinuria:
   - Autosomal dominant type
   - Due to deficiency of parahydroxyphenylpyruvate oxidase.

4. a. Enumerate the liver function tests and how van den Bergh test distinguishes different types of jaundice.

The tests used to diagnose liver disease are called liver function tests. They are:

Tests based on hepatic excretory function:
a. Serum bilirubin—total, conjugated and unconjugated
b. Urine bilirubin—bile pigments bile salts, urobilinogen
c. Fecal urobilinogen
d. Dye excretion test—bromosulphophthalein (BSP) test.

Markers of liver injury—estimation of liver enzymes:
a. Serum alanine aminotransferase (ALT)
b. Serum aspartate aminotransferase (AST)
c. Serum alkaline phosphatase (ALP)
d. Serum gamma glutamyltransferase (GGT).

Tests based on synthetic function (synthesis of plasma proteins)—estimation of:
a. Total plasma proteins
b. Serum albumin, globulin, A/G ratio
c. Prothrombin time.

Special tests—estimation of:
a. Ceruloplasmin
b. Ferritin
c. Alpha-1 antitrypsin (AAT)
d. Alpha-fetoprotein (AFP).

Tests based on detoxification function—estimation of:
a. Blood ammonia and bilirubin
b. Hippuric acid.

b. Importance of van den Bergh test in differentiating types of jaundice.

- The serum bilirubin estimation is based on van den Bergh reaction where diazotised sulfanilic acid reacts with bilirubin to form a purple colored complex, azobilirubin. Normal serum does not give a positive van den Bergh test
- When bilirubin is conjugated, the purple color is produced immediately on mixing with the reagent, the response is said to be van den Bergh direct positive

- When the bilirubin is unconjugated, the color appears only after addition of alcohol, so it is said to be van den Bergh indirect positive
- When both conjugated and unconjugated bilirubin are present, they produce an immediate color which intensifies on adding alcohol. It is then said to be biphasic
- In hemolytic jaundice, unconjugated bilirubin elevated so indirect positive
- In obstructive jaundice, conjugated bilirubin elevated so direct positive
- In hepatic jaundice, both conjugated and unconjugated.

5. **What are the components of mitochondrial electron transport chain. Describe the events and inhibitors of oxidative phosphorylation.**

Refer 2007 Essay Question 7.

6. **Explain the significance and reactions of hexose monophosphate shunt and disorders associated to it.**

Refer 2007 Short Note 5.

7. **With the help of a figure, describe the process by which DNA replication takes place in a cell.**

Refer 2007 Essay Question 9.

8. a. **What are the functions of sodium in the body?**

- Maintains osmotic pressure
- Maintains water balance
- Constituent of buffer and maintains acid–base balance
- Maintains muscle and nerve irritability
- Needed for maintaining muscle irritability and permeability of cell membrane.

b. **What is the reference range for levels of serum sodium?**

Normal serum Na levels—135-145 mmol/L.

c. **Describe the working of the renin-angiotensin-aldosterone system to maintain optimal amounts of sodium in the body.**

- **Renin-angiotensin system**—when there is fall in ECF volume, the renal blood flow decreases and this is sensed by the juxta- glomerular apparatus leading to secretion of renin. Renin stimulates production of angiotensin which gets converted to angiotensin II. Angiotensin II stimulates production of aldosterone (Fig. 4)
- **Aldosterone**—it acts on DCT and causes increased reabsorption of sodium and water.

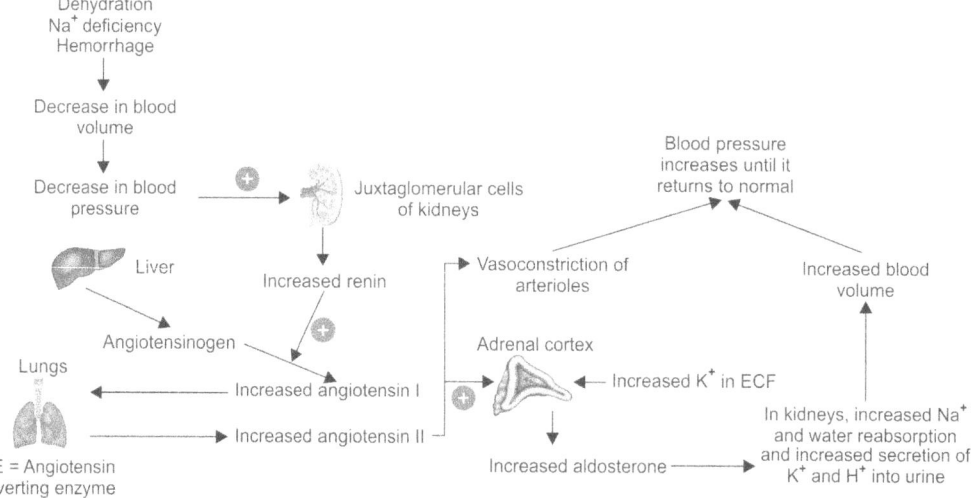

Fig. 4: Renin-angiotensin-aldosterone system.

d. **Briefly discuss disorders associated with derangements in sodium homeostasis.**

- **Hyponatremia**—decreased sodium level in blood is called hyponatremia.
  - **Causes**—vomiting, diarrhea, burns, Addison's disease, renal tubular acidosis, chronic renal failure, congestive cardiac failure, hyperglycemia, SIADH
  - **Drugs**—ACE inhibitors, lithium, NSAIDs, vasopressin and oxytocin. Pseudo-or dilutional hyponatremia-hyperproteinemia (myeloma) and mannitol
  - **Signs and symptoms**—dehydration, abdominal cramps, oliguria, tremors, and coma. May be asymptomatic
  - **Treatment**—administration of sodium under monitoring.
- **Hypernatremia**—increased sodium in blood is known as hypernatremia.
  - **Causes**—cushing's disease, prolonged cortisone therapy, pregnancy, dehydration, exchange transfusion with stored blood, primary hyperaldosteronism
  - **Drugs**—ampicillin, tetracycline, anabolic steroids, oral contraceptives, loop diuretics and osmotic diuretics
  - **Symptoms**—dry mucous membrane, fever, thirst, restlessness.

II. SHORT NOTES

1. Balanced diet.

Refer 2007 Short Note 14.

2. Causes of hypoglycemia.

Normal blood glucose level in fasting 70-110 mg/dL.

A fall in plasma glucose **less than 50 mg/dL is life-threatening.**

Causes

- **Drugs: Overdose of insulin**—this is the most common cause
- **Postprandial hypoglycemia**—2-3 hours after a meal, transient hypoglycemia is seen in some persons. This is due to over-secretion of insulin
- **Insulinoma**—insulin secreting tumor
- **Von Gierke's disease**—deficiency of glucose 6-phosphatase. Therefore, glucose-6-phosphate cannot be converted to glucose. Hypoglycemia occurs
- **Prolonged starvation**—excessive usage of diabetic drugs.

3. Allosteric inhibition.

Refer 2014 Short Note 46.
- Enzymes which have one catalytic site where the substrate binds and another separate site where the modifier binds are known as allosteric site [Greek: Allo = Other]
- Both the sites may or may not be nearer to each other
- If the binding of the regulatory molecule increases the activity of the enzyme, it is known as **allosteric activation,** and the regulatory molecule is known as positive modulator
- If the binding of regulatory molecule inhibits the activity of the enzyme it is known as **allosteric inhibition** and the regulatory molecule it is known as negative modulator
- Allosteric activation effect is said to be positive cooperativity and the allosteric inhibition effect is called negative cooperativity
- Combination of both is seen in most cases resulting in sigmoid curve
- Allosteric regulators are divided into two classes based on the influence of allosteric effector on k_m and V_{max}:
  a. K-class of allosteric enzymes—effector changes k_m but not V_{max}, e.g. phosphofructokinase
  b. V-class of allosteric enzymes—effector alters the V_{max}, but not K_m, e.g. acetyl-CoA carboxylase.

4. Obesity.

Refer 2017 Short Note 11.
- It is the most prevalent nutritional disorder. It is otherwise known as **overnutrition**
- It is a state in which excess fat has accumulated. There is an increase in number and size of adipocytes

- This is due to increased energy intake and decreased energy expenditure.

Obesity index or BMI Calculation

- BMI= W/H^2. [W= weight in kg; H = height in meters)^2
- It is used to assess obesity.

Major Causes

- Food habits—intake of calorie rich food in excess amounts
- Lack of exercise
- Genetic causes—due to mutation of leptin hormone secreted by adipocytes
- Effects of neuropeptide Y, ghrelin and nonesterified fatty acids can cause obesity.

Diseases Related to Obesity

- Effects on insulin:
  - Sensitivity of peripheral tissues to insulin is decreased
  - No. of insulin receptors are decreased in adipocytes
  - Plasma insulin level is elevated.
- Cardiovascular risk
- Diabetes mellitus
- Hypertension
- Metabolic syndrome
- Reduced life span.

Treatment

- Reduced intake of calories and fat
- Diet rich in vegetables
- Small frequent meals with lots of vegetables
- Controlled exercise.

5. Alkaptonuria.

Refer 2004 Short Note 11.

6. Functions of mitochondria.

Refer 2013 Short Answer Question 43.

7. Glycosylated hemoglobin (HbA1C).

Refer 2007 Short Note 15.

The best index of long-term control of blood glucose level is measurement of glycated-hemoglobin or glycosylated Hb (HbA1c).

When there is excess glucose in blood, it goes and binds with proteins especially Hb. When once attached, glucose is not removed from Hb. Therefore, it remains inside the RBC throughout the life span of RBC (120 days).

Interpretation

- It is used for monitoring the response to treatment
- Normal level—4-7%
- Diabetes—8-15%
- HbA1c level reveals the mean glucose level over previous 10-12 weeks
- It is not affected by recent food intake or recent changes in sugar level
- Elevated HbA1c indicates poor control of diabetes
- The risk of retinopathy and nephropathy are directly proportional to elevated HbA1c level.

8. Neoglucogenesis (gluconeogenesis).

Refer 2008 Essay Question 6.

9. Thalassemias.

Definition: Normal globin chains in Hb with abnormal proportions

Types: α-thalassemia, β-thalassemia and thalassemia syndromes.

α-thalassemia—rare

- Due to deletion of different types of genes. As there are 2 pairs of *alpha* genes per cell, the deletion of one gene in one chromosome and a pair of genes in the chromosome do not have much effect on chain production
- α globin chain synthesis is reduced or absent
- Excess of β chain and δ chain formation.

β-thalassemia—more common

- Due to deletion of genes. β globin chain synthesis is reduced or absent
- Two types:
  1. Beta (0)—due to base substitutions
  2. Beta (+)—due to defect in post-transcriptional modifications.

Thalassemia syndrome—seen in Asians, Africans and people from Mediterranean origin.

- Deficiency of HbA
- There will be hypochromic microcytic anemia
- Two types:
  i. Thalassemia major—homozygous; severe clinical manifestations. Nucleated RBCs seen in peripheral smears
  ii. Thalassemia minor—heterozygous; minimal clinical manifestations.
- Synthesis of unaffected chains occurs at normal rate. They get precipitated as they do not get complementary chains to bind. These precipitates or inclusion bodies damage the RBC membranes
- Homozygous beta thalassemia is characterized by anemia, hypersplenism and hepatosplenomegaly.

Treatment: Repeated blood transfusion, splenectomy, bone marrow transplant.

10. Purine salvage pathway.

Refer 2004 Short Note 15.

11. Post-translational modifications.

Refer 2006 Short Note 27.

12. Electrophoresis.

Refer 2006 Short Note 30.

13. Repair mechanism of DNA.

Refer 2003 Short Note 11.

14. Salvage pathway of purine synthesis.

Refer 2004 Short Note 15.

15. Functions of glucocorticoids.

Glucocorticoids are synthesized from the middle zone of adrenal cortex. Their functions are:

- **Carbohydrate metabolism**
  - Gluconeogenetic enzymes are stimulated
  - Glycolytic enzymes are suppressed
  - Decreased glucose uptake and all these leading to hyperglycemia.
- **Lipids metabolism**
  - Increased lipolysis leading to mobilization of fats and depositing in unusual sites
  - Increase in FFA by facilitating lipolytic hormones.
- **Proteins and nucleic acids**
  - Catabolism of both increased
  - Increased urea production
  - Amino acids go for gluconeogenesis.
- **Water and electrolytes**
  - Water excretion is promoted
  - Increased GFR and inhibition of ADH.
- **Bone**
  - Decreases serum calcium level by inhibiting osteoblasts function causing osteoporosis.
- **Immune system**
  - Suppresses immune system; lysis of lymphocytes. Anti-inflammatory and antiallergic.
- **Others**
  - Stimulates gastric acid secretion and induces acid peptic diseases.

16. Functions of albumin.

Refer 2009 Short Note 40.

17. Precipitation reactions of proteins.

Precipitation of proteins is needed to isolate proteins from the native solution. Precipitation is the loss of charge or loss of water of hydration from the proteins. It differs from denaturation. Many agents can precipitate the proteins.

- **Salting out**—when the protein solution is saturated with neutral salt like ammonium sulfate or sodium sulfate the shell of hydration is removed and protein precipitates. Albumin is precipitated by full saturation and globulins by half saturation with ammonium sulfate
- **Isoelectric precipitation**—isoelectric point or isoelectric pH is the pH of a protein at which level it carries equal number of positive and negative charges and the net charge is zero. At this pH, the protein does not move either to the anode or cathode in an electric field. Isoelectric point varies from protein to protein. Isoelectric pH of albumin is 4.88 and that of casein is 4.60
- **Organic solvents**—like ethanol removes hydration and precipitates the protein, e.g. ethanol is a disinfectant since it

precipitates bacterial and viral proteins when swabbed over the skin
- **Heavy metals** (positive charged), e.g. lead acetate, mercuric chloride, mercuric nitrate: In alkaline medium proteins have net negative charge (anions). When the positively charged heavy metals are added to this, the proteins get precipitated, e.g. using raw egg as an antidote for mercury poisoning
- **By negatively charged alkaloidal reagents**—for example, picric acid, trichloroacetic acid, phosphotungstic acid, sulphosalicylic acid, tannic acid. When proteins carry net positive charge these alkaloids will lower the pH and form thick flocculent precipitate, e.g. tanning

18. Renal tubular function tests.

Refer 2014 Short Answer Question 34.
- **Renal** tubules reabsorb or secrete certain substances, concentrate the urine and acidify the urine. So it is important for maintaining the specific gravity and osmolality of urine
- **The following are the tubular function tests:**
  - **Specific gravity (SG) of urine**—it is the simplest test. Specific gravity of urine depends on the concentration of the solutes. In early stages of renal failure SG may be low due to kidney's inability to excrete solutes
  - **Concentration test (fluid deprivation test):**
    - Fluid intake is restricted for 15 hours. The first urine sample in the morning is collected, SG and osmolality are measured
    - If the SG is more than 1.025 or the osmolality exceeds 850 mOsmol/kg the renal concentration capacity is said to be normal
    - Renal concentration ability is impaired due to tubular defect or in diabetes insipidus where there is decreased secretion of antidiuretic hormone.
- **Measurement of osmolality**—measurement of urine and plasma osmolality is done by using osmometer. **Normal urinary osmolality ranges from 60–1,200 mOsmol/kg. Normal plasma osmolality is 285–300 mOsm/kg.** The ratio between urine/plasma osmolality is calculated. Normal ratio is around 3-4.5. Urinary osmolality is decreased in diabetes insipidus
- **Dilution tests**—this is done to check whether kidneys can excrete an excess water load. After emptying the bladder 1,000 to 1,200 mL of water is given to the patient. Hourly urine is collected for next 4 hours. In each sample, volume specific gravity and osmolality are measured. A normal person will excrete all the water load within 4 hours. It is a more sensitive test
- **Urinary acidification test** (acid load test or ammonium chloride loading test).
  - This is used to diagnose renal tubular acidosis
  - Ammonium chloride is given orally in gelatin capsule (100 mg/kg body weight) to induce metabolic acidosis. HCl produced is excreted as acidified urine
  - Hourly urine collected for 2 to 8 hours, pH and acid excretion of each sample is noted
  - At least one sample should have pH lesser than 5.5. pH is not decreased in cases of renal tubular acidosis.
- **Fractional excretion of bicarbonate, sodium and phosphate in urine**—also help in assessing renal tubular functions.

19. Role of kidney in regulating the pH of blood.

Refer 2005 Essay Question 4.

20. Immunoglobulins.

Refer 2008 Short Note 11.

21. Isoenzymes of lactate dehydrogenase and their significance.

- Multiple molecular forms of an enzyme catalyzing the same reaction are isoenzymes

or isozymes, e.g. lactate dehydrogenase—5 isoenzymes (LDH 1, 2, 3, 4 and 5)
- They are synthesized from various tissues and hence useful to study the disorders of those organs
- Separation and identification of LDH isoenzyme by electrophoresis—depends upon the mobility in electrical field.

Isoenzymes of Lactate Dehydrogenase
- There are 5 isoenzymes. They are LDH1, LDH2, LDH3, LDH4, and LDH5
- LDH is a tetramer with 4 subunits. LDH1 (heart-H4), LDH2 (RBC-H3M1), LDH3 (brain-H2M2), LDH4 (lung, liver-H1M3), and LDH5 (liver, skeletal muscle-M4)
- Isoenzymes of LDH help in the diagnosis of heart and liver diseases
- Normally LDH2 level is higher in blood than LDH1. But this is reversed in myocardial infarction called as flipped pattern (LDH1 > LDH2)
- Increased activity of LDH5 is an indicator of liver diseases.

22. Functions, symptoms of vitamin thiamine deficiency.

Refer 2003 Essay Question 1.

23. Calcium homeostasis and its disorder. Disorders of calcium homeostasis.

Refer 2004 Essay Question 4 and 2007 Essay Question 6.

24. Metabolic adaptation in fed state.
- Fed state is 2-4 hours after ingestion of a normal meal
- During this period, there will be transient increase in plasma glucose, amino acids and triacylglycerol synthesized by intestinal mucosa
- There will be increased secretion of insulin and a drop in glucagon which leads to the increased synthesis of proteins
- There will be alterations in metabolism of liver, adipose tissues, muscle and brain
- Many metabolic fuels are interconvertible. Conversion of carbohydrates into fats and fats into carbohydrates, conversion of carbohydrates into proteins and proteins into carbohydrates, conversion of proteins into fats and fats into proteins can happen
- For example, glucose is metabolized into acetyl-CoA by glycolysis via pyruvate. Acetyl-CoA is the starting point for fatty acid synthesis, ketone bodies and cholesterol synthesis
- Glucose in excess can be stored as glycogen which can be broken down to glucose in fasting states
- Metabolic pathways are controlled by 4 mechanisms:
  1. Availability of substrates
  2. Allosteric regulations of enzymes, e.g. phosphofructokinase
  3. Covalent modifications of enzymes, e.g. glycogen phosphorylase
  4. Induction and repression of enzyme synthesis, e.g. HMG-CoA reductase.

Changes that Occur in Major Organs
- **Liver (center for distributing nutrient distribution)**—during fed state liver takes up carbohydrates, lipids and amino acids.
  a. Carbohydrates—maintenance of blood glucose level by:
    - Increased phosphorylation of glucose
    - Increased glycogen synthesis
    - Increased activity of HMP pathway
    - Increased glycolysis
    - Decreased gluconeogenesis.
  b. Lipids—increased fatty acid synthesis, ketogenesis, TAG and VLDL synthesis
  c. Amino acids—increased degradation of amino acids and synthesis of proteins.
- **Adipose tissues—storage of energy**
  a. Carbohydrates—increased glucose transport, increased glycolysis, increased activity of HMP pathway
  b. Lipids—increased fatty acid synthesis and increased TAG synthesis and degradation.
- **Skeletal muscle—resting**
  a. Carbohydrates
    - Increased glucose transport
    - Increased glycogen synthesis.

b. Lipids—fatty acids are released from chylomicrons and VLDL. They do not have primary importance in the source of energy
c. Amino acids—increased synthesis of proteins, increased uptake of branched chain amino acids.

- **Brain**
  a. Carbohydrates—complete oxidation of glucose to CO_2 and water. Glucose is the major fuel. No storage of glycogen
  b. Lipids—no storage of TAG. Energy is obtained from oxidation of fatty acids from blood.

25. What are the various mucopolysaccharides? Add a note on hyaluronic acid.

Refer Short Notes 30.

26. Lineweaver-Burk plot and its significance.

It is also called as double reciprocal plot. Sometimes the determination of enzyme activity needs very high substrate concentration which is impractical. A linear form of the Michaelis-Menten equation circumvents this difficulty and permits V_{max} and K_m to be extrapolated from initial velocity data obtained at lower concentrations of substrate.

$$V_i = \frac{V_{max}[S]}{K_m + [S]}$$

Invert,

$$\frac{1}{V_i} = \frac{K_m + [S]}{V_{max}[S]}$$

Factor

$$\frac{1}{V_i} = \frac{K_m}{V_{max}[S]} + \frac{[S]}{V_{max}[S]}$$

And simplify:

$$\frac{1}{V_i} = \left[\frac{K_m}{V_{max}}\right]\frac{1}{[S]} + \frac{1}{V_{max}}$$

This equation is got by taking the reciprocal of the Michaelis–Menten equation.

When $1/v_i$ is plotted against $1/[S]$ a straight line is obtained with the slope equal to K_m/V_{max}.

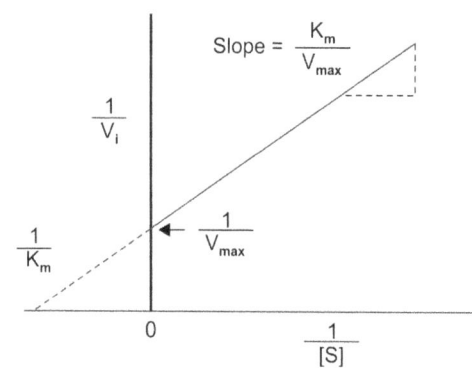

Fig. 5: Lineweaver-burk plot.

Such a plot is called a **double reciprocal** or **Lineweaver-Burk plot (Fig. 5)**.

Significance

- Double reciprocal or Lineweaver-Burk plot of $1/v_i$ versus $1/[S]$ is used to evaluate K_m and V_{max} values
- It can be used to determine the kinetic mechanisms of enzyme inhibitors.

27. Enzymes, coenzymes, inhibitors of pyruvate dehydrogenase reaction.

- Pyruvate which is the product of aerobic glycolysis in cytosol enters into the mitochondria
- Pyruvate is oxidatively decarboxylated to acetyl-CoA by the enzyme pyruvate dehydrogenase
- 5 coenzymes of this enzyme are—TPP (vitamin B1), coenzyme A, FAD (vitamin B2-riboflavin), NAD (niacin) and lipoamide (lipoic acid)
- This multienzyme complex is formed by 3 enzymes component namely:
  - Enzyme 1 (pyruvate dehydrogenase)—catalyzes oxidative decarboxylation for which TPP is the coenzyme-ethyl TPP is formed
  - Enzyme 2 (dihydrolipoyl transacetylase)—this oxidizes hydoxyethyl group to form acetyl lipoamide which joins with coenzyme A to form acetyl-CoA and reduced lipoamide is formed
  - Enzyme 3 (dihydrolipoyl dehydrogenase—catalyzes oxidation of lipoamide

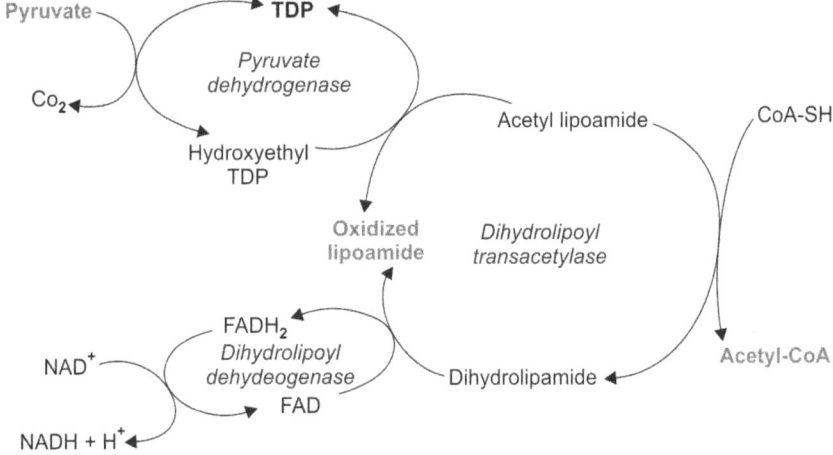

Fig. 6: Pyruvate dehydrogenase reaction.

to generate TPP, lipoamide. FAD and NAD help in this reaction.
- This is an irreversible process
- This enzyme is inhibited by the end product acetyl-CoA **(Fig. 6)**.

28. Alcohol metabolism.

- In stomach, alcohol is absorbed in small amount and in small intestines it is absorbed in larger amount
- Small amount is excreted through lungs
- Metabolism occurs in liver where ethanol is oxidized by the NAD-dependent cytoplasmic enzyme alcohol dehydrogenase to produce acetaldehyde

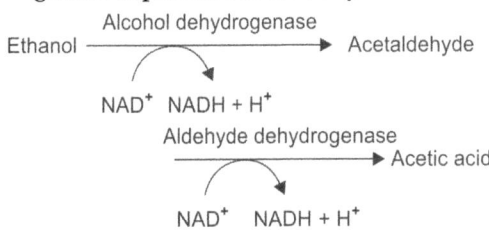

- Acetaldehyde is further oxidized to acetic acid by a mitochondrial NAD-dependent enzyme aldehyde dehydrogenase
- Acetic acid is then converted to acetyl-CoA
- Aldehyde is toxic and in excess it causes cell death
- Cytochrome P450 dependent—microsomal ethanol oxidising system (MEOS) detoxify alcohol
- Metabolic adaptations of alcoholism—lactic acidosis, hypoglycemia, ketogenesis, fatty liver, damage to mitochondria and apoptosis. Alcohol also causes CNS depression
- In pregnancy it leads to fetal alcohol syndrome.

29. Fredrickson classification of hyperlipoproteinemias.

Refer 2011 Short Notes 22.

30. Mention the types of heteropolysaccharides and their functions.

- Glycosaminoglycans (GAGs) or mucopolysaccharides are heteropolysaccharides containing the repeating units of disaccharides which is made up of uronic acid and amino sugars
- They are the essential components of connective tissue structure.

Structure of GAGs

- They are made up of repeating units of disaccharides which is made up of uronic acid and amino sugars
- This polymer is attached covalently to extracellular core proteins to form proteoglycans except hyaluronic acid. It looks like a bottle brush

- Proteoglycans join with one molecule of hyaluronic acid to form aggregates which is stabilized by link proteins
- Uronic acid present in GAGs are either glucuronic acid or its epimer iduronic acid. Keratan sulfate does not contain uronic acid
- The amino sugars are glucosamine or galactosamine
- Except hyaluronic acid all GAGs contain sulfates donated by the active sulfate—PAPS
- They are usually unbranched.

Common Glycosaminoglycans

- Hyaluronic acid
- Chondroitin sulfate
- Dermatan sulfate
- Heparin
- Heparan sulfate
- Keratan sulfate.

Hyaluronic Acid (Fig. 7)

- Anionic, nonsulfated glycosaminoglycan
- **Site of occurrence**—present in loose connective tissues, tendons, synovial fluid of joints, vitreous humor of eye
- **Repeating units**—composed of D-glucuronic acid and N-acetylglucosamine linked by β-1,4 and β-1,3 glycosidic bonds
- **Functions**—acts as lubricant and shock absorber. It helps in migration of cells, reproduction embryogenesis and in wound healing.

Chondroitin Sulfate (Fig. 8)

- **Site of occurrence**—it is present in ground substance of connective tissues present in cartilage, bone, tendons, cornea and skin
- **Repeating units**—it is made up of repeating units of glucuronic acid and N-acetylgalactosamine to which sulfate group is attached
- **Functions**—it provides an endoskeletal structure to maintain the structure and shape of the tissues like cartilage
- **Therapeutic uses**—it is used to treat osteoarthritis as anti-inflammatory agent, stimulating the synthesis of proteoglycans

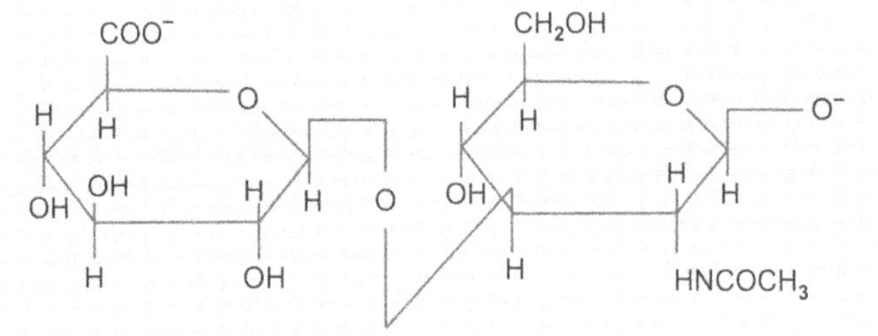

Fig. 7: Hyaluronic acid.

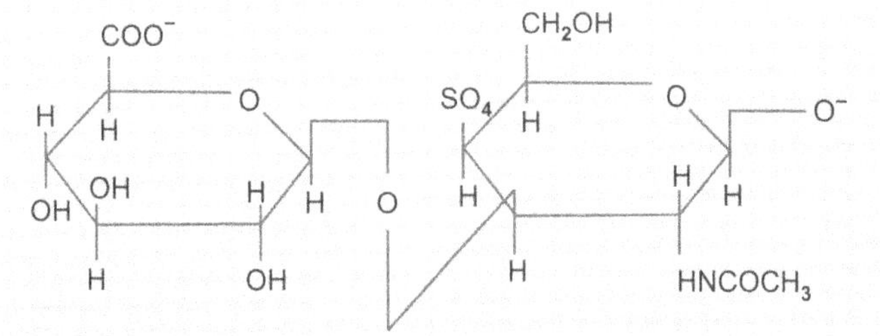

Fig. 8: Chondroitin sulfate.

Dermatan Sulfate

- **Site of occurrence**—it is present in connective tissues present in skin, blood vessels and heart valves
- **Repeating units**—it is made up of repeating units of L-iduronic acid and N-acetylgalactosamine to which sulfate group is attached
- **Functions**—it provides transparency to the cornea and maintains the shape of eye.

Heparin (Fig. 9)

Produced mainly by mast cells of liver.
- **Site of occurrence**—intracellular component of mast cells which line the arteries of liver, lung and skin
- **Repeating units**—highly sulfated glycosaminoglycan made up of glucosamine and glucuronic or iduronic acid
- **Functions**—it acts as an anticoagulant, causing release of lipoprotein lipase enzyme to act on the triglycerol.

Heparan Sulfate (Fig. 9)

- **Site of occurrence**—skin, aortic walls, fibroblast
- **Repeating units**—made up of glucosamine and glucuronic or iduronic acid like heparin. Glucosamine may be acetylated
- **Functions**—it acts as receptors in plasma membrane and mediates cell communications and cell growth. Responsible for charge selectiveness in glomerular filtration.

Keratan Sulfate

- **Site of occurrence**—loose connective tissue, cartilage, cornea.

- **Repeating units**—made up of N-acetylglucosamine and galactose. **No uronic acid**
- **Functions**—it provides transparency of the cornea.

31. Secondary structure of proteins/alpha helix.

Refer 2007 Short Note 25.

32. Structure of immunoglobulin with the help of a figure.

Refer 2008 Short Note 11.

33. Causes and manifestations of gout.

Refer 2005 Short Note 17.

34. Transamination reactions.

Refer 2008 Short Note 14.

35. Role of lungs in maintenance of pH of blood.

Refer 2007 Short Note 32.

36. Conjugation reactions involved in metabolism of xenobiotics.

Refer 2004 Short Note 14.

37. Principle and applications of electrophoresis.

Refer 2006 Short Note 30.

38. Functions of tyrosine in the body.

Refer 2015 Essay Question 6.

Products formed from Tyrosine

- Melanin pigments
- Catecholamines
- Thyroxine
- Tyramine.

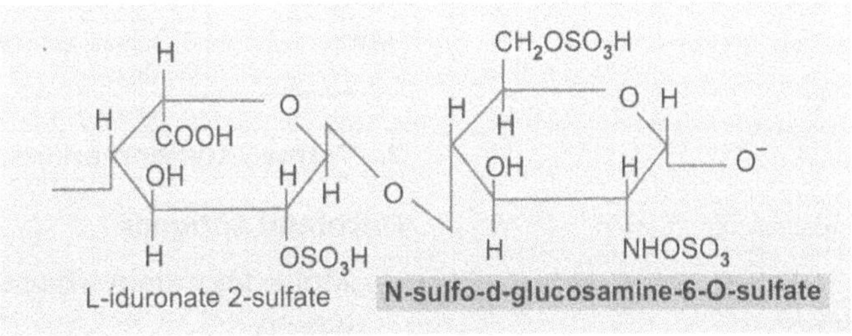

Fig. 9: Heparin and heparan sulfate.

Synthesis of Melanin (Fig. 10)

- Tyrosine is hydroxylated by tyrosinase to (dihydroxyphenylalanine) DOPA. It is a mono-oxygenase containing copper
- Tyrosinase acts again on DOPA to form DOPAquinone
- Decarboxylation and oxidation of DOPA-quinone converts it to indolequinone, which is polymerized to melanin.

Catecholamines (Fig. 11)

- Tyrosine is first hydroxylated to DOPA by tyrosine hydroxylase. It requires tetra-hydrobiopterin and NADPH
- DOPA is decarboxylated to form dopamine by DOPA decarboxylase, a PLP dependent enzyme. Dopamine is a catecholamine which is a neurotransmitter. In Parkinsonism, dopamine level is reduced. L-DOPA is used as a drug in Parkinsonism
- Dopamine is hydroxylated to norepinephrine by dopamine hydroxylase
- Norepinephrine is methylated to epinephrine by methyltransferase which needs SAM which is a methyl donor
- Epinephrine is methylated to metanephrine and oxidised to vanillyl mandelic acid (VMA) and excreted in urine. Normal level of excretion of VMA is 2-6 mg/day urine. This is elevated in pheochromocytoma and in neuroblastoma.

Thyroid Hormones

- Specific tyrosine molecules are iodinated to form mono, di, and tri-iodothyronine and thyroxine (T4)

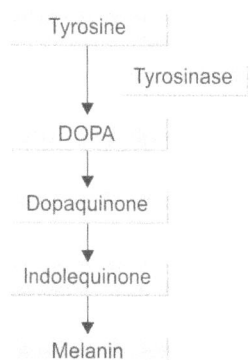

Fig. 10: Formation of melanin.

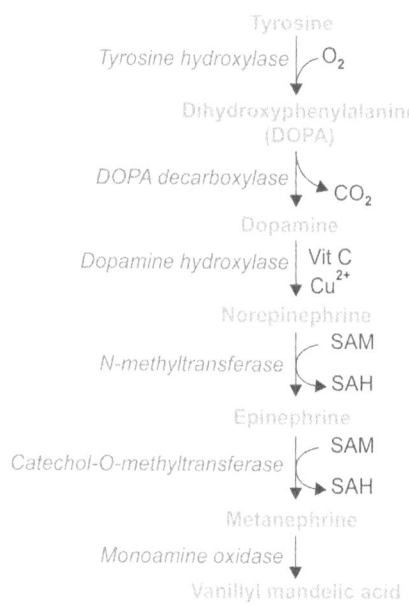

Fig. 11: Catecholemines.

Tyramine

- Tyrosine is decarboxylated to tyramine by intestinal bacteria which is one of the reasons for food allergy.

39. Tumor markers.
Refer 2003 Short Note 20.

40. Salvage pathway for purines and its importance in the body.
Refer 2004 Short Note 15.

III. SHORT ANSWER QUESTIONS

1. Markers of nucleus and mitochondria.

Organelles	Markers
Nucleus	Deoxyribonucleic acid (DNA)
Mitochondria	Glutamate dehydrogenase, ATP synthase

2. Name 2 tumor markers.

Oncofetal Antigens

- Alpha-fetoprotein—hepatoma, germ cell tumors
- Carcinoembryogenic antigen—colorectal and GI tumors

Enzymes
- Alkaline phosphatase—bone secondaries, liver secondaries
- Prostatic acid phosphatase—prostate cancer.

3. Functions of phospholipids.
Refer 2004 Short Note 1.
- Major structural component of membrane
- Regulating membrane permeability
- Second messenger in hormone action, e.g. phosphatidylinositol
- They help in fat absorption in the form of micelle
- They acts as emulsifying agents
- Important constituent of lipoproteins.
- Insulating nerve impulse, e.g. sphingomyelin
- They prevent fatty liver
- Dipalmitoylphosphatidylcholine is a pulmonary surfactant preventing respiratory distress syndrome.

4. Name the essential fatty acids.
Refer 2005 Short Note 10.

Essential fatty acids are those which cannot be synthesized by the body but have to be supplemented in the diet. They are polyunsaturated fatty acids. They are:
1. Linoleic acid (18 C)-ω6
2. Linolenic acid (18 C)-ω63
3. Arachidonic acid (20 C)-ω6—can be formed, if the dietary supply of linolenic acid is sufficient. So it cannot be strictly categorized under essential fatty acid.

5. Active forms of thiamine and riboflavin.
- Thiamine (B1)—active form (coenzyme).
  - thiamine pyrophosphate (TPP).
- Riboflavin (B2)—active coenzyme forms:
  - flavin mononucleotide (FMN)
  - flavin adenine dinucleotide (FAD and $FADH_2$).

6. Name the ketone bodies.
- The ketone bodies are mainly three, namely—**acetoacetate, β-hyroxybutyrate and acetone**
- Acetoacetate is the primary ketone body and the other two are secondary ketone bodies.

7. Significance of Rapaport–Leubering cycle.
Refer 2007 Short Note 18.
- No release of energy
- 2, 3 BPG combines with Hb and reduces the affinity towards oxygen. So, in the presence of 2, 3 BPG oxyHb unloads more O_2 so that the tissues get more O_2
- In hypoxia 2, 3 BPG level increases in RBCs and favors the release of oxygen to tissues even when pCO_2 is low
- 2,3 BPG level is increased in fetal circulation.

8. Name two glycogen storage diseases.

Type	Name	Defective enzyme	Clinical features
Type IA	Von-Gierke's disease	Glucose-6-phosphatase	Hypoglycemia; Hepatomegaly; ketosis, lactic acidosis; Hyperlipidemia; Hyperuricemia
Type II	Pompe's	Lysosomal maltase	Accumulation of abnormal glycogen in lysosomes of liver, heart and muscles; infantile form—early death

9. Significance of HMP shunt.
Refer 2005 Short Notes 2.
a. **Biochemical significance**
   - Biosynthesis of pentoses-ribose-5-phosphate for the synthesis of nucleotides and nucleic acids
   - Generation of NADPH reducing equivalents for:
     - Reductive synthesis of fatty acids, bile acids, cholesterol
     - NADPH is needed for the integrity of RBC membrane
     - Antioxidant—free radical scavenger.
b. **Clinical significance**—glucose-6-phosphate dehydrogenase deficiency.
   - X-linked recessive trait
   - Cells having the deficient enzyme have lower rate of NADPH production and deficiency of reduced glutathione leading to hemolysis

- This deficiency is manifested only when exposed to certain drugs, such as primaquine. Fava beans consumption and sulfa drugs also precipitate hemolysis
- Methemoglobinemia will be seen in circulation in glucose-6-phosphate deficiency.

10. Name the derivatives of cholesterol.
- Bile acids (BA) and bile salts (primary)—cholic acid and chenodeoxycholic acids; Secondary bile acids—lithocholic acid and deoxycholic acid and their conjugated Na and potassium salts
- Steroid and Sex hormones—steroid hormones—glucocorticoids and mineralocorticoids; Sex hormones from pregnenolone—progesterone, androgens–testosterone and estrogens
- Vitamin D and calcitriol.

11. Name the urea cycle disorders.
- Hyperammonemia type I autosomal recessive (AR)—enzyme deficient is carbamoyl phosphate synthetase I. Incidence is 1 in 100,000
- Hyperammonemia type II (X-linked)—enzyme deficient is ornithine transcarbamylase
- Citrullinemia (AR)—enzyme deficient is argininosuccinate synthetase
- Argininosuccinic aciduria—enzyme deficient is argininosuccinate lyase
- Hyperargininemia—enzyme deficient is arginase
- Hyperornithinemia (AR)—due to defective ornithine transport protein due to defect in *ORNT1* gene.

12. Causes of increased blood urea level.
- Normal blood urea level is 20-40 mg/dL. Urinary excretion of urea is 15-30 g/day
- Urea level may be increased due to high protein intake and inborn errors of urea cycle. Increased blood urea level leads to uremia
- Causes for elevation in urea level:
  a. Prerenal:
     - Increased protein breakdown after surgery, fever,
     - Diabetic coma, thyrotoxicosis,
     - Dehydration—vomiting, diarrhea,
     - Intestinal obstruction.
  b. Renal—acute glomerular nephritis, nephrosis, pyelonephritis, hypertension, polycystic kidney
  c. Postrenal: Obstruction—stones, stricture, enlarged prostate.

13. Name the derivatives of tryptophan.
a. Vitamin, niacin
b. Coenzymes, NAD, NADP,
c. Neurotransmitters, serotonin
d. Hormone, pineal—melatonin.

14. Fluorosis.
- Excessive intake of fluoride (more than 2 ppm) is toxic to the body
- The manifestations include mottling of enamel, stratification and discoloration of teeth (more than 5 ppm)—dental fluorosis
- In the advanced stages (more than 20 ppm), hypercalcification of limb bones and ligaments of spine get calcified leading to crippling of the individual—skeletal fluorosis
- These manifestations are collectively referred to as fluorosis
- A level more than 20 ppm is toxic leading to fluorosis which causes osteoporosis, osteosclerosis and brittle bones. Genu valgum is the characteristic feature. Fluorosis leads to blood concentration of fluoride of 50 µg/dL.

Prevention of Fluorosis
- To drink fluoride free water
- To avoid intake of jowar rich in fluoride
- To restrict in using fluoride containing toothpaste
- Vitamin C supplementation.

15. Parameter for the assessment of nutritive value of proteins.
a. **Biological value (BV) of proteins**—it is the ratio between the amount of nitrogen retained and nitrogen absorbed during a specific interval.

$$BV = \frac{\text{Retained nitrogen}}{\text{Absorbed nitrogen}} \times 100$$

b. **Net protein utilization (NPU)—**
   NPU = Retained nitrogen/intake of nitrogen × 100
   NPU is a better index than BV to denote nutritional quality and availability of a protein
c. **Net dietary protein value (NDPV)—**this value assesses the quantity and quality of proteins in the diet
   NDPV = Intake of N × 6.25 × NPU
d. **Protein efficiency ratio (PER)—**it is the weight gain per gram of protein intake
e. **Chemical score—**it is the content of essential amino acid (mg of amino acid per gram of protein).

16. Restriction endonucleases.
Refer 2007 Short Notes 28.

17. Mutagens.
- Mutagens are agents that can cause DNA damage thereby leading to mutation, e.g. X-rays, gamma rays, UV rays, benzopyrene in cigarette smoke, etc.
- They increase the rate of mutation and enhance the rate of incidence of cancer
- They may get into the body by means of occupation (aniline), diet (aflatoxins) and lifestyle (smoking).

18. Lesch-Nyhan syndrome.
Refer 2013 Short Answer Question 40.
- It is a X-linked inborn error of purine metabolism due to complete deficiency of HGPRTase which acts in purine salvage pathway
- It affects mainly males
- So the salvage pathway is stopped and PRPP accumulates which will go for increased purine synthesis and catabolism of purines to uric acid
- Hyperuricemia leads to nephrolithiasis and gout
- It is also characterized by self-mutilation, mental retardation.

19. Denaturation of proteins.
Refer 2009 Short Note 31.

20. Differences between DNA and RNA.
Refer 2008 Short Note 35.

S. No.	Characteristics	DNA	RNA
1.	Monomeric units	A, G, C, and thymidylate	A, G, C, and uridylate
2.	Sugar	Deoxyribose	Ribose
3.	Nature of strand/s	Double-stranded helix	Single-stranded
4.	Base pairs	$A=T; G\equiv C$	$A=U; G\equiv C$
5.	Types	A-DNA; B-DNA; Z-DNA	mRNA, tRNA, rRNA, snRNA
6.	Function	Carry genetic information, synthesis of RNA—transcription	Involved in the synthesis of proteins—translation
7.	Alkali hydrolysis	Not possible	Possible due to presence of OH group in 2' position

21. What are the enzymes required for DNA replication?
- DNA-dependent DNA polymerase—different in bacteria and mammals
  i. Bacterial (prokaryotic) DNA polymerase
     - DNAP-I (Pol I) (kornberg enzyme)—repair enzyme
     - DNAP-II (Pol II)—proofreading and repair
     - DNAP-III (Pol III)—synthesizing leading and lagging strands.
  ii. Mammalian (Eukaryotic) DNA Polymerase—5 types—α, β, γ, δ and ε. Alpha—gap filling, beta—DNA repair, gamma—mitochondrial DNA synthesis, delta—synthesis of leading and lagging strand and Epsilon—proofreading and DNA repair.
- Primase
- DNA topoisomerase—type I and II
- Helicase
- DNA gyrase—type II topoisomerase.

22. What is the principle of affinity chromatography?
- This is based on the specific and noncovalent affinity of substances like proteins and carbohydrates to a specific ligands like cofactor or substrates which is attached to the gel matrix, e.g. Ag-Ab, ligand-receptor, etc.

- The ligands get attached to an inert porous matrix in a column. This immobilized ligand helps to pick up the desired protein while all the protein is passing through the column
- The desired protein captured in the ligand is eluted and separated
- Thus coenzymes like NAD⁺ is used to separate and purify enzymes
- This procedure helps to separate vitamins, nucleic acids, drugs, hormone receptors, antibodies, immunoglobulins and membrane receptors.

23. What are the causes of respiratory acidosis?

Refer 2013 Short Note 17.
- Pneumonia
- Bronchitis
- Asthma
- COPD
- Sedatives
- Paralysis of respiratory muscles
- Brain tumor, head injury
- Ascites, peritonitis
- Sleep apnea
- Respiratory acidosis is due to primary excess of carbonic acid due to hypoventilation caused by retention of CO_2
- Ratio of bicarbonate to carbonic acid will be less than 20.

24. Maple syrup urine disease.
Refer 2009 Short Answer Question 31.

25. Urea clearance.

Measurement of GFR provides the most useful general index for the assessment of the severity of the renal damage. A decrease in renal function is assumed due to the loss of functional nephrons rather than decrease in the function of individual nephrons. GFR is a measure of number of functional nephrons.

Clearance is defined as the quantity of blood or plasma completely cleared off a substance per unit time and is expressed mL/min.

Urea clearance is the mL of blood which is cleared of urea per minute. Patient is asked to empty the bladder and 200 mL of water is given to drink. After 1 hour the volume of voided urine is measured, blood urea and urine urea are estimated.

Urea clearance = UV/P (where U = mg of urea/mL of urine, P = mg of urea/mL of plasma, V = volume of urine excreted)

Normal value is about 75 mL/min. Values below that shows a deteriorating renal function (progression to renal failure).

26. Bence Jones protein.

Refer 2009 Short Answer Question 28.
- Monoclonal light chains are excreted in urine in conditions like multiple myeloma. They are called Bence Jones protein. This is due to asynchronous production of H and L chains or due to deletion of portions of L chains
- The Bence Jones proteins precipitate when heated between 45-60° C and redissolve above 80° or below 45° C. Bradshaw test is also positive
- These proteins will block renal tubules leading to renal failure
- **Bradshaw test**—this is a positive test for multiple myeloma to show the presence of Bence Jones protein. Few mL of concentrated hydrochloric acid is taken in a test tube and few mL of urine is layered over it. A white ring of precipitate is formed to give positive result for Bradshaw's test.

27. What are Oncogenes?

Refer 2007 Short Note 7.
- Oncogenes are genes capable of causing cancer. They have the potential to cause cancer
- Oncogenes were originally discovered in tumor-causing viruses. Viral oncogenes, e.g. Rous sarcoma virus which causes sarcoma in avians. A strain of virus deficient in particular gene cannot cause this disease and named as *sarcoma* (*Src*) gene
- These are similar to certain genes present in normal avian cells called as proto-oncogenes
- Viral genes are denoted as *V-src* and cellular genes as *C-src*

- They are the sequence of DNA which has been altered or mutated from the proto-oncogenes
- They encode for certain proteins known as oncoproteins
- Products of many oncogenes are polypeptide growth factors, e.g. *sis* gene produces platelet derived growth factor (PDGF) needed for wound healing
- Some of the products act as receptors for growth factors, e.g. Erb B—produces receptors for epidermal growth factor (EGF).

Activation of Oncogenes

Viruses, chemical carcinogens, chromosome translocations, gamma rays, spontaneous mutations may activate the oncogenes which lead to malignancy.

Examples for Oncogenes Causing Cancer

- ErbB1—lung cancer
- ErbB2—gastric tumors.

Proto-oncogenes

- Proto-oncogenes are normal regulatory genes of cells
- Their products are mostly:
  a. Growth factors for the cells, e.g. *sis* gene for PDGF needed for wound healing
  b. Receptors for growth factors, e.g. erbB receptor for EGF
  c. Those involved in intracellular growth signaling pathways, e.g. src products.
- C-oncogenes are under the control of these regulatory genes and expressed whenever needed
- When proto-oncogenes are mutated, they become oncogenes which can not be controlled and increased growth signaling leads to cancer, e.g. ras, src, etc.

Antioncogenes or Oncosuppressor Gene

- These are the genes which protect a person from getting cancer
- When the gene is deleted or mutated cancer results
- Antioncogenes are written in capital letters, whereas oncogenes are written in small letters, e.g. retinoblastoma—(RB) (antioncogene).

28. Beer–Lambert law.

Refer 2011 Short Answers Questions 48.
- **Beer law**— it states that the amount of light absorbed by a colored solution is proportional to the concentration of the solution, i. e. absorbance $\propto$ concentration. As per this law, the intensity of the color is directly proportional to the concentration of the colored particles in the solution
- **Lambert's law**—it states that the amount of light absorbed by a colored solution is proportional to the depth of the liquid through which the light passes through the solution
- **Transmittance (T)**—the ratio of emergent light to intensity of incident light (E/i)
- **Absorbance**—is expressed as log T
- **Optical density**—is calculated as log T.

29. What are the forces that stabilize secondary structure of proteins?

- Secondary structure of proteins is stabilized by noncovalent bonds, such as:
  - Hydrogen bond—weak
  - Electrostatic bonds—ionic bonds (salt bridges)
  - Hydrophobic bonds—weak
  - Van der Waals forces.

30. Name the basic amino acids.

Basic amino acids are diamino-monocarboxylic acids. They have a positive charge on the functional group. They are: Lysine, arginine and histidine.

31. Cardiolipin.

- Cardiolipin is diphosphatidylglycerol made up of 2 molecules of phosphatidic acid connected by glycerol
- It is a major lipid of mitochondrial membrane which is necessary for the function of electron transport chain
- Commercially it is extracted from myocardium

- Deceased level of cardiolipin leads to mitochondrial dysfunction and it is implicated in heart failure, hypothyroidism and in certain types of myopathies
- It is antigenic and recognized by antibodies raised against *Treponema pallidum* which causes syphilis.

32. Mention the types of fatty acid oxidation.

- **Alpha oxidation of fatty acid:**
  - Removal of one carbon unit at a time by the oxidation of alpha carbon atom of fatty acids from the carboxyl end
  - There is no involvement of coenzyme A and no energy is produced.
- **Beta oxidation of fatty acid**
  - It is the process of oxidation and splitting of 2 carbon units which are sequentially removed at the beta carbon of fatty acids from the carboxyl end.
- **Omega oxidation of fatty acid**
  - Minor pathway occur in microsomes with the help of hydroxylase enzyme involving NADPH and cytochrome P450
  - This occurs when beta oxidation is defective
  - The end methyl group is converted to CH_2OH to produce dicarboxylic acid which is excreted in urine—dicarboxylic aciduria.
- **Peroxisomal oxidation**
  - Peroxisomes are the site of metabolism of H_2O_2 and they are able to conduct oxidation of long chain fatty acids (20 to 26 carbon) to acetyl-CoA and H_2O_2
  - This is a modified form of beta-oxidation found in peroxisomes
  - This dehydrogenation is not linked to phosphorylation and generation of ATP.

33. What are the products of arachidonic acid?

- Eicosanoids are derived from arachidonic acid
- Prostaglandin, prostacycline and thromboxanes are produced thorough cyclo-oxygenase pathway
- Leukotriens and lipoxins are formed via lipoxygenase pathway.

34. Carnitine.

- Long chain fatty acyl-CoA cannot pass through inner mitochondrial membrane. Hence activated fatty acids are transported to the mitochondria by carnitine shuttle
- Carnitine is synthesized from lysine and methionine in liver and kidney, and it is β-hydroxy-γ-trimethylammonium butyrate
- It is abundant in muscles
- Requirement of carnitine is more during growth and pregnancy
- The enzymes carnitine-acyltransferase I and II and carnitine-acylcarnitine translocase help in transport of carnitine through carnitine shuttle across the inner mitochondrial membrane
- Carnitine deficiency is reported in preterm infants in whom there is impaired fatty acid oxidation is noted. There will be hypoglycemia due to the utilization of more glucose
- During aging process carnitine concentration in cells is diminished. There will be osteoporosis in old people who needs carnitine therapy
- Primary carnitine deficiency has hepatomegaly, elevated transaminases and hyperammonemia. Secondary deficiency is associated with organic acidurias and due to certain drugs like valproic acid, zidovudine.

35. Anomerism.

Alpha and Beta Anomers (Fig. 12)

- Sugar can exist in 2 forms represented by α and β anomers
- C1 is called as anomeric carbon
- In alpha form the hydroxyl group is attached to C1 below the plane of the ring and in beta form OH group is above the plane of the ring

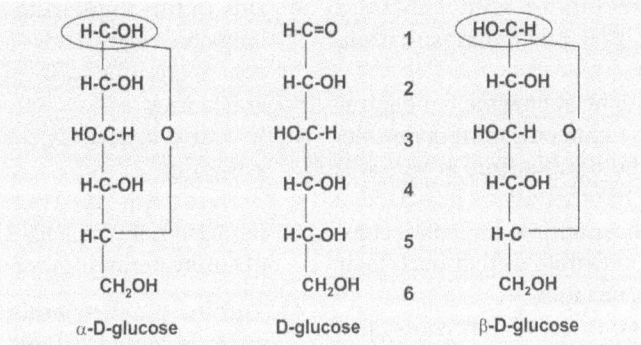

Fig. 12: Alpha and beta anomers.

36. How hemoglobin binds to oxygen.

- Oxygen binds to the ferrous atoms of Hb to form oxyhemoglobin
- Hydrogen is bound to the side chains of histidine residues in α and β chains
- CO_2 is bound to the alpha amino group of N terminal end of each polypeptide chain of Hb to form carbaminoHb
- The 'T' structure or tight form (tense form/taut form) of deoxyHb takes up 4 oxygen atoms to form oxyHb having R structure—relaxed form. This is done by **conformational changes** in the quaternary structure of Hb
- Oxygen **binds cooperatively** to Hb which enables the binding of more oxygen to Hb easily and to help in transport of oxygen.
- Because of this the O_2 binding curve of Hb is sigmoidal (S) in shape. This shape indicates that the affinity of Hb for binding of first molecule of oxygen is low and the subsequent oxygen molecules are bound with higher affinity **(Fig. 13)**.

37. K_m value and its significance.

Refer 2003 Short Note 8

According to Michaelis theory, the formation of enzyme substrate complex is a reversible, while the breakdown of complex to enzyme and product is irreversible:

$$V_i = \frac{V_{max}[S]}{K_m + [S]}$$

- K_m value is substrate concentration at half maximal velocity means 50% of enzyme

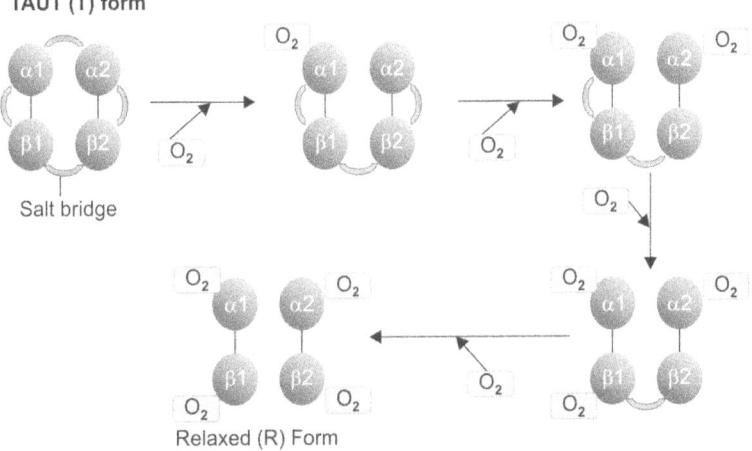

Fig. 13: Oxygen binding with hemoglobin.

molecules are bound with substrate molecules at that particular substrate concentration
- K_m is independent of enzyme concentration. If enzyme concentration is double, the V_{max} will be double, but ½ V_{max} will remain same. In other words irrespective of enzyme concentration, 50% molecules are bound to substrate at that particular substrate concentration
- K_m is the signature of enzymes and characteristic feature of a particular enzyme for a specific substrate
- K_m is a constant
- K_m denotes the affinity of enzyme for substrate and it is inversely related to the dissociation constant
- It denotes the affinity of enzyme for substrate. The lesser the value of K_m, the affinity of the enzyme for the substrate is more.

38. Bronze diabetes.
- Hemochromatos is a disease in which iron is directly deposited in the tissues (liver, spleen, pancreas and skin)
- The manifestations are bronzed pigmentation of the skin, cirrhosis of liver, and pancreatic fibrosis
- The triad of cirrhosis, hemochromatosis, and diabetes are referred to as **bronze diabetes**.

39. WHO criteria for diagnosis of diabetes mellitus.
- Fasting blood glucose should be more than 126 mg/dL for more than 2 occasion OR
- If 2-hours postglucose level of OGTT more than 200 mg/dL (even at one occasion) OR
- Both fasting and 2-hour values above these levels (on the same occasion)
- Random plasma glucose level is more than 200 mg/dL, on more than one occasion
- Glycated Hb (HbA1C) level more than 6.5% at any occasion—preferred method.

40. Zellweger's syndrome.
- It is a rare disorder characterized by the absence of peroxisomes in all tissues
- Due to this there will be no oxidation of long chain fatty acids (C26 to C38) which gets accumulated in brain tissues, liver and kidney
- It is also known as cerebrohepatorenal syndrome
- Proteins are not transported into the peroxisomes which leads to the formation of empty peroxisomes or ghost cells.

41. Outline the distribution of water in the various compartments of the body.
- Water is present both inside and outside cells and in GIT and GUT
- Two compartments—ECW and ICW
- ECW—water external to cell membranes
- ECW—intravascular (plasma) and extravascular (interstitial fluid)

Compartment	%TBW	Vol (L)
Total body water (TBW)	60%	42
Extracellular water (ECW)	20%	14
a. Intravascular	4%	2.8
b. Extravascular	16%	11.2
Intracellular water (ICW)	40%	28

42. What is the mechanism of action of steroid hormones?
- Steroid hormones are lipid soluble derivatives of cholesterol synthesized from adrenal cortex—cortical hormones, androgens (male sex hormones), estrogens—(female sex hormones) and calcitriol (vitamin D3). They belong to group I
- Their action is mediated by hormone receptor complex which acts as second messengers to communicate with intracellular reactions through intermediary molecules
- They act by regulation of gene expression
- Hormone response elements on DNA regulate transcription of genes.

43. List four features of the genetic code.
Refer 2005 Short Note 19.
- The letters A, G, T, and C correspond to the nucleotides found in DNA
- Within the protein coding genes these nucleotides are organized into three-letter code words called codons, and the

collection of these codons makes up the genetic code
- The code provides a foundation for explaining the way in which protein defects may cause genetic disease and for the diagnosis and perhaps the treatment of these disorders
- A triplet sequence of nucleotide on the mRNA is the codon for each amino acid.

Salient Features

- **Triplet codons**—each codon is consecutive sequence of three bases on the mRNA, e.g. UUU codes for phenylalanine
- **Nonoverlapping**—the codons are read one after another in a continuous manner, e.g. AUG, GAU, GCA, etc.
- **Nonpunctuated**—there is no punctuation in-between codons.
- **Degenerate**—61 codon codes for 20 amino acids so one amino acid has more than one codons, e.g. serine has 6 codons and glycine has 4 codons this is called degeneracy of code
- **Unambigous**—codons are unambiguous that means one codon stands only for one amino acids
- **Universal**—the codons are same for same amino acids in all species.

44. Explain the clinical relevance of serum creatinine levels.

- Normal serum level of creatinine is 0.7-1.4 mg/dL; Serum creatine is 0.2-0.4 mg/dL
- Serum creatinine is a **marker of renal failure**. Level of creatinine is increased in prerenal, renal and postrenal failures
- Creatinine clearance test is used to measure GFR
- Creatine kinase has many isoenzymes and is elevated in muscular dystrophies and myocardial infarction. It is the first enzyme to be elevated in myocardial infarction.

45. What is meant by the polymerase chain reaction? List two of its applications.

Refer 2010 Short Note 13

- It is an in vitro DNA amplification procedure in which millions of a particular sequence of DNA can be produced within few hours
- Two primers of about 20-30 nucleotides with complementary sequence of the flanking region are needed-
  - Step 1: Separation—DNA strands are separated by heating at 95°C for 15 seconds to 2 minutes
  - Step 2: Annealing—the primers are annealed by cooling to 50°C for 0.5 to 2 minutes. Then they hybridize with their complementary single-stranded DNA separated already
  - Step 3: Polymerization—new DNA strands are synthesized by Taq polymerase. This enzyme is derived from bacteria *Thermus aquaticus* that is found in hot springs. The polymerase reaction is allowed to take place at 72°C for 30 seconds in the presence of dNTPs of adenine, guanine, cytosine and thymine to duplicate both strands of DNA
  - Step 4: Steps 1, 2 and 3 are repeated to double up the DNA strands. After 20 cycles one million times amplifications will occur
- These cycles are repeated by automated instrument tempcycler.

Clinical Applications

1. Detection of infectious diseases—tuberculosis and viral diseases like HIV and hepatitis. PCR detects even one bacillus present in the specimen. Any other bacteria could also be detected similarly. This technique is widely used in the diagnosis of viral infections like hepatitis C and HIV
2. Medicolegal cases—PCR allows the DNA in a single cell or in a hair follicle to be analyzed. This is highly useful in forensic medicine to identify the criminal.

46. What are the reference levels of glucose and protein in cerebrospinal fluid? How are they affected in bacterial meningitis?

- Normal glucose level in CSF is 50–70 mg/dL and protein level is 50–70 mg/dL
- In bacterial meningitis, there will be marked increase in protein concentration and marked decrease in glucose concentration of CSF.

47. What is meant by quaternary structure of a protein? Name a protein abundantly found in blood that has a quaternary structure.

Quaternary Structure (Fig. 14)

- This occurs only in proteins which have more than one polypeptide chain—polymeric proteins
- These polypeptides aggregate to form quaternary structure to get one functional protein
- Each polypeptide chain is termed as subunit or monomer. Depending on the number of polypeptide chains, the proteins are dimer (2 chains), trimer (3 chains), and tetramer (4 chains) and so on
- If the protein has two copies of the same polypeptide chains they are termed as homodimer and if it has two different polypeptide chains they are called as heterodimer
- For example, **hemoglobin** is a hetero-tetramer having 2 alpha chains and 2 beta chains

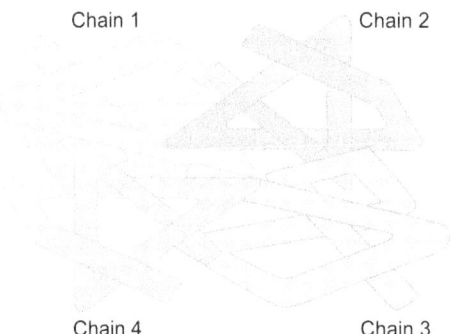

Fig. 14: Quatenary structure—hemoglobin.

- Quaternary structures are maintained by hydrogen bonds, electrostatic bonds, hydrophobic bonds and weak Van der Waal's forces.

48. Name the bases found in nucleic acids.

- The bases present in DNA—adenine, guanine, cytosine and thymine
- Bases present in RNA—adenine, guanine, cytosine and uracil.

49. List four causes of respiratory acidosis.

- Respiratory acidosis—primary excess of carbonic acid with ↑pCO_2. This is compensated by increase in bicarbonate:
  Causes: This occurs in chronic obstructive airways diseases, asthma, emphysema, paralysis of respiratory muscles, respiratory depressant toxic drugs.

50. What are the functions of glutathione?

Refer 2009 Short Answer Question 12.

- Glutathione is γ-glutamyl-cysteinyl-glycine. It is a tripeptide of biochemical importance. Glutamate combines with cysteine to form gamma-glutamylcysteine which combines with glycine to form glutathione. Each step needs one ATP.

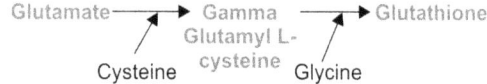

Functions of Glutathione

- **Role in absorption of amino acids in intestines, kidney tubules and in brain**—glutathione is involved in Meister cycle which is needed for absorption and transport of neutral amino acids in intestines, kidney tubules and brain
- **Coenzyme role**—glutathione is needed as a cofactor for:
  - maleylacetoacetate isomerase, converting maleylacetoacetate to fumarylacetoacetate
  - Cysteic acid → taurine
- **To maintain the integrity of RBC membrane**—glutathione present in the RBC is needed for inactivation of free radicals formed inside. Glutathione peroxidase

and glutathione reductase enzymes play important role in keeping glutathione in reduced state
- **Conversion of metHb**—metHb cannot transfer oxygen. Glutathione helps in the reduction of MetHb to normal Hb
- **Conjugation reactions**—glutathione (GSH) acts as a conjugation agent in detoxification reactions
- **Activation of enzymes**—glutathione keeps certain enzymes with -SH groups in their active site in reduced form.

MBBS Examination 2013

ANSWER ALL QUESTIONS

I. **Essay questions** (10/15 Marks each)

1. What is the normal blood sugar level? Describe in detail how it is maintained within normal limits?
2. Mention the source, daily requirement of vitamin B12. Describe its absorption, biochemical function and deficiency manifestations.
3. Name the aromatic amino acids. Add a note on physiologically important derivatives of tyrosine.
4. Explain protein synthesis in detail. Add a note on drugs that inhibit protein synthesis.
5. a. Classify enzymes.
   b. Describe in detail the various factors affecting enzyme action.
   c. Add a note on enzyme regulation.
6. Name the ketone bodies? How are they formed and utilized in the body? Add a note on the metabolic changes in diabetic ketoacidosis.
7. a. Describe the catabolism of heme in the body.
   b. Explain the different types of jaundice. How do you investigate a case of jaundice?
8. What is the normal pH of blood? Describe the various mechanisms which maintain it. Mention the acid base disorders.
9. Describe how bilirubin is formed and excreted in the body.
10. Describe the process by which ATP is synthesized in the body.
11. List the parameters that are commonly used in clinical practice as indicators to assess the functions of the liver. Explain the basis of the use of these parameters in assessment of liver function. Briefly discuss medical conditions in which these parameters become abnormal.
12. a. Describe the role of the kidney to maintain the pH of blood.
    b. What are the compensatory mechanisms the kidney will adopt to maintain pH in the presence of metabolic acidosis?

II. **Short notes** (5 Marks each)

1. Fatty liver and lipotropic factors.
2. Digestion and absorption, transport of iron.
3. Isoenzymes and their diagnostic importance.
4. Define biological oxidation and mechanism of ATP synthesis.
5. Principles of balanced diet.
6. Transport mechanism across cell membrane. Explain.
7. Cytochrome P450.
8. Galactosemia.
9. Prostaglandins and their importance.
10. Ketosis.
11. Thyroid function tests.
12. Recombinant DNA technology.
13. Structure of DNA (Watson-Crick model).
14. Post-transcriptional modifications.
15. Functions of albumin.
16. Electrophoresis and its applications.
17. Causes for respiratory acidosis.
18. Renal mechanism of maintaining acid-base balance.
19. Purine salvage pathway.
20. Lac operon concept.

21. 2,3 BPG—formation and its role.
22. Mechanism of synthesis of ATP in ETC.
23. Explain 'methyl folate trap'.
24. Carnitine shuttle.
25. What are dietary fibers and explain their importance in human nutrition with respect to the prevention of diseases.
26. Write briefly about the significance of HMP shunt pathway.
27. Sources, RDA and biological role of vitamin C.
28. Describe the energetics of complete oxidation of 1 mole of glucose to CO_2 and H_2O under aerobic conditions.
29. Bile salts—synthesis and biological role.
30. Write briefly about calcium homeostasis.
31. Active form of methionine and its function.
32. Inhibitors of protein biosynthesis.
33. Porphyria.
34. LAC operon.
35. Transcription and Post-transcriptional modification.
36. Cyclic AMP.
37. Detoxification by conjugation.
38. Renal function tests.
39. Tumor markers.
40. Different mechanisms involved in hormone action.
41. Role of carnitine in beta-oxidation of fatty acids.
42. Covalent modification of enzymes in regulation of enzyme activities.
43. Lactose intolerance.
44. What is the importance of the pentose phosphate pathway in the body?
45. Gluconeogenesis with reference to definition, substrates, sites and importance in the body.
46. Role of vitamin D in the body.
47. Causes of iron deficiency and its manifestations.
48. Isoenzymes with reference to definition, examples and clinical importance.
49. Glycated hemoglobin, with to its formation, reference value in blood and its clinical importance.
50. Thiamine with reference to its functions in the body, dietary sources and deficiency manifestations.
51. Denaturation of proteins.
52. Types of mutations.
53. Post-transcriptional modifications of RNA.
54. Restriction endonucleases and their uses.
55. Specialized products derived from tyrosine.
56. Principle and applications of electrophoresis.
57. Cell cycle.
58. Causes and clinical features of dehydration.
59. Consequences of hyperuricemia.
60. Structure of DNA. (Watson–Crick model).

III. Short answer questions
(2/3 Marks each)

1. Key enzyme of cholesterol synthesis and its regulation.
2. Formaminoglutamic acid (FIGLU).
3. Refsum's disease.
4. Comparison between prokaryotic and eukaryotic cells.
5. Glycosides.
6. Metal cofactors of enzymes.
7. Beriberi.
8. Lipid profile.
9. Limiting amino acids.
10. Glucose-6-phosphate dehydrogenase enzyme.
11. Enzyme defect in a) Phenylketonuria b) Alkaptonuria.
12. DNA polymerase enzyme.
13. Types of mutations.
14. Reverse transcriptase.
15. Inhibitors of RNA synthesis.
16. Features of genetic code.
17. Gout.
18. Name two renal function tests.
19. Denaturation of proteins.
20. Name two enzymes that are increased in hepatic jaundice.
21. What are zymogens? Give an example.
22. Mention two inhibitors of ETC with their site of action.

23. What is specific dynamic action and importance in calculating caloric requirements of an individual?
24. What are trace minerals? Give RDA of any 2 of them.
25. What is steatorrhea?
26. What is suicide inhibition? Give an example.
27. Laboratory criteria for diagnosis of diabetes mellitus.
28. Name the insulin dependent glucose transporters and their tissue distribution.
29. What is pulmonary surfactant and its clinical importance?
30. What is the biochemical basis of development of cataract in diabetes mellitus?
31. ELISA.
32. Hyperkalemia.
33. Okazaki fragments.
34. Thyroid function tests.
35. Creatinine clearance.
36. Gamma-aminobutyric acid (GABA).
37. Isoelectric pH of proteins.
38. Maple syrup urine disease.
39. Multiple myeloma.
40. Lesch-Nyhan syndrome and orotic aciduria.
41. List the vitamins that are required for the functioning of the citric acid cycle.
42. Give two examples of drugs that act as inhibitors of enzyme and name the enzyme that each one inhibits.
43. What is the function of mitochondria in a cell?
44. What is the mechanism of action of statins? What is the therapeutic use of this group of drugs?
45. List two dietary sources and two biochemical functions of vitamin C in the body.
46. Explain the mechanism of action of cyanide as a poison.
47. List two good dietary sources of iodine. What is the function of this mineral in the body?
48. Enzyme defect and most common clinical feature in Von Gierke disease?
49. What is meant by glycemic index of food?
50. List two differences between marasmus and kwashiorkor.
51. What is multiple myeloma? Which laboratory test can be used to confirm diagnosis of this condition?
52. List four functions of nucleotides.
53. Which amino acid gives rise to nitric oxide in the body? What is the enzyme that catalyzes this process?
54. What is the biochemical basis of the encephalopathy that can develop in patients who have liver cirrhosis?
55. List the biochemical abnormalities seen in phenylketonuria.
56. Give examples of four conjugating agents in the body that are involved in the metabolism of xenobiotics.
57. What is the role of gamma-aminobutyric acid in the body? Name the amino acid from which it is derived.
58. What is the principle of radioimmunoassay?
59. List the different types of immunoglobulins.
60. List four causes of respiratory acidosis.

I. ESSAY QUESTIONS

1. **What is the normal blood sugar level? Describe in detail how it is maintained within normal limits.**

Refer 2005 Essay Question 6.

2. **Mention the source, daily requirement of vitamin B12. Describe its absorption biochemical function and deficiency manifestations.**

Refer 2006 Short Note 8.

3. **Name the aromatic amino acids. Add a note on physiologically important derivatives of tyrosine.**

Refer 2012 Short Note 38.

Aromatic amino acids are phenylalanine, tyrosine, tryptophan and histidine

4. Explain protein synthesis in detail. Add a note on drugs that inhibit protein synthesis.

Refer 2014 Essay Question 8.

Definition: This is a process of synthesizing proteins by adding of amino acids sequentially in specific number and sequence determined by specific codons in mRNA by deciphering of genetic code.

- Differ in prokaryotes and eukaryotes
- **Site of translation:**
  - Prokaryotes-Cytoplasm (Ribosomes)
  - Eukaryotes-Cytoplasm-rough endoplasmic reticulum and mitochondria.

Requirements

- Amino acids—EAA
- mRNA to be translated
- tRNAs—adopter molecules
- Functional ribosomes
- Energy sources—ATP, GTP
- Enzymes
- **Protein factors**—for initiation, elongation and termination of polypeptide chain
  - Initiation
  - Elongation
  - Release factor.

Energy Sources

- 4 high energy bonds
- 2 from ATP, 2 from GTP.

Direction of Synthesis

From amino terminal end to carboxyl end.

TRANSLATION IN PROKARYOTES

Steps of Translation

1. Activation of amino acid and charging
2. Initiation
3. Elongation
4. Termination.

Steps are same in pro and eukaryotes.

Difference: Initiation—methionine in eukaryotes and N-formylmethionine in prokaryotes

- Initiation sequences
- Factors (pro)
- Inhibitory action of drugs.

Activation of Amino acid and Charging (Fig.1)

- Each enzyme recognizes a specific amino acid
- Two steps reaction of attachment of carboxyl group of amino acid to 3'end of tRNA by aminoacyl tRNA synthetase enzyme
- One ATP is needed.

Initiation (Fig. 2)

- Initiator sequence—Shine-Dalgarno sequence
- Initiator codon—N-formylmethionine
- Factors (Pro)—IF-1, IF-2, IF-3
- Generation of initiator—N-formylmethionyl tRNA
  - Donor of formyl group –N10 formyl H4 folate
  - Removed before protein synthesis is completed.

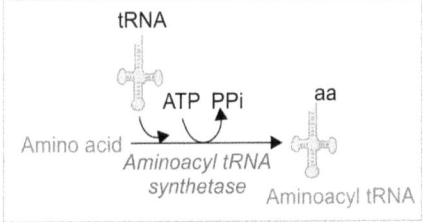

Fig. 1: Activation and charging of amino acid.

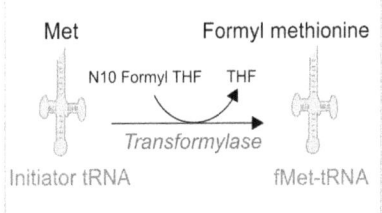

Fig. 2: Initiation.

Elongation (Fig. 3)

- Multistep process—3 steps
- Cyclic processes
- Factors—elongation factors EF-Tu and EF-Ts (EUK-Eef)
- Addition of amino acid to carboxyl end of chain:
  - Binding of aminoacyl tRNA to 'A' site
  - Peptide bond formation—peptidyl transferase—activity of 23S rRNA (50S)
  - **Translocation**—advancement of ribosome—3 nucleotides towards 3' end of mRNA (Both need–EF-G and GTP)
  - Movement of uncharged tRNA to empty (E site) and peptidyl tRNA into P site.

Termination

- Simple process
- Stop/nonsense codons UAG, UAA, UGA recognised by releasing factors- RF-1,2,3
- Releasing factor –RF-1 recognizes UAA and UAG; RF-2 recognizes UAA and UGA
- RF-3 promotes termination in association with GTP
- Peptidyl transferase is induced by these releasing factors and it causes hydrolysis of bond between peptide and tRNA at P site. Polypeptide chain is released from P site
- Dissociation of ribosomal units done by GTP hydrolysis
- Release of mRNA.

TRANSLATION IN EUKARYOTES (FIG. 4)

Steps

- **Activation of amino acid** and charging of amino acid to 3' end of tRNA **(similar to prokaryotes)**
  - Each enzyme recognizes a specific amino acid
  - Two steps reaction of attachment of carboxyl group of amino acid to 3'end of tRNA by aminoacyl tRNA synthetase enzyme
  - ATP needed.

Amino acid + ATP + Amono acyl tRNA synthetase

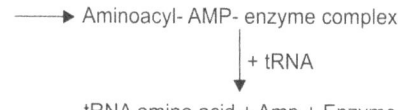

$\longrightarrow$ Aminoacyl- AMP- enzyme complex

$\downarrow$ + tRNA

tRNA amino acid + Amp + Enzyme

Initiation

- EUK–40S ribosome—binds to cap structure at 5' end of mRNA
- Initiator sequence—Marker sequence, Kozak consensus sequence
- Initiator codon—eukaryotes-AUG-methionine
- Factors (pro)-EUK-10 factors–eIF1 to eIF10.

Four Steps of Initiation

1. Ribosomal dissociation—80S to 40S and 60S subunits
2. Formation of 43S preinitiation complex—40S + ternary complex with Met-tRNA + eIF2
3. Formation of 48S initiation complex—43S + activated mRNA with eIF4
4. Formation of 80S initiation complex.

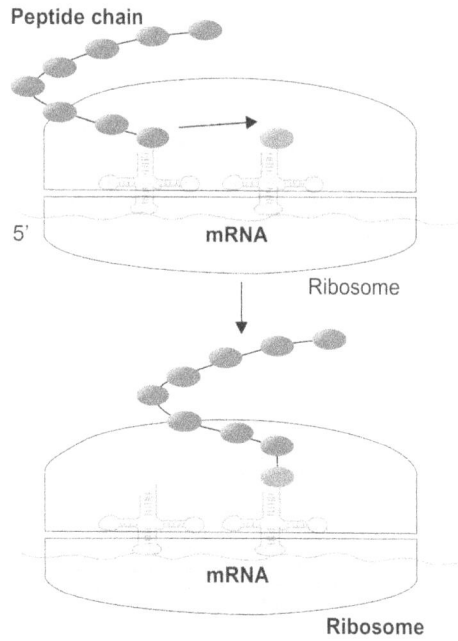

Fig. 3: Elongation.

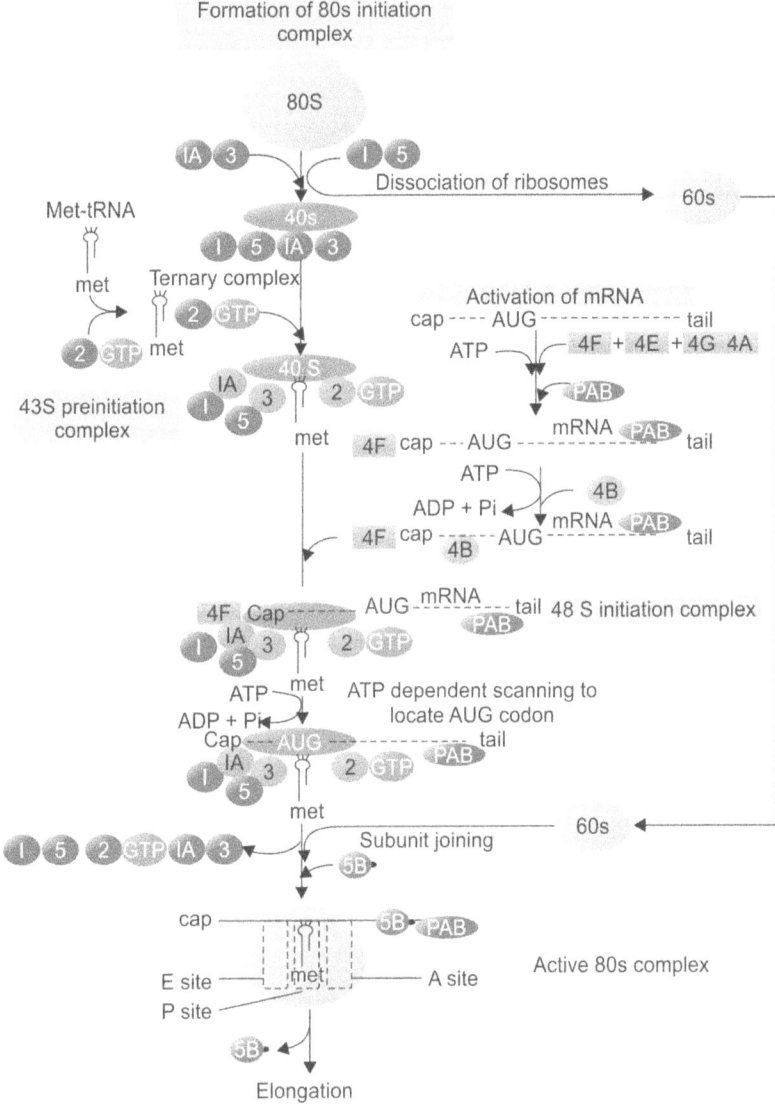

Fig. 4: Translation - Eukaryotes.

Elongation—3 Steps
1. Binding of aminoacyl tRNA to A site
2. Peptide bond formation—peptidyl transferase—28S RNA of 60S unit (ribozyme) needs 2 ATP and 2 GTP
3. Translocation—movement of growing peptide chain from A to P site then to E-exit site or empty site
- Factors - eEF1 and eEF2
- Translocation—needs eEF2 and GTP

- 6 amino acids/seconds are synthesized (prokaryotes—many in 18 seconds).

Termination
- Simple process
- Stop/nonsense codon—(UAG, UAA, UGA)—recognized by releasing factors - ERF
- GTP, peptidyl transferase promotes hydrolysis of bond between peptide and tRNA (in P site)

- Dissociation of 80S ribosome and Release of mRNA.

Post-translational modifications: Refer 2014 Short Note 14

Once the protein is synthesized by the process of translation by the ribosomes, it undergoes various modifications to become a fully functional protein. Those processes are called post-translational modification or post-translational processing of proteins. They are:
- Trimming
- Covalent modifications
  - Phosphorylation
  - Glycosylation
  - Hydroxylation
  - Carboxylation
  - Addition of groups—methyl, acetyl, farnesyl, amide.
- Subunit aggregation
- Protein folding.

Cleaving of Large Precursor Molecules (Trimming)–ER/Golgi/Secretory Vescicles

- Proteins like insulin are secreted as pre-pro-proteins. Proteinases cleave the N-terminal and C-terminal portions of pre-proinsulin. Then it undergoes disulfide bond creation to form mature insulin and get released
  - Pre-proinsulin → proinsulin → insulin
  - Cleaved after secretion, e.g. collagen
  - Zymogens (inactive proenzymes) → active enzymes, e.g. trypsinogen → trypsin.
- **Proteolytic cleavage** of 'N'-terminal methionine by hydrolysis
- **Removal of signal sequences:** Signal peptides—endoplasmic reticulum.

Protein Folding

- Chaperons are heat shock proteins. It facilitates and favor interactions on polypeptide surfaces to get specific confirmation of a protein. They irreversibly bind to hydrophobic regions of unfolded proteins and folding intermediates and stabilize them.

Covalent Modifications

- **Gamma carboxylation**—the gamma carbon of glutamic acid in clotting factors (II, VII, IX, XI) under the influence of vitamin K is needed for them to become active clotting factors
- **Hydoxylation**—of lysine and proline in alpha chain of collagen are needed for making bonds between them to increase the strength of collagen. Vitamin C acts as a cofactor in this
- **Phosphorylation**—of ser/thr/tyr in many regulatory enzymes like phosphorylase are important for the regulation of metabolic pathways
- **Glycosylation**—many proteins are glycoproteins. Carbohydrates are attached to ser/thr residues to the OH group or to the amide N of asparagine, e.g. proteins of plasma membrane and lysosomes occurs in ER/Golgi used to target proteins specific organelles, e.g. lysosomal enzymes modified by addition of mannose-6-phosphate
- **Methylation**—of lysine/histidine/arginine, e.g. histones
- **Acylation**—myelin proteolipids or transferrin receptor help in stable anchorage of protein in lipid bilayer of membranes.

Subunit Aggregation

Occurs in:
- Immunoglobulin
- Hemoglobin
- Maturation of collagen.

Clinical Applications

- Defective hydroxylation in collagen leads to collagen disorders like Ehlers-Danlos syndrome
- Defective protein folding may lead to dangerous prion diseases like bovine spongiform encephalopathy and Crueztfolt Jacob disease.

Inhibitors of Protein Synthesis

I. Reversible inhibitors in prokaryotes:
- **Antibiotics-Bacteriostatic:**
  - Tetracyclins—bind to 30S prevents attachment of aminoacyl tRNA to the A site
  - Chloromycetin—inhibits peptidyl transferase
  - Erythromycin and clindamycin—prevents translocation.
- **Bactericidal Antibiotics:**
  - Aminoglycosides:
    - Streptomycin is irreversible inhibitor of 30S ribosomes
    - Low concentration—misreading mRNA
    - Pharmacological concentration—prevents initiation complex; total inhibition of translation.

II. Inhibitors—Eukayotes
- Cycloheximide—inhibits both human and bacterial peptidyl transferase (60S)
- Diphtheria toxin—inactivates eEF2 by attaching ADP to eEF2; prevents translocation
- Ricin toxin (Castor bean seed)—inactivates 28S rRNA.

III. Inhibitors—Prokaryotes and Eukaryotes
- Puromycin: Structural analogue of tyrosinyl tRNA incorporated into the peptide chain causing inhibition of elongation in both prokaryotes and eukaryotes It acts as a research tool.

---

5. a. Classify enzymes. b. Describe in detail the various factors affecting enzyme action. c. Add a note on enzyme regulation.

a. Refer 2006 Short Note 22.

Definition

Enzymes are biocatalysts which are proteins in nature (except ribozymes). They are specific in their reaction. They are heat liable and colloidal which are required in small quantities for their action.

Classification

As per the site of location
- Intracellular enzymes within the cellular organelles, e.g. cytosol—enzymes of glycolysis, mitochondria—enzymes of TCA cycle
- Extracellular enzymes secreted from the cells but function outside the cells, e.g. digestive enzymes—pepsin, trypsin.

As per the diagnostic use—plasma enzymes
- Plasma specific or plasma functional enzymes—they have definite functions in plasma found in high concentration than in tissues mostly synthesized in liver, e.g. lipoprotein lipase, pseudocholinesterase
- Plasma nonspecific or plasma non-functional enzymes—they have no definite function in plasma; they may be absent or present in low amounts in plasma. During the damage of tissues of its origin, its level is elevated in plasma, e.g. amylase, acid phosphatase.

As per the types of reaction catalyzed
- For example, dehydrogenases—removes hydrogen atom. Proteases—hydrolase proteins.

IUB systems of classification
- As per this system enzymes are represented as EC number with 4 digits (IUB system). First digit represent the class, second for the subclass, third for the sub-subclass, and fourth represents specific enzyme in list.

CLASSES: (OTHLIL)
- Oxidoreductases—these class of enzymes catalyze oxidations and reductions.
  - $AH_2+B \rightarrow A+BH_2$
    For example, alcohol dehydrogenase, oxidases, reductases
- Transferases—these classes of enzymes catalyze transfer of moieties between substrate, such as amino acids, glycosyl, methyl, or phosphoryl group
  - $A\text{-}R+B \rightarrow A+B\text{-}R$
    For example, hexokinase, transaminase

- Hydrolases—these classes of enzymes catalyze hydrolytic cleavage of C-C, C-O, C-N, and other bonds by adding of water
  - A-B + H_2O → A-OH + B-H
    For example, acetylcholine + H_2O → choline + acetate catalyzed by acetylcholine esterase
- Lyases—these classes of enzymes catalyze cleavage of C-C, C-O, C-N, and other bonds by elimination, leaving double bonds without adding water-
  - For example, fructose 1,6, bisphosphate $\xrightarrow{Aldolase}$ glyceraldehyde-3-phosphate + DHAP
- Isomerases—these class of enzymes catalyze geometric or structural changes within a molecule, for example, racemases, epimerase, cis-trans isomerases
- Ligases—these class of enzymes catalyze the joining together of two molecules coupled to the hydrolysis of ATP. For example, acetyl-CoA + ATP → malonyl-CoA+ ADP+ Pi.

b. **Various factors which affect the enzyme activity.**

- Enzyme concentration
- Substrate concentration
- Product concentration
- Temperature
- pH (H^+ ion concentration)
- Presence of activators
- Presence of inhibitors
- Presence of repressor or derepressor
- Covalent modification.

Enzyme Concentration
- Rate of enzyme reaction or velocity is directly proportional to enzyme concentration. When the velocity is plotted against enzyme concentration a straight line is obtained. This property is used in estimating the level of enzyme in plasma by end point method (**Fig. 5**).

Substrate Concentration (Fig. 6)
- When the substrate concentration is increased the velocity is also increased initially and after subsequent addition of substrate it leads to loss of enzyme activity and velocity causing a flattened curve afterwards. A rectangular hyperbolic curve is obtained
- The maximum velocity obtained at substrate saturation level is called as V_{max}.

K_m-**Michaelis-Menten constant**
- According to Michaelis theory, the formation of enzyme substrate complex is a reversible reaction, while the breakdown of complex to enzyme and product is irreversible

$$V_i = \frac{V_{max}[S]}{K_m + [S]}$$

- K_m value is substrate concentration at half maximal velocity. It means 50% of enzyme molecules are bound with substrate molecules at that particular substrate concentration.

Effect of Temperature (Fig. 7)
- The velocity of an enzyme catalyzed reaction increases upto a particular temperature and slowly falls in higher

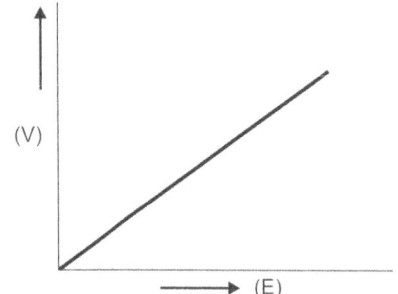

Fig. 5: Effect of enzyme concentration.

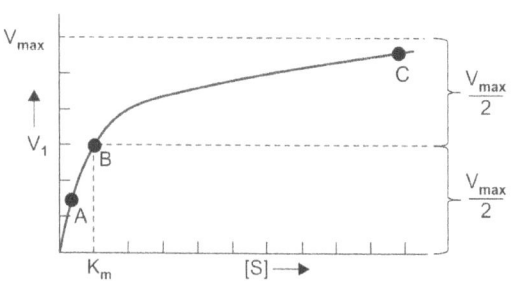

Fig. 6: Substrate concentration.

temperature due to degradation of enzyme molecule
- The temperature at which maximum amount of the substrate is converted to the product per unit time is called the optimum temperature. Most of the enzymes have the optimal temperatures ranges between 37–50°C, except some enzymes, e.g. thermobacillus (Taq pol II) present in bacteria living in hot springs
- When we draw the plot on a graph for velocity against temperature, a bell-shaped curve is obtained
- Temperature coefficient or Q_{10} is the factor by which the rate of catalysis is increased by a rise of 10°C.

Effect of pH (Fig. 8)
- Each enzyme has a unique pH range for maximal activity, beyond these ranges enzyme velocity will slowdown. This is known as optimum pH

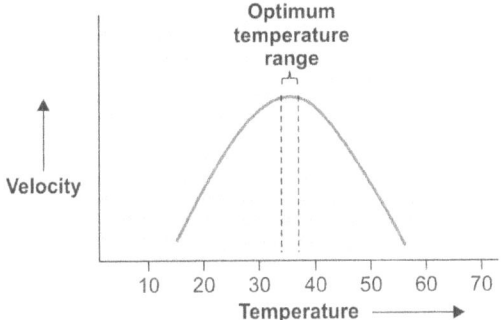

Fig. 7: Effect of temperature.

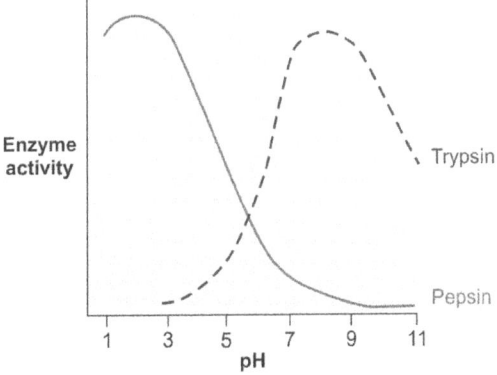

Fig. 8: Effect of pH.

- The velocity of the reaction declines above and below that pH
- When the velocity is plotted against pH a bell-shaped curve is obtained
- Change in pH may denature the enzyme
- The optimal pH for most of the enzymes is pH 6-8 except pepsin with optimum pH of 1-2 and ALP has pH of 9-10 and acid phosphatase has pH 4-5.

Presence of Activators
Enzymes can be activated by:
- Inorganic ions—chloride ions can activate salivary amylase enzyme; lipases is activated by calcium
- Conversion of inactive proenzyme or zymogen to active enzyme, e.g. trypsinogen to trypsin.

Presence of Inhibitors
- Inhibitors can bind reversibly or irreversibly to specific enzymes and reduce their activity, e.g. drugs, toxins, etc. The types of inhibition are: (a) Competitive inhibition; (b) Noncompetitive inhibition; (c) Uncompetitive inhibition; (d) Suicide inhibition; (e) Allosteric inhibition; (f) Feed-back inhibition.

Competitive Inhibition
- Enzyme inhibition in which the inhibitor competes with the normal substrate for the active site of the enzyme. Inhibitor closely resembles the substrate (substrate analogue)
- It may be overcome by increasing substrate concentration and is usually reversible
- K_m is increased but no change in V_{max}
  - For example, in TCA cycle malonate inhibits succinate dehydrogenase (SDH) by competing with succinic acid.

Noncompetitive Inhibition
- Enzyme activity is inhibited by substances that combine with the enzyme at a site other than the active site. This is known as noncompetitive inhibition
- There is no competition between substrate and inhibitor
- It is not relieved by increasing the substrate concentration and is irreversible
- V_{max} is reduced but K_m is not changed

- Increase of substrate concentration will not abolish noncompetitive inhibition, e.g. cyanide inhibits cytochrome oxidase, action of fluoride on enolase.

Uncompetitive Inhibition
- Here the inhibitors have no affinity for free enzyme but it binds with enzyme substrate complex
- V_{max} and K_m are decreased
- For example, inhibition of placental alkaline phosphatase by phenylalanine.

Suicide Inhibition
- It is also known as suicide inactivation or mechanism-based inhibition
- It is a form of irreversible enzyme inhibition
- Here the inhibitor gets more activated with the help of the enzyme to be inhibited. The activated product irreversibly inhibit further reaction
- For example, allopurinol inhibitor of xanthine oxidase (allopurinol gets converted to alloxanthine, a more effective inhibitor of xanthine oxidase).

Allosteric Regulation
- Enzymes which have one catalytic site where the substrate binds and another separate site where the modifier binds are known as allosteric enzymes. [Greek: Allo = Other], e.g. phosphofructokinase
- If the regulatory molecule enhance the activity of the enzyme it is known as allosteric activator (positive modulator) and if it inhibits the enzyme activity it is known as allosteric inhibitor (negative modulator)
- Allosteric regulators are divided into two classes based on the influence of allosteric effector on k_m and V_{max}
  1. K-class of allosteric enzymes—effector changes k_m but not V_{max}, e.g. phosphofructokinase
  2. V-class of allosteric enzymes: effector alters the V_{max}, but not K_m, e.g. acetyl-CoA carboxylase.

Key Enzymes (rate-limiting or regulatory enzymes)
- Allosteric enzyme which regulates a particular metabolic pathway is called a regulatory/rate-limiting/key enzyme of a reaction, e.g. ALA synthase in heme biosynthesis.

Feedback inhibition (end point inhibition): The activity of the enzyme is inhibited by the final product of the biosynthetic pathway, e.g. heme inhibits ALA synthase enzyme by allosteric feedback regulation.

Presence of Repressor or Derepressor
- Repressors act at the gene level and reduce the number of enzyme molecule, e.g. in heme synthesis, the rate-limiting enzyme ALA synthase is autoregulated by heme by repression
- Derepressors will relieve the repression on the operator site and remove the block in the synthesis of the molecule, e.g. glucokinase is induced by insulin.

c. Regulation of enzyme activity.
- Regulation of enzyme activity occurs at different stages and in different ways in an enzyme-catalyzed reaction
- There are regulatory enzymes in each metabolic pathway to regulate overall sequences and also to increase or decrease the catalytic activities. They act in the following ways:
  - Allosteric or noncovalent regulation
  - Covalent regulation
  - Activation of latent enzyme
  - Induction and repression of enzyme synthesis
  - Enzyme degradation
  - Isoenzymes.

Regulation by Allosteric Regulation (Noncovalent Regulation)
- If the effectors inhibit the enzyme activity, they are called as negative effectors
- Allosteric enzymes do not obey the Michaelis-Menton behavior
- When the substrate itself serves as an effector, the effect is called as homotropic
- If the effector is different from the substrate, the effect is said to be heterotropic
- Allosteric enzymes act at other sites than the active site of enzymes or catalytic

site. The allosteric sites are for binding regulatory metabolites which are called effectors or modulators.

Feedback Allosteric Inhibition

- The process of inhibiting the first step of a metabolic pathway by the final product is called feedback inhibition or end product inhibition

$$A \xrightarrow{E1} B \xrightarrow{E2} C \xrightarrow{E3} D \xrightarrow{E4} Product.$$

- For example, aspartate transcarbamoylase is an allosteric enzyme in pyrimidine synthesis. The product CTP inhibits this enzyme by feedback inhibition
- The rate-limiting enzyme of heme synthesis, ALA synthase is inhibited by heme which is the final product by the mechanism.

Covalent Regulation

Reversible regulation by addition of phosphate group (phosphorylation) or removal of phosphate group by dephosphorylation, e.g. glycogen phosphorylase—phosphorylation increased the activity.

Activation of Latent Enzymes

Inactive precursor form of enzymes is called proenzymes or zymogens. They get activated by proteolytic cleavage of one or more peptide bonds.
e.g. Chymotrypsinogen $\longrightarrow$ chymotrypsin
Pepsinogen $\longrightarrow$ pepsin.

Induction and Repression of Enzyme Synthesis

- Most of the enzymes are present in very small concentration and they have short half lives.
- Two types:
  1. **Constitutive enzymes**—housekeeping enzymes which cannot be controlled and their levels are always constant
  2. **Adaptive enzymes**—their concentration increases or decreases as per the body needs.
- Induction—means increased synthesis of enzyme while repression indicates the decreased synthesis. This occurs at the gene level through the mediation of hormones and other substances
  - For example, glycogen synthase is induced by the hormone insulin
  - Pyruvate carboxylase is repressed by glucose.

6. **Name the ketone bodies. How are they formed and utilized in the body. Add a note on the metabolic changes in diabetic ketoacidosis.**

Refer 2005 Essay Question 2.

- The ketone bodies are three in number namely—**acetoacetate, β-hyroxybutyrate and acetone**. Acetoacetate is primary ketone bodies and the other 2 are secondary ketone bodies
- Acetyl-CoA formed from fatty acids can enter and get oxidized in TCA cycle only when carbohydrates are available. During starvation and in uncontrolled diabetes mellitus, the acetyl-CoA takes the alternate fate of formation of ketone bodies
- Level of KB in blood is **less than 1 mg/dL**.
  Site of formation: Liver—mitochondrial matrix of liver cells
  Site of utilization of KB: Extrahepatic tissues
  Uses: During starvation, it is the major fuel for brain, heart and muscles. Brain gets 75% of energy from KB during starvation
- **Precursor:** Acetyl-CoA.

Synthesis of Ketone Bodies (Ketogenesis) Reactions (Fig. 9)

- **Condensation**—two molecules of acetyl-CoA condense to form acetoacetyl-CoA, this reaction is catabolized by thiolase
- **Production of HMG-CoA**—acetoacetyl-CoA condenses with another molecule of acetyl-CoA to produce β-hydroxy-β-methylglutaryl-CoA (HMG-CoA) by the enzyme HMG-CoA synthase. This is the key regulatory enzyme of ketogenesis
- **Lyase reaction**—HMG-CoA is cleaved to acetoacetate and acetyl-CoA by the action of HMG-CoA lyase present only in liver.

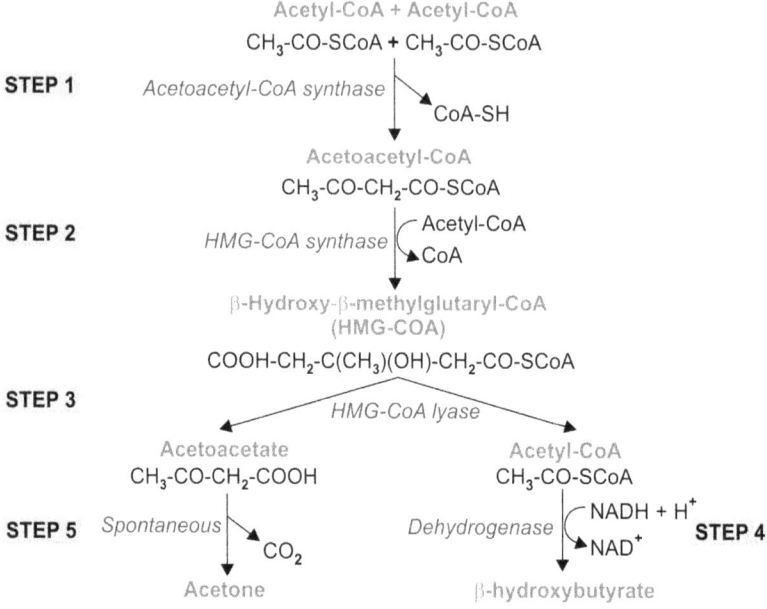

Fig. 9: Synthesis of ketone bodies.

- **Reduction and spontaneous decarboxylation**—acetoacetate is reduced by dehydrogenase to beta-hydroxybutyrate in the presence of NADH or it undergoes spontaneous decarboxylation to form acetone.

Utilization of Ketone Bodies

Ketone body utilization takes place in extrahepatic tissues for energy production. Tissues like heart, renal cortex prefer ketone bodies than glucose for energy production.

Ketolysis Reactions

Acetoacetate is activated to acetoacetyl-CoA by thiophorase enzyme
- Acetoacetate + succinyl-CoA → acetoacetyl-CoA + succinate
- Then acetoacetyl-CoA enters into beta-oxidation pathway to produce energy.

Conditions which Lead to Elevated Ketone Bodies: Ketosis

- Diabetic ketoacidosis
- Prolonged fasting
- Muscle wasting disease.

When the blood level of ketone bodies is more than 1 mg/dL that will lead to ketonemia, ketonuria excretion of KB in urine and smell of acetone in breath.

Features of Ketosis

- Metabolic acidosis
- Kussmaul's respiration—acidotic breathing due to compensatory hyperventilation
- Breath—smells of acetone
- Osmotic diuresis
- Dehydration
- Sodium loss
- Coma.

Laboratory Evaluation of Ketoacidosis

Ketone bodies appear in urine under pathological conditions, such as uncontrolled diabetes mellitus, persistent vomiting, Von Gierke' disease. The major ketone bodies are three—acetoacetic acid, β-hydroxybutyric acid and acetone.

Ketone bodies in urine are analyzed by Rothera's test, rapid tests, such as ketostix strips and acetest tablets.

Rothera's Test

Principle—freshly prepared sodium nitroprusside reacts with ketone bodies and form a purple colored ferropentacyanide complex. This test is specific for acetoacetate and β-hydroxybutyrate.

Procedure: 5 mL of urine is saturated with solid ammonium sulfate. 3 drops of sodium nitroprusside is added and then strong ammonia is poured along the sides of the tube to get a purple ring.

---

7. a. Describe the catabolism of heme in the body. b. Explain the different types of jaundice. How do you investigate a case of jaundice?

Refer 2005 Short Note 3.
- Normal value of total bilirubin is 0.2–0.8 mg/dL; unconjugated bilirubin is 0.2–0.6 mg/dL and conjugated bilirubin is 0–0.2 mg/dL
- If the levels are increased the person becomes jaundiced
- There are 3 types of jaundice—hemolytic (prehepatic) jaundice, hepatocellular (hepatic) jaundice and obstructive (post hepatic).
- Various types of test for diagnosis of jaundice **(Table 1)**:
  - van den Bergh (indirect)—unconjugated bilirubin in blood, positive for prehepatic and hepatic jaundice
  - Direct van den Bergh test—conjugated bilirubin in blood is positive and helps in detection of posthepatic jaundice
  - ALP—normal range: 40–125 U/L, increases slightly in hepatic jaundice and more in posthepatic jaundice
  - Hay's test—this test is specific for identification of urine bile salts—positive for posthepatic jaundice
  - Fouchet's test (conjugated bilirubin in urine)—this test gives positive result for both hepatic and posthepatic
  - Ehrlich test (for urobilinogen)—positive in prehepatic and positive in early stages of hepatic jaundice.

8. What is the normal pH of blood. Describe the various mechanisms which maintain it? Mention the acid-base disorders.

Refer 2005 Essay Question 4.

9. Describe how bilirubin is formed and excreted in the body.

Refer 2005 Short Note 3.

10. Describe the process by which ATP is synthesized in the body.

Refer 2007 Essay Question 7.

11. List the parameters that are commonly used in clinical practice as indicators to assess the functions of the liver. Explain the basis of the use of these parameters in assessment of liver function. Briefly discuss medical conditions in which these parameters become abnormal.

Refer 2005 Short Notes 32.
The tests used to diagnose liver disease are called liver function tests. They are:
- **Tests based on hepatic excretory function:**
  - Serum bilirubin

Table 1: Function tests for differential diagnosis of jaundice.

S.no	Tests	Hemolytic jaundice	Hepatic jaundice	Obstructive jaundice
1.	Serum total bilirubin	Increased	Increased	Increased
2.	Serum conjugated bilirubin / Unconjugated bilirubin	Normal / High	Increased / Increased	Increased / Normal
3.	Van den Bergh	Indirect +	Biphasic	Direct +
4.	Alkaline phosphatase	Normal	Increased	Highly increased
5.	Urine–bile salts (Hay's test)	Nil	Nil	Present
6.	Urine—conjugated bilirubin	Nil	Present	Present
7.	Urine—urobilinogen	Increased	Nil	Nil
8.	Fecal stercobilinogen	Increased	Decreased	Absent

- Urine - Bile pigment, bile salt, urobilinogen
- Fecal urobilinogen
- Dye excretion test—bromosulphthalein (BSP) test.
- **Markers of liver injury—estimation of Liver enzymes:**
  - Serum alanine aminotransferase (ALT)
  - Serum aspartate aminotransferase (AST)
  - Serum alkaline phosphatase (ALP)
  - Serum gamma-glutamyl transferase (GGT).
- **Tests based on synthetic function—(synthesis of plasma proteins)**—estimation of:
  - Total plasma proteins
  - Serum albumin, globulin, A/G ratio
  - Prothrombin time.
- **Special tests**—estimation of:
  - Ceruloplasmin
  - Ferritin
  - Alpha-1 antitrypsin (AAT)
  - Alpha-fetoprotein (AFP)—levels decreased.
- **Tests based on detoxification function**—estimation of:
  - Blood ammonia and bilirubin
  - Hippuric acid.

Abnormal Test Results

Van Den Bergh Test (Hepatic Excretory Function)—Estimation of Bilirubin

- The serum bilirubin estimation is based on van den Bergh reaction where diazotised sulfanilic acid reacts with bilirubin to form a purple colored complex, azobilirubin. Normal serum does not give a positive van den Bergh test
- When bilirubin is conjugated, the purple color is produced immediately on mixing with the reagent, the response is said to be van den Bergh is direct positive
- When the bilirubin is unconjugated, the color appears only after addition of alcohol, so it is said to be van den Bergh is indirect positive
- When both conjugated and unconjugated bilirubins are present, it produces an immediate color which intensifies on adding alcohol. It is then said to be biphasic.
- In hemolytic jaundice—unconjugated bilirubin elevated so it is indirect positive
- In obstructive jaundice—conjugated bilirubin elevated so it is direct positive
- In hepatic jaundice—both conjugated and unconjugated bilirubin elevated so it is biphasic.

Markers of Liver Injury

- Serum alanine aminotransferase—normal 10–35 IU/L, elevated in hepatic diseases, viral and toxic
- Serum aspartate aminotransferase—elevated in liver diseases but lesser than ALT. Ratio of AST/ALT is more than 2 in alcoholic liver disease
- Serum alkaline phosphatase highly elevated in obstructive liver diseases mainly in obstructive jaundice. It is a marker for obstructive jaundice
- Serum gamma-glutamyl transferase-increased in alcoholic liver diseases.

Synthetic Function-Albumin

- Almost all plasma proteins with exception of immunoglobulins are synthesized by liver. Normal total serum proteins level is 6–8 g/dL
- Albumin is quantitatively the most important protein synthesized by the liver, and reflects the extent of functioning liver cell mass. Normal albumin level is 2.5–3.5 g/dL
- In hepatocellular diseases hypoalbuminemia occurs
- Normal serum globulin level is 2 to 3.5 g/dL. In chronic inflammatory disorders, such as hepatitis and in cirrhosis of liver hyperglobulinemia will be present
- A/G ratio—since albumin has a half life of 20 days, in all chronic diseases of liver, the albumin level is decreased. A reversal of A/G ratio is seen in cirrhosis of liver. Normal A/G ratio is 1.2:1 and 1.5:1.
- **Prothrombin time (Synthetic function)**
  - Since prothrombin is synthesized by the liver, it is a useful indicator of liver function.

- The half life of prothrombin is 6 hours only. Therefore prothrombin time (PT) indicates the recent function of liver
- PT is prolonged only when more than 80% of liver function is lost
- In vitamin K deficiency PT is prolonged. To differentiate liver dysfunction from that of vitamin K deficiency, vitamin K is given to the patient and PT is measured. Elevated PT even after administration of vitamin K indicates liver dysfunction.

4. Special tests: Estimation of
- Ceruloplasmin—reduced in Wilson's disease
- Alpha-1 antitrypsin—deficiency causes emphysema
- Alpha-fetoprotein—tumor maker for hepatocellular carcinoma levels decreased.

---

12. a. Describe the role of the kidney to maintain the pH of blood.
b. What are the compensatory mechanisms the kidney will adopt to maintain pH in the presence of metabolic acidosis?

Refer 2005 Essay Question 4.

Metabolic Acidosis
- Primary change is decrease in plasma bicarbonate concentration which is compensated by ↓pCO_2 by hyperventilation
- This occurs in diabetic ketoacidosis, lactic acidosis, renal failure, renal tubular acidosis, etc.

High Anion Gap Metabolic Acidosis
- In metabolic acidosis, due to accumulation of acid anions will make the anion gap between 15 and 20
- This anion gap is increased when there is a decrease in cations as in hypokalemia, hypocalcaemia. When the cations are increased anion gap is altered as in hypoalbuminemia
- High anion gap metabolic acidosis (HAGMA) is seen in (a) Renal failure—the excretion of H^+ and generation of bicarbonate both are deficient; (b) Diabetic ketoacidosis; (c) Lactic acidosis—lactic acid is increased in tissue hypoxia, circulatory failure. (Normal lactic acid is less than 2 mmol/L).

Normal Anion Gap Metabolic Acidosis
- When there is a loss of both anion and cation, the anion gap is normal but acidosis may prevail
- Causes of normal anion gap metabolic acidosis (NAGMA) are:
  - Diarrhea—loss of intestinal secretion leads to acidosis. Bicarbonate, sodium and potassium are lost
  - Hyperchloremic acidosis—occurs in renal tubular acidosis, acetazolamide therapy and in ureteric transplantation.

Decreased anion gap—it is seen in hypoalbuminemia, multiple myeloma, and in hypercalcemia.

Compensation
Metabolic acidosis is compensated by:
- Respiratory compensation—hyperventilation so that pCO_2 comes down. There will be Kussmaul respiration, low pH, bicarbonate will be low. pCO_2 starts decreasing
- Renal compensation—increased excretion of acid and conservation of base occurs. This sets within 2–4 days.

II. SHORT NOTES

---

1. Fatty liver and lipotropic factors.

Refer 2009 Short Answer Question 2.

---

2. Digestion and absorption, transport of iron.

- Iron is mainly absorbed in the stomach and duodenum
- Iron is found in ferric forms in foods which is bound to proteins or organic acids
- Gastric HCl releases the iron from foods
- Reducing substances, such as ascorbic acid and cysteine convert ferric (Fe^{3+}) to ferrous (Fe^{2+}) form. Ferrous iron is easily soluble and readily absorbed.

Factors Affecting Iron Absorption

- Acidity, ascorbic acid and cysteine promote iron absorption
- Iron absorption is increased in iron deficiency anemia
- Small peptides and amino acids favor iron uptake
- Phytate (found in cereals) and oxalates (leafy vegetables) interfere with iron absorption
- High dietary phosphate content decreases iron absorption, while low phosphate promotes
- Iron absorption is impaired in malabsorption syndromes and in total/partial gastrectomy.

Iron in the Mucosal Cells (Fig. 10)

- Iron (Fe^{2+}) entering the mucosal cells is oxidized to ferric form (Fe^{3+}) by the enzyme ferroxidase
- Fe^{3+} combines with apoferritin to form ferritin (storage form of iron)
- From the mucosal cells iron either enters into the bloodstream or lost when the cells are desquamated according to the body needs.

Transport of Iron in the Plasma

- Iron enters the plasma in ferrous state with the help of a transport protein called ferroprotein
- Again it is oxidized to ferric form by a copper containing protein, ceruloplasmin which possesses ferroxidase activity
- Ferric iron then binds with a transport protein, transferrin. Each transferrin molecule can bind with two atoms of ferric iron (Fe^{3+})
- Plasma transferrin (250 mg/dL) can bind with 400 mg of iron/dL of plasma. This is known as total iron binding capacity (TIBC) of plasma.

3. **Isoenzymes and their diagnostic importance.**

Refer 2003 Short Note 5.

4. **Define biological oxidation and mechanism of ATP synthesis.**

Refer 2007 Essay Question 7.
Definition: The transfer of electrons from the reduced coenzymes through the electron transport chain to oxygen is known as biological oxidation.

5. **Principles of balanced diet.**

Refer 2007 Short Note 14.

6. **Transport mechanism across cell membrane. Explain (Flowchart 1).**

- Biological membrane is a semipermeable membrane
- It allows the passage of small uncharged particles but does not allow large polar particles

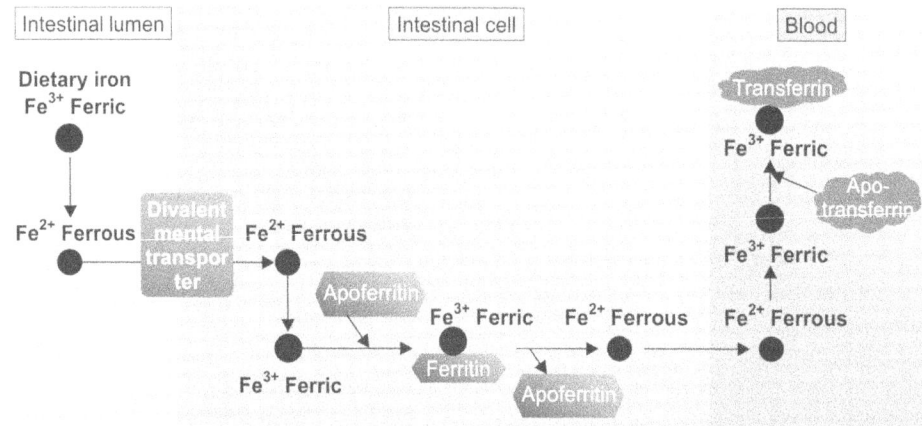

Fig. 10: Iron absorption and transport.

Flowchart. 1: Transport mechanism.

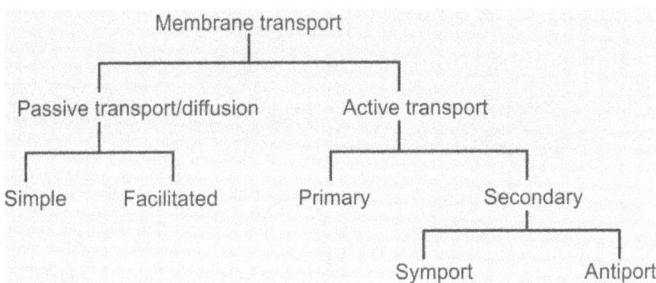

- Membrane proteins are called as carrier proteins or channel proteins. They are highly selective in transport of large molecules
- There are two types of transport mechanisms:
  1. Passive transport/passive diffusion
  2. Active transport.

Passive Diffusion or Transport

- This is the simple process of passive transport of a particular substance across the membrane which depends upon concentration gradient. This does not require energy, e.g. passage of water and gases across the membrane
- The direction is from a region of higher concentration to lower concentration
- Two types—simple diffusion and facilitated diffusion.

Simple Diffusion

- It occurs from higher to lower concentration
- Very slow process
- Does not require energy
- For example, diffusion of gases and transport of lipophilic molecules.

Facilitated Diffusion

- This is a type of passive transport
- It is a carrier mediated process which can operate bidirectionally
- This mechanism is similar to the V_{max} of enzymes
- The entry of the solutes will be competitively inhibited by similar solutes
- No energy is needed
- The rate of transport is more rapid than simple diffusion process

Active Transport

- Movement of molecules across the membrane against concentration gradient with the help of energy is known as active transport.

Salient Features

- It requires energy in the form of ATP
- Transport is unidirectional
- It requires transporters which are integral proteins
- Saturated at higher concentration of solutes
- For example, sodium pump, calcium pump.

Two types of active transport. They are:
1. Primary active transport—sodium pump, calcium pump
2. Secondary active transport—cotransport (symport) and counter transport (antiport).

Primary Active Transport (Fig. 11)

For example, sodium pump—cell has low sodium and high potassium. This is maintained by Na^+K^+ activated ATPase called sodium pump. It continually pumps sodium ions out of the cell and potassium ions from outside to inside generating an electrochemical gradient.

Physiological importance of sodium/potassium pump

- Cell volume is controlled by this pump
- Excitability of neurons and muscles is rendered by this process

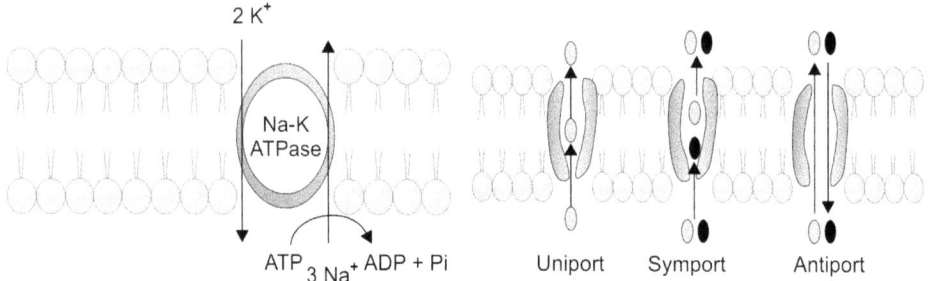

Fig. 11: Primary active transport. **Fig. 12:** Secondary active transport.

- Sugars and amino acids are transported by this pump.

Clinical Significance

Cardiac glycosides like digitonin and ouabain inhibit ATPase enzyme by inhibiting dephosphorylation. Digitalis is hence used in the treatment of congestive failure by enhancing the contractility of cardiac muscle.

Secondary Active Transport (Fig. 12)

- Here energy is provided by ATP indirectly for active transport of ions or molecules against concentration gradient
- Three types of secondary active transport:
  1. Symport or cotransport
  2. Antiport or counter-transport
  3. Uniport system.

1. **Symport/cotransport system (Fig.13)**—transfer of one molecule depends on the simultaneous transfer of another molecule in the same direction, e.g. glucose and many amino acids are transported against concentration gradient by this mechanism

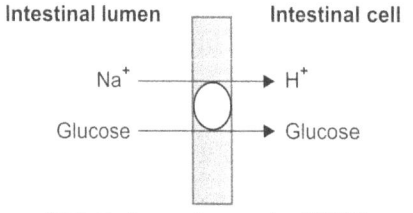

Fig. 13: Symport system.

2. **Antiport or counter-transport system**—transport of two solutes or ions in opposite direction, e.g. sodium—calcium counter transport, sodium—hydrogen counter transport, chloride—bicarbonate exchange in RBC
3. **Uniport system**—transport of single solute across the membrane, e.g. glucose transporters, calcium pump.

7. Cytochrome P450.

Refer 2004 Short Note 20.

8. Galactosemia.

Refer 2005 Short Note 7.

9. Prostaglandins and their importance.

Refer 2005 Short Note 13.

Prostaglandins are a type of eicosanoids which are 20 carbon compounds derived from arachidonic acid.

Synthesis of Prostaglandins (Fig. 14)

- **Cyclo-oxygenase pathway**—in this pathway all the prostaglandins, prostacyclines and thromboxanes are produced except LTs
- Phospholipids in the membranes are acted by phospholipases to release arachidonic acid
- Arachidonic acid is acted by cyclo-oxygenase enzyme to produce PGG2,H2 which are converted to PGD2,E2,F2
- It is also diverted to synthesize PGI2 by prostacycline synthase and TXA2 by thromboxane synthase.

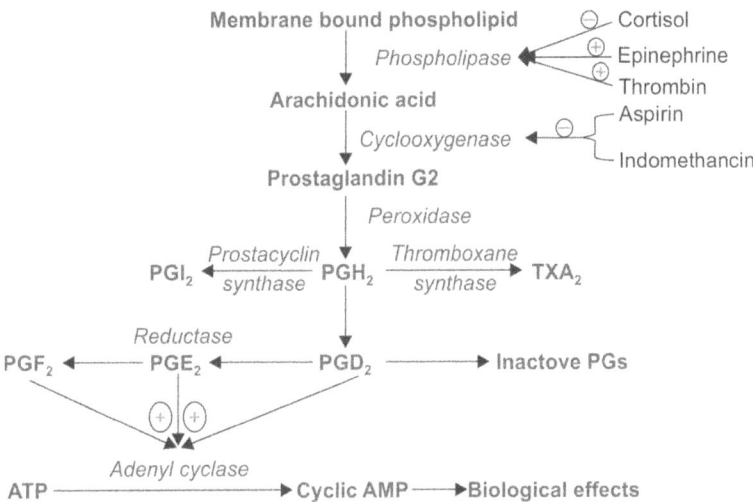

Fig. 14: Synthesis of prostaglandins.

Functions of Prostaglandins and Related Compounds

- **On CVS:**
  - PGI_2 is a powerful vasodilator, hence used in treatment of hypertension. PGI_2 inhibits vasodilatation and inhibits platelet aggregation to promote thrombus formation
  - TXA_2 produced by platelets are vasoconstrictors and cause platelet aggregation. PGI and TX are having opposite actions.
- **On ovary and uterus:** PGF_2 induces termination of pregnancy and induction of labor by stimulating uterine muscles. So it is used in medical termination of pregnancy and to arrest postpartum bleeding.
- **On respiratory tract:**
  - PGE is a potent bronchodilator, whereas PGF is bronchoconstrictor
  - PGE 1 and 2 are used in the treatment of asthma.
- **On immunity and inflammation:** PGE_2 and D_2 induce inflammation by increasing the permeability of capillaries.
- **On gastrointestinal tract (GIT):** PGE inhibit gastric secretion so it is used for treating the gastric ulcers.
- **Metabolic effects:** PGE_2 stimulates glycogenesis, induces calcium mobilization form bones and inhibits lipolysis.

10. Ketosis.

- The ketone bodies are mainly three, namely—acetoacetate, β–hyroxybutyrate and acetone
- Conditions which lead to elevated ketone bodies (ketosis)
- Diabetic ketoacidosis, prolonged fasting, muscle wasting disease.

When the blood level of ketone bodies is more than 1 mg/dL that will lead to ketonemia, ketonuria is excretion of KB in urine and smell of acetone in breath.

Features of Ketosis

- Metabolic acidosis
- Kussmaul's respiration—acidotic breathing due to compensatory hyperventilation
- Breath—smells of acetone
- Osmotic diuresis
- Dehydration
- Coma.

Laboratory Evaluation of Ketoacidosis

Ketone bodies appear in urine under pathological conditions, such as uncontrolled diabetes mellitus, persistent vomiting, Von Gierke disease. The major ketone bodies are acetoacetic acid, β-hydroxybutyric acid and acetone.

Ketone bodies in urine are analyzed by Rothera's test, rapid tests, such as ketostix strips and acetest tablets.

Rothera's Test

Principle—freshly prepared sodium nitroprusside reacts with ketone bodies and form a purple colored ferropentacyanide complex. This test is specific for acetoacetate and acetone. β-hydroxybutyrate will not answer this test.

Procedure—5 mL of urine is saturated with solid ammonium sulphate. 3 drops of sodium nitroprusside is added and then strong ammonia is poured along the sides of the tube to get a purple ring at the junction of two liquids.

11. Thyroid function tests.
Refer 2003 Short Note 16

12. Recombinant DNA technology.
Refer 2007 Short Note 23.

13. Structure of DNA (Watson–Crick model).
Refer 2006 Essay Question 10.

14. Post-transcriptional modifications.
Refer 2011 Essay Question 3 and also refer Short Notes 35 and 53 of this year

Transcription is the process of synthesis of RNA and the changes that occur after transcription is known as post-transcriptional modification.

15. Functions of albumin.
Refer 2009 Short Note 40.

16. Electrophoresis and its applications.
Refer 2006 Short Note 30.

17. Causes for respiratory acidosis.
- Pneumonia
- Bronchitis
- Asthma
- COPD
- Sedatives
- Paralysis of respiratory muscles
- Brain tumor, head injury
- Ascites, peritonitis
- Sleep apnea.

Respiratory acidosis is due to primary excess of carbonic acid due to hypoventilation caused by retention of CO_2. Ratio of bicarbonate to carbonic acid will be less than 20.

18. Renal mechanism of maintaining acid base balance.
Refer 2005 Essay Question 4. Also refer Essay Questions 8 and 12.

19. Purine salvage pathway.
Refer 2004 Short Note 15.

20. Lac operon concept.
Refer 2004 Short Note 19.

21. 2,3 BPG—formation and its role.
Refer 2007 Short Note 18.
Other names bisphosphoglycerate shunt (BPG shunt), Rapoport-Leubering cycle.

22. Mechanism of synthesis of ATP in ETC.
Refer 2007 Essay Question 7.
- Coupling of oxidation with phosphorylation is known as oxidative phosphorylation. Oxidative phosphorylation is explained by chemiosmotic theory by Peter Mitchell
- The transport of protons from inside to outside of the inner mitochondrial membrane of electron transport chain is accompanied by the generation of proton gradient across the membrane
- Protons (H^+ ions) accumulate outside the membrane to create an electrochemical potential difference and this force drives the synthesis of ATP by ATP synthase V complex.

There is also the creation of pH gradient on either side of the membrane.

COMPLEX V OF ETC–ATP SYNTHASE
- It is a proton assembly in the inner mitochondrial membrane
- It has 2 functional subunits–F_1 and F_0 and looks like a lollipop. F_0 is embedded in the membrane and water insoluble. Both F_0 and F_1 are connected by a protein

stalk. Protons enter through' F_0 subunit and it acts as a proton channel. F_1 unit projects into the matrix and catalyzes ATP synthesis
- As per Boyer's hypothesis, there will be a conformational change in the mitochondrial membrane proteins which leads to ATP synthesis. This is considered as Rotary motor or energy driving model or binding-change model
- ATP synthase enzyme has a central gamma unit surrounded by alternating α3 and β3 subunits. Due to the proton flux γ subunit rotates and that induces conformational changes in the β3 subunits which releases ATP. One β subunit has open (O) conformation, second has loose (L) conformation and third has tight (T) conformation
- Protons induce the rotation of γ subunit which in turn induces conformational changes in β subunits. ADP and Pi bind to β subunits in L conformation to form ATP by changing O site to L conformation and then T to O conformation and 3 ATP are generated for each revolution. So ATP synthase is considered as world's smallest molecular motor.

REGULATION OF ATP SYNTHESIS

- Availability of ADP—respiratory or acceptor control
- Source of NADH and $FADH_2$ from TCA cycle.

23. Explain 'methyl folate trap'.
Refer 2010 Short Note 2.

24. Carnitine shuttle.
Refer 2012 Short Answer Question 34.

25. What are dietary fibers and explain their importance in human nutrition with respect to the prevention of diseases.
Refer 2008 Short Note 10.

26. Write briefly about the significance of HMP shunt pathway.
Refer 2005 Short Note 2.

- Other name—pentose phosphate pathway or HMP pathway; Warburg-Dickens-Horecker pathway, phosphogluconate oxidative pathway
- It is an alternative pathway to glycolysis and TCA cycle for oxidation of glucose.

27. Sources, RDA and biological role of vitamin C.
Refer 2005 Essay Question 5.

28. Describe the energetics of complete oxidation of 1 mole of glucose to CO_2 and H_2O under aerobic conditions.

- **Total ATP synthesis in aerobic glycolysis = 7**
  - Glyceraldehyde-3-phosphate dehydrogenase (oxidative phosphorylation through ETC) = 2.5 × 2 = 5 ATP
  - 1,3-bisphosphoglycerate kinase (substrate level phosphorylation) = 1 × 2 = 2 ATP
  - Pyruvate kinase (substrate level phosphorylation) = 1 × 2 = 2 ATP
  - Total utilization of ATP glycolysis = 2 (hexokinase step and phosphofructokinase step)
  - **Net production of ATP in aerobic glycolysis = 9 - 2 = 7**
- Pyruvate to acetyl-CoA—Pyruvate Dehydrogenase—NADH – 5 ATP
- TCA cycle

Reactions	Coenzyme	ATP (old calculation)	ATP (new calculation)
Isocitrate to α-KG	NADH	3	2.5
α-KG to succinyl-CoA	NADH	3	2.5
Succinyl-CoA to succinate	GTP	1	1
Succinate to fumarate	FADH2	2	1.5
Malate to oxaloacetate	NADH	3	2.5
From 2 acetyl-CoA		12 12 × 2 = 24	10 10 × 2 = 20
Total ATP = 7 + 5 + 20 = 32 ATP			

29. Bile salts—synthesis and biological role.
Refer 2004 Short Note 9.

30. Write briefly about calcium homeostasis.

Refer 2004 Essay Question 4.

31. Active form of methionine and its function.

Refer 2007 Essay Question 4.

32. Inhibitors of protein biosynthesis.

Refer 2013 Essay Question 4.

Reversible Inhibitors in Prokaryotes

- Antibiotics–Bacteriostatic:
  - Tetracyclines—bind to 30S prevents attachment of aminoacyl tRNA to the ribosomal acceptor site
  - Chloramphenicol—inhibits peptidyl transferase
  - Erythromycin and clindamycin prevents translocation process.
- Bactericidal antibiotics:
  - Aminoglycosides:
    - Streptomycin is irreversible inhibitor of 30S ribosomes
    - Low concentration and of misreading mRNA
    - Pharmacological concentration—prevents initiation complex; total inhibition of translation.

Inhibitors—Eukaryotes

- Cycloheximide—inhibits both human and bacterial peptidyl transferase (60S)
- Diphtheria toxin—inactivates eEF2 by attaching ADP to eEF2; prevents translocation
- Ricin toxin—inactivates 28S rRNA.

Inhibitors—Prokaryotes and Eukaryotes

Puromycin structural analog of tyrosin tRNA incorporated into the peptide chain causing inhibition of elongation in both prokaryotes and eukaryotes. It acts as a research tool.

33. Porphyria.

Refer 2009 Essay Question 5.

34. LAC operon.

Refer 2004 Short Note 19.

35. Transcription and post-transcriptional modification.

Refer 2011 Essay Question 3.

36. Cyclic AMP.

Refer 2005 Short Note 8.

37. Detoxification by conjugation.

Refer 2004 Short Note 14.

38. Renal function tests.

Classification of Renal Function Test

To screen for Kidney Diseases

- Urine analysis—physical, chemical and microscopic examination
  - **Physical examination**
    - Volume (24-hours urinary output)
    - Appearance—color
    - pH
    - Specific gravity
    - Osmolality
    - Smell
  - **Chemical examination**:
    - Qualitative analysis for abnormal constituents of urine mainly glucose, protein and blood
  - **Microscopic examination of the centrifuged sediment of urine:**
    - For RBC, WBC, pus cells, crystals—to rule out urinary stones and casts.

Estimation in Blood

- **Blood urea**—blood urea is elevated in renal conditions like acute glomerular nephritis, early stages of nephrosis, malignant hypertension, and pyelonephritis. Elevation of blood urea is known as uremia.
- **Serum creatinine**—this is a better marker of renal function than blood urea. It is elevated in renal failure cases.

To assess Glomerular Function

- Glomerulus acts as a sieve in filtering blood but it retains cells and proteins thus forming a glomerular filtrate normally 170 to 180 L/day. Out of this only 1.5 L of

fluid is excreted as urine and the rest are reabsorbed through the tubules
- **Glomerular filtration rate (GFR)**—normal GFR is 120-125 mL/min. This is reduced in renal failure
- **Clearance tests**—done to assess the glomerular filtration and renal blood flow
- **Renal clearance of a substance is the volume of plasma from which the substance is completely cleared by the kidney in 1 minute**
- Clearance = mg of substance excreted per min/mg of substance per mL of plasma; $C = U \times V/P$, where C = clearance of the substance; U = concentration of the substance in urine; P = Concentration of the substance in plasma; V= Volume of urine passed per minute
- Clearance is expressed as milliliter of plasma per unit time
- Clearance tests—this test is done by using either endogenous markers, such as urea or creatinine or exogenous markers like Inulin, ^{51}Cr labeled EDTA, ^{99}Tec-labeled EDTA, etc. Out of all creatinine clearance test is the best
- Creatinine clearance test—it is based on the rate of excretion of metabolically produced creatinine which is excreted through urine. Creatinine is freely filtered by the glomeruli but not reabsorbed by the tubules. A small amount of creatinine is secreted by the tubules
- 24-hours urine is collected and blood is also collected for the estimation of creatinine. Urinary volume is measured (V) and the concentration of creatinine in urine (U) and plasma (P) are estimated and by using the formula $C = U \times V/P$ the creatinine clearance is calculated
- Normal range for creatinine clearance is 90-129 mL/min
- Reduced creatinine clearance indicates chronic renal damage and reduced blood flow to glomeruli.

To Assess Tubular Functions

- Renal tubules reabsorb or secrete certain substances, concentrate the urine and acidify the urine. So it is important for maintaining specific gravity and osmolality of urine.
- **The following are the tubular function tests:**
  - **Specific gravity (SG) of urine**—it is the simplest test. Specific gravity of urine depends on the concentration of the solutes. In early stages of renal failure SG may be low due to kidney's inability to excrete solutes
  - **Urine concentration test (fluid deprivation test)**
    - Fluid intake is restricted for 15 hours. The first urine sample in the morning is collected and SG and osmolality are measured
    - If the SG is more than 1.025 or the osmolality exceeds 850 mOsmol/kg the renal concentration capacity is said to be normal
    - Renal concentration ability is impaired due to tubular defect or in diabetes insipidus where there is decreased secretion of antidiuretic hormone.
  - **Measurement of Osmolality**—measurement of urine and plasma osmolality is done by using osmometer. Normal urinary osmolality ranges from 60-1200 mOsmol/kg. Normal Plasma osmolality is 285-300 mOsm/kg. The ratio between urine/plasma osmolality is calculated. Normal ratio is around 3-4.5. Urinary osmolality is decreased in diabetes insipidus
  - **Dilution tests**—this is done to check whether kidneys can excrete an excess water load. After emptying the bladder 1000-1200 mL of water is given to the patient. Hourly urine is collected for next 4 hours. In each sample, volume, specific gravity and osmolality are measured. A normal person will excrete all the water load within 4 hours. It is a more sensitive test
  - **Urinary acidification test** (acid load test or ammonium chloride loading test)
    - This is used to diagnose renal tubular acidosis

- Ammonium chloride is given orally in gelatin capsule (100 mg/kg body weight) to induce metabolic acidosis. HCl produced is excreted as acidified urine
- Hourly urine collected for 2-8 hours pH and acid excretion of each sample noted
- Atleast one sample should have pH lesser than 5.5. pH is not decreased in cases of renal tubular acidosis.
- **Fractional excretion of bicarbonate, sodium and phosphate in urine**—also help in assessing renal tubular functions.

Markers of Glomerular Permeability: Proteinuria

- Glomerular sieve will not permit bigger molecules having molecular weight more than 67,000D. But in glomerular damage which occurs in diseases like diabetic nephropathy the higher molecular weight proteins are also filtered and appeared in urine
- Albumin is one of the first protein to appear in urine due to glomerular damage
- Types of proteinuria are: Glomerular proteinuria, microalbuminuria, overflow proteinuria, tubular proteinuria, etc.

39. Tumor markers.

Refer 2003 Short Note 20.

40. Different mechanisms involved in hormone action.

As per the mechanism of action, hormones are grouped as Group I and II. Group II has 5 subgroups–IIA, IIB, IIC, IID, IIE
- Group I—hormones with intracellular receptors, e.g. glucocorticoids, androgen, estrogen, calcitriol, thyroxine
- Group II—hormones binding with cell surface receptors
- It has 5 sub groups depending on the second messenger:
  - **Group IIA**—acting through **Cyclic AMP as second messenger,** e.g. ACTH, FSH, glucagon, calcitonin
  - The cAMP (second messenger) in turn activates the enzyme protein kinase
  - This kinase is a tetrameric molecule having two regulatory and two catalytic subunits
  - This complex has no activity. But cAMP bind to the regulatory and catalytic subunits.
  - **Group IIB**—hormones binding with cell surface receptors and acting through **Cyclic GMP as second messenger**, e.g. atrial natriuretic peptide (ANP) and nitric oxide
  - **Group IIC**—hormones binding with cell surface receptors and acting through **calcium or phosphatidyl-inositol (PIP$_2$) as second messenger,** e.g. TRH, oxytocin, vasopressin, catecholamines
  - **Group IID**—hormones having cell surface receptors and mediating through **tyrosine kinase**—e.g. insulin, somatomedin, IGF
  - **Group IIE**—hormones having cell surface receptors and their intracellular messenger is a kinase or utilizing phosphatase cascade, e.g. GH, interleukin.

41. Role of carnitine in beta-oxidation of fatty acids.

Refer 2008 Essay Question 1.

42. Covalent modification of enzymes in regulation of enzyme activities.

- It is one of the regulations of enzyme activity
- Covalent modification is mostly done by addition or removal of phosphate groups from seine/tyrosine/threonine residues of the enzyme **(Fig. 15)**
- Reversible regulation is done by addition of phosphate group (phosphorylation) or removal of phosphate group (dephosphorylation)
  - For example, glycogen phosphorylase—phosphorylation increases the activity

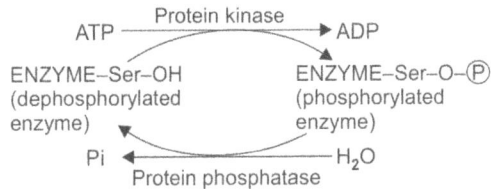

Fig. 15: Covalent modification.

and dephosphorylation decreases the activity of phosphorylase
- Glycogen synthase—phosphorylation decreases the activity of glycogen synthase, whereas dephosphorylation increases the activity of glycogen synthase.

43. Lactose intolerance.

Refer 2011 Short Answer Question 8.

44. What is the importance of the pentose phosphate pathway in the body?

Refer 2005 Short Note 2.

45. Gluconeogenesis with reference to definition, substrates, sites and importance in the body.

Refer 2008 Essay Question 6.

Definition: Synthesis of glucose from non-carbohydrate substrates (sources)
- Sites: Organs—liver and kidney (Cortex)
- Substrates—pyruvate, lactate, amino acids (glucogenic), propionate, glycerol.

Key Enzymes in Gluconeogenesis

- **Pyruvate carboxylase**—pyruvate in the cytoplasm enters the mitochondria. Then, carboxylation of pyruvate to oxaloacetate is catalyzed by pyruvate carboxylase. It needs biotin and ATP
- **Phosphoenolpyruvate carboxykinase (PEPCK)**—It converts oxaloacetate to phosphoenolpyruvate by removing CO_2. GTP donates the phosphate
- **Fructose 1,6-bisphosphatase:**
  - Fructose 1, 6-bisphosphate → fructose-6-phosphate + Pi
  - This step will bypass PFK step.
- **Glucose-6-phosphatase**—it is active in liver and absent in muscle.
  - Glucose-6- phosphate + H_2O → glucose + Pi

Importance of Gluconeogenesis

- Whenever carbohydrate source is insufficient, gluconeogenesis meets the needs of the body to maintain blood glucose homeostasis
- It is a continuous source of glucose to tissues like brain, RBC, lens, cornea of eyes, and renal medulla.

46. Role of vitamin D in the body.

Refer 2003 Short Note 1.

47. Causes of iron deficiency and manifestations of such deficiency.

Causes of Deficiency of Iron

- Deficient dietary intake of iron
- Defective absorption—malabsorption syndrome after surgery
- Hookworm infestation
- Repeated pregnancies
- Chronic blood loss as in piles, peptic ulcer and uterine bleeding
- Nephrosis, subtotal gastrectomy and lead poisoning are other causes of iron deficiency.

Clinical Features

- Microcytic hypochromic anemia ensues
- In anemia body cells lack oxygen and the person becomes apathic
- Severe iron deficiency leads to heart failure
- Chronic deficiency leads to achlorhydria, impaired attention, irritability, lower memory, poor scholastic performance.

48. Isoenzymes with reference to definition, examples and clinical importance.

Refer 2003 Short Note 5.
- Multiple molecular forms of an enzyme catalyzing the same reaction are isoenzymes or isozymes, e.g. lactate dehydrogenase—5 isoenzymes—(LDH 1,2,3,4 and 5), creatine kinase—3 isoenzymes (CK-1, 2,3) and alkaline phosphatase

- They are physically distinct forms of the same enzyme activity
- They are synthesized from various tissues and hence useful to study the disorders of those organs
- They are made up of different subunits. If the subunits are the same they are known as homomultimer. They are represented by same gene. If the subunits are different they are known as heteromultimer produced by different gene
- Separation and identification of isoenzymes:
  - Electrophoresis—depends upon the mobility in electrical field
  - Heat stability—some gets denatured by heat, e.g. bone isoenzyme of ALP
  - Inhibitors—tartrate labile ACP
  - Substrate specificity or K_m value—different for each isoenzyme, e.g. glucokinase and hexokinase
  - Localization—LDH-H4 form is present in heart; LDH-M4 in skeletal muscle.

Lactate Dehydrogenase

- LDL catalyzes the conversion of pyruvate to lactate and vice versa. LDL is concentrated in RBC cell; therefore minor hemolysis causes the false value. Normal values ranges from 100-200 U/L
- Elevation of LDH is seen in hemolytic anemia, hepatocellular damage, muscular dystrophy, cancer, etc.
- LDH is tetramer made up of two H (heart) bands and two M(muscle) bands. Both of these are same molecular weight and with minor amino acid variations
- There are 5 isoenzymes. They are LDH1, LDH2, LDH3, LDH4, and LDH5
- With two different polypeptide chains therefore 5 combinations of H and M are possible namely H4, H3M, H2M2, M3H, M4. The tissue specificity and diagnostic importance of these 5 isoenzymes is as follows:
  - H4 form found in heart which is useful for diagnosing heart disease
  - M4 form found in muscle, hence it is useful in diagnosing muscle diseases
  - Isoenzymes of LDH help in the diagnosis of heart and liver diseases
  - Flipped pattern is observed in myocardial infarction (LDH1 > LDH2)
- Increased activity of LDH5 is an indicator of liver diseases.

Creatine Kinase

- It catalysis the synthesis of creatine phosphate from creatine and ATP
- Normal blood ranges from 15-100 IU/L
- It is made up of 2 polypeptides namely M and B, therefore 3 combinations of isoenzymes are possible. They are MM found in skeletal muscle, MB found in heart and BB found in brain
- Creatine kinase (CK) subform is highly elevated in muscular dystrophies, acute cerebrovascular injuries. It is most reliable factor in diagnosing AMI
- Three isoenzymes—CK BB(1), CK MB(2), CK MM(3):
  - CK BB (1) present in brain
  - CK MB (2) is the earliest reliable marker of myocardial infarction
  - CK MM (3) is elevated in muscle diseases.

Alkaline Phosphatase

- It is nonspecific enzyme which hydrolyses aliphatic, aromatic and heterocyclic compounds at pH 9-10 in the presence of Mn and Mg. Zinc is a constituent ion of alkaline phosphatase (ALP)
- ALP produced by osteoblasts for the calcification process
- Normal serum levels are 40-125 U/L. Moderate increase seen in hepatic diseases, and very high levels are seen in hepatic obstruction and in bone diseases
- ALP has nearly 6 types of Isoenzymes which are:
  - Alpha-1 ALP, alpha-2 heat labile ALP, alpha-2 heat stable ALP, pre-beta ALP, Gamma- ALP, leukocyte ALP (LAP). They are due to the difference in the carbohydrate content
  - Alpha-1 ALP—it is about 10% total ALP and is increased in obstructive jaundice
  - Alpha-2 ALP—it is about 20% of total ALP and heat llabile increased in hepatitis.

- Alpha 2 heat stable ALP—it is about 1% of total ALP. It is heat stable above 65°C
- Pre-beta ALP—it is about 50% of total ALP. It is elevated in bone diseases
- Gamma ALP—it is about 10%, it is increased in ulcerative colitis
- Leukocyte ALP (LAP)—it is increased in lymphomas and decreased in chronic myeloid leukemia.

Acid Phosphatase

- It acts at a pH between 4 and 6
- Normal value in serum is 2.5–12 U/L
- Secreted by prostate cells, RBCs, WBCs and platelets
- The value of acid phosphatase (ACP) is increased in prostate cancer and it is an important tumor marker for prostate cancer
- It has got a tartrate labile isoenzyme which is helpful in follow-up of prostate cancer. Its normal level is 1U/L.

49. Glycated hemoglobin with reference to its formation, reference value in blood and its clinical importance.

Refer 2007 Short Note 15.

50. Thiamine with reference to its functions in the body, dietary sources and deficiency manifestations.

Refer 2003 Essay Question 1 and 2007 Essay Question 8.

51. Denaturation of proteins.

Refer 2009 Short Note 31.

52. Types of mutations.

Refer 2008 Short Note 34.

53. Post-transcriptional modifications of RNA.

Refer 2011 Essay Question 3.

54. Restriction endonucleases and their uses.

Refer 2007 Short Note 28.

55. Specialized products derived from tyrosine.

Refer 2012 Short Note 38.

56. Principle and applications of electrophoresis.

Refer 2006 Short Note 30.

57. Cell cycle.

Refer 2011 Short Note 36.

58. Causes and clinical features of dehydration.

Refer 2010 Short Note 35.

59. Consequences of hyperuricemia.

Refer 2008 Short Note 18.

- Uric acid is the catabolic end product of purine nucleotides
- Normal blood level of uric acid is 2–5 mg/dL for females and 3–7 mg/dL for males When uric acid level is increased in blood it is known as hyperuricemia
- Because of increased level of uric acid in blood, it tends to get deposited as crystals in synovial fluid of joints leading to inflammation and acute arthritis. This disease is called gout
- Two types of gout—primary and secondary gout
- Uric acid gets deposited in the cooler areas of body like distal joints to form tophi
- Hyperuricemia leads to increased excretion of uric acid through kidneys, so uric acid crystals gets deposited in the urinary tract leading to renal calculi.

60. Structure of DNA (Watson–Crick model).

Refer 2006 Essay Question 10.

- In 1953 James Watson and Francis Crick deduced the double helical structure of DNA
  Right handed double helix—DNA consists of 2 helical polynucleotide chains twisted around in right handed double helix. Purine and pyrimidine bases are inside the helix. Phosphate and deoxyribose units are on the outside. The planes of bases are perpendicular to the helical axis. Sugars are kept at right angles to the bases
- **Base pairing rule (Chargaff's rule)**
  - In DNA, the 2 strands are complementary to each other

- The number of adenine molecules are equal to thymine molecules (A=T) and number of cytosine molecules are equal to guanine molecules (C=G)
- Adenine pairs with thymine by 2 hydrogen bonds (A=T); guanine pairs with cytosine by 3 hydrogen bonds (GC). This is called Chargaff's rule.
- **Hydrogen bonding**—adenine pairs with thymine by 2 hydrogen bonds (A=T); guanine pairs with cytosine by 3 hydrogen bonds (GC). GC bond is stronger than AT bond
- **Antiparallel**—the 2 strands of DNA run antiparallel to each other. One strand runs in 5' to 3' direction, while the opposite strand runs in 3' to 5' direction.

Structure of Helix (Fig. 16)

- Diameter or width of the helix is 20Å (1.9 to 2.0 nm)
- It has a pitch of 3.4 nm per turn
- Within a single turn 10 base pairs are seen
- Adjacent pairs are separated by 0.34 nm
- It has a major groove (1.2 nm) and a minor groove (0.6 nm) which wind along the molecule parallel to the phosphodiester backbone
- Proteins interact with the bases in these grooves.

Different forms of DNA Double Helix

DNA exists in six structural forms. They are: A-DNA, B-DNA, C-DNA, D-DNA, E-DNA and Z-DNA. Out of these A, B, and Z forms are important.

- **B-DNA**—it has the classic Watson–Crick model. It is the most common form
- **A-DNA**—is right handed helix having 11 base pairs per turn
- **Z-DNA**—is a left handed helix containing 12 base pairs per turn. The polynucleotide strands of DNA move in a zigzag fashion.

S. No.	Property	A-DNA	B-DNA	Z-DNA
1.	Shape	Broadest	Medium	Narrow
2.	Type of helix	Right handed	Right handed	Left handed
3.	Base pairs per turn	11	10	12
4.	Helix diameter	25.5Å	23.7Å	18.4Å
5.	Pitch per turn of helix	25.3Å	35.4Å	45.6Å
6.	Major groove	Narrow	Wide	Flat
7.	Minor groove	Very broad	Narrow	Very narrow

III. SHORT ANSWER QUESTIONS

1. **Key enzyme of cholesterol synthesis and its regulation.**

- Key enzyme of cholesterol synthesis—HMG-CoA reductase
- HMG-CoA is reduced by a NADPH-dependent enzyme to form mevalonate (6C)
- Statin group of drugs like lovastatin, compactin competitively inhibit HMG-CoA reductase enzyme.

2. **Formaminoglutamic acid (FIGLU).**

Refer 2010 Short Answer Question 28.

3. **Refsum disease.**

- This is due to defect in the alpha oxidation due to the deficiency of the enzyme phytanic acid alpha oxidase
- So phytanic acid is not degraded and gets accumulated in the nervous tissue
- It is a rare neurological disorder characterized by cerebral ataxia and peripheral neuropathy, retinitis pigmentosa, and nerve deafness

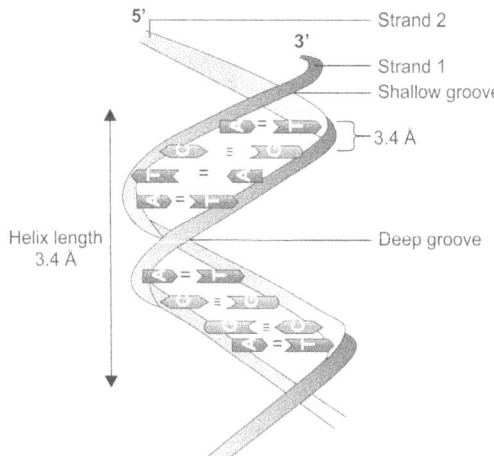

Fig. 16: Structure of helix.

- Symptoms get regressed with restricted intake of phytanic acid
- Milk contains more phytanic acid and it has to be avoided.

4. Comparison between prokaryotic and eukaryotic cells.

Refer 2006 Short Note 26.
- Prokaryotic cells do not have typical nucleus, e.g. bacteria and algae
- Eukaryotic cells have nucleus surrounded by nuclear membrane
- The anatomical and physiological differences between prokaryotic and eukaryotic cells are tabulated as follows:

S. No.	Characteristics	Prokaryotic cells	Eukaryotic cells
1.	Size	Small (1–10 µm)	Large (10–100 µm)
2.	Cell membrane	Rigid cell wall	Flexible plasma membrane
3.	Subcellular organelles	Absent	Distinct organelles seen (mitochondria, nucleus, lysosomes)
4.	Nucleus	Not well defined; no nuclear membrane	Well defined nucleus surrounded by nuclear membrane; DNA present with histones
5.	Mitochondria	Absent. Enzymes of energy metabolism bound to membrane	Present. Energy in the form of ATP synthesized in mitochondria
6.	Cytoplasm	Organelles and cytoskeletons are absent	Contains organelles and cytoskeletons
7.	Cell division	By fission; no mitosis	Mitotic division
8.	Examples	Unicellular organisms—bacteria, algae	Multicellular organisms—higher animals and plant cells

5. Glycosides.

- Glycosidic linkages or bonds are formed when the hemiacetal or hemiketal OH group of anomeric carbon (C-1) reacts with a hydroxyl group of another carbohydrate or noncarbohydrate (like alcohol—glycerol or phenol)
- Noncarbohydrate units are called aglycones. The bonds may be O- glycosidic if they form disaccharides, oligosaccharides or polysaccharides
- The bonds may be N-glycosidic which are found in nucleotides, e.g. ATP
- The resulting compounds are called glycosides. If the sugar is glucose the compound is called glucosides
- Glycosides do not reduce Benedict's reagent as there is no free aldehyde or keto group but they may be hydrolyzed with boiling with dilute acids to release free sugar to reduce Benedict's reagent.

Glycosides of medical importance (All are of plant origin)
- Antibiotics like streptomycin is a glycoside
- Cardiac glycosides like ouabain and digoxin which increase the heart muscle contraction and used in the treatment of congestive heart failure. They inhibit Na^+/K^+ ATPase system
- Anticancer drugs, such as daunorubicin and doxirubicin are anthracycline glycosides.

6. Metal cofactors of enzymes.

- Metalloenzymes are enzymes which require metal ions for their activity. These enzymes hold the metals tightly and are not readily exchanged, e.g. carbonic anhydrase—zinc, phenol oxidase—copper
- Metal activated enzymes—in this type the metal is not tightly held by the enzyme and can be exchanged easily with other ions, e.g. ATPase—Mg^{2+} and Ca^{2+}, enolase-Mg^{2+}.

7. Beriberi.

Refer 2009 Short Note 26.
- The deficiency of thiamine leads to disease called beriberi, its features are depending on its type which are as follows:

Wet Beriberi

Affects cardiovascular system
- It is related to edema of face, trunk, and serous cavities.

- Breathlessness, palpitation, swollen calf muscles, elevated systolic pressure, fast and bouncing pulse are seen
- The heart becomes weak.

Dry Beriberi

Affects nervous system

- It is mostly related to degeneration of nervous system (peripheral neuritis)
- Muscles are weak and unable for movement and patients are become bedridden.

Infantile Beriberi

The child has symptoms like sleeplessness, restlessness, vomiting, convulsions, and death.

Deficiency is Assessed by

- Assay of thiamine in biological samples
- Assessment of transketolase activity in erythrocyte is the key indicator of TPP deficiency.

8. Lipid profile.

- Total plasma lipids—400-600 mg/dL
- Total cholesterol—150-200 mg/dL
- HDL cholesterol—30-60 mg/dL (male); 35-75 mg/dL (female)
- LDL cholesterol—60-150 mg/dL
- Triglycerides—50-200 mg/dL (male); 40-150 mg/dL (female)
- Phospholipids—150-200 mg/dL
- Free fatty acids—10-20 mg/dL.

9. Limiting amino acids.

Refer 2009 Short Answer Question 9.
- Some of the proteins do not contain one or more essential amino acids. These limit the weight gain or growth of the animals when those proteins are fed to the animals. They are known as limiting amino acids for that particular protein
- Limiting amino acids in:
  - Rice and wheat: Lysine and threonine—rectified by feeding pulse proteins
  - Zein: Tryptophan and lysine meat proteins rectify this
  - Bengal gram: Cysteine and methionine—rectified by cereals.

Protein	Limiting amino acids	Proteins has to be supplemented
Rice	Lys, thr	Pulse proteins
Zein	Tyr, lys	Meat proteins
Tapioca	Phe, tyr	Fish
Bengal gram	Cys, met	Cereals

10. Glucose-6-phosphate dehydrogenase enzyme. Explain.

Refer 2009 Short Answer Question 37.
- Hexose monophosphate pathway is an alternate pathway in carbohydrate pathway
- It has two phases of reactions:
  1. Phase I (oxidative phase)—irreversible phase
  2. Phase II (nonoxidative phase)—reversible phase.

Oxidative Phase

- **Step 1:** Rate-limiting step catalyzed by glucose-6-phosphate dehydrogenase enzyme which is NADP-dependent. One NADPH is produced.

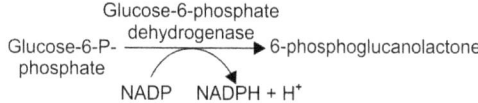

Glucose-6-phosphate dehydrogenase deficiency—Congenital

- It is the most common inborn error of metabolism. It is X-linked recessive trait
- This will lead to drug induced hemolytic anemia
- The deficiency is manifested only when exposed to certain oxidant drugs or toxins like primaquine for malaria or ingestion of toxic glycosides in fava beans (favism)
- Sulfa drugs may also precipitate hemolysis. This leads to jaundice and severe anemia
- This disease offers resistance to plasmodium infection and protects the individual from malaria since the parasite requires reduced glutathione which is not available in the G6PD deficiency.

11. Enzyme defect in: (a) Phenylketonuria; (b) Alkaptonuria.

- It is due to deficiency of phenylalanine hydroxylase in phenylalanine metabolism

- So phenylalanine is not converted into tyrosine and it gets accumulated-condition which is known as hyperphenylalaninemia
- The excess of phenylalanine is converted to phenylpyruvate, phenyllactate, and phenylacetate and phenylacetylglutamine. Phenylpyruvate, phenyllactate, phenylacetate are excreted in urine.

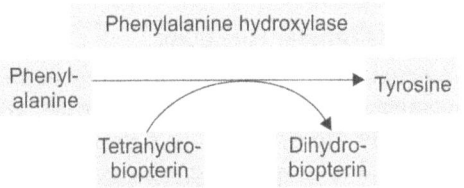

- **Alkaptonuria:** It is an autosomal recessive condition affecting 1:250,000 births in tyrosine metabolism
  - It is due to the defect in homogentisate oxidase enzyme
  - Homogentisate gets accumulated and oxidized to benzoquinone acetate and forms alkaptone bodies.

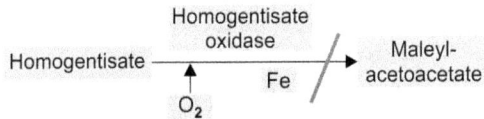

12. DNA polymerase enzyme.

Refer 2012 Short Answer Question 21.

DNA—dependent DNA polymerase-different in bacteria and mammals
- Bacterial (prokaryotic) DNA polymerase
  - DNAP—I (Pol I) (Kornberg enzyme)—repair enzyme
  - DNAP—II (Pol II)—proofreading and repair
  - DNAP—III (Pol III)—synthesizing leading and lagging strands.
- Mammalian (eukaryotic): DNA polymerase—5 types: $\alpha, \beta, \gamma, \delta$ and ε
  - Alpha—gap filling
  - Beta—DNA repair
- Gamma—mitochondrial DNA synthesis
- Delta—synthesis of leading and lagging strand
- Epsilon—proofreading and DNA repair.

13. Types of mutations.

Refer 2008 Short Note 34.

14. Reverse transcriptase.

Refer 2009 Short Note 32.
- Synthesis of DNA from RNA by reverse transcriptase enzyme is known as reverse transcription
- Genetic material for many living organisms is in DNA.
- Reverse transcriptase is RNA-dependent DNA polymerase
- DNA-dependent RNA polymerase is involved in transcription (production of mRNA from DNA)
- But some viruses and other organisms have only RNA as their genetic material. Retro viruses are RNA viruses, e.g. HIV
- The enzyme reverse transcriptase will make DNA strand from RNA. Usually transcription is the production of mRNA from DNA. So this process of making DNA from RNA is named as reverse transcription
- Once the virus infects human cells, the viral RNA is converted into DNA by reverse transcription and this DNA is known as complementary DNA (cDNA)
- The single-stranded DNA acts as template to produce double-stranded (ds) DNA. This DNA is incorporated into human genome and it leads to the production of viral proteins and RNA.

15. Inhibitors of RNA synthesis.

Refer 2017 Short Notes 35.

PROKARYOTES

- **Rifampicin**—inhibits initiation by binding to β subunit of RNAP, no formation of phosphodiester bond, used in the treatment of TB and leprosy
- **Actinomycin D–chemotherapy**—binds to DNA template and interferes in the movement of RNAP.

OTHER INHIBITORS

- Alpha-amanitin—toxin from mushroom, inactivates RNA polymerase II
- 3'-deoxyadenosine—causing chain termination.

16. Features of genetic code.

Refer 2005 Short Note 19.
- The letters A, G, T, and C correspond to the nucleotides found in DNA
- Within the protein coding genes these nucleotides are organized into three-letter code words called codons, and the collection of these codons makes up the genetic code
- The code provides a foundation for explaining the way in which protein defects may cause genetic disease and for the diagnosis and perhaps for the treatment of these disorders
- A triplet sequence of nucleotide on the mRNA is the codon for each amino acid
- There are four different bases they can generate 64 codons.

SALIENT FEATURES

Refer 2005 Short Note 19.

17. Gout.

Refer 2005 Short Note 17.

18. Name two renal function tests.

To Assess Glomerular Function

- Glomerulus acts as a sieve in filtering blood but it retains cells and proteins thus forming a glomerular filtrate normally 170 to 180 liters/day. Out of this only 1.5 liters of fluid is excreted as urine and the rest are reabsorbed through the tubules
- **Glomerular filtration rate (GFR)**—normal GFR is 120–125 mL/min. This is reduced in renal failure
- **Clearance tests**—done to assess the glomerular filtration and renal blood flow
- **Renal clearance of a substance is the volume of plasma from which the substance is completely cleared by the kidney in 1 minute**
- **Clearance** = mg of substance excreted per min/mg of substance/mL of plasma
- C = U x V/P, where C = Clearance of the substance; U = Concentration of the substance in urine; P = Concentration of the substance in plasma; V= Volume of urine passed/minute.

To Assess Tubular Functions

- Renal tubules reabsorb or secrete certain substances, concentrate the urine and acidify the urine. So it is important for maintaining specific gravity and osmolality of urine
- **The following are the tubular function tests:**
  - **Specific gravity (SG) of urine**—it is simplest test
  - **Urine concentration test (fluid deprivation test):**
    - Fluid intake is restricted for 15 hours. The first urine sample in the morning is collected, SG and osmolality are measured.
  - **Measurement of osmolality**—measurement of urine and plasma osmolality are done by using osmometer
  - **Dilution tests**—this is done to check whether kidneys can excrete an excess water load
  - **Urinary acidification test** (acid load test or ammonium chloride loading test)—
    - This is used to diagnose renal tubular acidosis
    - Ammonium chloride is given orally in gelatin capsule (100 mg/kg body weight) to induce metabolic acidosis. HCl produced is excreted as acidified urine.

19. Denaturation of proteins.

Refer 2009 Short Note 31.

20. Name two enzymes that are increased in hepatic jaundice.

- Alanine transaminase
- Aspartate transaminase
- GGT
- Alkaline phosphatase.

21. What are zymogens? Give an example.
Refer 2009 Short Answer Question 4.

22. Mention two inhibitors of ETC with their site of action.

Inhibitors of ETC (Fig. 17)

Site Specific Inhibitors
- **Complex I to coenzyme Q (CoQ) specific inhibitors:**
  - Barbiturates—amobarbital
  - Antibiotic—piercidin
  - Rotenone an insecticide, fish poison
  - Alkylguanides—hypotensive drugs.
- **Complex II to coenzyme Q**
  - Carboxin
- **Complex III to cytochrome c inhibitors:**
  - Antimycin
  - British anti-Lewisite (BAL)
  - Naphthoquinone.

23. What is specific dynamic action and importance in calculating caloric requirements of an individual?

Refer 2010 Short Answer Question 9.
- It is represented as thermogenic effect of food
- This refers to increased heat production or increased metabolic rate following the intake of food
- The heat is produced after intake of food which is due to energy expenditure for digestion and absorption of food from reserved energy (diet induced thermogenesis)
- Specific dynamic action (SDA) can be considered as the activation of energy needed for various chemical reactions. This activation energy is to be supplied initially. This activation energy is varied to different food
- For example, for carbohydrate—5%, for proteins—30% and for fat—15% etc.
- If a person takes 250 g of carbohydrates, SDA is calculated as follows:
  - Actual calories from 250 g carbohydrate = $250 \times 4 = 1{,}000$ kcal

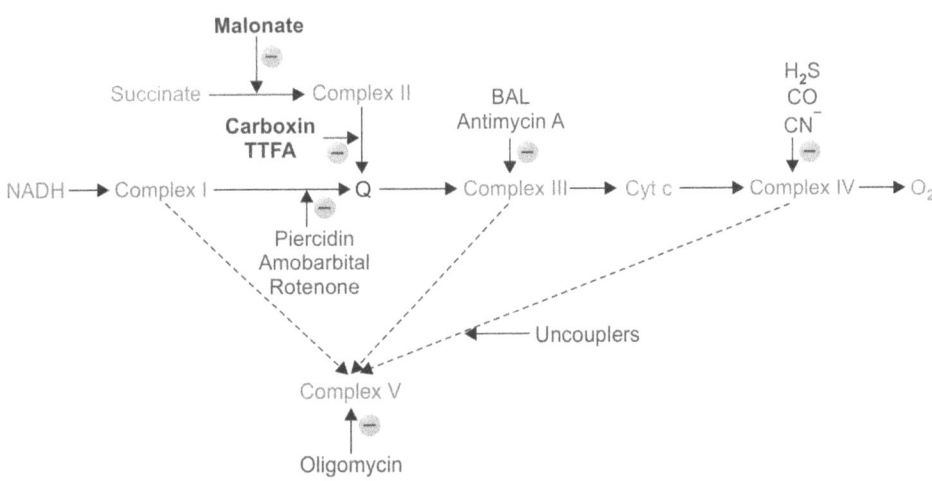

Fig. 17: Inhibitors of electron transport chain.

- SDA of CHO = 5%, i.e. about 100 kcal is drawn from our reserve energy, thus net generation of energy from 250 g is 900 kcal.
- Hence an extra calorie should be provided to account for the loss of energy as SDA
  - Energy requirement of an individual depends upon—occupation, physical activity and lifestyle which can be divided into 3 groups—sedentary, moderate and heavy. Heavy workers need high BMR
  - Energy requirement is calculated by the energy required for—1. Basal metabolic rate (BMR), 2. Specific dynamic action (SDA), 3. Extra energy expenditure for physical activities.

24. What are trace minerals? Give RDA of any two of them.

Trace elements are the minerals whose requirement is less than 100 mg/day. They are iron, iodine, copper, manganese, zinc, molybdenum, selenium and fluoride.
- **RDA of ninc:** For adults is 10 mg/day; children 10 mg/day
- RDA of Selenium : 50-100 µg/day
- RDA of iodine : 150-200 µg/day.

25. What is steatorrhea?

- This condition is due to defective digestion of lipids
- Daily excretion of fat in feces is more than 6 g/day. Unsplit fat is seen in feces
- It is due to:
  - Defect in the secretion of bile or pancreatic juice into the intestine
  - Chronic diseases of pancreas
  - Impairment in the lipid absorption by the intestinal cells.

26. What is suicide inhibition? Give an example.

- It is also known as suicide inactivation or mechanism-based inhibition
- It is a form of irreversible enzyme inhibition
- Here the inhibitor gets more activated with the help of the enzyme to be inhibited. The activated product irreversibly inhibit further reaction
- For example, allopurinol inhibitor of xanthine oxidase (allopurinol gets converted to alloxanthine, a more effective inhibitor of xanthine oxidase).

27. Laboratory criteria for diagnosis of diabetes mellitus.

Refer 2012 Short Answer Question 39.
- Fasting blood glucose—should be more than 126 mg/dL for more than two occasion OR If 2-hours post-glucose level of OGTT—more than 200 mg/dL (even at one occasion)
OR
- Both fasting and 2 hour values above these levels on the same occasion
- Random plasma glucose level is more than 200 mg/dL on more than one occasion
- Glycated Hb (HbA1c) more than 6.5% at any occasion—this is the preferred method for initial diagnosis of diabetes mellitus (DM).

28. Name the insulin dependent glucose transporters and their tissue distribution.

- Type 4 (GluT4)—it is the only transporter under the control of insulin. It is distributed in skeletal muscle, heart muscle and adipose tissues
- In type II diabetes mellitus there is reduction in membrane. GluT4 to produce insulin resistance in muscle cells and in adipocytes.

29. What is pulmonary surfactant and its clinical importance?

Refer 2011 Short Answer Question 25.
- Dipalmitoyl lecithin, phosphatidylglycerol, cholesterol and surfactant proteins A, B and C are the constituents of lung surfactant produced from the lung epithelium
- This is needed for the normal functioning of lungs. It decreases the surface tension of the aqueous layer of lung and prevents collapse of lung alveoli

- Low levels of lung surfactant in newborn children leads to respiratory distress syndrome (RDS) which is the most common cause for neonatal mortality
- Administration of natural or artificial surfactants is of therapeutic benefit.

30. What is the biochemical basis of development of cataract in diabetes mellitus?

- In diabetes mellitus, the increased glucose present in the body will be converted to high level of sorbitol through polyol pathway
- This sorbitol concentration increases in the lens causing osmotic damage and cataract. Galactitol also gets deposited over the lens to develop cataract.

31. ELISA.

Refer 2009 Short Note 15.
- Enzyme-linked immunosorbent assay (ELISA)
- It is a nonisotope immunoassay
- ELISA is used widely to measure hormone, growth factors, tumor markers, bacterial and viral antigens, etc.
- Here the antigen is labeled with a stable enzyme, whereas in radioimmunoassay a radioisotope is used.

Principle

- Enzymes used as labels catalyze color change in the substrate which is then detected
- The amount of enzyme labeled antigen bound is inversely proportional to the amount of antigen in the serum being analyzed
- Commonly used enzyme substrate combinations are: Alkaline phosphatase with substrate, p-nitrophenyl and horseradish peroxidase with tetramethylbenzidine
- Two types of ELISA:
  1. Antibody detection—indirect ELISA (single antibody)
  2. Antigen detection—sandwich ELISA (double antibody).

Antibody Detection: Indirect ELISA

- This is used to detect small quantities of antibodies
- HIV antibody is detected by this method. Specific antigen to the antibody coated well is taken.
- Then the sample (serum) is added and incubated. The antibody in patient's sample binds to the antigen and fixed.

32. Hyperkalemia.

Refer 2014 Short Answer Question 32.
- The normal plasma potassium level is 3.5 to 5.2 mmol/L
- Plasma potassium level above 5.5 mmol/L is known as hyperkalemia
- Hyperkalemia is life-threatening. It is characterized by flaccid paralysis, bradycardia, and cardiac arrest
- ECG—elevated T-wave, widening of QRS complex, lengthening of PR interval.

Causes

- Decreased renal excretion of potassium—urinary tract obstruction, renal failure, deficient aldosterone, heart failure
- Entry of potassium to extracellular space—increased hemolysis, tissue necrosis, burns, tumor lysis, crush injury
- Redistribution of potassium to extracellular space—metabolic acidosis, diabetes mellitus, tissue hypoxia
- Hyperkalemic periodic paralysis
- Drugs—spironolactone, ACE inhibitors, beta-blockers, cyclosporine, digoxin
- Pseudohyperkalemia—seen in hemolysis, improper blood collection, thrombocytosis, leukocytosis or polycythemia.

Treatment

When potassium level >6.5 mmol/L, intravenous glucose and insulin should be given. Continuous ECG monitoring should be done.

33. Okazaki fragments.

Refer 2015 Short Answer Question 40.

34. Thyroid function tests.

Refer 2003 Short Note 16.
- Thyroid gland synthesize the thyroid hormones—thyroxine (T3 and T4) and calcitonin

- Thyroid function tests are useful in assessing the functioning of thyroid gland and to diagnose the hyper- and hypothyroidism.

In Vitro TFT

Assay of Hormones

a. **Serum Total T3 and T4 by immunoassay—RIA/ELISA**
   - Normal T3 = 70-200 ng/dL; T4 = 5-12.5 µg/dL
   - In hyperthyroidism, thyroid hormone levels—both T3 and T4 levels are increased but TSH levels decreased
   - In hypothyroidism, T3 and T4 are reduced in serum but TSH level is increased.

b. **Free T3 and T4 (fT3 and fT4)**
   - More reliable test
   - Normal value of free T4 = 10-27 pmol/L; T3 = 3-9 pmol/L
   - Values increased in hyperthyroidism, thyrotoxicosis and decreased in hypothyroidism.

c. **Thyroid binding proteins—thyroid binding globulin (TBG)**
   - Normal level of TBG = 12-28 µg/mL
   - TBG—increased in hypothyroidism, pregnancy and in estrogen therapy
   - Level decreased in hyperthyroidism, nephrotic syndrome.

d. **Resin uptake test (T_3RU or T_3U)**
   - Indirect estimate of binding capacity of plasma TBG
   - Radioactive iodine labeled—^{125}I-T_3 is added to the patient's serum which will occupy the free binding sites on TBG. Excess unattached $_{125}I$-T_3 is removed and the amount taken up by the resin is estimated
   - Normal value of T_3U is 25-35%
   - Values increased in hyperthyroidism and decreased in hypothyroidism.

e. **Plasma TSH (RIA method)**
   - Normal value = 2 to 6 µU/mL
   - In primary hyperthyroidism, TSH level is elevated due to lack of feedback but in secondary hyperthyroidism, TSH, T3 and T4 levels are low.

f. **Thyroid antibodies**
   - To detect autoimmune disorders of thyroid gland caused due to the antibodies against thyroid tissues.

In Vivo Tests

- **Thyroid iodine uptake test**—tracer amounts of radioactive iodine ^{131}I is given to the patient and its uptake by the thyroid gland is measured. Normal value—1-13% absorbed after 2 hours and 15-45% is absorbed after 24 hours
- **TRH stimulation test:** An abnormal response is observed in hyperthyroidism and hypopituitrism
- **TSH stimulation test:** IV administration of TSH will increase blood thyroid hormone level
- **Thyroid scanning**—ultrasonography.

35. Creatinine clearance.

- Renal clearance of a substance is the volume of plasma from which the substance is completely cleared by the kidney in 1 minute
- Clearance = mg of substance excreted per min/mg of substance per/mL of plasma; C = U x V/P, where C = Clearance of the substance; U = Concentration of the substance in urine; P = Concentration of the substance in plasma; V = Volume of urine passed/minute. Clearance is expressed as milliliter of plasma/unit time
- Creatinine clearance test—it is based on the rate of excretion of metabolically produced creatinine which is excreted through urine. Creatinine is freely filtered by the glomeruli but not reabsorbed by the tubules. A small amount of creatinine is secreted by the tubules
- 24-hours urine is collected and blood is also collected for the estimation of creatinine. Urinary volume is measured (V) and the concentration of creatinine in urine (U) and plasma (P) are estimated and by using the formula C = U x V/P the creatinine clearance is calculated
- Normal range for creatinine clearance is 90-120 mL/min

- Reduced creatinine clearance indicates chronic renal damage and reduced blood flow to glomeruli.

36. Gamma-aminobutyric acid (GABA).
Refer 2010 Short Answer Question 38.

37. Isoelectric pH of proteins.
Refer 2006 Short Note 11.

38. Maple syrup urine disease.
Refer 2009 Short Answer Question 31.

39. Multiple myeloma.
Refer 2013 Short Answer Question 51 also.
- It is otherwise known as plasmacytoma.
- In this condition Ig secreting cells are transformed into malignant cells due to the proliferation of one clone which is seen as M band or monoclonal band or myeloma band on electrophoresis
- Multiple myeloma is characterized by paraproteinemia, anemia, lytic bone lesions and proteinuria. Pathological fracture of weight bearing bones, ribs and vertebrae are commonly seen
- Excretion of monoclonal light chains in urine—Bence Jones proteinuria
- Laboratory findings:
  - Bone marrow examination—large number of malignant plasma cells
  - X-ray—punched out osteolytic lesions in bones and more in skull
  - Hypercalcemia and hypercalciuria
  - Electrophoresis—raised beta-2 microglobulin, M band
  - Bradshaw test—positive (few mL of urine layered over few mL of concentric HCl shows white ring of precipitate).

40. Lesch-Nyhan syndrome and orotic aciduria.
Refer 2015 Short Answer Question 60.
A. Lesch-Nyhan syndrome
- It is a X-linked inborn error of purine metabolism and it is due to complete deficiency of HGPRTase which acts in purine salvage pathway
- It affects mainly males

- So the salvage pathway is stopped and PRPP accumulates which will go for increased purine synthesis and catabolism of purines to uric acid
- Hyperuricemia leads to nephrolithiasis and gout
- It is also characterized by self-mutilation, mental retardation.

B. Orotic aciduria: (autosomal recessive condition)
- This condition results from the absence of either or both the enzymes ORPTase, OMP decarboxylase of pyrimidine synthetic pathway
- There are 2 types—type I and II
  - **Type I orotic aciduria:** The condition results from the absence of either or both of the enzyme orotate phosphoribosyl transferase (ORPTase)and OMP decarboxylase—the enzyme of pyrimidine synthesis
  - **Type II orotic aciduria:** The condition results from the absence of the enzyme OMP decarboxylase.

Clinical Features
- Growth is retarded and megaloblastic anemia is present
- Orotic acid crystalluria.

41. List the vitamins that are required for the functioning of the citric acid cycle.
- Only the coenzymes of B-complex group of vitamins play important role in TCA cycle
- Five coenzymes help in α-ketoglutarate dehydrogenase step; TPP from B1 or thiamine, NAD from niacin, FAD from riboflavin, CoA from pantothenic acid and lipoic acid
- NAD—helps as coenzyme for:
  - Isocitrate dehydrogenase
  - α-ketoglutarate dehydrogenase
  - Malate dehydrogenase
- FAD—acts as coenzyme for α–ketoglutarate dehydrogenase and succinate dehydrogenase steps
- CoA, lipoic acid and TPP—in α-ketoglutarate dehydrogenase reaction.

42. Give two examples of drugs that act as inhibitors of enzyme and name the enzyme that each one inhibits.

- Usually they are structural analogue of the substance
- They bind and compete to the substrate binding site of the enzyme forming an enzyme inhibitory complex (EI)
- K_m value is increased but no change in V_{max}

Examples:
1. Many drugs act as competitive inhibitors, e.g. sulfonamide is an analogue of PABA and inhibits pteroid synthetase in the folic acid synthesis
2. Allopurinol inhibits xanthine oxidase.

43. What is the function of mitochondria in a cell?

Structure of Mitochondria (Fig. 18)

- It is rod like or spherical double membrane structure having diameter of 0.5–1 μm and length of 7 μm
- Outer membrane is permeable to small molecules. The inner membrane is folded inside to form cristae which increase the surface area. Inner mitochondrial membrane contains enzymes of electron transport chain (ETC)
- Space between two membranes is called the intermitochondrial space which contains enzymes like adenylate kinase
- Space within the inner membrane is mitochondrial matrix which contains enzymes of citric acid cycle, beta-oxidation of fatty acids.

Functions of Mitochondria

- It helps in oxidative phosphorylation
- It is called **power house of cell** because it synthesizes ATP through electron transport chain. Energy released from oxidation of foodstuffs is trapped as chemical energy in the form of ATP. Inner mitochondrial membrane has the ETC which has got 4 complexes through which electrons are transferred from metabolic reactions to synthesize ATP at the 5th complex by oxidative phosphorylation.
- Important metabolic pathways occur only in the mitochondria and the enzymes of those pathways are located in various parts of the mitochondria, e.g. TCA cycle, beta-oxidation of fatty acids, ketone body synthesis
- Some of the metabolic pathways occur partly in mitochondria and partly in cytosol, e.g. urea cycle, gluconeogenesis, heme synthesis and pyrimidine synthesis.
- **Cytochrome P450** enzyme systems present in inner mitochondrial membrane is involved in steroidogenesis
- Mitochondria have specific DNA. Message from the DNA can synthesize mitochondrial proteins by the ribosome of mitochondria. Hence, mitochondria are considered as the evolutionary remnant of parasites
- They play important role in initiating apoptosis.

44. What is the mechanism of action of statins? What is the therapeutic use of this group of drugs?

- Statin group of drugs like lovastatin, mevastatin, compactin, etc. are structural analogues of intermediates in the conversion of HMG-CoA to mevalonate by the enzyme HMG-CoA reductase which is the rate-limiting enzyme of cholesterol synthesis
- So these drugs competitively inhibit HMG-CoA reductase enzyme and interfere with the synthesis of cholesterol
- The synthesis of cholesterol will be inhibited and they act as hypocholesterolemic drugs.

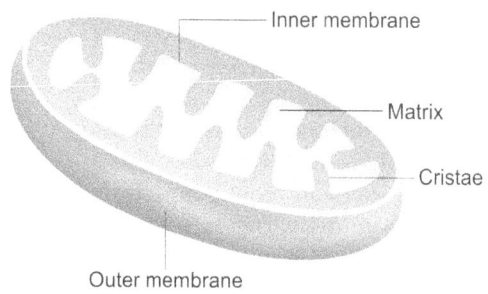

Fig. 18: Structure of mitochondria.

45. List two dietary sources and two biochemical functions of vitamin C in the body.

- Vitamin C is a water-soluble vitamin
- Other name—**ascorbic acid,** antiscorbutic vitamin
- **Sources: Vegetables and fruits**
  Rich sources: Gooseberry (amla), citrus fruits, guava, green vegetables, tomatoes, potato.

Biochemical Functions of Vitamin C

Vitamin C is the coenzyme for hydroxylase.
  - **Hydroxylation of proline and lysine—** post-translational hydroxylation of proline and lysine residues are necessary for the formation of cross-links in collagen to give strength to the fibers
  - **Tyrosine metabolism:**
    a. **Dopamine-β-hydroxylase** is a copper-containing enzyme involved in the synthesis of the catecholamines like norepinephrine and epinephrine from tyrosine in the adrenal medulla and central nervous system
    b. Vitamin C helps in oxidation of para-hydroxyphenylpyruvate to homogentisic acid.
- **Hydroxylation of tryptophan** to 5 hydroxytryptophan (serotonin) by hydroxylase enzyme needs vitamin C.

46. Explain the mechanism of action of cyanide as a poison.

Refer 2015 Short Answer Question 27.
- Complex IV of respiratory chain is inhibited by classic poisons like cyanide (others are H2S and CO)
- Cyanide inhibits the enzyme cytochrome oxidase and prevents transfer of electrons from cytochrome aa3 to molecular oxygen and thereby arrests respiration
- It causes tissue anoxia by chelating the ferric ions of the intracellular respiratory enzyme cytochrome oxidase and stops cellular respiration
- It is present in air as HCN which comes from vehicle exhaust
- Cyanide in large quantity affects CNS which may lead to convulsion, coma and death and in low dose it leads to headache, dizziness and numbness.

47. List two good dietary sources of iodine. What is the function of this mineral in the body?

- Sources: Seafood, drinking water, iodized table salt, onions, vegetables
- RDA: 150–200 µg/day

Functions

- Only biological role of iodine helps in the formation of thyroxine (T4) and tri-iodo thyronine (T3) and help in a large number of metabolic functions
- About 80% of body iodine is stored in thyroglobulin as iodothyroglobulin in thyroid glands
- Radioactive iodine is useful in thyroid scanning I^{131}.

48. Enzyme defect and most common clinical feature in Von Gierke disease?

Refer 2003 Short Note 6.

49. What is meant by glycemic index of food?

- It is assessed by GTT (glycemic response) after a particular diet and compare it with a reference meal 50 g of glucose

$$\text{Glycemic index} = \frac{\text{Incremental area under glucose tolerance curve after 50 g test meal}}{\text{Incremental area under glucose tolerance curve after 50 g of glucose (reference meal)}} \times 100$$

- Simple carbohydrates like glucose or sugar will have high glycemic index
- But the same amount of complex carbohydrates like starch or dietary fibers have lower glycemic index as the digestion and absorption of these carbohydrates are slow
- Glycemic index of carbohydrates is lowered if it is combined with proteins fat or fibers

For example, potato chips have high GI (85-90) whereas ice cream has lower GI (around 35) as it has lots of fats.

50. List two differences between marasmus and kwashiorkor.

Marasmus—this is due to severe deficiency of both dietary energy and proteins—primary calorie insufficiency and secondary protein deficiency. Marasmus means to waste.

Kwashiorkor—this is due to isolated deficiency of proteins with sufficient calorie intake. Kwashiorkor means sickness the older child gets when the next child is born.

The differences between these two malnutrition conditions are tabulated.

	Marasmus	Kwashiorkor
Age of onset	Below 1 year	1–5 years
Deficiency of	Calorie and proteins	Proteins alone
Cause	Early weaning and repeated infection	Starchy diet after weaning. Precipitated by acute infection
Growth retardation of child	Marked	Severe

51. What is multiple myeloma? Which laboratory test can be used to confirm diagnosis of this condition?

Refer 2013 Short Answers Question 39.
- It is otherwise known as plasmacytoma
- In this condition Ig secreting cells are transformed into malignant cells due to the proliferation of one clone which is seen as M band or myeloma band on electrophoresis
- Multiple myeloma is characterized by paraproteinemia, anemia, lytic bone lesions and proteinuria. Pathological fracture of weight bearing bones.

Laboratory Findings
- Bone marrow examination—large number of malignant plasma cells
- X-ray–punched out osteolytic lesions
- Hypercalcemia and hypercalciuria
- Raised beta-2 microglobulin and M band in gamma region of serum electrophoresis
- Bradshaw test—positive.

52. List four functions of nucleotides.

Refer 2014 Short Note 20.
- Nucleotides are nitrogenous base + pentose sugar + phosphate group
- They are the phosphorylated nucleosides
- The phosphate group is attached to the hydroxyl group of pentoses by an ester linkage
- Depending on the nature of the pentoses, the nucleotides are of 2 types: (1) Ribonucleotides; (2) Deoxyribonucleotides
- Depending upon the number of phosphate groups added they are known as: 1P—monophosphates (MP), 2P—diphosphates (DP) and 3P—triphosphates (TP).

Ribonucleotides

a. Adenosine ribonucleotides:
   - AMP-Cyclic AMP—Major metabolic regulator and second messenger in hormonal action
   - ATP—energy currency of cell; high energy phosphate. It helps in the formation of active methionine (SAM) involved in transmethylation; it is also needed for the synthesis of certain coenzymes like NAD, FAD, etc.
b. Guanosine ribonucleotides–GMP, GDP and GTP
   - Cyclic GMP—it is also a second messenger for hormonal action
   - GTP—involved in protein synthesis as energy source.
c. Uridine ribonucleotides—UMP, UDP and UTP
   - UDP sugars act as donors of sugar for the synthesis of glycogen (UDP- glucose)
   - UDP-galactose—for the synthesis of glycoproteins and proteoglycans
   - UDP-glucuronate is a conjugating agent for conjugation of bilirubin, drugs, etc.
d. Cytosine ribonucleotides—CDP, CDP and CTP
   - CDP choline is needed for the synthesis of sphingomyelin.
e. Hypoxanthine nucleotide
   - Ionosine monophosphate (IMP)—precursor or parent nucleotide of purine ribonucleotides.

Deoxyribonucleotides

dAMP, dGMP, dCMP, dthymidine (dTMP)—they are present in DNA.

53. Which amino acid gives rise to nitric oxide in the body? What is the enzyme that catalyzes this process?

- Amino acid—arginine
- Enzyme—nitric oxide synthase contains heme, FAD, FMN, tetrahydrobiopterin, NADPH.

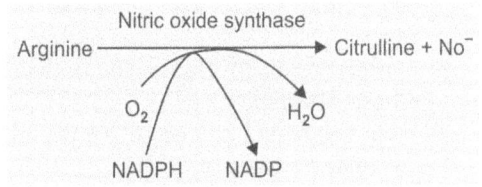

54. What is the biochemical basis of the encephalopathy that can develop in patients who have liver cirrhosis?

- Proteins are degraded in liver to produce ammonia which is toxic to the body especially affects brain
- Ammonia is detoxified in the liver to produce urea and excreted through kidney
- Liver cirrhosis is a common cause of hyperammonemia
- In cirrhosis there will be collateral circulation around the liver
- Portal blood is shunted directly into systemic circulation and so ammonia level in serum will be elevated above 5-35 micromole/liter
- Ammonia has direct neurotoxic effect on the CNS causing symptoms like slurred speech, drowsiness, vomiting, cerebral edema and blurred vision causing hepatic encephalopathy
- In very high concentration ammonia causes coma and death.

55. List the biochemical abnormalities seen in phenylketonuria.

Refer 2010 Short Note 39.

56. Give examples of four conjugating agents in the body that are involved in metabolism of xenobiotics.

Refer 2004 Short Note 14.

57. What is the role of gamma-aminobutyric acid in the body? Name the amino acid from which it is derived.

Refer 2010 Short Answer Question 38.

58. What is the principle of radioimmunoassay?

- Radioimmunoassay is based on the competition between the labeled and unlabeled antigens to bind with antibody to form antigen-antibody complexes which may be labeled or unlabeled
- The antigen-antibody reaction is allowed to take place and at the end of incubation period, the tube will contain free and bound antigen
- Then these two forms are separated by the protein precipitating agents
- The radioactivity of the bound form in the precipitate is measured
- The specificity of antibody and the sensitivity of radioactivity are combined in this technique.

59. List the different types of immunoglobulins.

- The different classes of Ig are IgG, IgM, IgA, IgD and IgE IgG depending on the type of heavy chains
- IgG -Gamma heavy chains (γ), IgM-Mu (μ) chains, IgA-Alpha (α) chains, IgD-Delta heavy chains (δ), and IgE-Epsilon (ε) heavy chains
- The light chains of immunoglobulins are either kappa (κ) or lambda (λ) in all classes.

60. List four causes of respiratory acidosis.

Respiratory Acidosis

- Primary excess of carbonic acid with $\uparrow pCO_2$. This is compensated by increase in bicarbonate
- This occurs in chronic obstructive airways diseases, asthma, emphysema, paralysis of respiratory muscles, respiratory depressant toxic drugs
- Other causes are—pneumonia, bronchitis, status asthmaticus, brain tumor, head injury, ascites, peritonitis.

MBBS Examination 2014

ANSWER ALL QUESTIONS

I. Essay questions   (10/15 Marks each)

1. Describe the synthesis of glucose from alanine and mention its regulation.
2. How are low-density lipoproteins (LDL) produced in the body? Describe, with the help of a diagram, their metabolic fate. What determines this process of their metabolic fate? Explain the clinical significance of this lipoprotein.
3. What is the reference range for serum uric acid? What is the source of uric acid in the body? What is its ultimate fate? Discuss causes of abnormalities in levels of serum uric acid.
4. Describe recombinant DNA technology. Explain the different techniques with its application.
5. Describe the beta oxidation of palmitic acid and its regulation.
6. Discuss in detail the replication of DNA. Mention the inhibitors of replication.
7. Describe in detail about the metabolic changes and complications in diabetes mellitus. Add a short note on the biochemical investigations to be done in diabetes mellitus.
8. Describe in detail the steps in protein synthesis. Add a note about post-translational modification and inhibitors of protein synthesis.

II. Short notes   (5 Marks each)

1. Name 5 enzymes, serum levels of which are increased in disease conditions along with the corresponding disease condition where such changes are seen.
2. Briefly explain the chemiosmotic hypothesis of Mitchell.
3. What is meant by dietary fiber? Explain its importance in one's diet.
4. Explain the folate trap hypothesis.
5. What is surfactant? Explain its importance in the body in health and disease.
6. Explain with a diagram the fluid mosaic model of cell membranes.
7. What are good dietary sources of iron? Explain how iron is absorbed from the gastrointestinal tract.
8. Explain how the activity of an enzyme is affected by the pH of the medium.
9. What are the functions of calcium in the body?
10. Describe the functions and deficiency manifestations of vitamin A.
11. Essential amino acids.
12. Structure of tRNA.
13. Restriction endonucleases.
14. Post-translational modifications of proteins.
15. What is creatine clearance? Write the normal value of it.
16. Sources of ammonia in the body and its metabolism.
17. Functions of glycine in the body.
18. Heavy metal poisonings.
19. Disorders associated with potassium homeostasis.
20. Functions of nucleotides.
21. Coenzymic role of pyridoxine.
22. Factors regulating blood calcium.

23. Transamination reaction and its significance.
24. Homocystinurias.
25. Write in detail about compounds which affects electron transport chain and oxidative phosphorylation (Inhibitors of ETC).
26. Write about the biological actions and clinical applications of prostaglandins.
27. What is blotting technique? Write in detail about southern blot technique.
28. Give a detailed account of how bilirubin is formed and excreted.

16. What are the compensatory changes that occur in response to respiratory acidosis?
17. Outline the mechanism of action of glucagon.
18. What is reference range of sodium? Write two causes of hyponatremia.
19. What is the function of cytochrome P450 in the body?
20. Name two tumor suppressor genes and the malignancy that is specifically associated with abnormalities in each of these genes.
21. Wilson's disease.
22. Define isoenzymes and give two examples.
23. Specific dynamic action.
24. Chemiosmotic theory.
25. Von Gierke disease.
26. Pyruvate dehydrogenase complex.
27. Ionophores.
28. Oral glucose tolerance test.
29. Deficiency manifestations of vitamin D.
30. Biochemical functions of iron.
31. Bicarbonate buffer system.
32. Hyperkalemia.
33. Define electrophoresis and mention its applications.
34. Renal tubular function tests.
35. Urinary findings in jaundice.
36. Methemoglobin.
37. Structure of immunoglobulin.
38. Regulation of heme synthesis.
39. Operon concept.
40. Define PCR and mention its four applications.
41. Therapeutic uses of enzymes.
42. Types of lipases
43. Lipotropic factors.
44. Metabolism of propionyl-CoA.
45. Prevention of atherosclerosis.
46. Allosteric regulation.
47. Significance of multienzyme complexes with example.
48. Functions of phosphate.
49. What is saponification and iodine number? Write its importance.

III. Short answer questions (3/4 Marks each)

1. Explain the mechanism of action of cyanide as a poison.
2. List two differences between hexokinase and glucokinase.
3. Give two examples of drugs that act as inhibitors of enzyme and name the enzyme that each one inhibits.
4. Explain the role of 2, 3, bisphosphoglycerate in supply of oxygen to tissue.
5. List two differences between fetal and adult forms of hemoglobin.
6. Why do patients with cholelithiasis often pass clay-colored stools?
7. What is meant by the metabolic syndrome? What is the significance of this condition?
8. Write two functions and RDA of pyridoxine.
9. List two differences between marasmus and kwashiorkor.
10. Give two examples of substrate level phosphorylation.
11. List two applications of electrophoresis in medicine.
12. List the different types of immunoglobulins.
13. Outline the reaction by which deoxynucleotides are formed in a cell from ribonucleotides.
14. Explain the anti-neoplastic effect of methotrexate.
15. List the biochemical abnormalities seen in phenylketonuria.

50. Write about glycine cleavage systems and mention the derivatives of glycine.
51. Polyamines.
52. Types of chromatography. Write in brief about any one type of chromatography.
53. Metabolic alkalosis.
54. Histamine.
55. Telomere and telomerase.
56. Write about protein targeting and its disorders.
57. Methemoglobinemia.
58. Normal serum electrolyte values.
59. Nitric oxide.

I. ESSAY QUESTIONS

1. **Describe the synthesis of glucose from alanine and mention its regulation.**

Refer 2008 Essay Question 6 for alanine to glucose.

2. **How are low-density lipoproteins (LDL) produced in the body? Describe with the help of a diagram their metabolic fate. What determines this process of their metabolic fate? Explain the clinical significance of this lipoprotein.**

Refer 2003 Short Note 7.

3. **What is the reference range for serum uric acid? What is the source of uric acid in the body? What is its ultimate fate? Discuss causes of abnormalities in levels of serum uric acid.**

- Reference range of uric acid in serum— 2–5 mg/dL, in females, 3–7 mg/dL in males
- Source of uric acid in the body: Breakdown of purine nucleotides:
  - **Exogenous:** Dietary purines derived by the digestion of nucleic acids
  - **Endogenous purines:** Synthesized in the body—de novo synthesis and purine Salvage pathway.
- **Synthesis of uric acid (Fig. 1):**
  - Purine catabolism leads to the production of uric acid
  - **Step 1:** Adenosine monophosphate (AMP) is converted to adenosine by **nucleotidase** by the removal of phosphate. GMP is also converted to guanosine by nucleotidase
  - **Step 2: Adenosine deaminase** converts adenosine to inosine by the removal of ammonia
  - **Step 3:** By the addition of one phosphate, **nucleoside phosphorylase** enzyme removes ribose-1-phosphate from inosine and guanosine to form hypoxanthine and guanine, respectively

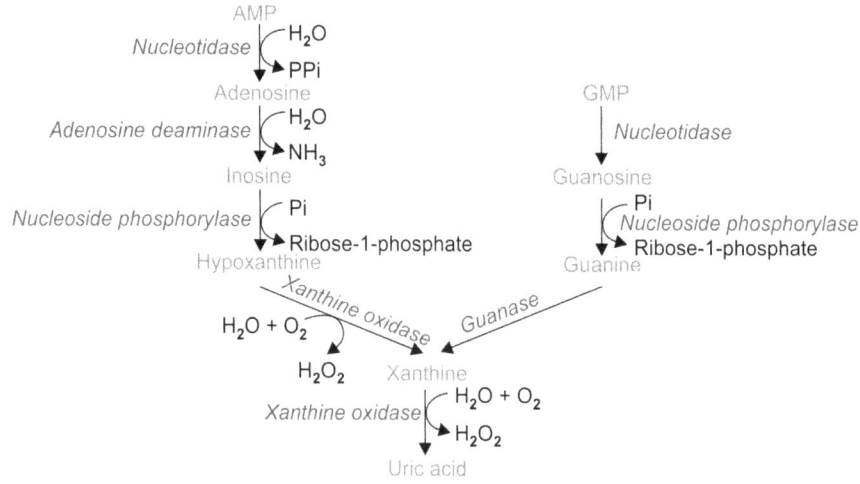

Fig. 1: Synthesis of uric acid.

- **Step 4:** Guanine is converted to xanthine by guanase enzyme hypoxanthine is acted by xanthine oxidase to form xanthine. Hydrogen peroxide is released
- **Step 5:** Xanthine is converted to uric acid by the enzyme xanthine oxidase. Hydrogen peroxide is released which is decomposed to water and oxygen by catalase enzyme canthine oxidase is a metalloenzymes containing molybdenum (Mo) and iron. It is competitively inhibited by allopurinol.

Fate of Uric Acid

Uric acid (UA) is excreted in urine. Normal urinary excretion of uric acid is 500–700 mg/day
Normal blood level of uric acid is 2–5 mg/dL for females and 3–7 mg/dL for males.

Causes of Abnormalities in Uric Acid Level

Disorders connected with these metabolic pathways are either increased or decreased production of uric acid—namely hyper-and hypouricemia.

I. **Hypouricemia:** Decreased level of uric acid less than 2mg/dL is known as hypouricemia.
   Conditions in which there is hypouricemia:
   - Immunodeficiency disorders of purine metabolism:
     a. Adenosine deaminase (ADA) deficiency
     b. Purine nucleoside phosphorylase deficiency.
   - Xanthinuria: Complete deficiency of xanthine oxidase which converts xanthine to uric acid
   - Renal lithiasis: Adenosine phosphoribosyl transferase—complete deficiency.

II. **Hyperuricemia:** When uric acid levels is increased in blood it is known as hyperuricemia.
   Causes of hyperuricemia:
   - Normal production and excretion of urates—due to renal disorders
   - Increased production and excretion of UA:
     a. Primary causes: Enzyme defects
     b. Secondary to other diseases: Cancer, trauma, psoriasis, pre-eclamptic toxemia (PET), renal insufficiency
     c. Unrecognised defects.
   - Decreased excretion of uric acid: Mostly due to secondary causes.

- **Primary causes: Due to inherited enzyme defects**
  1. Gout—due to:
     a. Abnormal superactive PRPP synthetase—X-linked recessive
     b. Active phosohoribosyl amido transferase—X-linked recessive
     c. Partial deficiency of HGPRTase (Salvage pathway enzyme) is X-linked recessive
        * Abnormal superactive phosphoribosylpyrophosphate (PRPP) synthetase—X-linked recessive
        * 5-phosphoribosyl amidotransferase—X-linked recessive
  2. Von Gierke disease: Due to glucose-6-phosphatase (G6P deficiency)
  3. Lesch-Nyhan syndrome: It is X-linked inborn error of purine metabolism due to complete deficiency of HGPRTase which is an enzyme of purine salvage pathway.

- **Secondary causes: Secondary to other diseases.** This may be seen in:
  - Increased diet intake, alcohol consumption
  - Increased production of uric acid: Due to increased turnover of cells as in malignancy lymphomas, leukemia, polycythemia, psoriasis, after treatment of cancer, trauma and starvation
  - Reduced excretion of uric acid: Renal failure, thiazide diuretics, lactic acidosis and ketoacidosis.

4. **Describe recombinant DNA technology. Explain the different techniques with its application.**

Refer 2007 Short Note 23.

5. **Describe the β-oxidation of palmitic acid and its regulation.**

Refer 2006 Essay Question 5.

6. **Discuss in detail the replication of DNA. Mention the inhibitors of replication.**

Refer 2007 Essay Question 9.

7. **Describe in detail about the metabolic changes and complications in diabetes mellitus. Add a short note on the biochemical investigations to be done in diabetes mellitus.**

- The metabolic disorder associated with insulin deficiency is **diabetes mellitus (DM)**
- It is a syndrome of impaired metabolism of carbohydrate, lipid and protein.

Two types: Type I DM—insulin dependent DM (IDDM); Type II—noninsulin dependent (NIDDM)

- **TYPE I**—it is due to decreased insulin production. This may be due to destruction of beta cells of pancreas due to congenital, viral or autoimmune causes. This type occurs below 30 years. It is common during adolescence. These patients are more prone to ketosis
- **TYPE II: Common. 95%**—due to insulin resistance. Seen in individuals above 40 years. They are less prone for ketosis. 60% cases are obese.

Metabolic Changes in Diabetes

- Glucosuria
- Hyperglycemia
- Polyurea
- Polydipsia
- Ketoacidosis if not treated properly
- Hypertriglyceridemia
- Poor wound healing.

Complications of Diabetes Mellitus

- **Acute:**
  - Diabetic ketoacidosis: More in type I. The level of ketone bodies exceeds 1 mg/dL and the utilization of ketone bodies is less, there will be ketonemia and ketonuria and the breath smells of acetone. Patient may be dehydrated. Rothera's test confirms the presence of ketone bodies in urine
  - Lactic acidosis: Due to overproduction of lactic acid, due to increased glycolysis and underutilization of lactic acid as in impaired TCA cycle. This also occurs in patients treated by biguanides.
- **Chronic:** Due to hyperglycemia, there will be glycation of circulating body proteins like Hb, albumin, LDL and extracellular proteins to produce advanced glycation end products which get deposited in various tissues to cause chronic complications of diabetes mellitus. They are:
  - **Vascular diseases:** Atherosclerosis, intravascular thrombosis may occur. If it affects cerebral vessels it results in paralysis. In coronary vessels it causes myocardial infarction. In smaller vessels it causes microangiopathy which will result in diabetic retinopathy and nephropathy
  - **Eye complications:** Hyperglycemia ends in increased production of sorbitol which gets deposited on the lens to produce diabetic cataract. Retinal microvascular abnormalities will end in retinopathy and blindness
  - **Neuropathy:** Decreased glucose utilization and the conversion of glucose to sorbitol in Schwann cells and the production of advanced glycation end products are the causes for peripheral neuropathy with paresthesia. Foot ulcers and gangrene may occur due to this neuropathy and so diabetic patients should take care of their feet
  - **Kimmelsteel-Wilson syndrome:** This occurs due to nephrosclerosis resulting in proteinuria and renal failure. This occurs due to glycation of basement membrane proteins
  - In **diabetic mothers**, as insulin is an anabolic hormone they may deliver big babies, or end in abortion or intrauterine death.

Diagnosis of Diabetes Mellitus

- Blood glucose level
  - Fasting: More than 126 mg/dL
  - Two hours after glucose: More than 200 mg/dL
- Fasting and postprandial blood glucose estimation: Once in 3 months for monitoring
- Complete lipid profile: Total cholesterol, TAG, HDL and LDL cholesterol—once in 6 months
- Kidney function tests: Blood urea and serum creatinine—twice a year
- Microalbuminuria and frank albuminuria—once in a year.
  - Microalbuminuria: Presence of 50-300 mg/day albumin in urine—predictor of renal damage;
  - Albumin: >300 mg/day in urine—overt diabetic nephropathy.
- Glycated Hb: Best index of long-term control of DM HbA1C levels reveal mean glucose level over the previous 10-12 weeks
- Fructosamines
- Advanced glycation end products.

Diagnostic Criteria for Diabetes Mellitus (WHO)

- Fasting blood glucose—should be more than 126 mg/dL for more than 2 occasion. OR
- Two hours post-glucose value of OGTT is more than 200 mg/dL (even at one occasion) OR
- Both fasting and 2 hour values above these levels—on the same occasion
- Random plasma glucose level is more than 200 mg/dL on more than one occasion
- Glycated Hb-HbA1c—more than 6.5% at any occasion. This is the preferred method for initial diagnosis of DM.

8. **Describe in detail the steps in protein synthesis. Add a note about post translational modification and inhibitors of protein synthesis.**

Refer 2013 Essay Question 4.

II. SHORT NOTES

1. **Name 5 enzymes, serum levels of which are increased in disease conditions along with the corresponding disease condition where such changes are seen.**

Clinically important enzymes are grouped into 2. They are:

1. **Plasma specific or plasma functional enzymes:** They have definite functions in plasma found in high concentration than in tissues mostly synthesized in liver, e.g. lipoprotein lipase, pseudocholinesterase
2. **Plasma nonspecific or plasma nonfunctional enzymes:** They have no definite function in plasma; they may be absent or present in low amounts in plasma. During the damage of tissues of its origin, its level is elevated in plasma, e.g. amylase, acid phosphatase.

Enzymes of clinical interest are given below:

- **Aspartate aminotransferase (AST/SGOT)**
  - Normal serum level of AST—8-20 U/L
  - Its coenzyme is pyridoxal phosphate (PLP)
  - It is a marker of liver injury and its level is increased in hepatitis and in cancer of liver
  - It is also a marker of myocardial infarction.
- **Alanine transaminase (ALT/SGPT)**
  - Normal serum level of ALT—13-35 U/L for males and 10-30 U/L for females
  - Its coenzyme is pyridoxal phosphate (PLP)
  - It is highly increased in toxic or viral hepatitis and moderately increased in cirrhosis and chronic hepatitis.
- **Gamma-glutamyl transferase (GGT)**
  - GGT has 11 isoenzymes
  - It is seen in liver, kidney, pancreas, intestinal cells and prostate glands
  - Normal level is 10-30 U/L
  - It is increased in infective hepatitis and prostate cancers

- It is a marker of alcohol abuse. GGT is increased in alcoholics when other liver functions are within normal limits. It is decreased rapidly within few days of stopping alcohol. Increase in GGT is proportional to the amount of alcohol consumed.
- **Acid phosphatase (ACP)**
  - It acts at a pH between 4 and 6
  - Normal value in serum is 2.5–12 U/L
  - Secreted by prostate cells, RBCs, WBCs and platelets
  - The value of ACP is increased in prostate cancer and it is an important tumor marker for prostate cancer.
  - It has got a tartrate labile isoenzyme which is helpful in follow-up of prostate cancer. Its normal level is 1U/L.
- **Lactate dehydrogenase:**
  - There are 5 isoenzymes. They are LDH1, LDH2, LDH3, LDH4, and LDH5
  - LDH is a tetramer with 4 subunits. LDH1 (heart-H4), LDH2 (RBC-H3M1), LDH3 (hrain-H2M2), LDH4 (lung, liver-H1M3), and LDH5 (liver, skeletal muscle-M4)
  - Isoenzymes of LDH help in the diagnosis of heart and liver diseases. LDH 2 level is higher in blood than LDH 1. But this is reversed in myocardial infarction called as flipped pattern (LDH 1 > LDH 2)
  - Increased activity of LDH-5 is an indicator of liver diseases.

2. **Briefly explain the chemiosmotic hypothesis of Mitchell.**

Refer 2006 Short Note 5.

3. **What is meant by dietary fiber? Explain its importance in one's diet.**

Refer 2008 Short Note 10.

4. **Explain the folate trap hypothesis (Fig. 2).**

Refer 2010 Short Note 2.
- B_{12} coenzyme methylcobalamin acts as the coenzyme in the conversion of homocysteine to methionine

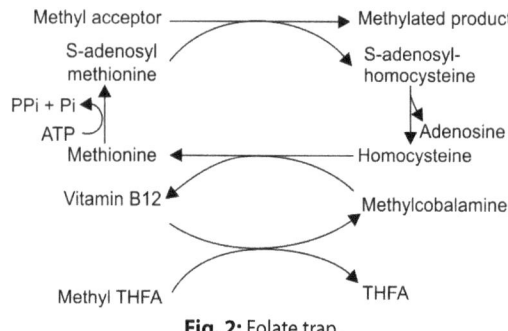

Fig. 2: Folate trap.

- Folic acid also plays important role in it. In the folic acid metabolism H_4F is reversibly converted to N^5, N^{10}-methylenetetrahydrofolate by serine hydroxymethyltransferase enzyme which is then irreversibly reduced to N_5 methyltetrahydrofolate
- This methyl THF donates its methyl group to cobalamin which is converted to methylcobalamine
- This methyl B_{12} then supplies the methyl group to homocysteine to form methionine
- In the case of B_{12} deficiency this transfer of methyl group is not possible and so methyl THF is trapped inside the cells and there is no formation of methionine from homocysteine. This is called **folate trap.**

5. **What is surfactant? Explain its importance in the body in health and disease.**

Refer 2011 Short Answers Question 25.
- Dipalmitoyl lecithin is effective surface active agent and it is a precursor of lung surfactant
- It reduces surface tension in the alveoli and prevents alveolar collapse
- When there is insufficient lung surfactant, it leads to respiratory distress syndrome (RDS)
- Acute respiratory syndrome is due to the deficiency of dipalmitoyl lecithin which is the lung surfactant
- In its absence the lungs tend to collapse causing respiratory distress syndrome

6. **Explain with a diagram the fluid mosaic model of cell membranes.**

Refer 2008 Short Note 5.

7. **What are good dietary sources of iron? Explain how iron is absorbed from the gastrointestinal tract.**

Refer 2006 Essay Question 8 and 2011 Essay Question 4.

8. **Explain how the activity of an enzyme is affected by the pH of the medium (Fig. 3).**

- Each enzyme has a unique pH range for maximal activity, beyond these ranges enzyme velocity will slowdown. This is known as optimum pH
- The velocity of the reaction declines above and below that pH
- When the velocity is plotted against pH a bell-shaped curve is obtained
- Change in pH may denature the enzyme
- The optimal pH for most of the enzymes is pH 6–8 except pepsin with optimum pH of 1–2 and ALP has pH of 9–10 and acid phosphatase has pH 4–5.

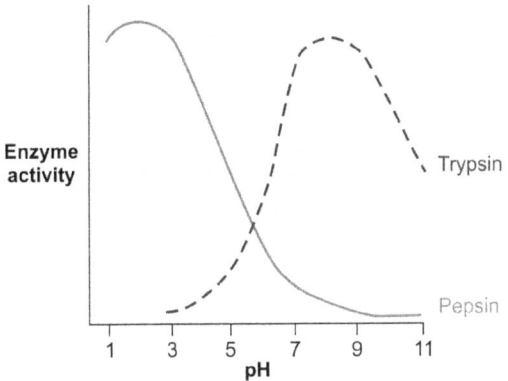

Fig. 3: Effect of pH on enzyme velocity.

9. **What are the functions of calcium in the body?**

Refer 2007 Essay Question 6.

10. **Describe the functions and deficiency manifestations of vitamin A.**

Refer 2006 Essay Question 7.

11. **Essential amino acids.**

Refer 2005 Short Note 40.

12. **Structure of tRNA.**

Refer 2004 Short Note 12.

13. **Restriction endonucleases.**

Refer 2007 Short Note 28.

14. **Post-translational modifications of proteins.**

Refer 2006 Short Note 27.

15. **What is creatine clearance? Write the normal value of it.**

- **Clearance tests:** Done to assess the glomerular filtration and renal blood flow
- **Renal clearance of a substance is the volume of plasma from which the substance is completely cleared by the kidney in 1 minute**
- Clearance = mg of substance excreted/min/mg of substance/mL of plasma; C = U × V/P where C = Clearance of the substance; U = Concentration of the substance in urine; P = Concentration of the substance in plasma; V= Volume of urine passed per minute
- Clearance is expressed as milliliter of plasma/unit time
- Clearance tests: This test is done by using either endogenous markers such as, urea or creatinine or exogenous markers like Inulin, ^{51}Cr-labelled EDTA, ^{99}Tec-labelled EDTA, etc. Out of all creatinine clearance test is the best
- Creatinine clearance test: It is based on the rate of excretion of metabolically produced creatinine which is excreted through urine. Creatinine is freely filtered by the glomeruli but not reabsorbed by the tubules. A small amount of creatinine is secreted by the tubules
- 24-hours urine is collected and blood is also collected for estimation of creatinine. Urinary volume is measured (V) and the concentration of creatinine in urine (U) and plasma (P) are estimated and by using the formula C = U × V/P the creatinine clearance is calculated

- **Normal range for creatinine clearance is 90–120 mL/min**
- Reduced creatinine clearance indicates chronic renal damage and reduced blood flow to glomeruli.

16. Sources of ammonia in the body and its metabolism.

Refer 2005 Essay Question 7.

17. Functions of glycine in the body.

Glycine is the simplest amino acid.

Metabolic Products

- Methylenetetrahydrofolate by glycine cleavage system to join one-carbon pool
- Glucose: It is glucogenic.

Special Products Formed from Glycine (Fig. 4)

- Creatine, creatine phosphate and creatinine
- Heme
- Purine nucleotides.
- Glutathione
- Conjugating agent
- Constituent of most of the proteins—more in collagen.

Creatine Production from Glycine (Fig. 5)

- Creatine and creatinine are the non-protein nitrogenous substances present in normal urine. They are synthesized by 3 amino acids—arginine, glycine and methionine. The synthesis occurs in kidney, liver and muscles
- Normal serum level of creatinine is (0.7–1.4 mg/dL); serum creatine is 0.2–0.4 mg/dL
- Serum creatinine is a marker of renal failure. Creatinine clearance test is used to measure GFR.

Production of Heme (Fig. 6)

- Succinyl CoA combines with glycine catalyzed by the enzyme ALA synthase in the presence of the coenzyme pyridoxal phosphate in the mitochondria to form alpha-amino-beta-keto-adipic acid which is converted by the same enzyme to delta-aminolevulinic acid. It is the rate-limiting step in heme synthesis.

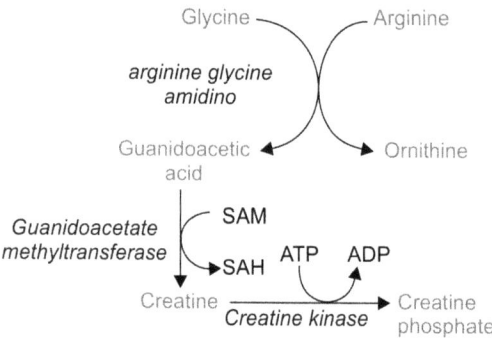

Fig. 5: Synthesis of creatine.

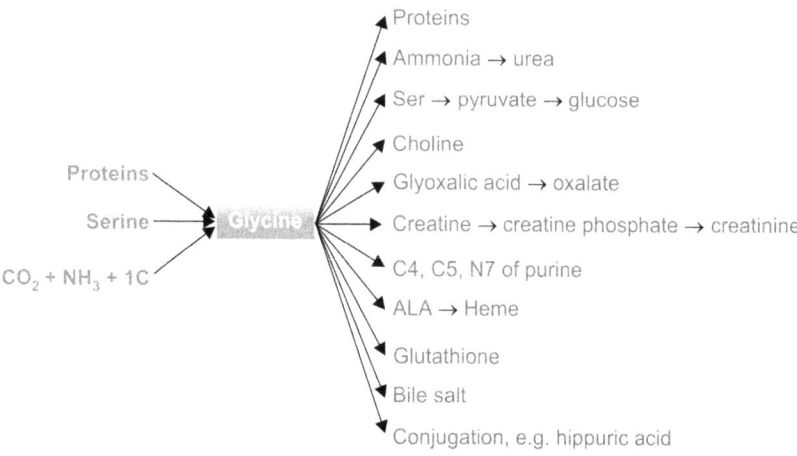

Fig. 4: Metabolic fate of glycine.

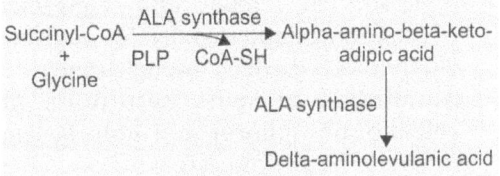

Fig. 6: Role of glycine in heme synthesis.

Synthesis of Purine (Fig. 7)

Whole molecules of glycine are contributed for the formation of C4, C5 and N7 of purine ring.

Conjugating Agent

Glycine acts as a conjugating agent
- It conjugates bile acids to produce conjugated bile acids which are less toxic. Glycocholic acid and glycochenodeoxycholic acid are the conjugated primary bile acids
- In the liver glycine conjugates benzoic acid and detoxifies it to form hippuric acid which is easily excreted from urine.

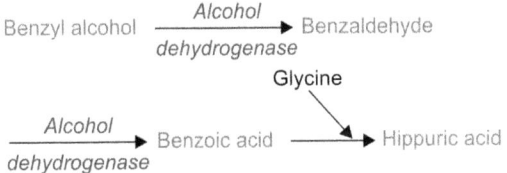

Neurotransmitter

- Glycine acts as an inhibitory neurotransmitter by opening chloride specific channels. It causes over-excitation in high concentration.

Glutathione Formation

- Glutathione is gamma-glutamyl-cysteinyl-glycine. It is a tripeptide of biochemical importance. Glutamate combines with cysteine to form gamma-glutamylcysteine which combines with glycine to form glutathione. Each step needs one ATP.

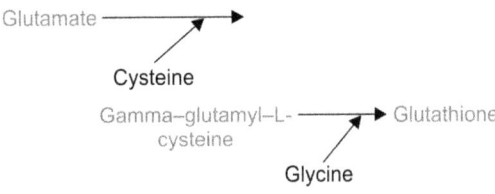

18. Heavy metal poisonings.

Heavy metal poisons are lead, mercury, aluminium, arsenic, etc.

Lead Poisoning

- It is a cumulative poison and is accumulated in tissues. 90% lead is seen in bones, 9% in blood, and 1% in brain and kidneys
- There is no safe level. More than 25 µg/dL in adults and more than 10 µg/dL in children lead to toxicity
- It crosses the placenta and causes miscarriage, stillbirth and premature delivery
- Permanent neurological defects, cerebral palsy and optic atrophy may be seen
- In children, mental retardation, learning disabilities, behavioral problems and seizures, etc.

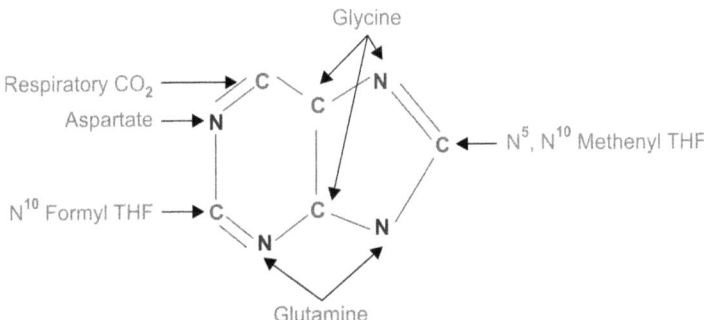

Fig. 7: Contribution of glycine to purine.

- Anemia, abdominal colic and loss of appetite are common
- Discoloration and blue line among the gums are features of acute lead poisoning
- Lead inhibits heme synthesis by inhibiting the enzymes ALA dehydratase and ferrochelatase. Lifespan of RBC shortened. Anemia is predominent due to reduced heme synthesis and also lead inhibits iron absorption
- Treatment: Calcium dodecyl edentate, pencillamine and BAL—dimercaprol and dimercaptosuccinic acid are used as antidotes.

Arsenic Toxicity

- The oxides of arsenic are commonly used as fruit sprays, pesticides, rat poisons, etc.
- It acts on sulfhydryl enzymes and interferes with cell metabolism
- It may also cause intravascular hemolysis which leads to hemoglobinuria
- There will be anaphylactic reactions
- Later complications are agranulocytosis, hepatitis, jaundice and encephalitis.

Mercury Poisoning

- It is one of the commonest industrial poison
- It occurs due to inhalation of elementary mercury vapor from broken thermometer, sphygmomanometer
- In acute poisoning pulmonary edema and encephalopathy may result
- In chronic poisoning, there will be a classical triad of oral lesions, tremor and psychological changes may result—called erethism
- Organic mercury poisoning is called Minamata disease which is characterized by dysarthria, ataxia and visual problems.

Aluminium Toxicity

- Common in paint workers and exposure from packing, building materials, cosmetics, antacids and aluminium cooking vessels
- A person can tolerate upto 1 mg/day of aluminium and usually 100 mg/day aluminium is excreted through urine
- Aluminium prevents absorption of calcium, phosphorus and iron. It also interferes heme synthesis
- Aluminium toxicity may lead to Alzheimer's disease and Parkinson's disease and also implicated in degeneration of dendrites.

19. Disorders associated with potassium homeostasis.

- Potassium is the major intracellular cation and maintains intracellular osmotic pressure. Normal serum potassium level—3.5-5.2 mEq/L.

Hypokalemia

Plasma potassium level below 3 mEq/L is hypokalemia.
- Signs and symptoms: Muscular weakness, fatigue, muscle cramps, hypotension, decreased reflexes, palpitation, cardiac arrhythmias, and cardiac arrest. ECG waves are flattened, T wave is inverted. This may be corrected by oral feeding of orange juice.
- **Causes:**
  - Increased renal excretion: Cushing's syndrome, hyperaldosteronism, hyperreninism, hypomagnesemia, renal tubular acidosis
  - Shift/redistribution of potassium: Alkalosis, insulin therapy, thyrotoxic periodic paralysis, hypokalemic periodic paralysis
  - Gastrointestinal loss: Diarrhea, vomiting, aspiration, deficient intake, malabsorption
  - Intravenous saline infusion in excess
  - Drugs: Insulin, salbutamide, osmotic diuretics, thiazides, corticosteroids.
- Treatment: Adequate supplementation of potassium. About 100 mmol KCl/day in 3-4 divided doses.

Hyperkalemia

Plasma potassium level above 5.5mmol/L is known as hyperkalemia.

Refer 2013 Short Answers Question 32.

20. Functions of nucleotides.
Refer 2013 Short Answers Question 52.
- Nucleotides are nitrogenous base + pentose sugar + phosphate group
- They are the phosphorylated nucleosides
- The phosphate group is attached to the hydroxyl group of pentoses by an ester linkage
- Depending on the nature of the pentoses, the nucleotides are of 2 types—(1) Ribonucleotides: (2) Deoxyribonucleotides
- Depending upon the number of phosphate groups added they are known as—1P-Monophosphates (MP), 2P-Diphosphates (DP) and 3P-Triphosphates (TP).

Ribonucleotides
a. Adenosine ribonucleotides:
   - AMP—cyclic AMP: Major metabolic regulator and second messenger in hormonal action
   - ATP: Energy currency of cell; high energy phosphate. It helps in the formation of active methionine (SAM) involved in transmethylation; it is also needed for the synthesis of certain coenzymes like NAD, FAD, etc.
b. Guanosine ribonucleotides: GMP, GDP and GTP
   - Cyclic GMP: Major metabolic regulator and second messenger in hormonal action
   - GTP: Involved in protein synthesis as energy source
c. Uridine ribonucleotides: UMP, UDP and UTP
   - UDP sugars act as donors of sugar for the synthesis of glycogen (UDP-glucose);
   - UDP-galactose—for the synthesis of glycoproteins and proteoglycans
   - UDP-glucuronate is a conjugating agent for conjugation of bilirubin, drugs, etc.
d. Cytosine ribonucleotides: CDP, CDP and CTP
   - CDP choline is needed for the synthesis of sphingomyelin
e. Hypoxanthine nucleotide:
   - Ionosine monophosphate (IMP): Precursor or parent nucleotide of purine ribonucleotides

Deoxyribonucleotides
d-AMP, d-GMP, d-CMP, deoxythymidine monophosphate (dTMP): They are present in DNA.

21. Coenzymic role of pyridoxine.
Pyridoxine (B6) is a water-soluble vitamin. Its coenzyme is pyridoxal phosphate (PLP)
- Sources: Yeast, rice polishing, wheat germs, cereals, legumes (pulses), oil seeds, egg, milk, meat, fish and green leafy vegetables
- **RDA:** Related to protein intake
Adults—1-2 mg/day; Pregnancy—2. 5 mg/day; Infants—0. 5 mg/day.

Biochemical Functions
- **Transamination:** PLP acts as a coenzyme for transaminase enzymes—AST and ALT forming schiff base **(Fig. 8)**
- PLP acts as a coenzyme for **decarboxylation of amino acids to form biologically important amines**, e.g.

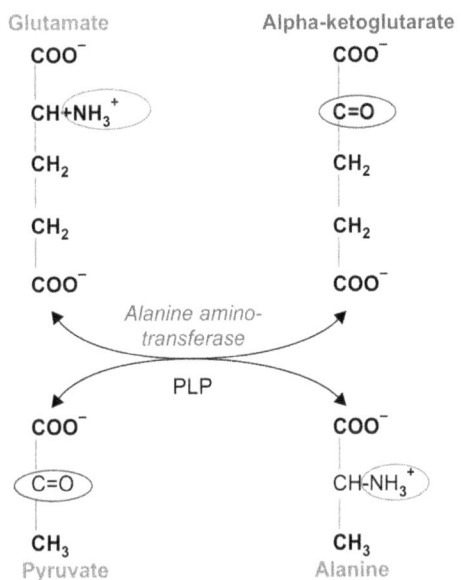

Fig. 8: Transamination.

Glutamate → GABA + CO_2
Histidine → histamine + CO_2
Cysteine → taurine + CO_2

- PLP plays important role in **methionine and cysteine metabolism** in the reactions catalyzed by cystathionine synthase, Cystathionase—desulphhydrase and Transsulphuration reactions
- **Heme synthesis:** ALA synthetase is a PLP-dependent enzyme
- **For the synthesis of Niacin:** Kyneurinase needs PLP as coenzyme
- **Glycogen phosphorylase:** This enzyme contains PLP.

Deficiency Manifestations

- Neurological ↓ Biological amines: Serotonin, GABA Epinephrine
  Convulsions: Children
  Demyelination: Low sphingomyelin
  Peripheral neuritis
  Carpal tunnel diseases
- Dermatological: Low niacin from tryptophan—pellagra
- Hematological ↓ heme synthesis.

22. Factors regulating blood calcium.

Refer 2004 Essay Question 4 and 2005 Essay Question 8.

Normal Blood Level of Calcium

- Total calcium level—9-11 mg/dL
- Three forms of calcium in blood are:
  1. Ionized calcium (active form)—5 mg/dL.
  2. Protein bound Ca—4 mg/dL
  3. Protein complexed with phosphate, HCO_3^-, citrate—1 mg/dL.

Factors Regulating Calcium Level

1. Hormonal Regulation

A. Vitamin D (Calcitriol 1, 25-dihydroxycholecalciferol):
   - The active vitamin D (calcitriol) acts as a steroid hormone. It is synthesized in kidney.
     - **Effect on intestine:** Calcitriol binds to specific cytoplasmic receptors which interacts with DNA and induces the synthesis of mRNA for specific proteins. Calbindin which is a calcium binding protein which helps in the absorption of calcium and phosphorus from the intestines
     - **Effects on bone:** Calcitriol stimulates the activity of osteoblasts which help in mineralization of bones. They secrete alkaline phosphatase enzyme which in turn increases the ionic concentration of phosphate and calcium
     - **Effects on kidney:** Calcitriol increases the reabsorption of calcium and phosphorous from the renal tubules there by conserving both minerals.

B. **Parathyroid hormone:**
   - Parathyroid hormone (PTH) is secreted by four parathyroid glands present at the posterior aspect of thyroid gland
   - Decreased serum calcium level leads to release of PTH from parathyroids. PTH activates the enzyme adenyl cyclase in target cells and increases intracellular calcium concentration
   - **PTH and bones:** PTH causes demineralization of bones. It activates pyrophosphatase in osteoclasts leading to bone resorption and decalcification. Calcium is released into the bloodstream and increases blood calcium level. This leads to loss of bone matrix
   - **PTH and kidneys:** PTH causes decreased renal excretion of calcium and increased excretion of phosphates and increased reabsorption of calcium leading to increased blood calcium level
   - **PTH and intestines:** PTH stimulates increased production of calcitriol which acts on intestine to absorb more calcium leading to increased calcium level in blood.

C. **Calcitonin:**
   - Secreted by parafollicular cells of thyroid gland
   - It is a polypeptide of 32-34 amino acids and its secretion is stimulated by serum calcium, gastrin, glucagon and biological amines

- It decreases serum calcium level by inhibiting resorption of bone and decreases the activity of osteoclasts and increases the activity of osteoblasts
- Calcitonin and PTH are antagonistic to each other but both together promote growth and remodeling of bone
- In kidney: Calcitonin increases excretion of phosphates in urine like PTH.

2. Other factors

Phosphorus
- There is a reciprocal relationship of calcium with phosphorus
- Ionic product of Ca × P is kept as a constant;
- Normally-(Ca) 10 mg/dL × (P) 4 mg/dL = 40; ionic product is 40
- In renal insufficiency ↓ excretion of P ↑ level of P in blood ↓ level of calcium—tetany.

Serum Proteins
- Total calcium level is decreased in hypoalbuminemia: For reduction of each 1 g/dL of albumin there will be reduction of 0.8 mg/dL of calcium
- Ionized calcium level will be normal and so no deficiency manifestations will be present.

Alkalosis and Acidosis
- Alkalosis favors binding of more calcium with proteins by lowering of ionized calcium but the total calcium level is normal. Calcium deficiency is manifested
- Acidosis favors ionization of calcium.

Renal Threshold for Calcium

Renal threshold for calcium is 10 mg/dL and calcium gets excreted at this level

Children

In children the normal calcium level will be near the upper limit and the ionic product of calcium × P = 50 (adult-40).

23. Transamination reaction and its significance.

Refer 2008 Short Note 14.

24. Homocystinurias.

Refer 2011 Short Note 12.

25. Write in detail about compounds which affects electron transport chain and oxidative phosphorylation. (Inhibitors of ETC).

Refer 2005 Short Note 24.

26. Write about the biological actions and clinical applications of prostaglandins.

Refer 2005 Short Note 13.
- The precursor molecule for eicosanoids is arachidonic acid
- They are 4 types of eicosanoids—1. Prostaglandins (PGs), 2. Prostacyclins (PGI), 3. Thromboxanes (TXs), 4. Leukotrienes (LTs)
- According to the attachment of different substituent groups to the ring prostaglandins are classified as A, B, D, E, F, G and H. PGI—prostacyclins
- **Cyclo-oxygenase pathway:** In this pathway all the prostaglandins, prostacyclines and thromboxanes are produced except LTs.

Functions of prostaglandins and related compounds:

- **On CVS:**
  - PGI_2 is a powerful vasodilator, hence used in treatment of hypertension
  - PGI_2 inhibits platelet aggregation to promote thrombus formation
  - TXA_2 produced by platelets are vasoconstrictors and cause platelet aggregation. PGI and TX are having opposite actions.
- **On ovary and uterus:** PGF_2 induces termination of pregnancy and induction of labor by stimulating uterine muscles. So it is used in medical termination of pregnancy and to arrest postpartum bleeding
- **On respiratory tract:** PGE is a potent bronchodilator whereas PGF is bronchoconstrictor. PGE 1 and 2 are used in the treatment of asthma
- **On immunity and inflammation:**
  - PGE_2 and D_2—induce inflammation by increasing the permeability of capillaries.
  - PGE_2—reduces T and B cell functions

- PGE—↑ Erythema, wheal production—allergy
- **On gastrointestinal tract:**
  - PGE—inhibits gastric secretion
  - Increase intestinal motility
  - Treatment—acid peptic disease
  - Stimulates pancreatic secretion—increase intestinal motility, causing diarrhea.
- **Metabolic effects:**
  - Metabolic effect: Through cAMP-PGE_2—decreases lipolysis, ↑ glycogenesis and calcium mobilization from bone
  - PGE_2 stimulates glycogenesis, induces calcium mobilization from bones and inhibits lipolysis.
  - PGE_2—vasodilatation, smooth muscle relaxation.

27. What is blotting technique? Write in detail about southern blot technique.

Refer 2005 Short Notes 38.
- Blotting is a technique for transferring DNA, RNA and proteins on to a carrier so they can be separated, and often follows the use of a gel electrophoresis **(Fig. 9)**
- The southern blot is used for transferring DNA, the northern blot for RNA and the western blot for protein.
- **Southern blotting (Fig. 10):** This technique was found out by EM Southern
  - This technique is based on DNA hybridization technique
  - Used to detect specific DNA segment
- **Steps:**
  - DNA is extracted from the tissues
  - It is fragmented by using restriction endonucleases
  - The cut fragments are electrophoresed in agarose gel
  - It is then treated with NaOH to convert DNA to single-stranded DNA

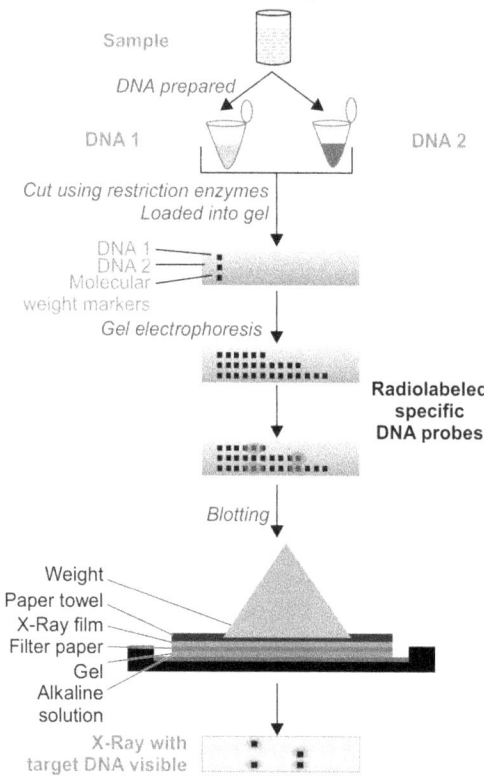

Fig. 10: Southern blotting.

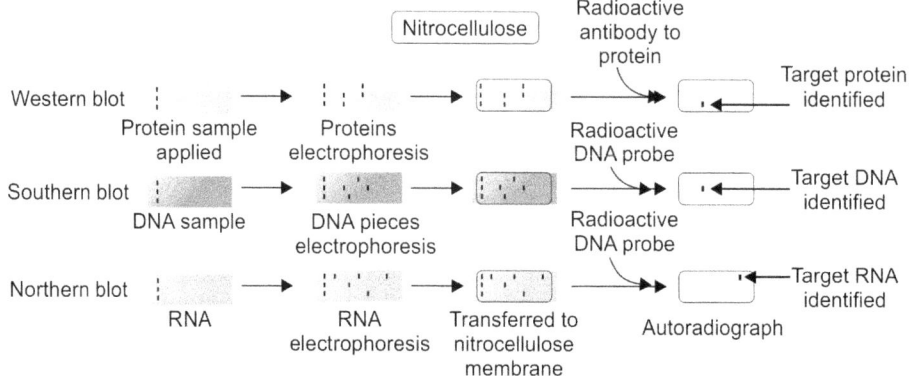

Fig. 9: Blotting techniques.

- The gel is then blotted over a nitrocellulose membrane
- An exact replica of the pattern in the gel is reproduced in the membrane. The DNA gets attached to the membrane
- The DNA is fixed to the membrane at 80°C.
- A radioactive DNA probe which is complementary to the desired DNA fragment is applied
- This probe gets attached to the desired DNA (DNA hybridization)
- The membrane is washed and a radiographic film is exposed on the membrane
- The X-ray is developed to identify the DNA.

28. Give a detailed account of how bilirubin is formed and excreted.

Refer 2005 Short Note 3.

III. SHORT ANSWER QUESTIONS

1. Explain the mechanism of action of cyanide as a poison.

Refer 2013 Short Answer Question 46.

2. List two differences between hexokinase and glucokinase.

- Both the enzymes catalyze phosphorylation of glucose to glucose-6-phosphate in glycolysis in an irreversible reaction. It needs ATP and Mg. Both are isoenzymes.

S. No.	Particulars	Hexokinase	Glucokinase
1.	Site	In all tissues	In liver only
2.	Specificity	Phosphorylation of hexoses	Phosphorylation of only glucose
3.	K_m	Low K_m for substrates	High K_m for glucose
4.	Substrate affinity	High	Low
5.	Inhibitor	Glucose-6-phosphate	Nil
6.	Induction	Not induced	By insulin and glucose

3. Give two examples of drugs that act as inhibitors of enzyme and name the enzyme that each one inhibits.

Competitive inhibitors (Substrate analogue inhibitors):

- Many drugs act as competitive inhibitors. For example, **sulfonamide** is an analog of para-aminobenzoic acid (PABA) and inhibits pteroid synthetase in the folic acid synthesis
- **Allopurinol** inhibits xanthine oxidase. Usually they are structural analog of the substrate—hypoxanthine
- They bind and compete to the substrate binding site of the enzyme forming an enzyme inhibitory complex (EI)
- K_m value is increased but no change in V_{max}.

4. Explain the role of 2, 3-bisphosphoglycerate in supply of oxygen to tissue.

Refer glycolysis in RBC 2007 Short Note 18.

5. List two differences between fetal and adult forms of hemoglobin.

- The **adult hemoglobin** is represented as HbA
- It is made up of 2 alpha chains and 2 beta chains and each polypeptide contain a nonprotein part/prosthetic group called heme
- Fetal Hb (HbF): Made up of 2 alpha and 2 gamma chains
- Normal adult blood contains 97% HbA, 2% HbA_2 and 1% HbF.
- Differences in physicochemical properties of HbF and HbA are:
  - Solubility of deoxy-HbF is increased than HbA
  - HbF has slower electrophoretic mobility
  - Interaction with 2, 3-bisphosphoglycerate (BPG) is decreased in HbF.

6. Why do patients with cholelithiasis often pass clay-colored stools?

- Color of feces is due to stercobilinogen
- In complete obstruction of biliary tract, due to extrahepatic causes like stones in

gallbladder, biliary atresia (cholelithiasis) and also due to intrahepatic cholestasis bile will not enter the intestine
- So no stercobilinogen is entering into the gut, and the stools become clay-colored
- This is one of the important markers of obstructive jaundice.

7. What is meant by the metabolic syndrome? What is the significance of this condition?

- Metabolic syndrome (MetS) is a combination of abdominal obesity, atherogenic dyslipedemia (low HDL cholesterol and hypertriglceridemia), high blood pressure and increased blood glucose
- It is also called insulin resistant syndrome as there will be insulin resistance and decreased glucose tolerance
- **Significance**: People with MetS are having high-risk of coronary heart disease and type II diabetes
- Management of MetS: Weight loss, moderate exercise, reduced intake of saturated fats, transfatty acids and cholesterol.

8. Write two functions and RDA of pyridoxine.

- Pyridoxine or vitamin B_6: Coenzymes forms—pyridoxine (pyridoxol), pyridoxal-aldehyde form and pyridoxamine
- Active coenzyme is pyridoxal phosphate (PLP)
- Functions: PLP acts as a coenzyme for:
  - Transamination—aspartate aminotransferse (AST) and alanine aminotransferase (ALT), e.g. alanine + alpha-ketoglutarate (α-KG) $\rightarrow$ pyruvate + glutamate
  - Decarboxylation-to form biologically important amines, e.g. histidine to histamine.
- Recommended daily allowance (RDA) for pyridoxine: Adults—1-2 mg/day; Pregnancy and lactation—2.5 mg/day.

9. List two differences between marasmus and kwashiorkor.

Refer 2004 Short Notes 4.

Disorders of malnutrition commonly manifested as protein-energy malnutrition (PEM). There are two major types of malnutritional diseases:
1. **Marasmus:** This is due to severe deficiency of both dietary energy and proteins—primary calorie insufficiency and secondary protein deficiency. Marasmus means "to waste".
2. **Kwashiorkor:** This is due to isolated deficiency of proteins with sufficient calorie intake. Kwashiorkor means sickness the older child gets, when the next child is born.

The differences between these two malnutrition conditions are tabulated.

Particulars	Marasmus	Kwashiorkor
Age of onset	Below 1 year	1–5 years
Deficiency of	Calorie and proteins	Proteins alone
Cause	Early weaning and repeated infection	Starchy diet after weaning. Precipitated by acute infection
Growth retardation of child	Marked	Severe
Attitude	Irritable and fretful	Lethargic and apathetic
Appearance	Shrunken skin and bones, dehydrated	Looks plump due to edema of face and lower limbs

10. Give two examples of substrate level phosphorylation.

- It is the production of ATP at the substrate level of certain metabolic pathways without the involvement of electron transport chain (ETC)
- Energy is trapped directly from the substrate, without the help of the ETC.
- **Glycolysis:**
  a. Energy of 1, 3-BPG is trapped to synthesize 1 ATP molecule with the help of bisphosphoglycerate kinase.

Phosphoglycerate kinase
1, 3-bisphosphoglycerate $\xrightarrow{\text{ADP} \quad \text{ATP}}$ 3-phosphoglycerate

  b. Energy of PEP trapped to synthesize 1 ATP with the help of pyruvate kinase.

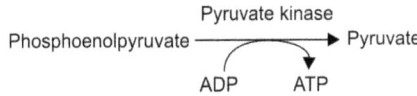

- **TCA cycle:**
  - Energy of succinyl-CoA is trapped to synthesize 1 ATP with the help of succinate thiokinase

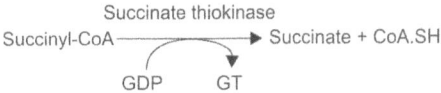

11. List two applications of electrophoresis in medicine.

- Separation of serum proteins, lipoproteins and other classes of macromolecules
  - **Normal bands (Fig. 11):**
    - 5 bands: Albumin (55–65%), Alpha 1-globulin (2–4%), Alpha-2 globulin (6–12%), Beta globulin (8–12%) and Gamma globulin (12–22%)
    - Albumin has maximum and gamma globulin has minimum mobility.
  - **Abnormal bands:** To diagnose (Fig. 11)
    - Nephrotic syndrome: Globulin is produced more by liver in compensation of renal loss of albumin. So alpha 2 band is prominent

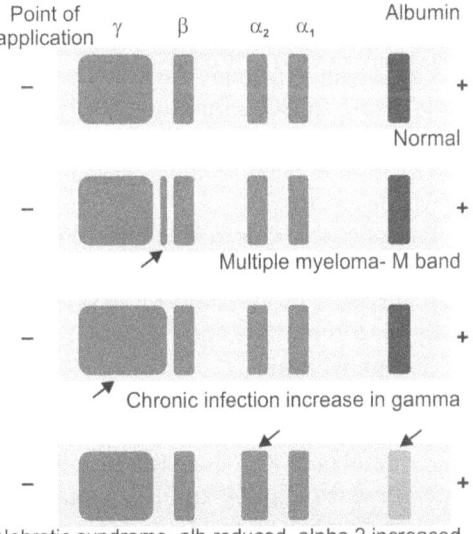

Fig. 11: Electrophoretic pattern of plasma proteins—normal and abnormal.

- Cirrhosis: Albumin synthesized in liver is decreased due to cirrhosis and so albumin band is thin and less prominent
- Multiple myeloma: Light chain immunoglobulins are produced more so there will be a prominence in gamma globulin region (M band).
- **Hemoglobin electrophoresis**
  - S band is seen in sickle cell anemia
  - Various hemoglobinopathies and thalassemias can be diagnosed.

12. List the different types of immunoglobulins.

- The different classes of Ig are IgG, IgM, IgA, IgD and IgE IgG—depending on the type of heavy chains
- Gamma (γ), IgM-Mu (μ), IgA-Alpha (α), IgD-Delta (δ), IgE-Epsilon (ε)
- The light chains of immunoglobulins are either kappa (κ) or lambda (λ).

13. Outline the reaction by which deoxynucleotides are formed in a cell from ribonucleotides.

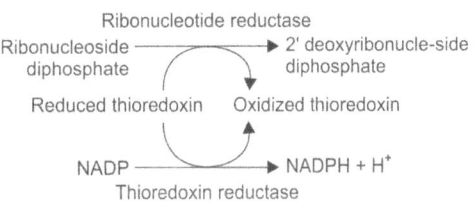

- Deoxyribonucleotides of purines and pyrimidines are formed by the reduction at the 2' carbon of the corresponding nucleoside diphosphate by the enzyme ribonucleotide reductase which contains nonheme iron
- This enzyme needs a cofactor—thioredoxin and NADP.

14. Explain the antineoplastic effect of methotroxeate (Fig. 12).

- Methotrexeate is a synthetic pyrimidine analog
- It is a competitive inhibitor of dihydrofolate reductase as it has structural similarity to folic acid

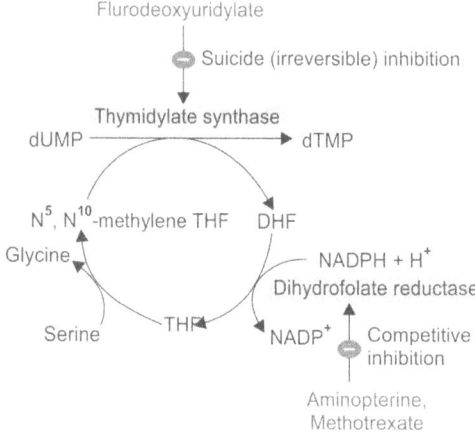

Fig. 12: Competitive inhibition by methotroxeate.

- It inhibits the enzyme dihydrofolate reductase thereby reduces the regeneration of tetrahydrofolate which is needed for the incorporation of C_2 and C_8 of purines and C_5 methyl group in thymidine
- Subsequently DNA synthesis is inhibited and also cell division
- Methotrexeate is an anticancer agent used to treat choriocarcinoma and acute leukemia.

15. List the biochemical abnormalities seen in phenylketonuria.

- Phenylketonuria is the inborn error of metabolism in phenylalanine metabolism

$$\text{Phenylalanine} \xrightarrow[\text{Tetrahydrobiopterin} \to \text{Dihydrobiopterin}]{\text{Phenylalanine hydroxylase}} \text{Tyrosine}$$

- It is an autosomal recessive disease with an incidence of 1: 10, 000 births
- It is due to deficiency of phenylalanine hydroxylase
- So phenylalanine is not converted into tyrosine and it accumulates hyperphenylalaninemia
- The excess of phenylalanine is converted to phenylpyruvate, phenyllactate, and phenylacetate and phenylacetylglutamine. Phenylpyruvate, phenyl-lactate, phenylacetate are excreted in urine.

Clinical Manifestations

- The child is mentally retarded
- Convulsions, tremors, agitation, hyperactivity may be present
- The child often has hypopigmentation due to reduced availability of tyrosine for melanin production
- Phenyl-lactate in sweat causes mousy body odor.

Laboratory Diagnosis

- Blood level of phenylalanine is elevated: Normal level is 1mg/dL, which is elevated to >20 mg/dL
- This is confirmed by Tandem mass spectroscopy
- Guthrie's test is confirmative
- Urine ferric chloride test is positive
- DNA probes—to diagnose the defects in phenylalanine hydroxylase and dihydrobiopterin reductase.

Treatment

- Early detection
- Low phenylalanine diet: Tapioca based diet which has low phenylalanine is the treatment of choice
- Gene therapy is under trial.

16. What are the compensatory changes that occur in response to respiratory acidosis?

- There will be primary excess of carbonic acid due to CO_2 retention as a result of hypoventilation
- The ratio of bicarbonate to carbonic acid will be less than 20
- Excess of carbonic acid is buffered by Hb and protein buffer system which cause slight rise in bicarbonate. Kidneys respond by conserving base and excrete H^+ as NH_4^+
- **Compensation**
  - In acute conditions: For every 10 mm rise in pCO_2 there will be increase of 1 mmol of HCO_3. There will be fall of pH, increase of pCO_2 and HCO_3 may be N or reduced
  - In chronic cases: HCO_3 increases by 3.5 mmol/L. There will be fall of pH, increase of pCO_2 and HCO_3 is highly in-

creased. Kidneys respond by conserving HCO_3^- and excreting H^+ as NH_4^+
- Chronic cases will be compensated well unlike acute cases. Renal compensation occurs generating more bicarbonate and excreting more H^+.
- Causes of respiratory acidosis:
  - Pneumonia
  - Bronchitis
  - Asthma
  - Chronic obstructive bulmonary diseases (COPD).

17. Outline the mechanism of action of glucagon.

- It is a hyperglycemic hormone produced from α-cells of islets of Langerhans of pancreas
- Its functions are agonist to the insulin actions—anti-insulin action
- It stimulates gluconeogenesis, glycogenolysis and increases blood glucose level
- Glucagon combines with a membrane bound receptor which activates G protein and adenylate cyclase
- ATP is converted to cAMP which activates glycogen phosphorylase and inactivates glycogen synthase thereby increasing the level of glucose.

18. What is reference range of sodium? Write two causes of hyponatremia.

- Normal level of sodium in plasma is 136–145 mEq/L
- **Hyponatremia:** Decreased sodium level in blood is called hyponatremia
- Causes: Vomiting, diarrhea, burns, Addison's disease, renal tubular acidosis, chronic renal failure, congestive cardiac failure, hyperglycemia, SIADH
- Drugs: ACE inhibitors, lithium, NSAIDs, vasopressin and oxytocin.

19. What is the function of cytochrome P450 in the body?

Refer 2004 Short Note 20
- In liver microsomes, cytochromes P450 are found together with cytochrome b_5 and have an important role in detoxification
- Benzpyrene, aminopyrine, aniline, morphine, and benzphetamine are hydroxylated, increasing their solubility and aiding their excretion
- Many drugs, such as phenobarbital have the ability to induce the formation of microsomal enzymes and of cytochromes P450
- Mitochondrial P 450 system is involved in steroidogenesis.

20. Name two tumor suppressor genes and the malignancy that is specifically associated with abnormalities in each of these genes.

- These are the genes which protect the body from getting cancer
- Cancer results when this gene is deleted or mutated
- Antioncogenes are written with capital letters and the oncogenes are represented by small letters
- For example, *retinoblastoma (RB) oncosuppressor gene* in chromosome 13
- Familial breast cancer gene—*BRCA 1* gene in chromosome 17

21. Wilson's disease.
Refer 2007 Short Note 24.

22. Define isoenzymes and give two examples.
Refer 2003 Short Note 5.

23. Specific dynamic action.
Refer 2010 Short Answer Question 9.

24. Chemiosmotic theory.
Refer 2003 Short Note 4.

25. Von Gierke's disease.
Refer 2003 Short Note 6.

26. Pyruvate dehydrogenase complex (Fig. 13).

- Pyruvate which is the end product of aerobic glycolysis is converted to acetyl coA by the multienzyme complex pyruvate dehydrogenase complex
- The three enzymes present in pyruvate dehydrogenase complex are:

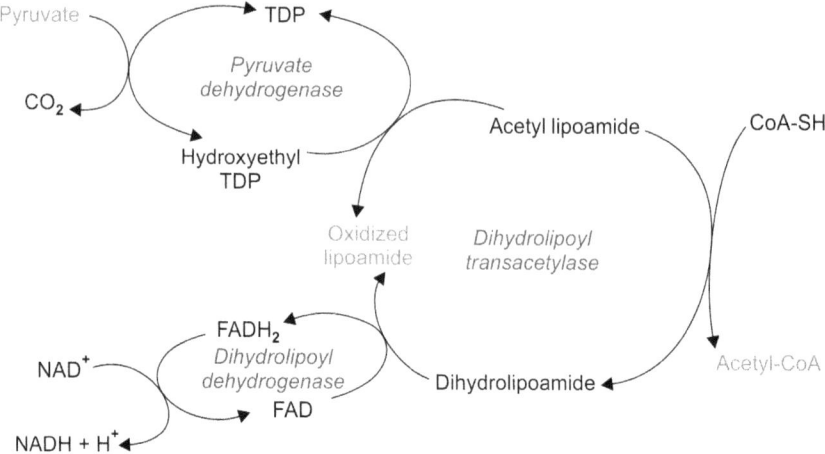

Fig. 13: Action of pyruvate dehydrogenase complex.

1. **Pyruvate decarboxylase (enzyme I):** It catalyzes oxidative decarboxylation with the help of TPP—its coenzyme. Hydroxylethyl-TPP is formed
2. **Dihydrolipoyl transacetylase (enzyme-2):** The hydroxyethyl group of TPP is oxidized to acetyl group by this enzyme and then acetyl group is transferred from TPP to lipoamide to form acetyl lipoamide
3. **Dihydrolipoate dehydrogenase (enzyme 3):** This enzyme oxidizes lipoamide and at the end all the cofactors are reformed.

- The coenzymes of pyruvate dehydrogenase are 5 coenzymes—NAD, FAD, CoA, lipoic acid and TPP.

Thus pyruvate is converted to acetyl-CoA and enters into TCA cycle.

27. Ionophores.

- They are membrane shuttles for specific ions
- They transport antibiotics produced by certain microorganisms
- They increase the permeability of membranes to ions by acting as channel formers
- There are 2 types of ionophores:
  1. Mobile ion carriers (e.g. valinomycin)
  2. Channel formers (e.g. gramicidin)
- In higher organisms, ion gradient is dissipated by ionophores which abolishes the proton gradient. This results in uncoupling of oxidative phosphorylation.

28. Oral glucose tolerance test.

Refer 2008 Short Note 30.

29. Deficiency manifestations of vitamin D.

Refer 2014 Short Answer Question 48.
- Vitamin D is a fat-soluble vitamin
- Deficiency of vitamin D causes: a) Rickets in children and b) Osteomalacia in adults.

Rickets (Children)

- Because of the poor mineralization of bones, they become soft and pliable
- Main features are—bossing of frontal bones, pigeon chest, knock knees, bow legs and rickety rosary—enlargement of epiphysis at the lower end of ribs and costochondral junction causing beading of ribs
- Harrison's sulcus—a transverse depression from the costal cartilage to axilla due to indentation of lower ribs to diaphragm.

Osteomalacia (Adult)

- There will be softening of bones due to poor mineralization and increased osteoporosis which leads to fractures

- Calcium and phosphorus values are low in blood
- Serum alkaline phosphatase level is increased.

30. Biochemical functions of Iron.

- Iron is an important trace element. Serum iron concentration is 120 µg/dL
- It is the integral part of hemoglobin and myoglobin and is required for transport of oxygen
- Cytochromes and nonheme proteins of electron transport chain and oxidative phosphorylation need iron
- Peroxidase contains iron which is required for the phagocytosis of bacteria by neutrophils
- It is needed for the immune competence of body
- It helps in the transport, storage and utilization of oxygen in the body.

31. Bicarbonate buffer system.

Refer 2006 Short Note 29.
Buffers resist changes in pH when small quantities of an acid or an alkali are added.
Various buffers in body are: Bicarbonate buffer system, phosphate buffer system and protein buffer system.

Bicarbonate Buffer System

- It is the most important buffer in plasma and is formed by ($NaHCO_3/H_2CO_3$)
- It accounts for 65% of buffering capacity in plasma and 40% of buffering action in the whole body
- The base HCO_3^- is the metabolic component as it is regulated by kidney and the acid H_2CO_3 is called respiratory component since it is regulated by the lungs.
  - The normal bicarbonate level in plasma is 24 mmol/L
  - The normal carbonic acid concentration in blood is 1.2 mmol/L and it has a pKa of 6.1
  - The normal pCO_2 of arterial blood is 40 mm of Hg.
- Substituting these values in the Henderson-Hasselbalch equation:
  - $pH = pKa + \log[HCO_3]/[H_2CO_3]$
  - $pH = 6.1 + \log 24/1.2$
  - $pH = 6.1 + \log 20$
  - $pH = 6.1 + 1.3 = 7.4$
- Under physiological conditions with a plasma pH 7.4, the ratio of bicarbonate to carbonic acid (HCO_3/H_2CO_3) is 20:1. In blood the concentration of bicarbonate is 20 times higher than carbonic acid in blood
- This is referred as alkali reserve and this is responsible for effective buffering of H^+ ions produced in the body.

32. Hyperkalemia.

Refer 2013 Short Answers Question 32.
- The normal plasma potassium level is 3.5–5.2 mmol/L
- Plasma potassium level above 5.5 mmol/L is known as hyperkalemia
- Hyperkalemia is life-threatening. It is characterized by flaccid paralysis, bradycardia, and cardiac arrest
- ECG: Elevated T-wave, widening of QRS complex, lengthening of PR interval.

Causes

- Decreased renal excretion of potassium: Urinary tract obstruction, renal failure, deficient aldosterone, heart failure
- Entry of potassium to extracellular space: Increased hemolysis, tissue necrosis, burns, tumor lysis, crush injury
- Redistribution of potassium to extracellular space: Metabolic acidosis, diabetes mellitus, tissue hypoxia
- Hyperkalemic periodic paralysis
- Drugs: Spironolactone, ACE inhibitors, beta-blockers, cyclosporine, digoxin.

Pseudohyperkalemia: Seen in hemolysis, improper blood collection, thrombocytosis, leukocytosis or polycythemia.

Treatment: When potassium level >6.5 mmol/L, intravenous glucose and insulin should be given. Continuous ECG monitoring should be done.

33. Define electrophoresis and mention its applications.

Refer 2006 Short Note 30.

34. Renal tubular function tests.

Refer 2012 Short Notes 18.
- **Renal** tubules reabsorb or secrete certain substances, concentrate the urine and acidify the urine. So it is important for maintaining specific gravity and osmolality of urine.
- **The following are the tubular function tests:**
  - **Specific gravity (SG) of urine—** simplest test: Specific gravity of urine depends on the concentration of the solutes. In early stages of renal failure SG may be low due to kidney's inability to excrete solutes.
  - **Urine concentration test (fluid deprivation test):**
    - Fluid intake is restricted for 15 hours. The first urine sample in the morning is collected, SG and osmolality measured
    - If the SG is more than 1.025 or the osmolality exceeds 850 mOsmol/kg the renal concentration capacity is said to be normal
    - Renal concentration ability is impaired due to tubular defect or in diabetes insipidus where there is decreased secretion of antidiuretic hormone.
  - **Measurement of osmolality:** Measurement of urine and plasma osmolality are done by using osmometer. **Normal urinary osmolality ranges from 60–1200 mOsmol/kg. Normal plasma osmolality is 285–300 mOsm/kg.** The ratio between urine/plasma osmolality is calculated. Normal ratio is around 3–4.5. Urinary osmolality is decreased in diabetes insipidus
  - **Dilution tests:** This is done to check whether kidneys can excrete an excess water load. After emptying the bladder 1,000–1,200 mL of water is given to the patient. Hourly urine is collected for next 4 hours. In each sample volume, specific gravity and osmolality are measured. A normal person will excrete all the water load within 4 hours. It is a more sensitive test
  - **Urinary acidification test** (acid load test or ammonium chloride loading test):
    - This is used to diagnose renal tubular acidosis
    - Ammonium chloride is given orally in gelatin capsule (100 mg/kg body weight) to induce metabolic acidosis. HCl produced is excreted as acidified urine
    - Hourly urine collected for 2 to 8 hours and pH and acid excretion of each sample noted
    - At least one sample should have pH lesser than 5.5. pH is not decreased in cases of renal tubular acidosis.
  - **Fractional excretion of bicarbonate, sodium and phosphate in urine** also help in assessing renal tubular functions.

35. Urinary findings in jaundice.

- Jaundice or icterus is a condition in which there is yellowish discoloration of the skin and sclera due to hyperbilirubinemia
- Bilirubin is the catabolic end product of heme
- According to the site and causes of jaundice it is classified as:
  - Prehepatic or hemolytic jaundice
  - Hepatic or hepatocellular jaundice and
  - Posthepatic or obstructive jaundice
- The types of jaundice can be identified depending on the laboratory tests.

Urinary Findings

S. No.	Urinary tests	Hemolytic jaundice	Hepatic jaundice	Obstructive jaundice
1.	Urine–bile salts (Hay's test)	Nil	Nil	Present
2.	Urine–conjugated bilirubin	Nil	Present	Present
3.	Urine–urobilinogen	Increased	Nil	Nil

- Hay's test: This test is specific for identification of urine bile salts—positive for posthepatic jaundice
- Fouchet's test (conjugated bilirubin in urine): This test gives positive result for both hepatic and posthepatic
- Ehrlich test (for urobilinogens): Positive in prehepatic jaundice and positive in early stages of hepatic jaundice.

36. Methemoglobin.
Refer 2009 Short Answer Question 36.

37. Structure of immunoglobulin.
Refer 2008 Short Note 11.

38. Regulation of heme synthesis.
Refer 2008 Essay Question 2.

Regulation of Heme Synthesis

1. **Rate-limiting enzyme ALA synthase** is regulated:
   a. By repression: Heme inhibits the synthesis of ALA synthase enzyme as a co-repressor
   b. By allosteric inhibition by hematin.
2. **Compartmentalization of the enzymes:** Rate-limiting enzyme is in mitochondria. Steps 1, 5, 6, and 7 take place in mitochondria and steps 2, 3, and 4 occur in cytoplasm
3. **Drugs/poisons:**
   - Barbiturates induce heme synthesis
   - Isoniazide decreases the availability of PLP and so decreases heme synthesis
   - Lead—inhibits ferrochelatase and ALA dehydratase.
4. **Glucose:** High concentration of glucose in the cells prevents induction of ALA synthase.

39. Lac operon concept.
Refer 2004 Short Note 19.

40. Define PCR and mention its four applications.
Refer 2010 Short Note 13.

41. Therapeutic uses of enzymes.
- Streptokinase and urokinase: Myocardial infarction (to lyse the intravascular clot)
- Pepsin and trypsin: Indigestion
- Asparaginase: Acute lymphoblastic leukemia
- Alpha-1 antitrypsin: Emphysema
- Papain: Anti-inflammatory.

42. Types of lipases.
1. Digestive lipases:
   a. Stomach:
      - Lingual lipase: It acts on short chain TAG present in milk, butter and ghee
      - Gastric lipase: It is acid stable, pH 5.4 and it digests 30% of TAG.
   b. Intestinal level
      - **Pancreatic** lipase with colipase hydrolyses the fatty acids in 1st and 3rd carbon atoms of glycerol forming 2 monoacylglycerol and 2 fatty acids
      - **Colipase** is secreted from pancreas. It binds to TAG at the oil water interface. It is activated by trypsin
      - **Intestinal** lipase—acts with bile acids on TAG with medium chain fatty acids to give 3 FFA and glycerol
      - **Phospholipases**—phospholipases A2 + BA—acts on phospholipids having unsaturated fatty acids in position-2 to give unsaturated fatty acid + lysolecithin.
2. **Non-digestive lipases:**
   - **Capillary walls: Lipoprotein lipase:** Acts on TAG of CM and VLDL and gives rise to FFA + glycerol. It is stimulated by insulin
   - **Adipocytes:** Hormone sensitive lipase: Acts on stored TAG to release FFA + DAG/MAG.

43. Lipotropic factors.
Fatty liver refers to the deposition of excess fat—TGL in the liver cells. Progression of fatty liver ends in cirrhosis of liver
- Fatty liver can be prevented by taking lipotropic factors, such as choline, lecithin, methionine, vitamin E, selenium and omega-3 fatty acids.

Lipotropic factors: They are choline, lecithin, methionine, vitamin E, selenium and omega-3 fatty acids. They are required for the normal mobilization of fat from liver. When they are deficient fat gets deposited in liver causing fatty liver.

Mode of Actions

- Choline: It reverses fatty changes in liver
- Lecithin and methionine: They help to synthesize apoproteins and choline
- Selenium and vitamin E: Antioxidants—give protection
- Omega-3 fatty acids: Present in marine oils and also has protective action.

44. Metabolism of propionyl-CoA.

Synthesis of Propionyl-CoA

- Oxidation of odd chain fatty acid produces propionate
- Metabolic end products of valine, isoleucine and methionine
- Glycolytic end product of glucose in ruminants.

Fate of Propionyl-CoA (Fig. 14):

i. Propionyl-CoA is carboxylated to D-methylmalonyl-CoA by carboxylase enzyme which needs biotin, CO_2 and one molecule of ATP
ii. D-methylmalonyl-CoA is acted by racemase enzyme to give L-malonyl-CoA
iii. L-methylmalonyl-CoA is rearranged to form succinyl-CoA by mutase enzyme for which deoxyadenosyl cobalamine acts as coenzyme
iv. Succinyl-CoA then enters TCA cycle and converted to fumarate, malate and finally to oxaloacetate
v. Oxaloacetate comes out of mitochondria to the cytosol to the gluconeogenic pathway by reversal of glycolysis through phosphophenol pyruvate to form glucose.

45. Prevention of atherosclerosis.

a. **Atherosclerosis:**
   - Hardening of the arteries due to deposition of cholesterol and other lipids in the arterial wall which leads to the formation of plaque and causes narrowing of blood vessel lumen
   - Atherosclerosis leads to ischemic heart disease and cardiovascular diseases.
b. **Prevention:**
   a. Change of lifestyle—regular exercise, balanced diet, stop smoking, maintaining proper weight
   b. Control of hypertension, diabetes and dyslipidemia
   c. To reduce total cholesterol below 180 mg/dL
   d. To decrease LDL cholesterol below 130 mg/dL
   e. To keep HDL cholesterol above 35 mg/dL.

46. Allosteric regulation.

- Enzymes which have one catalytic site where the substrate binds and another separate site where the modifier binds, are known as allosteric site [Greek: Allo = Other]
- Both the sites may or may not be nearer to each other
- If the binding of the regulatory molecule increases the activity of the enzyme, it is known as **allosteric activation,** and the regulatory molecule is known as positive modulator

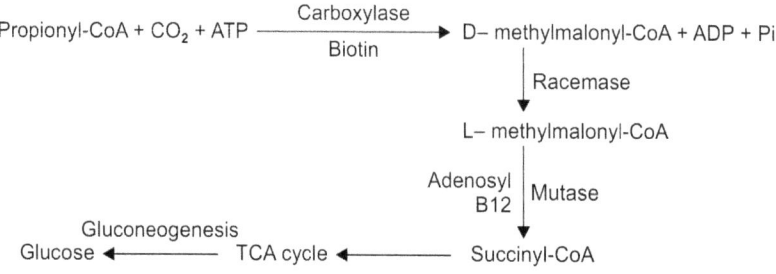

Fig. 14: Fate of propionyl-CoA.

- If the binding of regulatory molecule inhibits the activity of the enzyme it is known as **allosteric inhibition** and the regulatory molecule it is known as negative modulator
- Allosteric activation effect is said to be positive cooperativity and the allosteric inhibition effect is called negative cooperativity.
- Combination of both are seen in most cases resulting in sigmoid curve
- Allosteric regulators are divided into two classes based on the influence of allosteric effector on K_m and V_{max}. They are as follows:
  1. K-class of allosteric enzymes: Effector changes K_m but not V_{max}, e.g. phosphofructokinase
  2. V-class of allosteric enzymes: Effector alters the V_{max}, but not K_m, e.g. acetyl-CoA carboxylase.

47. Significance of multienzyme complexes with example.

Many enzymes combine together to act on a particular substrate as a single enzyme complex with variable actions are called multienzyme complex.

Examples for Multienzyme complex
1. Pyruvate dehydrogenase
2. Alpha-ketoglutarate dehydrogenase
3. Glycine cleavage system
4. Fatty acid synthase complex.

Enzymes 1 and 4 are explained here:
1. Pyruvate dehydrogenase complex:
   - This multienzyme catalyzes conversion of pyruvate to acetyl-CoA connecting aerobic glycolysis and TCA cycle. It is an irreversible process
   - Pyruvate + CoA. SH + TPP+ lipoic acid + NAD + FAD
     $$\xrightarrow{\text{Pyruvate dehydrogenase}}$$
     Acetyl-CoA + CO_2 + NADH + H^+ + $FADH_2$
   - This multienzyme consists of 3 enzymes—1. Pyruvate dehydrogenase which decarboxylates pyruvate 2. Dihydrolipoyl transacetylase 3. Dihydrolipoyl dehydrogenase
   - It needs 5 coenzymes—TPP, lipoic acid, coenzyme A, NAD, FAD
   - It is the committed step for complete oxidation of glucose and produces 5 ATP from one molecule of glucose
   - This is analogous to alpha-keto glutarate dehydrogenase multienzyme complex of TCA cycle.
2. Fatty acid synthase multienzyme complex (Fig. 15):
   - It is the multienzyme complex. It catalyses the synthesis of fatty acid from acetyl-CoA.

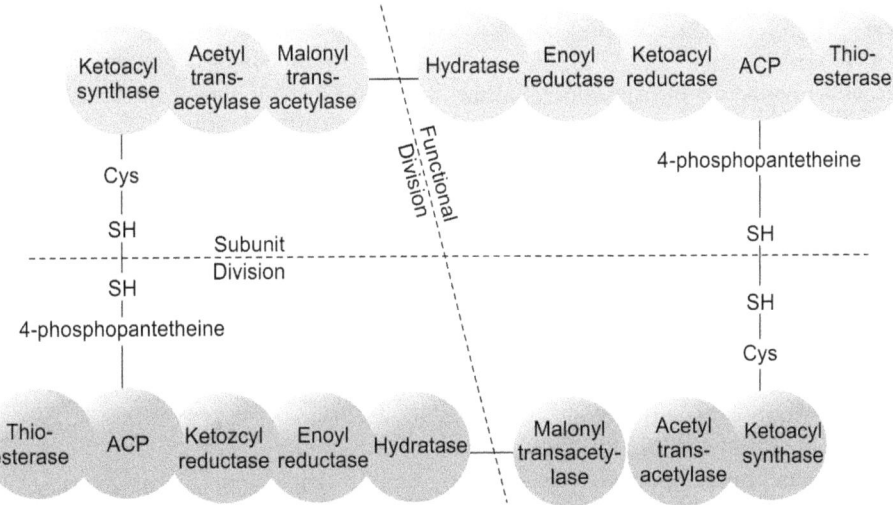

Fig. 15: Fatty acid synthase multienzyme complex.

- It is a dimer with identical subunits. Each subunit is organized into 3 domains with 7 enzymes.

Domain 1: Other name: Condensing unit:
- It is the initial substrate binding site.
- Enzymes are: i) Beta-ketoacyl-acyl carrier protein synthase; ii) Acetyl transferase; iii) Malonyl transacylase.

Domain 2: Other name: Reduction unit
- It contains dehydratase, enoyl reductase, beta-ketoacyl reductase and acyl carrier protein (ACP).

Domain 3: Other name: Releasing unit
- It contains thioesterase or deacylase.
- **Advantage of multienzyme complex:**
  - Intermediates of the reaction can easily interact with the active site of enzyme.
  - One gene codes for all the enzymes, so they are equimolecular in concentration
  - Efficiency of the synthetic process is enhanced.

48. Functions of phosphate.

- **Formation of bone and teeth:** Vitamin D stimulates osteoblasts to produce alkaline phosphatase which leads to the formation of calcium phosphate hydroxyapatite crystals which is deposited on the bone causing mineralization
- **Production of high energy phosphates like:**
  a. ATP—energy currency of the cell
  b. CTP—needed for phosphatidylcholine and other compound synthesis
  c. GTP—is needed for G proteins
  d. UTP—bilirubin conjugation and glycogen metabolism.
- Synthesis of coenzymes like NAD and NADP
- DNA and RNA synthesis—phosphodiester bond links the sugar units which forms backbone of nucleic acids
- Esters: Formation of G6P, F6P, etc.
- Phospholipids like lecithin formation
- Formation of phosphoproteins like casein
- Activation of enzymes by phosphorylation
- Phosphate buffer: It is made of Na_2HPO_4/NaH_2PO_4. It has a pKa of 6.8.

49. What is saponification and iodine number? Write its importance.

A. Saponification number:
- It is defined as number of miligrams of KOH needed to saponify one gm of fat. It is an indicator of molecular weight of fat.
- It is inversely proportionate to the molecular weight of fat. It is high in fats with short chain fatty acid.
- Saponification number of butter = 220; coconut oil = 260.

B. Iodine number:
- It is defined as number of grams of iodine needed to saturate 100 g of given fat. It is an indicator of degree of instauration of fat
- High iodine number indicates higher degree of unsaturation
- It also helps to identify adulteration
- Iodine number of butter =27; coconut oil = 8.

50. Write about glycine cleavage systems and mention the derivatives of glycine.

Refer 2014 Short Notes 17—functions of glycine.
- This is a multienzyme complex (**Fig. 16**)
- It is the reversal of the glycine synthase reaction
- This consists of 3 enzymes and one H-protein that has a covalently attached dihydrolipoyl moiety

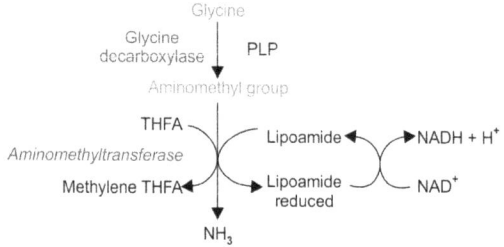

Fig. 16: Glycine cleavage system.

- This system consists of:
  - Glycine decarboxylase
  - Aminomethyltransferase
  - Methylene H_4F synthase and lipoamide dehydrogenase.
- This multienzyme complex reacts with CO_2, NH_3 and one carbon unit to form glycine.
- NAD, lipoamide, PLP and THFA are the coenzymes of this step.

Glycine + H_4 folate + NAD → CO_2 + NH_2 + N^5, N^{10} methylene H_4 folate + NADH + H^+

Metabolic Products
- Methylenetetrahydrofolate by glycine cleavage system to join one-carbon pool
- Glucose: It is glucogenic.

Special Products (Fig. 17)
- Creatine, creatine phosphate and creatinine by the combination of glycine, arginine and active methionine at liver, kidney and muscles
- Heme: ALA synthase condenses glycine with succinyl-CoA to form delta-aminolevulinic acid—rate-limiting step
- Purine nucleotides: Glycine contributes all its atoms for the formation of purine ring—C4, 5 and N7
- Glutathione: It is formed by the combination of glutamate, cysteine and glycine
- Conjugating agent: Glycine conjugates bile acids to form glycocholic acid
- Constituent of most of the proteins—more in collagen—every third amino acid is glycine
- Glycine—it is a neurotransmitter.

51. Polyamines (Fig. 18).
- A polyamine is an organic compound having two or more primary amino groups—NH_2
- Polyamines are putrescine, spermidine and spermine

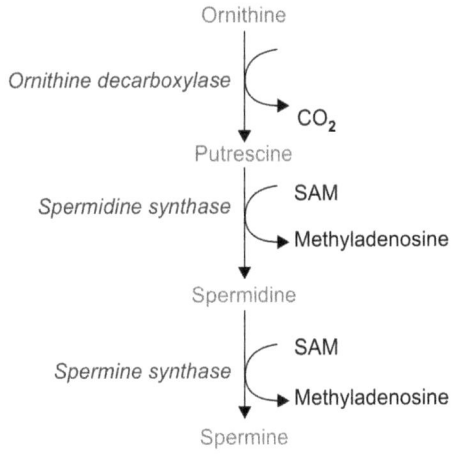

Fig. 18: Polyamine synthesis.

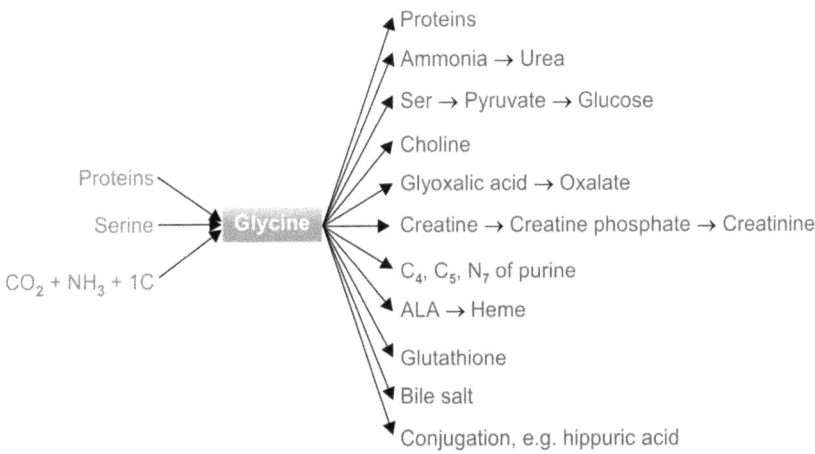

Fig. 17: Products derived from glycine.

- They are aliphatic amines synthesized from Ornithine (arginine)
- Functions:
  - The polyamines help in protein synthesis
  - Polyamines are involved in cell proliferation, stabilization of ribosomes and DNA, synthesis of DNA and RNA, protection of DNA against deprivation
  - Polyamine concentration is increased in cancer cells
  - Polyamines are growth factors in cell culture systems.

Inhibitors: Difluromethyl ornithine (DFMO) is a powerful inhibitor of polyamine synthesis by suicidal inhibition. Trypanosomes are parasites that are destroyed by DFMO since polyamines are needed for their reproduction.

52. Types of chromatography. Write in brief about any one type of chromatography.

Definition: It is a separative procedure for separating components of a solution by differences in migration rate as the solution (mobile phase) is passed through a stationary phase. The term is derived from the Greek word chroma means color. This is used to separate almost all biological substances including proteins, carbohydrates, lipids and nucleic acids.

Types of Chromatography

1. **Adsorption chromatography**
2. **Partition chromatography**
3. **Gel infiltration (size exclusion) chromatography**
4. **High pressure liquid chromatography**
5. **Ion exchange chromatography**
6. **Affinity chromatography**

Partition Chromatography is Discussed here

Partition chromatography:
- This is a technique of chromatography which includes different types depending on the phases between which the components are partitioned, e.g. solid-liquid, liquid–liquid, gas-liquid, etc.
- This is used for the separation of mixtures of amino acids and peptides
- There is a stationary phase which may be either solid or liquid and a mobile phase which may be liquid or gas
- The components of mixture to be separated are partitioned between the two phases depending on the partition coefficient (solubility) of the particular substances
- The types of partition chromatography are: i) Paper chromatography; ii) Thin layer chromatography.

  i. **Paper chromatography:**
     - In this type the stationary phase is water held on a solid support of filter paper (cellulose)
     - The mobile phase is a mixture of immiscible solvents like water, a nonpolar solvent and an acid or base, e.g. butanol-acetic acid-water, phenol-water-ammonia
     - Chromatography can be done with the mobile phase applied from top—descending type or bottom—ascending type
     - A few microliters of the mixture to be separated is applied as a small spot at one end of the paper 1" away from the edges. In ascending type the paper is placed in a glass trough containing the solvent and allowed to move in the paper
     - It takes 14–16 hours
     - The distance to which each component moves depends on its partition coefficient.

  ii. **Thin layer chromatography:**
     - This is liquid-liquid chromatography
     - Thin layer of silica gel is spread on a glass plate
     - Sample is applied as small spots
     - The plates placed in a trough containing the solvent. It takes 3–4 hours.

Visualization of Chromatography

- After the run is over, the paper or the plate is dried

- Location reagents, such as ninhydrin will be sprayed for amino acids and proteins; sulfuric acid sprayed for phospholipids and diphenylamine for sugars
- Spots are identified and the distance traveled by the solute and solvent are marked and retardation factor (Rf) value calculated

Importance of Rf Value

Rf value is the ratio of distance traveled by substance to distance traveled by the solvent. It is a constant for a particular solvent system.

Applications of Chromatography

- To separate mixtures of amino acids, proteins and carbohydrates
- To purify proteins, enzymes, nucleic acids
- To determine the molecular weight of proteins
- To analyze drugs, hormones, vitamins
- To analyze certain substances qualitatively and quantitatively
- To identify sugar, amino acids and drugs in urine or serum.

53. Metabolic alkalosis.

Alkalosis

Loss of acid or accumulation of bases causing increased pH. There are 2 types of alkalosis—metabolic and respiratory alkalosis.

Metabolic Alkalosis

- It is due to primary excess of bicarbonate which is compensated by ↑pCO_2 by hypoventilation
- This is seen in vomiting, hypokalemia, Cushing, syndrome, diuretic therapy
- This occurs when excess base is added or during defective base excretion or due to loss of acid
- Ratio of bicarbonate to carbonic acid will be more than 20
- This is subclassified to: a. Chloride responsive and b. Chloride resistant types

a. Chloride responsive metabolic alkalosis: Seen in prolonged vomiting, nasogastric aspiration or administration of diuretics
b. Chloride resistant metabolic alkalosis: Seen in hypertension, hyperaldosteronism, severe potassium depletion, Cushing's syndrome
- In metabolic alkalosis there is hypokalemia as there is an attempt to conserve hydrogen ions by kidney in exchange of potassium. This potassium loss will lead to hypokalemia.

54. Histamine.

- Histamine is a biological amine–derived from histidine
- It is a decarboxylated product of histidine by histidine decarboxylase which needs PLP

$$\text{Histidine} \xrightarrow[\text{PLP}]{\text{Histidine decarboxylase}} \text{Histamine} + CO_2$$

- Histamine is produced in the body from platelet mast cells and basophils
- Effects of histamine are—smooth muscle contraction, enhanced vascular permeability, increased acid secretion
- It causes fall of BP
- Along with slow reacting substances (SRS) it produces allergic reactions against drugs like penicillin. There will be fall of BP and vasodilatation
- Antihistamine drugs block the histamine receptors and control allergic reactions
- Histamine acts on H_2 receptors and stimulates gastric acid secretion. H_2 receptor antagonists are used in the treatment of acid peptic ulcers of stomach.

55. Telomere and telomerase.

- The end pieces of chromosomes are called as telomeres
- Replication will not take place upto these ends—3' or 5' ends

- Telomerases or telomere terminal transferases do the job of replicating at these end pieces of chromosomes
- Telomerase acts as a reverse transcriptase to synthesize this small DNA strand
- In old age telomerase activity is lost leading to chromosomal instability and cell death
- Drugs which prevent expression of gene for telomerase act as anticancer agents.

56. Write about protein targeting and its disorders.

- This is also called as 'protein sorting' or 'protein localization'
- The secreted proteins, integral proteins of plasma membrane, membrane proteins of endoplasmic reticulum and lysosomal enzymes are synthesized from rough endoplasmic reticulum
- The newly synthesized proteins are then delivered to the destined compartment
- The secretory proteins contain a signal peptide (SP) region of about 15–35 amino acids present in the amino terminal region
- This signal peptide helps in anchoring of ribosomes on ER
- Signal recognition particle (SRP) is attached to SP region and blocks protein synthesis
- The newly formed nascent protein is passed through the membranes into the channels of ER
- During this process carbohydrate moieties are added at particular region by specific enzymes. This is called co-translational glycosylation
- According to the destination of the protein inside the cells, the proteins carry an address which is present in the carboxy terminal end of proteins.

Disorders due to Defective Protein Targeting

- **Zellweger syndrome:**
  - This is due to defective oxidation of very long chain fatty acids (VLCFA)
  - Here the correct address is not printed on the protein pockets and so it could not be delivered to the correct destination
  - Peroxisomal enzymes which are produced cannot enter into the peroxisomes
  - Because of this, there is insufficient oxidation of VLCFA which leads to accumulation of VLCFA in CNS causing neurological impairment and death in childhood.
- **Primary hyperoxaluria:** This is due to protein targeting defect by which the enzyme alanine glyoxalate aminotransferase is seen in mitochondria instead of peroxisomes which is its normal destination
- **Familial hypercholesterolemia:** This is due to deficient transport signals
- **Cystic fibrosis:** Caused due to improper localization of proteins
- **Inclusion cell disease: (I-cell disease):** This is due to nonentry of normal enzymes into lysosomes. Mannose 6-phosphate—the marker to target enzymes to lysosomes is absent in this condition.

57. Methemoglobinemia.

Refer 2009 Short Answers Question 36.
- Methemoglobin (MetHb) is a type of Hb variant. The iron in the heme is in ferrous form normally. When it is oxidized to ferric form then it is called methemoglobin
- Normally the MetHb level in blood is less than 1%. It has decreased capacity of transporting oxygen
- Small quantities of MetHb formed are reduced by MetHb reductase systems using NADH and Cytochrome b_5. Remaining is reduced using NADPH-dependent enzyme. Glutathione dependent metHb reductase system is also present
- **Methemoglobinemia:** Increase in MetHb level in blood is known as methemoglobinemia. It is manifested as cyanosis.
- Two types—congenital and acquired

1. Congenital methemoglobinemia: Cytochrome b5 reductase deficiency is the cause for this. Oral administration of methylene blue reduces the symptoms.
2. Acquired methemoglobinemia: May be due to Intake of: a) Water containing nitrates; b) Absorption of aniline dyes; c) Drugs like acetaminophen, sulfanilamides amyl nitrate ingestion.

- G6PD deficiency causes reduced availability of NADPH for the RBCs. At that time the NADPH-dependent methemoglobin reductase will be inactive leading to methemoglobinemia.

58. Normal serum electrolyte values.

- Sodium = 136–145 (140) mEq/L
- Potassium = 3.5–5 (4) mEq/L
- Chloride = 96–106 (105) mEq/L
- Bicarbonate = 24 mEq/L.

59. Nitric oxide.

Refer 2011 Short Note 11.

MBBS Examination 2015

ANSWER ALL QUESTIONS

I. Essay questions (10/15 Marks each)
1. Write in detail about the dietary sources, daily requirement and biochemical functions of thiamine. Add a note on the deficiency manifestations.
2. What is a buffer? Describe in detail about the renal regulation of blood pH.
3. Structure and functions of phospholipids.
4. Describe in detail about the formation and transport of ammonia in our body. Add a note on urea cycle.
5. Write a note on the metabolism of vitamin D.
6. Describe in detail about the synthesis of tyrosine and its metabolic end products.

II. Short notes (2/5 Marks each)
1. Apolipoproteins.
2. Metabolism of adipose tissue in fasting condition.
3. Purine salvage pathway.
4. Metabolism of methionine.
5. Glycolysis in RBC (2, 3-bisphosphoglycerate cycle/2, 3 BPG shunt). Rapoport-Luebering cycle.
6. Shuttle pathways across mitochondrial membrane.
7. Laboratory investigations in different types of jaundice.
8. Structure of DNA (Watson–Crick model).
9. Competitive enzyme inhibition.
10. Carnitine.
11. Structure of messenger RNA (mRNA).
12. Liver function tests.

III. Short answer questions (4/5 Marks each)
1. Fate of oxaloacetate.
2. Liver enzymes.
3. Functions of magnesium.
4. Dietary fibers.
5. Cytochrome P450.
6. Functions of phospholipids.
7. Suicide inhibition of enzymes.
8. Causes for abnormal GTT curves.
9. Biologically important peptides.
10. Biological value of protein.
11. Gout.
12. Define transcription. Name four post-transcriptional modifications.
13. Primary structure of proteins.
14. Metabolic functions of glycine.
15. Maple syrup urine disease.
16. Hartnup's disease.
17. Adaptation to high altitude.
18. Genetic code.
19. Types of mutations.
20. Structure of tRNA.
21. Ocular changes in vitamin A deficiency.
22. Amphipathic lipids.
23. Kwashiorkor.
24. Enzymes in diagnosis of myocardial infarction.
25. Biochemical functions of zinc.
26. Hormones that regulate blood calcium level. Explain.
27. Mechanism of cyanide poisoning.
28. Metabolism of glucose-6-phosphate.
29. Lipoprotein lipase.
30. Cori cycle (lactic acid cycle).
31. Paper chromatography.
32. Transmethylation reactions.
33. Pancreatic function tests.

34. Alkaptonuria.
35. Acute intermittent porphyria.
36. Sickle cell disease.
37. Bile salts.
38. Renal glomerular function tests.
39. Anion gap.
40. Okazaki fragments.
41. Fatty liver.
42. Inhibitors of citric acid cycle.
43. Cholesterol lowering action of fibrates.
44. One carbon compound.
45. Functions of copper.
46. Biochemical alteration in protein-energy malnutrition (PEM).
47. Conjugations/phase II reactions of detoxifications.
48. Stereoisomerism.
49. Actions of insulin.
50. Hyperglycemic hormones.
51. ELISA.
52. Isoelectric pH of proteins.
53. Wilson's disease.
54. Laboratory diagnosis of phenylketonuria.
55. Chloride shift.
56. DNA repair mechanism.
57. Plasma buffers.
58. Gene therapy.
59. Functions of albumin.
60. Orotic aciduria.

I. ESSAY QUESTIONS

1. Write in detail about the dietary sources, daily requirement and biochemical functions of thiamine. Add a note on the deficiency manifestations.

Refer 2003 Essay Question 1.

2. What is a buffer? Describe in detail about the renal regulation of blood pH.

Refer 2003 Essay Question 4—mechanisms 1 and 2011 Essay Question 8.

3. Structure and functions of phospholipids.

Refer 2004 Short Note 1.

4. Describe in detail about the formation and transport of ammonia in our body. Add a note on urea cycle.

Refer 2005 Essay Question 7.

5. Write a note on the metabolism of vitamin D.

Refer 2003 Short Note 1 and 2011 Short Note 1. Cholecalciferol or Vitamin D is a derivative of cholesterol and the ultimate precursor for cholecalciferol is 7-dehydrocholesterol (7-DHC) in animals. Ergocalciferol is the precursor form of vitamin D in plants—vitamin D2.

Biosynthesis of Active Vitamin D

Refer 2011 Short Note 1.

7-dehydrocholesterol $\xrightarrow{\text{Light}}$ Provitamin D

$\xrightarrow{\text{Thermal Isomerization}}$ Cholecalciferol

- 7-DHC is rich in malphigian layer of epidermis. The bond between 9 and 10 of 7-DHC is cleaved and converted into cholecalciferol by the action of UV light. That is why this is called as sunshine vitamin
- Vitamin D is a prohormone. Activation of provitamin D (cholecalciferol) into active vitamin D (calcitriol) takes place at two different sites.

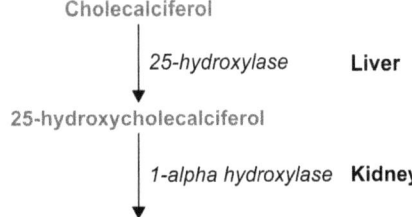

- **25 hydroxylation of cholecalciferol in liver**—cholecalciferol through blood reaches the liver cells and undergoes hydroxylation at 25th carbon. This reaction is catalyzed by 25-hydroxylase to form 25-hydroxycholecalciferol
- **In plasma**—25 HCC is bound to vitamin D binding protein

- **1 hydroxylation in kidney:** the active form of vitamin D is synthesized at kidney. 25-hydroxycholecalciferol is hydroxylated at 1st position and converted into 1, 25-dihydroxycholecalciferol/calcitriol. It is the **active form of vitamin D.**

Sources: Exposure to sunlight produces cholecalciferol. Other dietary sources include—fish liver oil (cod, eel), meat, egg, milk.

RDA: Children, pregnancy and lactation—10 µg/day (400 IU), adults—5 µg/day (200 IU). Adults above 60 years - 600 IU/day.

Biochemical functions of calcitriol

Refer 2011 Short Note 1.

The active form of vitamin D is calcitriol which is 1, 25-dihydroxycholecalciferol.

Biochemical Functions of Calcitriol

Calcitriol acts as steroid hormone. It binds to specific cytoplasmic receptors which interacts with DNA and induces the synthesis of mRNA for specific proteins called Calbindin which is a calcium-binding protein which will lead to biological actions.

- **Effect on intestine:** Calcitriol induces the synthesis of calbindin and helps in the absorption of calcium and phosphorus from the intestines **(Fig. 1)**
- **Effects on kidney:** Calcitriol increases the reabsorption of calcium and phosphorous from the renal tubules thereby conserving both the minerals
- **Action on bones:** Calcitriol increases the activity of osteoblasts and hence mineralization of bones is increased. It remodels the activity of osteoclasts and osteoblasts. It prevents rickets and osteomalacia.

Deficiency manifestations: Deficiency of vitamin D causes rickets in children and osteomalacia in adults.

Rickets (Children)

- Because of the poor mineralization of bones, they become soft and pliable
- Main features are—bossing of frontal bones, pigeon chest, knock knees, bow legs and rickety rosary—enlargement of epiphysis at the lower end of ribs and costochondral junction causing beading of ribs
- Harrison's sulcus—a transverse depression from the costal cartilage to axilla due to indentation of lower ribs to diaphragm.

Osteomalacia (Adults)

- There will be softening of bones due to poor mineralization and increased osteoporosis which leads to fractures

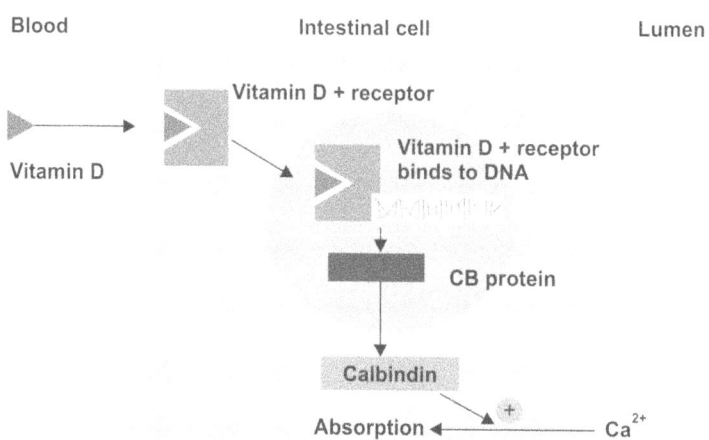

Fig. 1: Absorption of calcium by calcitriol.

- Calcium and phosphorus values are low in blood
- Serum alkaline phosphatase level is increased.

Hypervitaminosis D

This is due to increased intake of vitamin D. The patient will be very weak having the symptoms of polyuria, increased thirst, increased blood pressure and weight loss. Increased level of calcium leads to calcification of vascular and kidney tissues.

6. Describe in detail about the synthesis of tyrosine and its metabolic end products.

Synthesis of tyrosine: Tyrosine is hydroxylated phenylalanine.

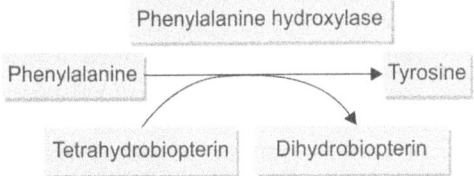

Conversion of Phenylalanine to Tyrosine by Hydroxylation (Fig. 2)

Step-1: Synthesis of tyrosine: Phenylalanine hydroxylase enzyme hydroxylates phenylalanine to tyrosine in the presence of the cofactor tetrahydrobiopterin, and coenzymes—NADPH and NADH. It is an irreversible reaction. Further tyrosine is catabolized by various steps to form fumarate (glucogenic pathway) and acetoacetate (ketogenic pathway).

- Tyrosine is an aromatic amino acid. It is synthesized from phenylalanine. It is both glucogenic and ketogenic.

Catabolism of Tyrosine (Fig. 2)

- **Step 2: Transamination:** Tyrosine is transaminated by tyrosine transaminase using PLP and alpha-ketoglutarate to form p-hydroxyphenylpyruvate and glutamic acid. This step is induced by glucocorticoids
- **Step 3: Synthesis of homogentisic acid (Dihydroxyphenyl acetate):** p-hydroxy-

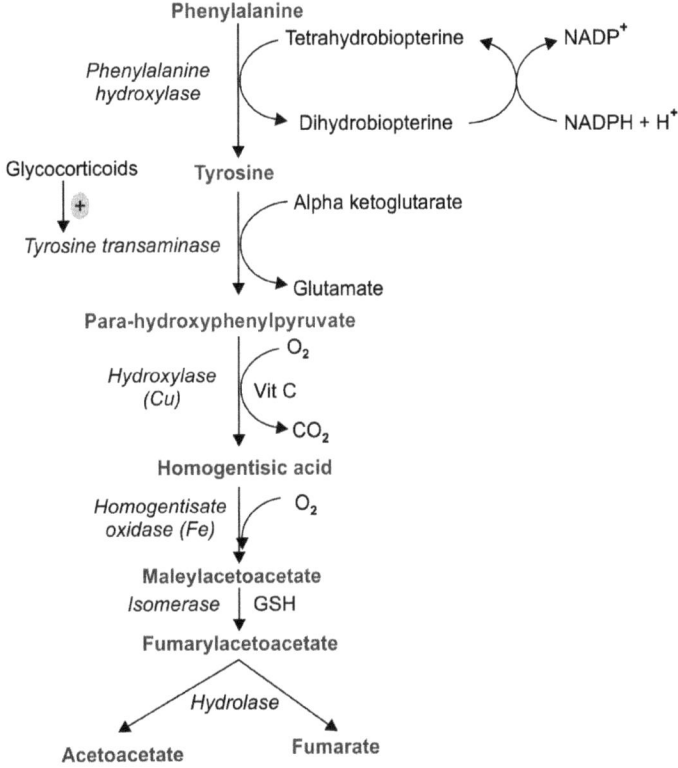

Fig. 2: Metabolism of phenylalanine and tyrosine.

phenylpyruvate is converted to homogentisate by hydroxylase enzyme. It is a copper containing enzyme. Ascorbic acid is required for this reaction
- **Step 4: Formation of maleylacetoacetate:** By the cleavage of aromatic ring homogentisate is converted to maleylacetoacetate by a dioxygenase called homogentisate oxidase which contains an iron atom at its active site
- **Step 5: Isomerisation of maleyl-to-fumaryl acetoacetate:** Maleylacetoacetate is converted to its isomer fumarylacetoacetate by isomerase using glutathione (GSH) as its cofactor
- **Step 6: Hydrolysis of fumarylacetoacetate:** Fumarylacetoacetate is cleaved into fumarate (glucogenic) and acetoacetate (ketogenic) by a hydrolase enzyme.

Other products formed from Tyrosine

Refer 2013 Short Note 55
- Melanin pigments
- Catecholamines
- Thyroxine
- Tyramine

Synthesis of Melanin (Fig. 3):
- Tyrosine is hydroxylated by tyrosinase to dihydroxyphenylalanine (DOPA). It is a mono-oxygenase containing copper
- Tyrosinase acts again on DOPA to form DOPAquinone
- Decarboxylation and oxidation of DOPA-quinone converts it to indolequinone, which is polymerized to melanin.

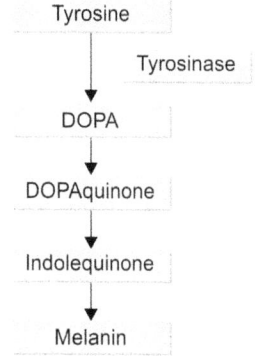

Fig. 3: Formation of melanin.

Catecholamines (Fig. 4):
- Tyrosine is first hydroxylated to DOPA by tyrosine hydroxylase. It requires tetrahydrobiopterin and NADPH
- DOPA is decarboxylated to form dopamine by DOPA decarboxylase, a PLP dependent enzyme. Dopamine is a catecholamine which is a neurotransmitter. In Parkinsonism, dopamine level is reduced. L-DOPA is used as a drug in Parkinsonism
- Dopamine is hydroxylated to norepinephrine by dopamine hydroxylase
- Norepinephrine is methylated to epinephrine by methyltransferase which needs SAM which is a methyl donor
- Epinephrine is methylated to metanephrine and oxidized to vanillylmandelic acid (VMA) and excreted in urine
- Normal level of excretion of VMA is 2-6 mg/day urine. This is elevated in pheochromocytoma and in neuroblastoma.

- **Thyroid hormones**

Specific tyrosine molecules are iodinated to form mono-, di and tri-iodothyronines and thyroxine (T4)

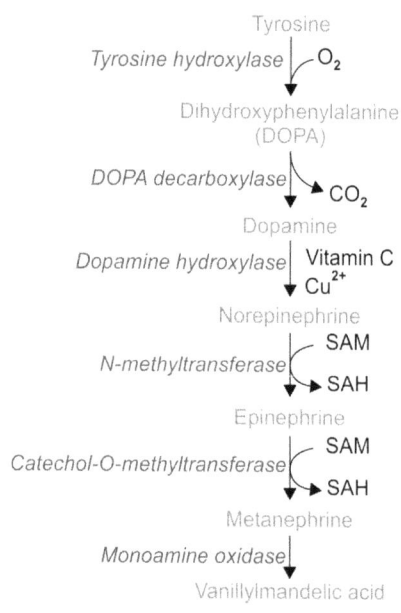

Fig. 4: Synthesis and degradation of catecholamines.

Tyramine

Tyrosine is decarboxylated to tyramine by intestinal bacteria which is one of the reasons for food allergy.

II. SHORT NOTES

1. **Apolipoproteins.**

Refer 2007 Short Note 21.

2. **Metabolism of adipose tissue in fasting condition.**

- Excess calories ingested are stored in adipose tissues as triacylglycerol
- This TAG undergoes turnover everyday by production of new TAG and degradation
- During fasting TAG from adipose tissues is mobilized under the effect of the hormones like glucagon and epinephrine
- The intracellular hormone sensitive lipase gets activated by cyclic AMP mediated cascade. The phosphorylated form of the enzyme is active
- This activated hormone sensitive lipase acts on TAG and liberates fatty acids
- During starvation and fasting when there is no intake of calories, lipolysis occurs under the influence of glucagon, ACTH, glucocorticoids and thyroxine
- TAG is broken down to free fatty acids and glycerol
- This free fatty acids are utilized by the peripheral tissues as fuel.

3. **Purine salvage pathway.**

Refer 2004 Short Note 15.

4. **Metabolism of methionine.**

Refer 2007 Essay Question 4.

5. **Glycolysis in RBC (2, 3-bisphosphoglycerate cycle/2, 3 BPG shunt). Rapoport-Luebering cycle.**

Refer 2007 Short Note 18.

6. **Shuttle pathways across mitochondrial membrane.**

Special shuttle systems carry the reducing equivalents from the cytoplasm to the mitochondria by an indirect route involving enzymatic processes. They are called as shuttle mechanisms. They are: 1. Malate-aspartate shuttle; 2. Glycerol phosphate shuttle; 3. Creatine phosphate shuttle.

1. Malate-Aspartate Shuttle (Fig. 5)

- It is the most active NADH shuttle mechanisms which carry reducing equivalents from cytosol to mitochondria by 2 carriers and 4 enzymes
- **Cytosolic malate dehydrogenase** converts cytosolic oxaloacetate to malate
- A **dicarboxylate transporter** system transfers malate across the membrane

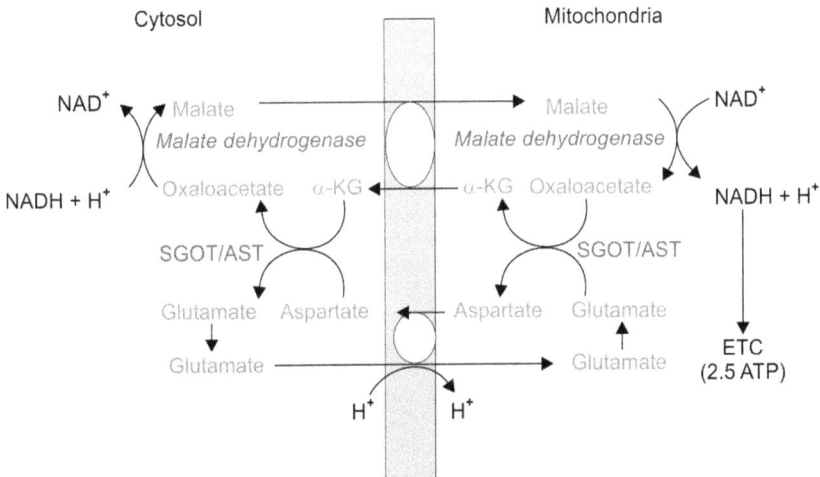

Fig. 5: Malate–aspartate shuttle.

- The reducing equivalents carried by malate are transferred to mitochondrial NAD by **mitochondrial malate dehydrogenase** and malate gets reoxidized to oxaloacetate
- NADH thus formed leads to the formation of 2.5 ATP/electron pair
- Oxaloacetate formed cannot pass through the membrane back to the cytosol and so it is converted to aspartate by **transamination** with glutamate and aspartate is transported to cytosolic side
- In the **cytosol, aspartate transaminase enzyme** converts aspartate to oxaloacetate and glutamate.

2. Glycerol Phosphate Shuttle (Fig. 6)
- It is one of the shuttle mechanisms which carry reducing equivalents from cytosol to mitochondria
- From cytosolic NADH, a pair of electrons are transferred to dihydroxyacetone phosphate (DHAP) to form glycerol-3-phosphate by the cytosolic enzyme glycerol-3-phosphate dehydrogenase
- Glycerol-3-phosphate diffuses through the outer mitochondrial membrane into the intermembrane space of mitochondria where it is oxidized to DHAP by a FAD containing isoenzyme of glycerol-3-phosphate dehydrogenase which is converted to FADH2
- In the inner mitochondrial membrane (METC) FADH2 produces 1.5 molecules of ATP
- DHAP returns back to cytosol to be used for the next shuttle
- This shuttle is predominant in muscles.

3. Creatine Phosphate Shuttle
- This shuttle facilitates transport of high energy phosphate from mitochondria
- This occurs mainly in the mitochondria of active tissues, such as heart and skeletal muscle
- An isoenzyme of creatine kinase (CK_m) found in the mitochondrial intermembrane space catalyzes the transfer of high energy phosphate.

7. Laboratory investigations in different types of jaundice.

Refer 2005 Short Note 32 and 2013 Essay Question 7 (b).
- Bilirubin is the end product of catabolism of heme
  - Normal value of total bilirubin is 0.2–0.8 mg/dL;
  - Unconjugated bilirubin is 0.2–0.6 mg/dL and
  - Conjugated bilirubin is 0–0.2 mg/dL.
- If the levels are increased the person becomes jaundiced
- There are 3 types of jaundice:
  1. Hemolytic (prehepatic) jaundice,
  2. Hepatocellular (hepatic) jaundice
  3. Obstructive (posthepatic).

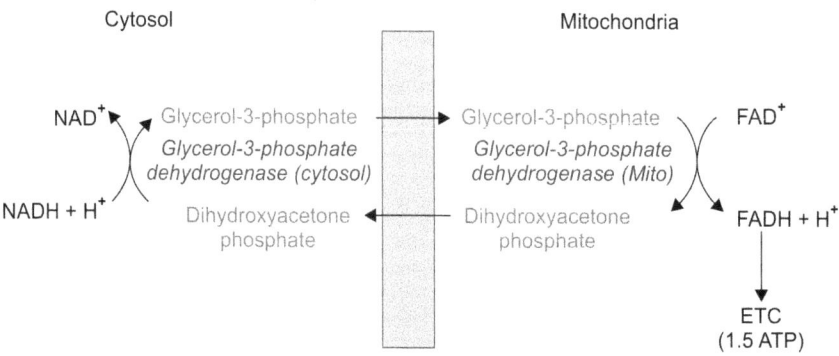

Fig. 6: Glycerol phosphate shuttle.

Function tests for differential diagnosis of jaundice

S. No.	Tests	Hemolytic jaundice	Hepatic jaundice	Obstructive jaundice
1.	Serum total bilirubin	Increased	Increased	Increased
2.	Serum conjugated bilirubin	Normal	Increased	Increased
	Unconjugated bilirubin	High	Increased	Normal
3.	Van den Bergh	Indirect +	Biphasic	Direct +
4.	Alkaline phosphatase	Normal	Increased	Highly increased
5.	Urine–bile salt (Hay's test)	Nil	Nil	Present
6.	Urine–conjugated bilirubin	Nil	Present	Present
7.	Urine–urobilinogen	Increased	Nil	Nil
8.	Fecal stercobilinogen	Increased	Decreased	Absent

- Van den Bergh (Indirect): Unconjugated bilirubin in blood, positive for prehepatic and hepatic jaundice
- Direct van den Bergh test: Conjugated bilirubin in blood is positive—helps in detection of posthepatic jaundice
- ALP: Normal range—40 -125 U/Lt—increases slightly in hepatic jaundice and more in posthepatic jaundice
- Hay's test: This test is specific for identification of urine Bile salts–positive for posthepatic jaundice, by the lowering of surface tension by bile salts
- Fouchet's test (conjugated bilirubin in urine): This test gives positive result for both hepatic and posthepatic
- Ehrlich test (for urobilinogen): Positive in prehepatic and positive in early stages of hepatic.

8. Structure of DNA (Watson–Crick model) (Fig. 7).

Refer 2006 Essay Question 10 and 2010 Essay Question 3.
- **Right handed double helix**—DNA consists of two helical polynucleotide chains twisted around in right handed double helix. Purine and pyrimidine bases are inside the helix. Phosphate and deoxyribose units are on the outside. The planes of bases are perpendicular to the helical axis. Sugars are kept at right angles to the bases
- **Base pairing rule—Chargaff's rule**
  - In DNA, the two strands are complementary to each other
  - The number of adenine molecules are equal to thymine molecules (A=T) and number of cytosine molecules are equal to guanine molecules (C=G)
  - Adenine pairs with thymine by two hydrogen bonds (A=T); guanine pairs with cytosine by 3-hydrogen bonds (G≡C). This is called Chargaff's rule.
- **Hydrogen bonding**—adenine pairs with thymine by two hydrogen bonds (A=T); guanine pairs with cytosine by 3 hydrogen bonds (G≡C). GC bond is stronger than AT bond
- **Antiparallel**—the two strands of DNA run antiparallel to each other. One strand runs in 5' to 3' direction while the opposite strand runs in 3' to 5' direction

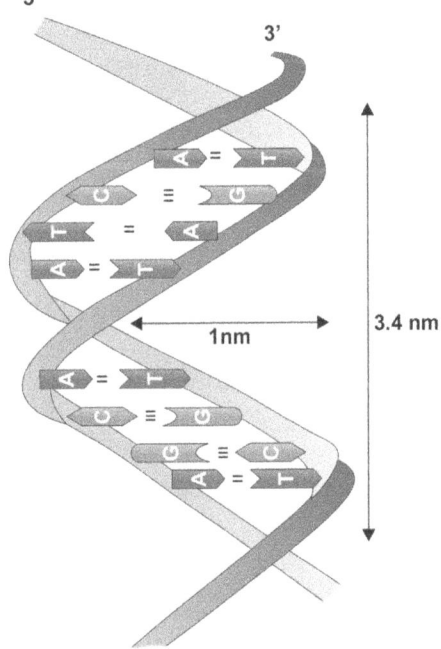

Fig. 7: Structure of DNA.

- **Structure of helix**
  - Diameter or width of the helix is 20Å (1.9–2.0 nm)
  - It has a pitch of 3.4 nm per turn
  - Within a single turn 10 base pairs are seen
  - Adjacent pairs are separated by 0.34 nm
  - It has a major groove (1.2 nm) and a minor groove (0.6 nm) which wind along the molecule, parallel to the phosphodiester backbone.
  - Proteins interact with the bases in these grooves.

Different forms of DNA Double Helix

DNA exists in three structural forms. They are: A-DNA, B-DNA and Z-DNA.
- **B-DNA**—it is the classic Watson–Crick model. It is the most common form. The DNA is a right handed helix. It has two polydeoxyribonucleotide strands twisted around each other. The two strands are antiparallel. One strand runs from 5' to 3' direction and other from 3' to 5' direction. The width of double helix is 2 nm. Each turn of helix is 3.4 nm with 10 pairs of nucleotides. The sugar forms the backbone to which base is attached. The bases in two strands form hydrogen bonds and they are arranged according to Chargaff's rule.
- **A-DNA**—it is right handed helix having 11 base pairs per turn
- **Z-DNA**—it is a left handed helix containing 12 base pairs per turn. The polynucleotide strands of DNA move in a zigzag fashion.

S. No.	Property	A-DNA	B-DNA	Z-DNA
1.	Shape	Broadest	Medium	Narrow
2.	Type of helix	Right handed	Right handed	Left handed
3.	Base pairs per turn	11	10	12
4	Helix diameter	25.5 Å	23.7 Å	18.4 Å
5.	Pitch per turn of helix	25.3 Å	35.4 Å	45.6 Å
6.	Major groove	Narrow	Wide	Flat
7.	Minor groove	Very broad	Narrow	Very narrow

9. Competitive enzyme inhibition.

Definition: Enzyme inhibitors are organic or inorganic substances which can bind reversibly or irreversibly with the enzymes and alter the catalytic activity of the enzyme, e.g. drugs, toxins, etc.
- **Reversible inhibition:** In this type, the inhibitors bind **noncovalently** with the enzymes and the inhibition will be reversed when the inhibitors are removed This is further classified into:
  - A. Competitive inhibitors (substrate analogue inhibitors)
  - B. Non competitive reversible inhibitors
  - C. Uncompetitive inhibitors.

A. Competitive inhibitors (substrate analog inhibitors)

- Usually they are structural analog of the substance
- They bind and compete to the substrate binding site of the enzyme forming an enzyme inhibitory complex (EI)
- K_m value is increased but no change in V_{max}
- For example, competitive inhibition of succinate dehydrogenase by malonate which resembles succinate (TCA cycle)
- Many drugs act as competitive inhibitors. For example, sulfonamide is an analog of PABA and inhibits pteroid synthetase in the folic acid synthesis
- Allopurinol inhibits xanthine oxidase.

10. Carnitine.

In β-oxidation the activated medium chain fatty acids have to be transported from cytoplasm to the mitochondria
- Activated fatty acids are transported to the mitochondria by carnitine shuttle (**Fig. 8**)
- Carnitine is synthesized from lysine and methionine in liver and kidney and it is beta-hydroxy-gamma-methyl ammonium butyrate
- Carnitine carries fatty acyl groups across the inner mitochondrial membrane. Transfer of acyl group to carnitine occurs by the enzyme carnitine acyltransferase

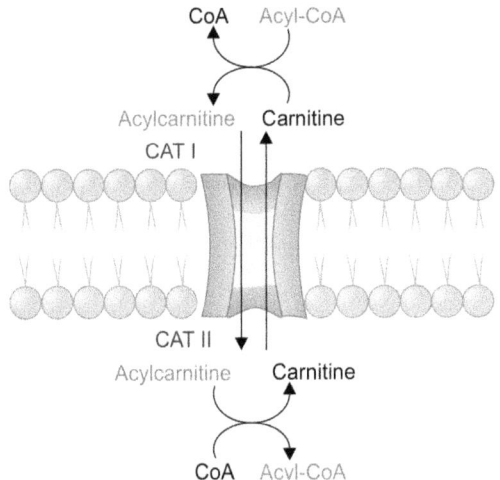

Fig. 8: Carnitine shuttle.

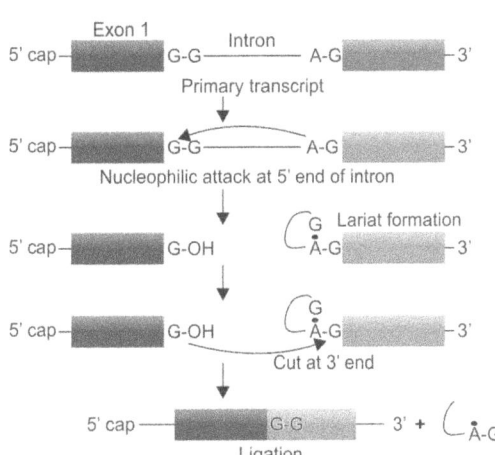

Fig. 9: Post-transcriptional modification of mRNA.

(CAT-1) at the cytosolic side of inner mitochondrial membrane to form acylcarnitine
- Translocase enzyme carries acylcarnitine across the membrane to the matrix of mitochondria where the second enzyme carnitine acyltransferase II (CAT II) transfers acyl group to coenzyme. Free carnitine will return back to cytosol by translocase
- Thus the fatty acids can enter into mitochondria for further oxidation.

11. Structure of messenger RNA (mRNA).

- It is synthesized from DNA by transcription. Its precursor is the heterogenous nuclear RNA (hnRNA) from which mRNA is synthesized by post-transcriptional modification
- It has a poly A tail at its 3' end and a cap at 5' end consisting of 7 methyl-GTP
- It contains the codons for protein synthesis which serve as a template for protein synthesis. It is attached to ribosome on which protein synthesis occurs
- mRNA formed and released from DNA template is known as primary transcript
- The primary transcripts are longer than the mRNA. They are known as the heterogeneous nuclear RNA or hnRNA
- They have to undergo certain processing to become mature RNA. This process is called post-transcriptional modifications, such as splicing, 5' capping, 3' tailing and methylation **(Fig. 9)**
- **Exons and introns:** The long primary transcripts have coding regions called exons and uncoding regions called introns. The introns are removed and the exons spliced together. This is done by using snRNA. This is called post-transcriptional modification
- **3' end-Poly A tail:** The 3' end of mRNA is attached with 20–250 adenine nucleotides. This is to protect the 3'end from the attack of 3' exonuclease present in the cytoplasm
- **5' end capping:** The 5' end is capped by 7-methylguanosine triphosphate. This will prevent the attack of cytoplasmic 5' exonuclease attack on mRNA
- **Methylation:** N_6 of adenine molecules and 2' hydroxy group of ribose are methylated.

12. Liver function tests.

The tests used to diagnose liver disease are called liver function tests. They are:
- **Tests based on hepatic excretory function:**
  a. Serum bilirubin: **Van den Bergh test**
  b. Urine bile pigments: Bilirubin, bile salts, urobilinogen
  c. Fecal urobilinogen

d. Dye excretion test: Bromosulpho-phthalein (BSP) test.
a. **van Den Bergh test (Hepatic excretory function)—estimation of bilirubin:**
   - The serum bilirubin estimation is based on van den Bergh reaction where diazotized sulfanilic acid reacts with bilirubin to form a purple colored complex, azobilirubin. Normal serum does not give a positive van den Bergh test
   - When bilirubin is conjugated, the purple color is produced immediately on mixing with the reagent, the response is said to be van den Bergh is direct positive
   - When the bilirubin is unconjugated, the color appears only after addition of alcohol, so it is said to be van den Bergh is indirect positive
   - When both conjugated and unconjugated bilirubins are present, it produces an immediate color, which intensifies on adding alcohol. It is then said to be biphasic
   - In hemolytic jaundice—unconjugated bilirubin elevated so indirect positive
   - In obstructive jaundice—conjugated bilirubin elevated so direct positive
   - In hepatic jaundice—both conjugated and unconjugated bilirubin elevated so biphasic.
- **Markers of liver injury—estimation of liver enzymes:**
  a. Serum alanine aminotransferase (ALT)—increased more than AST
  b. Serum aspartate aminotransferase (AST)
  c. Serum alkaline phosphatase (ALP)—highly increased in obstructive liver diseases
  d. Serum gamma-glutamyl transferase (GGT)—increased in alcoholic diseases.

- **Tests based on synthetic function (Synthesis of plasma proteins)—**

Estimation of Total Plasma Proteins, Serum Albumin, Globulins, A/G ratio

- Almost all plasma proteins with exception of immunoglobulins are synthesized by liver. Normal total serum proteins level is 6–8 g/dL
- Albumin is quantitatively the most important protein synthesized by the liver, and reflects the extent of functioning liver cell mass. Normal albumin level is 2.5–3.5 g/dL
- In hepatocellular diseases hypoalbuminemia occurs
- Normal serum globulin level is 2–3.5 g/dL. In chronic inflammatory disorders, such as hepatitis and in cirrhosis of liver hyperglobulinemia will be present
- A/G ratio: Since albumin has a half life of 20 days, in all chronic diseases of liver, the albumin level is decreased. A reversal of A/G ratio is seen in cirrhosis of liver. Normal A/G ratio is between 1.2:1 and 1.5:1.

Prothrombin Time

- Since prothrombin is synthesized by the liver, it is a useful indicator of liver function
- The half life of prothrombin is 6 hours only. Therefore PT indicates the recent function of liver
- PT is prolonged only when more than 80% of liver function is lost
  - In vitamin K deficiency PT is prolonged. To differentiate liver dysfunction from that of vitamin K deficiency, vitamin K is given to the patient and PT is measured. Elevated PT even after administration of vitamin K indicates liver dysfunction.
- **Special tests**
a. **Estimation of ceruloplasmin**—level increased in biliary cirrhosis, active

hepatitis, hemochromatosis and biliary obstruction. Level decreased in Wilson's disease
b. **Alpha-1 antitrypsin (AAT)**—acute phase protein. Levels are low in neonatal cholestasis, juvenile cirrhosis in children and micronodular cirrhosis in adults
c. **Alpha-fetoprotein (AFP)**—reference value—upto 1year <30 ng/mL; Adults <15 ng/mL. Increased in chronic hepatitis, hepatocellular. In maternal serum it is elevated in open neural tube defects carcinoma, germ cell tumor and teratoma of ovary.
- **Tests based on detoxification function**—estimation of:
a. Blood ammonia
b. Hippuric acid.

III. SHORT ANSWER QUESTIONS

1. Fate of oxaloacetate.

- Oxaloacetate is formed by the carboxylation of pyruvate by pyruvate carboxylase which requires biotin, CO_2 and ATP
- In TCA cycle malate is dehydrogenated by malate dehydrogenase enzyme in the mitochondria to form oxaloacetate in the presence of NAD to produce 3 ATP

Fate of oxaloacetate (Fig. 10):
a. Oxaloacetate (4C) acts as a catalyst entering into TCA cycle and helps in complete oxidation of acetyl-CoA and returns back without any change
b. It combines with acetyl-CoA to form 6 carboned tricarboxylic acid citrate by the enzyme citrate synthase
c. Oxaloacetate is transaminated by aspartate transaminase (AST) to give rise to aspartate—an acidic amino acid in the presence of pyridoxal phosphate. Aspartate is needed for the synthesis of purines and pyrimidines
d. Oxaloacetate is transported to cytosol from mitochondria by malate-aspartate shuttle through malate. In the cytosol oxaloacetate is converted to phosphoenolpyruvate by phosphoenolpyruvate carboxykinase (PEPCK) enzyme by the removal of CO_2, GTP donates the phosphate
e. Phosphoenolpyruvate by reversal of glycolysis by various steps is converted to glucose by gluconeogenic pathway.

2. Liver enzymes.

Hepatic enzymes: Alanine aminotransferase (ALT), Aspartate aminotransferase (AST), gamma-glutamyl transferase (GGT), alkaline phosphatase (ALP), nucleotide phosphatase (NTP).
1. Alanine transaminase (ALT/SGPT)
   - Normal serum level of ALT—35-45 U/L for males and 10-35 U/L in females
   - Its coenzyme is pyridoxal phosphate (PLP)
   - It is highly increased in toxic or viral hepatitis and moderately increased in cirrhosis and chronic hepatitis.
2. Aspartate aminotransferase (AST/SGOT)
   - Normal serum level of AST-<30 IU/L
   - Its coenzyme is pyridoxal phosphate
   - It is a marker of liver injury and its level is increased in hepatitis and in cancer of liver.

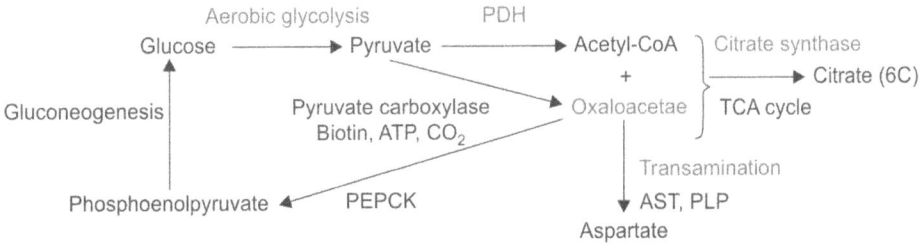

Fig. 10: Fate of oxaloacetate.

3. Gamma-glutamyl transferase (GGT)
   - GGT has 11 isoenzymes. It is seen in liver, kidney, pancreas, intestinal cells and prostate glands
   - Normal level is 10–30 U/L
   - It is increased in infective hepatitis and prostate cancers
   - It is a marker of alcohol abuse. GGT is increased in alcoholics when other liver functions are within normal limits. It is decreased rapidly within few days of stopping alcohol. Increase in GGT is proportional to the amount of alcohol consumed.
4. Alkaline phosphatase (ALP)
   - Marker enzyme for obstructive liver diseases
   - Normal value: 40 to 125 U/L
   - Six isoenzymes of alkaline phosphatase (ALP)
   - Alpha-1 ALP, Alpha-2 heat labile ALP, Alpha -2 heat stable ALP, Pre-beta ALP, Gamma- ALP, Leucocyte ALP (LAP)
   - They are classified based on the difference in the carbohydrate content
   - Increase in Alpha-1 ALP—obstructive jaundice; alpha-2 ALP—indicates hepatitis and pre-beta ALP—indicates bone diseases, Gamma-ALP—ulcerative colitis; LAP—increased in lymphomas.

3. Functions of magnesium.

Refer 2010 Short Answer Question 14.
- Magnesium is an important intracellular cation
- Total body Mg is 25 g, out of which 60% is complexed with calcium in bone
- RDA: 400 mg/day for men; 300 mg/day for women
- Normal serum level is 1.8 to 2.2 mg/dL
- Functions:
  a. Activator of many enzymes like alkaline phosphatase, hexokinase, fructokinase, phosphofructokinase, adenylyl cyclase. ATP is also needed for these reactions
  b. It prevents neuromuscular irritability
  c. It helps in insulin dependent uptake of glucose and Mg improves glucose tolerance.
- Deficiency of Mg leads to neuromuscular irritability
- Hypomagnesemia may be due to vomiting, diarrhea, PEM, cirrhosis and diuretic therapy
- Hypermagnesemia may be due to excessive intake, renal failure, rickets, hyperparathyroidism, etc.

4. Dietary fibers.
Refer 2008 Short Note 10.

5. Cytochrome P450.
Refer 2004 Short Note 20.

6. Functions of phospholipids.
Refer 2004 Short Note 1.

7. Suicide inhibition of enzymes.
- It is also known as suicide inactivation or mechanism-based inhibition
- It is a form of irreversible enzyme inhibition in which the inhibitor makes use of the enzyme's own reaction mechanism to inactivate it
- For example, allopurinol—inhibitor of xanthine oxidase (allopurinol gets converted to alloxanthine, a more effective inhibitor of xanthine oxidase)
- Aspirin inactivates the enzyme cyclooxygenase which catalyze the first reaction in the synthesis of prostaglandins from arachidonic acid. That is why aspirin is used as an anti-inflammatory, antipyretic and analgesic drug. Because of this effect it is also used to inhibit platelet aggregation and thrombosis.

8. Causes for abnormal GTT curves (Figs. 11A to D).
Refer 2008 Short Note 30.
- While conducting glucose tolerance test to diagnose a case of diabetes mellitus or in a suspected doubtful case, urine and blood samples are collected in the fasting and postglucose load states—every half hourly. The results are marked in a graph and interpreted.

A. Normal GTT (Fig. 11A)

- Fasting blood sugar value is between 80–100 mg%
- The glucose level rises sharply and a peak is reached at 1 hour
- The blood glucose level comes to normal in 2 hours
- All the urine samples are negative for glucose.

B. Renal Glycosuria (Fig. 11B)

- It resembles the normal curve
- Blood glucose level is not high but glucose is present in all the urine samples. This is due to the lowering of the renal threshold (180 mg%) which is seen physiologically in pregnancy, and pathologically in renal tubular defects.

C. Impaired Glucose Tolerance (IGT) (Fig. 11C)

- It is a condition when blood glucose values are above the normal level but below the diabetic level
- Fasting blood glucose level is less than 120 mg%
- Peak level is above the renal threshold, i. e. higher than 180 mg% at 1 hour
- The blood glucose level comes down in 2 hours to less than 180 mg%
- Urine glucose is positive at 1 hour
- IGT patients have associated problems like hypertension, lipid disorders, high uric acid level and obesity.

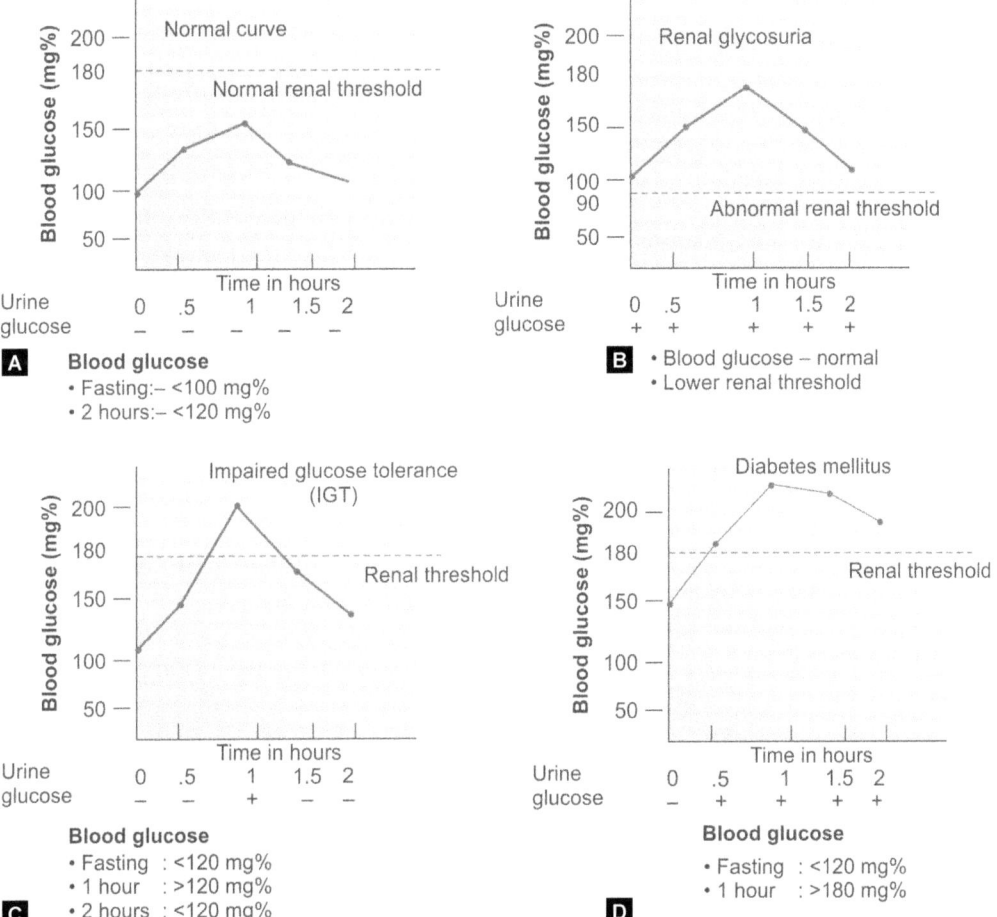

Figs. 11A to D: Different curves of glucose tolerance test.

D. Diabetes Mellitus (Fig. 11D)

- Fasting blood sugar is less than 180 mg% (below the renal threshold value—180 mg%)
- Peak value is above the renal threshold value
- Blood glucose level does not come to the fasting level in 2 hours and it is more than 180 mg%
- All the urine samples are positive for glucose except for the first sample (fasting).

9. Biologically important peptides.

Peptides are polymers of amino acids. Two amino acids are covalently joined to form a dipeptide by a peptide bond and three amino acids form tripeptide and so on.

Important Peptides

- **Dipeptides**-i) Aspartame—artificial sweetener containing aspartate and phenylalanine; ii) Carnosine and anserine-Pseudopeptides containing beta alanine and histidine
- **Tripeptide-**
  a. Glutathione (GSH)-Gamma-glutamyl-cysteinyl-glycine which contains glutamate, cysteine and glycine. It is involved in maintaining the integrity of erythrocyte membrane and it keeps certain enzymes in active state
  b. Thyrotropin releasing hormone (TRH) from hypothalamus—releases thyrotropin from anterior pituitary gland.
- **Nanopeptides:** Containing 9 amino acids. They are: a) Oxytocin and vasopressin from posterior pituitary; b) Bradykinin-powerful vasodilator
- **Deccapeptides**-10 amino acids. Angiotensin I—10 amino acids; antibiotic Gramicidin S—circular peptide
- Other peptides having **more than 10 amino acids:**
  - Pancreatic hormones—insulin (51 amino acids-2 chains of 30 +21 amino acids); glucagon (29 amino acids)
  - Corticotropin—from anterior pituitary (39 amino acids).

10. Biological value of protein.

- It is one of the indices of assessing the nutritional value of proteins. It is done by feeding the protein to an animal and assessing the weight gain
- Amount of protein ingested = 100 mg
- Amount absorbed (recovered in feces) = 100-4 = 96 mg
- Amount retained (amount seen in urine = 96-24 = 72 mg)
- Biological value (BV): It is the ratio between the nitrogen retained and nitrogen absorbed during a specific interval

$$BV = \frac{\text{Retained nitrogen}}{\text{Absorbed nitrogen}} \times 100$$

BV in this case = 72 × 100 ÷ 96.

11. Gout.

Refer 2005 Short Note 17.

12. Define transcription. Name four post-transcriptional modifications.

Refer 2011 Essay Question 3 and 2013 Short Note 53.

13. Primary structure of proteins (Fig. 12).

Refer 2003 Essay Question 3.

- The primary structure of proteins refers to the linear sequence of amino acids in the

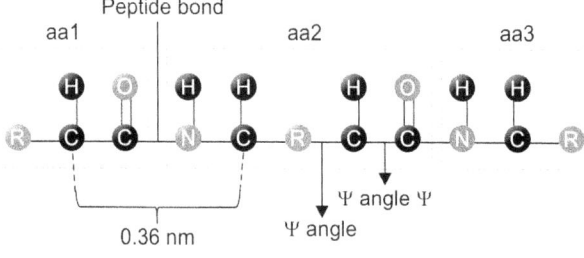

Fig. 12: Primary structure of proteins.

polypeptide chain. It denotes the number and sequence of amino acids in protein
- The primary structure is held together by covalent or peptide bonds
- The two ends of the polypeptide chain are referred to as the carboxyl terminus (C-terminus) and the amino terminus (N-terminus) based on the nature of the free group on each end
- The primary structure of a protein is determined by the gene corresponding to the protein.

14. Metabolic functions of glycine.
Refer 2004 and 2009 Essay Question 3 and also refer 2014 Short Note Question 17.

15. Maple syrup urine disease.
Refer 2007 Essay Question 10 and 2009 Short Answer Questions 31.

16. Hartnup's disease.
Refer 2010 Short Answer Question 39.
- It is an autosomal recessive disorder seen in tryptophan metabolism
- It is named after the family of Hartnup in whom the disorder was described first
- It is due to defective amino acid transport during absorption of amino acids from the intestines and also during reabsorption of amino acids from renal tubules
- This leads to the deficiency of tryptophan and nicotinic acid and NAD
- Neurological and pellagra like symptoms are present
- Aminoaciduria will be present due to failure of amino acid transport in renal tubules
- Increased excretion of indole compounds will be detected by Obermeyer test
- **Treatment:** Supplementation of niacin and high protein diet.

17. Adaptation to high altitude.
Physiologic changes which accompany exposure to high altitude are:
- Increase in number of erythrocytes
- Concentration of Hb within the erythrocytes
- Synthesis of 2, 3-bisphosphoglycerate (BPG) and elevated BPG lowers the affinity of HbA for oxygen (increases P50) which enhances the release of O_2 at peripheral tissues.

18. Genetic code.
Refer 2005 Short Note 19.

19. Types of mutations.
Refer 2013 Short Answer Question 13.

20. Structure of tRNA.
Refer 2004 Short Note 12.
Transfer RNA or Soluble RNA is a type of RNA
- It shows extensive internal base pairing
- It has clover leaf-like structure
- It contains unusual bases. They are dihydrouracil (DHU), pseudouridine (ψ) and hypoxanthine. Many bases are methylated
- It acts as an adapter molecule in carrying a specific amino acid for a particular codon in mRNA and helps in protein synthesis—translation
- It has an acceptor arm, anticodon arm, DHU arm and pseudouridine arm
  - **Acceptor arm is at 3′ end:** It carries the amino acids. It has seven base pairs. The end sequence is CCA-3′. The 3′ end hydroxyl group is bonded with carboxyl end of amino acids
  - **Anticodon arm of tRNA:** It is present at the opposite side of acceptor arm. It recognizes the triplet nucleotide codon present in mRNA
  - **DHU arm of tRNA:** It contains dihydrouridine. DHU arm serves as the recognition site for enzymes

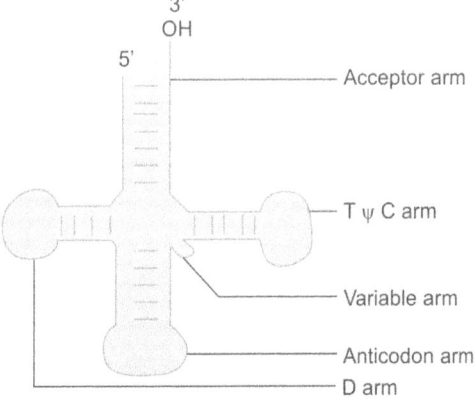

Fig. 13: Structure of transfer RNA.

- **Pseudouridine arm of tRNA:** It contains pseudouridine and it is involved in binding tRNA to ribosomes.

Functions of tRNA

- tRNA has got a major role in translation (protein synthesis)
- The tRNA molecules carry the specific amino acid at the CCA-3' end of the acceptor arm. There are about 20 tRNA molecules available, one specific for each amino acid
- The three nucleotide base sequences at the anticodon arm of the tRNA recognize the corresponding complimentary codons in the mRNA to form base pairs to continue protein synthesis.

21. Ocular changes in vitamin A deficiency.

Refer 2014 Short Note 10.

- **Vitamin A is a fat-soluble vitamin**
- **Night blindness or nyctalopia:** Earliest symptoms of vitamin A deficiency. Visual acuity is diminished in dim light. Dark adaptation time is increased
- **Xerophthalmia:** More prolonged deficiency leads to **xerophthalmia**—dryness of conjunctiva which may spread to cornea. Keratinization of corneal epithelium making it glazy and lustreless
- **Bitot's spots:** Grayish white triangular plaques are seen adherent to conjunctive due to increased thickness **(Fig. 14)**
- **All the above changes are reversible when vitamin is supplemented**
- **Keratomalacia:** When there is persistent xerophthalmia, it is progressed to keratomalacia—softening of cornea and keratinization which may lead to total blindness due to corneal opacity. There is degeneration of corneal epithelium which gets vascularized. Bacterial infection may lead to corneal ulceration, perforation of cornea and total blindness.

22. Amphipathic lipids.

- They are lipids containing both hydrophobic and hydrophilic groups
- Example—phospholipids, fatty acids, bile salts and cholesterol
- They have a polar or hydrophilic head with a nonpolar hydrophobic tail
- When they are mixed with water they form micelles
- Micelles are primarily molecular aggregates of amphipathic lipids
- Micelle formation facilitated by bile salts is essential for lipid digestion.

23. Kwashiorkor.

- This is due to the malnutrition of proteins with adequate energy intake. Kwashiorkor means sickness the older child gets, when the next child is born. This is the commonest nutritional disorder in many parts of the world
- Kwashiorkor is entirely preventable if children are given a well-balanced diet containing adequate amount of protein and the essential amino acids
- The salient features of kwashiorkor is tabulated:

	Kwashiorkor
Age of onset	1–5 years
Growth retardation of child	Mild retardation
Attitude	Lethargic and apathetic
Appearance	Edema on face (moon face) and limbs
Appetite	Anorexia
Skin	Crazy pavement, dermatitis
Hair	Sparse, soft and thin
Other	Angular stomatitis, cheilosis, watery diarrhea, muscle wasting, fatty liver
Serum albumin	<2 g (hypoalbuminemia)
Serum cortisol	Decreased

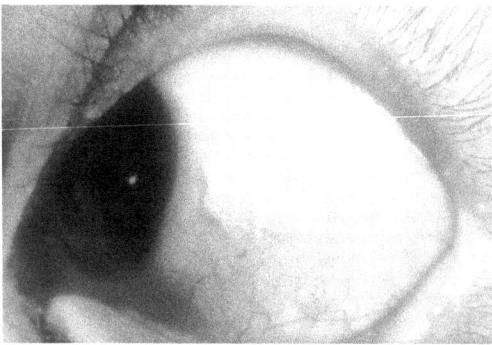

Fig. 14: Bitot's spots.

24. Enzymes in diagnosis of myocardial infarction.

Enzyme changes in acute myocardial infarction.

Enzymes elevated in myocardial infarction are creatine kinase MB, aspartate transaminase and lactate dehydrogenase 1.

Other markers are—myoglobin, cardiac troponin I and T.

Creatine Kinase

- CK MB is the first enzyme to be elevated in MI
- It is released into the circulation within 6-8 hours, reaches its peak value within 24-30 hours and returns to normal level by 2nd or 3rd day.

Aspartate Transaminase

- Rises sharply after CPK, and reaches a peak within 48 hours of MI
- It takes 4-5 days to return to normal level.

Lactate Dehydrogenase

- LDH has 5 isoenzymes—LDH-1, LDH-2, LDH-3, LDH-4, and LDH-5. LDH is a tetramer with 4 subunits
- LDH-1 rises from the second day after infarction, attains a peak by the 3rd or 4th day and takes about 10-15 days to reach normal level
- It is the last enzyme to rise and also the last enzyme to return to normal level in MI
- LDH-1 is more than LDH-2 in MI (flipped pattern). (LDH-1 > LDH-2).

Cardiac Troponins

Cardiac troponins are not enzymes but proteins highly useful in the diagnosis of MI. Troponin I (inhibitory element of actomyosin) and Troponin T (tropomysin binding element) are markers of MI. Troponin I (TnI) is released into the circulation within 4 hours after the onset of symptoms of myocardial ischemia. Peaks at 14-24 hours and remains elevated for 3-5 days postinfarction. Troponin T (TnT) increases within 6 hours of MI, peaks at 72 hours and remains elevated upto 7-10 days.

25. Biochemical functions of zinc.

Refer 2004 Short Note 13.

26. Hormones that regulate blood calcium level.

Refer 2004 Essay Question 4.
Normal serum calcium is 9-11 mg/dL.

Hormonal Regulation

A. Vitamin D—calcitriol
B. Parathyroid
C. Calcitonin.

A. Vitamin D (Calcitriol- 1, 25 dihydroxycholecalciferol)

The active vitamin D (calcitriol) acts as a steroid hormone. It is synthesized in kidney.

- **Effect on intestine:** Vitamin D helps in the absorption of calcium and phosphorus from the intestines
- **Effects on bone:** Calcitriol stimulates the activity of osteoblasts which help in mineralization of bones
- **Effects on kidney:** Calcitriol increases the reabsorption of calcium and phosphorous from the renal tubules thereby conserving both minerals.

B. Parathyroid Hormone (PTH)

- Decreased serum calcium level leads to release of PTH from parathyroids
- **PTH and bones**: PTH causes demineralization of bones. Calcium is released into the bloodstream and blood calcium level is increased. This leads to loss of bone matrix
- **PTH and kidneys**: PTH causes decreased renal excretion of calcium and increased excretion of phosphates and increased reabsorption of calcium
- **PTH and intestines**: PTH stimulates increased production of calcitriol which acts on intestine to absorb more calcium.

C. Calcitonin

It decreases serum calcium level by inhibiting resorption of bone and decreases the activity of osteoclasts and increases the activity of osteoblasts.

27. Mechanism of cyanide poisoning.

Refer 2013 Short Answer Questions 46.

28. Metabolism of glucose-6-phosphate.

- Glucose-6-phosphate is the central molecule connecting many metabolic pathways of carbohydrate metabolism
- **Synthesis of glucose-6-phosphate**: Glucose is phosphorylated to glucose-6-phosphate in the presence of glucokinase/hexokinase. It is an irreversible step **(Fig. 15)**.
- **Utilization of glucose-6-phosphate:**
  1. Glycolysis: Glucose-6-phosphate is isomerized to fructose-6-phosphate to get converted to pyruvate in aerobic glycolysis and lactate in anaerobic glycolysis
  2. Gluconeogenesis: Glucose-6-phosphate is converted back to glucose by glucose-6-phosphatase. This enzyme is absent in muscles
  3. Glycogenesis: Glucose-6-phosphate is converted to glycogen—the storage form of glucose in liver and muscle
  4. HMP pathway: Glucose-6-phosphate is oxidized by glucose-6-phosphate dehydrogenase to form NADPH and riboses
  5. Uronic acid pathway: Glucose-6-phosphate is converted to glucose-1-phosphate which is converted to UDP glucose, the active glucose which is dehydrogenated to the active glucuronic acid—UDP-glucuronate.

29. Lipoprotein lipase.

Lipoprotein lipase: It is located at the endothelial layers of capillaries of adipose tissue, muscle and heart and not in liver
- It is activated by Apo C-II of chylomicrons (CM)
- It hydrolyses TAG of CM and very low-density lipoproteins (VLDL) and gives rise to FFA + glycerol
- It is stimulated by insulin.

30. Cori cycle (lactic acid cycle) (Fig. 16).

Definition: Transferring lactate from muscle tissues to liver and re-synthesis of glucose in liver is known as Cori cycle. In this cycle,

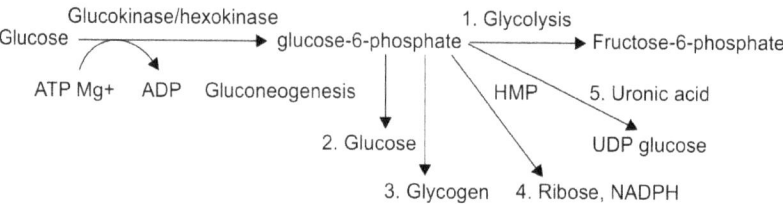

Fig. 15: Synthesis of glucose-6-phosphate.

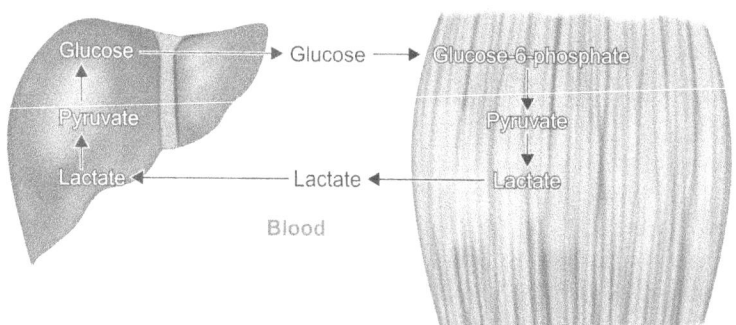

Fig. 16: Cori cycle.

glucose is converted to lactate in muscle and in liver this lactate is reconverted into glucose.
Effects: In contracting muscle, pyruvate is reduced to lactate which gets accumulated in muscle and may lead to muscular cramps in strenuous muscular exercise.
- It rescues lactate for further use (gluconeogenesis) and counteracts lactic acidosis
- It is of less importance in starvation but important in more normal situations especially in certain cells, such as matured RBC, medulla, retina which are lacking mitochondria and virtually anaerobic
- Lactate is carried from skeletal muscle to liver through blood. In the liver lactate is converted to pyruvate and by gluconeogenesis it is converted to glucose which is then transported to muscles for energy supply
- **Significance of Cori cycle:** Lactate produced in muscle is reutilized by the body. This is an energy expensive process. During exercise there is excessive production of lactate which is utilized by liver to produce glucose. This process needs ATP. The increased oxygen consumptions explains for oxygen debt after vigorous exercise.

31. Paper chromatography.

- This is one of the types of partition chromatography
- In this type the stationary phase is water held on a solid support of filter paper (cellulose)
- The mobile phase is a mixture of immiscible solvents like water, a nonpolar solvent and an acid or base. For example, butanol-acetic acid-water, phenol-water-ammonia
- Chromatography can be done with the mobile phase applied from top is called descending type or from bottom-ascending type
- A few microliters of the mixture to be separated is applied as a small spot at one end of the paper 1" away from the edge. In ascending type the paper is placed in a glass trough containing the solvent and allowed to move in the paper
- It takes 14–16 hours
- The distance to which each component moves depends on its partition coefficient.

32. Transmethylation reactions.

Refer 2007 Essay Question 4.
Transmethylation reaction is acceptance of a methyl group from a donor like S-adenosyl-methionine (SAM) by an acceptor resulting in the formation of a methylated compound.
- Transmethylation reaction requires SAM which is formed by accepting adenosyl group from ATP by methionine by methionine adenosyltransferase.

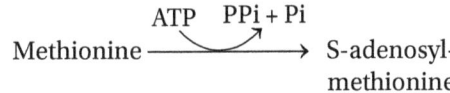

Methionine ⟶ S-adenosyl-methionine

The examples for transmethylation reactions are:

Methyl acceptor	Methylated product
Guanidoacetic acid	Creatine
Serine	Choline
Epinephrine	Metanephrine
Norepinephrine	Epinephrine
tRNA	Methylated tRNA

33. Pancreatic function tests.

- Exocrine pancreas secretes about 1,000–2,500 mL of pancreatic secretion which is alkaline. It contains bicarbonate and enzymes
- This secretion is under the control of the hormones secretin and cholecystokinin
- Enzymes present in pancreatic juice are—pancreatic amylase, lipase and proteolytic enzymes like trypsin, chymotrypsin, carboxypeptidase and elastase in their zymogen forms.

Pancreatic Function Tests
- **Measurement of pancreatic enzymes:**
  - **Serum amylase:** Normal level 28–100 IU. In acute pancreatitis this level increases within 5 hours of onset and reaches the peak within 12 hours. The level returns to normal within 2–4 days. When serum amylase level starts falling, urinary amylase level rises up

- Amylase is increased in cholecystitis, peptic ulcer, mesenteric diseases, in obstruction of intestines
- **Serum lipase:** Highly elevated in acute pancreatitis and it persists for 7–14 days.
- **Secretin–cholecystokinin test:** Duodenal content is aspirated first in fasting condition and then 1 unit/kg of secretin is given followed by CCK. Again duodenal content is aspirated for 80 minutes for each 10 minutes. Each sample analyzed for volume, bicarbonate content and amylase activity
- **Lundh test:** After aspirating the duodenal content, 500 mL of freshly prepared fluid meal is given. Further the duodenal secretions are collected at 30 minutes intervals for 2 hours and analyzed
- **Indirect tests:** Tumor markers like carcinoembryonic antigen, alpha-fetoprotein, pancreatic oncofoetal antigen; Fat balance studies and measurement of leucine aminopeptidase
- **Measurement of sweat electrolytes:** Estimation of sweat electrolytes–increased levels of N and chloride in sweat especially sweat chloride level more than 60 mmol/L is diagnostic of cystic fibrosis.

34. Alkaptonuria.

Refer 2004 Short Note 11.

35. Acute intermittent porphyria.

Refer 2006 Short Note 9 and 2006 Short Note 24.

36. Sickle cell disease.

Refer 2008 Short Note 23.

37. Bile salts.

Refer 2004 Short Note 9.
- Bile salts are derivatives of cholesterol
- **Synthesis of bile acids/bile salts:** Bile acids are synthesized in the liver from cholesterol. They contain 24 carbon atoms. Cholesterol is catabolized to bile acids and salts, vitamin D, sex and steroid hormones.

Bile Acids
- Types of bile acids are:
  1. Primary bile acids: Cholic acid and chenodeoxy cholic acid—synthesized in liver
  2. Secondary bile acids: Deoxycholic acid and lithocholic acid derived from primary bile acids in intestines by deconjugation and 7α-dehydroxylations.
- **Steps of synthesis:**
  - Cholesterol is hydroxylated at 7th position by 7α-hydroxylase enzyme which is the rate limiting enzyme which needs NADPH and vitamin C and converted into 7α-hydroxycholesterol
  - This in turn is acted by 12α-hydroxylase with the addition of CoA-SH in the presence of NADPH to form cholyl-CoA and chenodeoxycholyl-CoA with the removal of 3C propionate. This forms 24 carbon cholic acid or chenodeoxycholic acid (primary bile acids) with the removal of CoA-SH
  - The so formed 24C bile acids conjugated with glycine/taurine to produce glycocholic acid or taurocholic acid and glycochenodeoxycholic acid/taurochenodeoxy cholic acid
  - These primary bile acids are converted to secondary bile acids by intestinal bacteria by deconjugation and 7α-dehydroxylation to form deoxycholic acid and lithocholic acid, respectively.

Bile Salts
- They are the sodium or potassium salts of primary and secondary bile acids
- **Functions of Bile salts:**
  - They facilitate the lipid digestion
  - They act as detergent in the formation of lipid micelle
  - They emulsify the lipids into droplets to form mixed micelles and thereby increase the surface area of the particles and lower the surface tension
  - Micellar formation helps in absorption of lipids.

38. Renal glomerular function tests.

Renal function tests comprised of: a) Glomerular function tests and b) Tubular function tests.

- **Glomerular function tests:** Glomerulus acts as a sieve in filtering blood but it retains cells and proteins thus forming a glomerular filtrate—normally 170-180 L/day. Out of this only 1.5 L of fluid is excreted as urine and the rest are reabsorbed through the tubules
- **Glomerular filtration rate (GFR):** Normal GFR is 120-125 mL/min. This is reduced in renal failure
- **Clearance tests:** Done to assess the glomerular filtration and renal blood flow
- **Renal clearance of a substance is the volume of plasma from which the substance is completely cleared by the kidney in 1 minute**
- **Clearance** = mg of substance excreted per min/mg of substance/mL of plasma;
  $$C = U \times V/P$$
  C = Clearance of the substance; U = Concentration of the substance in urine; P = Concentration of the substance in plasma; V= Volume of urine passed/minute
- Clearance is expressed as milliliter of plasma per unit time
- Clearance tests: This test is done by using either endogenous markers, such as urea or creatinine or exogenous markers like Inulin, ^{51}Cr-labelled EDTA, ^{99}Tec-labelled EDTA, etc. Out of these creatinine clearance test is the best
- Creatinine clearance test: It is based on the rate of excretion of metabolically produced creatinine which is excreted through urine. Creatinine is freely filtered by the glomeruli but not reabsorbed by the tubules. A small amount of creatinine is secreted by the tubules
- Blood and 24-hours urine are collected for estimation of creatinine. Urinary volume is measured (V) and the concentration of creatinine in urine (U) and plasma (P) are estimated and by using the formula $C = U \times V/P$ the creatinine clearance is calculated
- Normal range for creatinine clearance is 90-129 mL/min
- Reduced creatinine clearance indicates chronic renal damage and reduced blood flow to glomeruli.

39. Anion gap.

Refer 2005 Short Note 33.
- The sum of cations and anions in ECF is always the same to maintain the electrical neutrality
- Sodium and potassium together form 95% of cations
- Chloride and bicarbonate form 86% of the anions. So these electrolytes are commonly measured
- Hence there is always a difference between the measured anions and cations
- **The unmeasured anions constitute the anion gap.** This is due to the presence of protein anions, sulfate, phosphate and organic acids
- **The normal value is 12 mmol/L.** It is increased in some forms of metabolic acidosis
- It is calculated as difference between $(Na^+ + K^+)$ and $(HCO_3^- + Cl^-)$.

High Anion Gap Metabolic Acidosis (HAGMA)

- In metabolic acidosis, accumulation of acid anions will make the anion gap between 15 and 20
- This anion gap is increased when there is a decrease in cations as in hypokalemia, hypocalcemia. When the cations are increased anion gap is altered as in hypoalbuminemia
- HAGMA is seen in: a) Renal failure—the excretion of H$^+$ and generation of bicarbonate both are deficient. b) Diabetic keto acidosis c) Lactic acidosis—lactic acid is increased in tissue hypoxia, circulatory failure. (normal lactic acid is less than 2 mmol/L).

Normal Anion Gap Metabolic Acidosis (NAGMA)

- When there is a loss of both anion and cation, the anion gap is normal but acidosis may prevail
- Causes of NAGMA:
  a. Diarrhea—loss of intestinal secretion leads to acidosis. There will be loss of bicarbonate, sodium and potassium

b. Hyperchloremic acidosis—occurs in renal tubular acidosis, acetazolamide therapy and in ureteric transplantation.

Decreased anion gap: It is seen in hypoalbuminemia, multiple myeloma, and in hypercalcemia.

40. Okazaki fragments (Fig. 17).

Refer 2013 Short Answer Question 33.
- During replication, the polymerase III holoenzyme binds to template DNA and synthesizes DNA in the 5' to 3' direction. On the leading (forward) strand, the DNA is synthesized continuously. On the lagging (retrograde) strand, the DNA is synthesized in short (1–5 kb) fragments
- RNA primer and the newly synthesized DNA molecules are called **Okazaki fragments**
- After many Okazaki fragments are generated, the replication complex begins to remove the RNA primers and the gaps are filled with the proper base paired deoxynucleotides
- The fragments of newly synthesized DNA are joined by the enzyme DNA ligases.

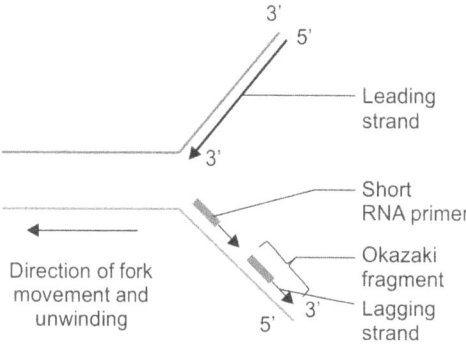

Fig. 17: Okazaki fragments.

41. Fatty liver.
Refer 2009 Short Answer Question 2.

42. Inhibitors of citric acid cycle.

The following enzymes of TCA cycle are inhibited as follows:
- Aconitase:
  - Inhibited by fluoroacetate
  - It is a noncompetitive inhibition.
- α-ketoglutarate dehydrogenase:
  - Inhibited by arsenite
  - It is a noncompetitive inhibition.
- Succinate dehydrogenase:
  - By malonate
  - It is a competitive inhibitor.

43. Cholesterol lowering action of fibrates.

- Fibrates (e.g. gemfibrozil, fenofibrate) are compounds derived from fibric acid
- They affect both triglyceride and cholesterol rich particles by the following mode of action:
  - Limitation of substrate availability for triglyceride synthesis in liver
  - Promotion of action of lipoprotein lipase and increases the level of HDL to promote VLDL turnover.
  - Modulation of LDL receptor/ligand interaction
  - In the liver it increases beta oxidation of fatty acids thereby decreasing the production of cholesterol rich VLDL and increased clearance of chylomicron remnants
  - Stimulation of reverse cholesterol transcription.

44. One-carbon compound.

- One-carbon compounds are organic molecules which contain a single carbon atom
- One carbon compounds donate carbon atoms for synthesis of different other compounds
- They are attached either to 5th/10th/both 5th and 10th N of tetrahydrofolic acid
- One carbon compounds are:
  a. Methyl–CH_3–N^5 methyl H_4 folate
  b. Methylene–CH_2–N^5N^{10} methylene H_4F
  c. Methenyl–=CH–N^5N^{10} methenyl H_4F
  d. Hydroxymethyl-CH_2OH-
  e. Formyl–CHO–N^{10} Formyl H_4F
  f. Formimino–CH=NH–N^5 Formimino H_4F.
- THFA is a carrier of one carbon groups. One-carbon groups play a vital role in donating carbon atoms for synthesis of different types of compounds

- **Different one-carbon compounds**

Group	Structure
Formimino	HN=CH-
Formyl	HCO
Methyl	$-CH_3$
Methylene	$-CH_2-$
Methenyl	=CH

[N^5 and N^{10} atoms of THFA carry the one-carbon groups]

S. No.	Folic acid derivative	One carbon group transferred	Compounds produced
1	N^5, N^{10} methylene THFA	Methylene (CH_2)	Serine—glycine interconversion—dTMP Glycine cleavage system
2	N^5, N^{10} methenyl THFA	Methenyl (=CH)	C_8 of purine ring
3	Formyl THFA	Formyl	C_2 of purine ring
4	N^5, N^{10} methylene THFA	Methylene (CH_2)	dTMP in DNA
5	N^5-methyl-THFA	Methyl (CH_3)	N^5- methyl $-H_4F-$ methylcobalamin homocysteine to methionine
6	N^5-formimino THFA	Formimino (-CH=NH)	Histidine -(FIGLU)

Except methyl group, other one-carbon groups are carried by THFA.

45. Functions of copper.

- Copper is a trace element. Iron present in muscles, liver, bone marrow, brain, kidney, hair and heart
- It is present in enzymes, such as ceruloplasmin, cytochrome oxidase, superoxide dismutase, etc.
- It helps in absorption and incorporation of iron into Hb
- It is necessary for the action of tyrosinase enzyme in tyrosine metabolism
- It acts as a cofactor for hydroxylation reactions done by vitamin C
- Normal requirement is 1.5-3 mg/day for an adult.

46. Biochemical alteration in protein-energy malnutrition (PEM).

Refer 2004 Short Note 4.

Disorders of malnutrition is commonly manifested as protein energy malnutrition. There are two major types of malnutritional diseases:

1. **Marasmus**—this is due to severe deficiency of both dietary energy and proteins. Primary calorie insufficiency and secondary protein deficiency. Marasmus means to waste.
2. **Kwashiorkor**—this is due to isolated deficiency of proteins with sufficient calorie intake. Kwashiorkor means sickness the older child gets, when the next child is born.

The differences between these two malnutrition conditions are tabulated below:

	Marasmus	Kwashiorkor
Age of onset	Below 1 year	1–5 years
Deficiency of	Calorie and proteins	Proteins alone
Cause	Early weaning and repeated infection	Starchy diet after weaning. Precipitated by acute infection
Growth retardation of child	Marked	Severe
Attitude	Irritable and fretful	Lethargic and apathetic
Appearance	Shrunken skin and bones, dehydrated	Looks plump due to edema of face and lower limbs
Appetite	Normal	Anorexia
Skin	Dry and atrophic	Crazy pavement dermatitis due to peeling and cracking of skin
Hair	No change	Sparse, soft and thin
Other features	Watery diarrhea, weakness and other nutritional deficiencies	Angular stomatitis, cheilosis, watery diarrhea, muscle wasting
Serum albumin	2–3 g/dL	< 2 g/dL
Serum cortisol	Increased	Decreased

47. Conjugations/phase II reactions of detoxifications.
Refer 2004 Short Note Question 14.

48. Stereoisomerism.
Refer 2011 Short Note 28.
Glucose with four asymmetric carbon atoms can form 16 isomers as per Vant Hoff's formula (2^n) where 'n' is the number of asymmetric carbon ($2^4 = 16$)

- **D-and L isomerism:** The designation of a sugar isomer as the D form or of its mirror image as the L form. It depends on the orientation of H and OH groups on the penultimate carbon (carbon adjacent to primary alcohol) **(Fig. 18)**.
- **Enantiomers:** In D and L isomerism, the groups attached to carbon atoms of glucose 2, 3, 4, and 5 are totally reversed to produce mirror images. These 2 forms –D and L isomers are known as **Enantiomers**.

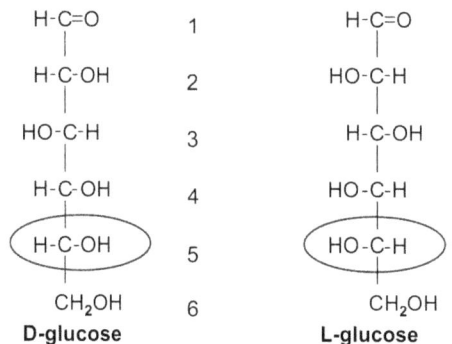

Fig. 18: D-and-L isomerism.

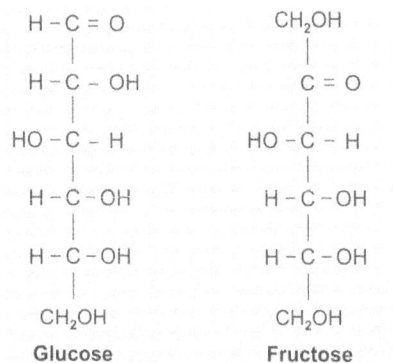

Fig. 19: Aldohexose-ketohexose isomers.

- **Aldose–ketose isomerism (Fig. 19):** Fructose has the same molecular formula as glucose but differs in structural formula. There is a potential keto group in position 2 of fructose whereas there is a potential aldehyde group in position 1 of glucose.

49. Actions of insulin.
Refer 2006 Short Note 20.

50. Hyperglycemic hormones.

- They increase the level of blood glucose acting against the action of insulin
- They are glucagon, epinephrine, thyroxine, glucocorticoids, growth hormones and ACTH. They are anti-insulin hormones:
- **Glucagon**
  - It is produced from α-cells islets of Langerhans of pancreas
  - Its functions are opposite to the insulin actions—anti-insulin action
  - It stimulates gluconeogenesis, glycogenolysis.
- **Epinephrine or adrenaline**
  - Synthesized from the amino acid tyrosine from adrenal medulla
  - It is released in response to flight, fright, exercise and hypoglycemia
  - It increases glycogenolysis and stimulates lipolysis.
- **Thyroxine**
  - Secreted by thyroid gland as T3 and T4
  - It increases gluconeogenesis and rapid absorption of glucose.
- **Glucocorticoids**
  - These hormones are hyperglycemic in nature secreted from zona fascicularis of adrenal cortex
  - They stimulate gluconeogenesis, and glycogenolysis and suppress glycolysis
  - Glucocorticoids stimulates protein metabolism.
- **Growth hormones (somatotropin)**
  - Secreted by anterior pituitary gland
  - It inhibits the glucose utilization by cells
  - It stimulates protein synthesis.

51. ELISA.
Refer 2009 Short Note 15.

52. Isoelectric pH of proteins.
- It is the pH at which a particular molecule or surface carries no net electrical charge or contain electric charges, negative as well as positive
- The pI is the pH value at which the amino acids exist as ampholytes or Zwitter ion in solution depending on the pH of the medium
- At this point there is no mobility in an electric field
- Solubility and buffering capacity will be minimum at this pH
- The net charge on the molecule is affected by pH of its surrounding environment and can become more positively or negatively charged due to the loss or gain of protons (H^+). In acidic solution they are cationic and in alkaline solutions they are anionic
- If we add hydrochloric acid to this solution drop by drop at a particular pH, 50% of the molecules are cations and 50% in zwitter ionic form. pH at this position is pK1
- If we titrate the solution with NaOH, molecules become anions. When 50% of molecules are anions, that pH is known as pK2
- Isoelectric pH of monoamino-monocarboxylic amino acids can be calculated as:

$$pI = \frac{pK1 + pK2}{2}$$

e.g.: pI of glycine = $\frac{2.4 + 9.8}{2} = 6.1$

- In amino acids with more than two ionizable groups, pK values are also more. For example, aspartic acid has pK1—2.1; pK2—9.8 and pK3—3.9. At physiological pH of 7.4, both the carboxyl and amino groups of amino acids are completely ionized.

53. Wilson's disease.
Refer 2007 Short Note 24.

54. Laboratory diagnosis of phenylketonuria.
- Blood level of phenylalanine is elevated—normal level is 1 mg/dL, which is elevated to >20 mg/dL
- This is confirmed by Tandem mass spectroscopy
- Guthrie's test is confirmative
- Urine ferric chloride test is positive
- DNA probes—to diagnose the defects in phenylalanine hydroxylase and dihydrobiopterin reductase.

55. Chloride shift (Fig. 20).
- Hb is the major blood buffer in RBCs and it acts along with bicarbonate system
- It has 38 histidine residues
- **In the tissue level:** OxyHb releases O_2 to the tissues which is facilitated by low pO_2, low pH and high pCO_2, CO_2 produced in the tissues is returned to the lungs carried by Hb where CO_2 is eliminated in expired air
- **In the RBC:** CO_2 is converted to carbonic acid by carbonic anhydrase. This results in lowering of pH and the formation of deoxy-Hb decrease in pH and the Hb becomes deoxy-Hb
- DeoxyHb neutralises carbonic acid to increase the pH and there will be increase in bicarbonate and decrease in pCO_2

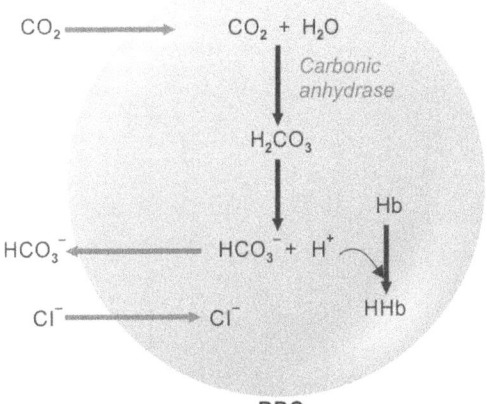

Fig. 20: Chloride shift.

- To maintain electroneutrality chloride ions enter into RBC for each bicarbonate leaves. This is called **Chloride shift**.

56. DNA repair mechanism.

Refer 2003 Short Note 11.

57. Plasma buffers.

Buffers resist changes in pH when small quantities of an acid or an alkali are added. Various buffers in blood are:
- **Bicarbonate buffer system (Bicarbonate—carbonic acid system)** ($NaHCO_3/H_2CO_3$):
  - It is the most important buffer in plasma and is formed by ($NaHCO_3/H_2CO_3$).
  - It accounts for 40% in whole body and 65% in plasma.
  - The base HCO_3^- is the **metabolic component** and it is regulated by kidney and the carbonic acid (H_2CO^3) is called **respiratory component** since it is regulated by the lungs
  - The **normal bicarbonate level** in plasma is 24 mmol/L
    - The normal pCO_2 of arterial blood is 40 mm of Hg.
    - The **normal carbonic acid concentration** in blood is 1.2 mmol/L.
  - Carbonic acid has a pKa of 6.1 so it is a poor buffer. But the high blood concentration and the ratio of base to salt is high (20:1), which makes it an effective buffer.
  - Under physiological conditions, with pH 7.4 the ratio of bicarbonate to carbonic acid is **20:1**
- **Phosphate buffer system**—it is an intracellular buffer with low concentration in plasma
  - It is made of Na_2HPO_4/NaH_2PO_4. It has a pK_a of 6.8. It is an effective buffer system because its pKa value 6.7 is nearer to physiological pH.
  - The ratio of $HPO_4 : H_2PO_4 = 4:1$
- **Protein buffer system:**
  - **Intracellular—Hb buffer system (KHb/HHb)**
    - Hb is the major blood buffer in RBCs and it acts along with bicarbonate system
    - It has 38 histidine residues
    - **In the tissue level:** OxyHb releases O_2 to the tissues which is facilitated by low pO_2, low pH and high pCO_2 and CO_2 produced is returned to the lungs, carried by Hb where CO_2 is eliminated in expired air **(Fig. 21A)**
    - **In the RBC:** CO_2 is converted to carbonic acid by carbonic anhydrase resulting in decrease in pH and the Hb becomes deoxy-Hb
    - DeoxyHb neutralizes carbonic acid to increase the pH and there will

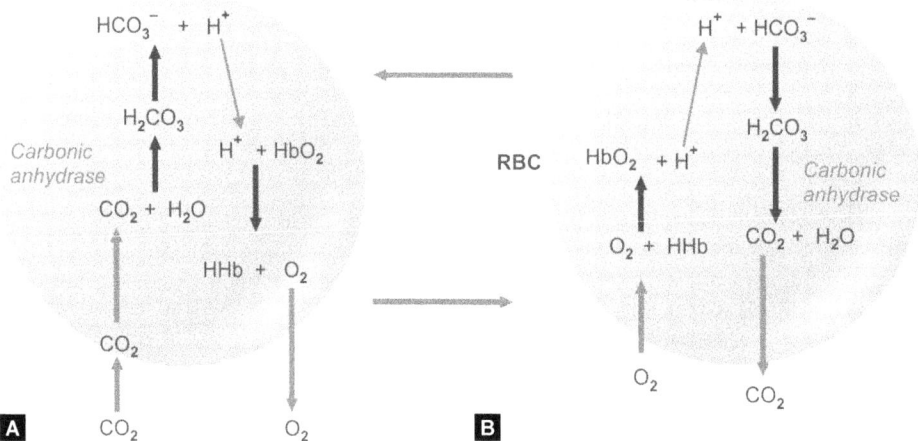

Figs 21A and B: Buffer action in tissue and lungs.

be increase in bicarbonate and decrease in pCO_2
- To maintain electroneutrality chloride ions enter into RBC for each bicarbonate leaves. This is called **chloride shift**
- **In the lungs:** OxyHb releases H^+ which is buffered by bicarbonate to form carbonic acid which is converted by carbonic anhydrase to CO_2 and water which get eliminated by ventilation **(Fig. 21B)**.
- **Extracellular-(Na protein/H protein)** Buffering capacity of proteins depend on the pKa value of ionizable side chains.
- The most effective buffer is imidazole group of **Histidine** molecules with a pKa value of 6.1.
- Albumin contains 16 histidine residues and so albumin accounts for the nonbicarbonate buffer system.

58. Gene therapy.

Refer 2010 Short Note 15.

59. Functions of albumin.

Refer 2009 Short Note 40.

60. Orotic aciduria.

Refer 2010 Short Note 37.

MBBS Examination 2016

ANSWER ALL QUESTIONS

I. Essay questions   (10/15 Marks each)

1. Describe the digestion and absorption of carbohydrates. Briefly write the metabolic fate of pyruvate.
2. Name the important buffer systems in the body. Describe in detail the role of lungs and kidneys in maintenance of acid-base balance.
3. Describe the sources, daily requirement, absorption, biochemical functions and deficiency manifestations and toxicity of iron.
4. What is polymerase reaction? Write a note on the steps involved in PCR and its applications.

II. Short notes   (4/5 Marks each)

1. Metabolism of LDL.
2. Mode of action of enzymes.
3. Write about post-transcriptional processing. Mention about post-transcriptional inhibitors.
4. Describe about the various patterns of diseases in protein electrophoresis.
5. Write about glycated hemoglobin, fructosamines, advanced glycation end products.
6. Pyruvate dehydrogenase complex.
7. Disorders of tyrosine metabolism.
8. Southern blot technique and its applications.

III. Short answer questions
     (2/3/4 Marks each)

1. Inhibition of ATP synthesis.
2. Wald's visual cycle.
3. Biochemical functions of vitamin C.
4. Functions of phosphorus.
5. Calcitonin.
6. Define BMR and mention the factors affecting it.
7. Consequences of diabetic ketosis.
8. Membrane proteins.
9. Coenzyme activity of biotin.
10. Lecithin-cholesterol acyltransferase.
11. Carcinoid syndrome (malignant carcinoid syndrome).
12. Write about urea cycle disorders.
13. Write about acute phase and negative acute phase protein.
14. What are the derivatives of aromatic amino acids? Write about serotonin.
15. High anion gap metabolic acidosis.
16. Write about alpha I antitrypsin and diseases associated with it.
17. Important functions of serine.
18. Types of DNA repair mechanism. Write in detail about any one repair mechanism.
19. Oxidative phosphorylation (OXPHOS) diseases.
20. Hybridoma technology and its application.
21. Functions of pyridoxal phosphate.
22. K_m value.
23. Write about amino sugar with example and its importance.
24. Lactose intolerance.
25. Diagnostic uses of enzymes.
26. Cahill and Cori cycle.
27. Vitamin K cycle.
28. Functions of copper.
29. Chylomicrons.
30. Nucleosomes.

31. Definition and importance of creatine clearance test.
32. Hyponatremia.
33. Telomerase.
34. Primary antioxidant enzymes and their activity.
35. Metabolic acidosis.
36. Specialized products of glycine.
37. Thyroid function tests.
38. Biochemical features of hemolytic jaundice.
39. Modes of gene therapy.

I. ESSAY QUESTIONS

1. **Describe the digestion and absorption of carbohydrates. Briefly write the metabolic fate of pyruvate.**

Digestion of Carbohydrates (Fig. 1)

Carbohydrates taken in the diet are:
- Polysaccharides like starch, glycogen
- Disaccharides like lactose (milk sugar), sucrose—cane sugar
- Monosaccharides—glucose, fructose.

Site and Enzymes

- Digestion in the **mouth**—digestion of carbohydrates starts in the mouth
  - Salivary alpha amylase (ptyalin)- mouth—acts on starch randomly and cleaves α -1,4 glycosidic bonds during mastication. It requires neutral pH and chloride ions
  - Products formed are—limit dextrins, maltotriose, maltose.
- **Stomach**—high acidity in stomach due to gastric HCl, inactivates salivary amylase

Small intestine:
- Bicarbonate present in the pancreatic juice neutralize the acidic pH
- Pancreatic alpha-amylase—acts on α -1,4 glycosidic bonds of starch to produce maltose, isomaltose and oligosaccharides
- At the mucosal lining of upper jejunum final digestion of di- and oligosaccharides occurs by disachharidases like maltase, sucrose and lactase and oligosachharidases.

Absorption of Carbohydrates

- The digested products of carbohydrates—the monosaccharides mainly glucose/galactose are absorbed from the lumen of duodenum and upper jejunum. Hexoses are absorbed more rapidly and galactose is absorbed more efficiently

a. **Active transport against concentration gradient (from low glucose concentration to higher concentration)—SGlut-1 and 2:**
  - This requires energy, specific transport proteins and sodium ions
  - It is a co-transport or symport mechanism
  - Absorption of glucose is carried through sodium dependent glucose trasporter-1(SGLUT-1) which is specific to intestine and SGLUT-2 which is specific to kidney
  - Energy is provided by the hydrolysis of ATP linked to sodium pump. By this Na^+ is expelled from the cell in exchange of K^+. So energy is needed indirectly.
  - This principle is applied in common treatment for diarrhea by **oral rehydration fluid** which **contains glucose and sodium**. Presence of glucose in fluid allows uptake of sodium to replenish body NaCl

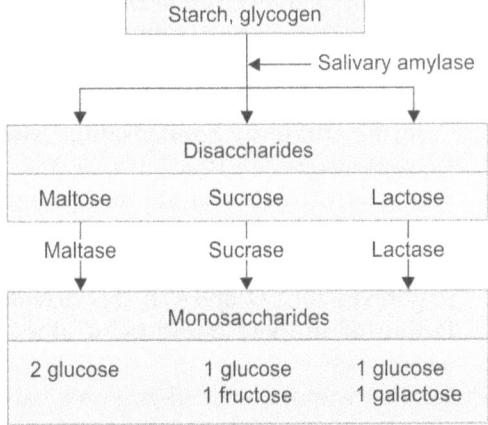

Fig. 1: Digestion of carbohydrates.

- Active transport is inhibited by the cardiac glycoside-Ouabain which inhibits sodium PUMP and phlorhizin which inhibits reabsorption of glucose in kidney tubules.
b. **Facilitated bidirectional transport with concentration gradient (GluT):**
    - Glucose is transported by this mechanism by various glucose transporters—Type 1,2,3,4,5,and 7
    - GluT1: It is the commonest transporter in brain, kidney, colon, placenta, retina and RBCs
    - Type 2 (GluT2) **(Fig. 2)**: It is an uniport and the delivery is by ping pong mechanism by the inversion of the transporter into the inner side of membrane—found in liver, beta cells of pancreas—glucose sensors, low affinity for glucose but high K_m for glucose
    - Type 3 (GluT3): High affinity for glucose present in neurons, brain, kidney
    - Type 4 (GluT4) **(Fig. 3)**: Major transporter in skeletal muscle, heart muscle and adipose tissues. It is the only transporter **under the control of insulin.** In type II diabetes mellitus there is reduction in membrane GluT4 to produce insulin resistance in muscle cells and adipocytes
    - GluT5: In intestines, testes, sperms and kidney—specific for fructose and mannose.

Metabolic Fate of Pyruvate (Fig. 4)

Formation of Pyruvate

- Pyruvate is derived from aerobic glycolysis of glucose

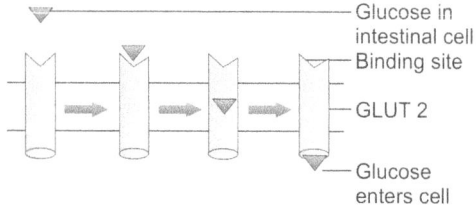

Fig. 2: GluT2.

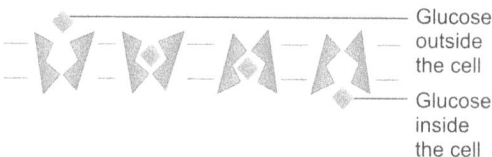

Fig. 3: GluT4.

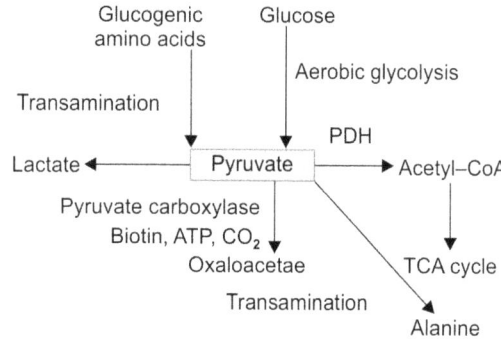

Fig. 4: Formation and fate of pyruvate.

- Some glucogenic amino acids like glycine, alanine, serine, threonine, tryptophan and cysteine are catabolized to form pyruvate which is converted to acetyl-CoA to enter into TCA cycle.

Fate of Pyruvate

- Formation of lactate in muscle and RBC by lactate dehydrogenase enzyme with NADH as coenzyme
    a. Formation of acetyl-CoA by oxidative decarboxylation done by pyruvate dehydrogenase enzyme with the help of five coenzymes—TPP, NAD, FAD, Coenzyme A and lipoic acid
    b. Acetyl-CoA enters into TCA cycle and forms citrate by condensation with oxaloacetate
- Formation of oxaloacetate by the carboxylation of pyruvate by the mitochondrial enzyme pyruvate carboxylase which requires biotin, CO_2 and ATP. This enzyme is one of the key enzymes of gluconeogenesis
- Pyruvate is transaminated by transaminase enzyme to give rise to amino acids like alanine (ALT enzyme).

2. **Name the important buffer systems in the body. Describe in detail the role of lungs and kidneys in maintenance of acid-base balance.**

Buffers in Body Fluids

Buffers are solutions which can resist changes in pH when small quantities of an acid or an alkali are added. Various buffer systems in blood are:
- **Bicarbonate buffer system**—It is the most important buffer in plasma and is formed by ($NaHCO_3/H_2CO_3$). It accounts for 40% in whole body and 65% in plasma
- **Phosphate buffer system**
- **Protein buffer system**

Role of Lungs in Maintenance of pH of Blood. (Second Line of Defence) (Figs. 5 and 6)

- When there is fall in pH (acidosis) the respiratory rate is stimulated resulting in hyperventilation. This would eliminate more CO_2 thereby lowering H_2CO_3.
- In tissues (**Fig. 6**), pCO_2 is high and pH is low to the formation of acids by the cells like lactate and production of CO_2 by cells. CO_2 diffuses into RBC. It combines with water to form carbonic acid by carbonic anhydrase and dissociates into H^+ and HCO_3^-. So RBC traps H^+ from the tissues. Some of the HCO_3^- diffuses out of the cell in exchange for chloride.
- In the lungs (**Fig. 5**), H^+ combines with HCO_3^- to form H_2CO_3 which becomes H_2O and CO_2. This CO_2 is released into the lungs. So lungs reduce the acid load of H_2CO_3 by excretion of CO_2.
- In metabolic acidosis lungs hyperventilate to excrete more acid. In metabolic alkalosis the reverse happens.

Renal Regulation of Acid Base Balance: (Third Line of Defence)

- Kidneys regulate pH of extracellular fluid
- Normal urine has pH around 6. This pH is lower than that of ECF (7.4). This is called **acidification of urine**

Steps of this Mechanism

- Excretion of H^+
- Reabsorption of bicarbonate
- Excretion of titratable acid
- Excretion of ammonia.
- **Excretion of H^+** (generation of bicarbonate) (**Fig. 7**)—in proximal convoluted tubular cells, CO_2 combines with water to form carbonic acid using carbonic anhydrase.

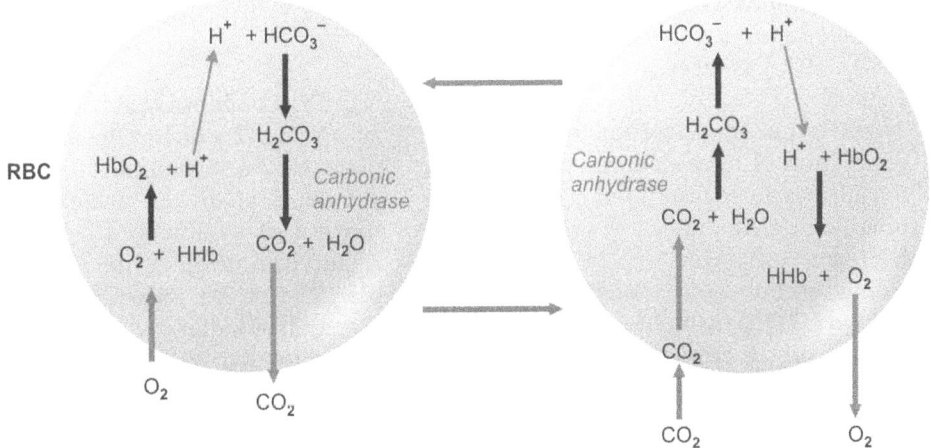

Fig. 5: Reactions in lungs.   **Fig. 6:** Reaction in tissues.

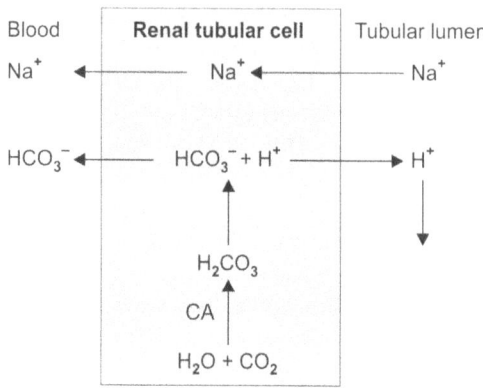

Fig. 7: Excretion of H⁺.

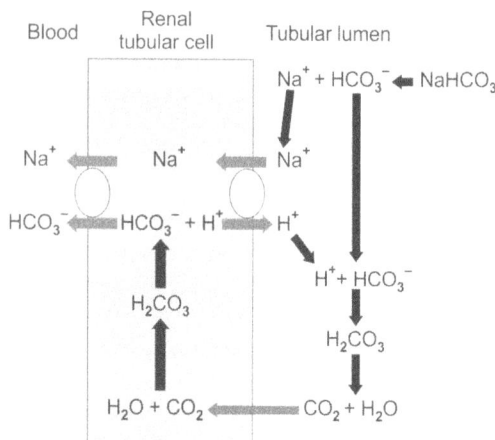

Fig. 8: Reabsorption of bicarbonate.

- Then it ionizes to H⁺ and HCO_3^-. This H⁺ is then secreted into the tubular lumen in exchange for Na⁺
- There is net excretion of hydrogen ions and net generation of bicarbonate. This increases the alkali reserve.
- **Reabsorption of HCO_3 (Fig. 8)**
  - Sodium bicarbonate in the lumen becomes sodium and bicarbonate
  - Sodium is taken up by PCT cells in exchange of hydrogen ions. H⁺ combines with HCO_3^- in the tubular lumen to form carbonic acid which forms CO_2 and water and both are diffused into the cell and converted back to carbonic acid
  - In the cell again it dissociates to H⁺ and HCO_3^-. HCO_3^- is taken into blood with sodium
  - There is no net excretion of H⁺ or generation of new bicarbonate. The net effect is the reabsorption of filtered bicarbonate mediated by sodium—hydrogen exchanger
  - By this reaction, base is conserved.
- **Excretion of H⁺ as titratable acid (Fig. 9)**
  - In the distal convoluted tubules, hydrogen ions are secreted into the tubular fluid in exchange of sodium
  - This sodium is obtained from Na_2HPO_4— disodium hydrogen phosphate which is a base

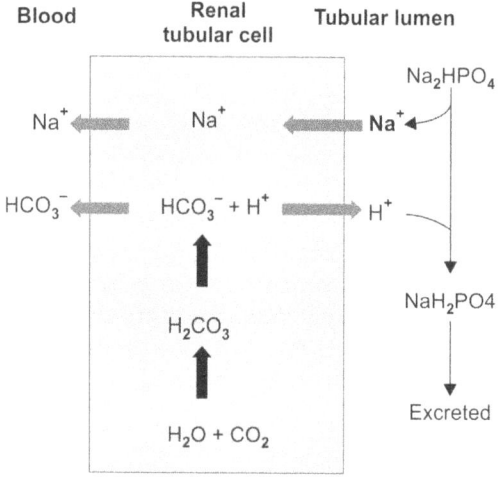

Fig. 9: Excretion of titratable acid as phosphate.

- Na_2HPO_4 combines with H⁺ to form the acid NaH_2PO_4 which is the major form of titratable acid in urine
- Titratable acidity of urine refers to number of milliliters of N/10 NaOH required to titrate 1 liter of urine to pH 7.4. This is a measure of net acid excretion by kidney
- As the tubular fluid moves down the renal tubules, more H⁺ ions are added causing more acidification of urine with fall in pH of urine up to pH 4.5
- The acid and basic phosphate pair is considered as urinary buffer.

- **Excretion of NH_4^+ (Fig. 10)**—occurs mostly at DCT. This helps to excrete H^+ and reabsorb HCO_3
  - This is another mechanism to buffer H^+ ion into the tubular fluid
  - H^+ ions combine with NH_3 to form ammonium ions (NH_4)
  - The enzyme glutaminase deamidates glutamine in DCT and converted it into glutamate and ammonia.

This ammonia is secreted into the lumen which combines with hydrogen ions to become ammonium ions and get excreted in urine.

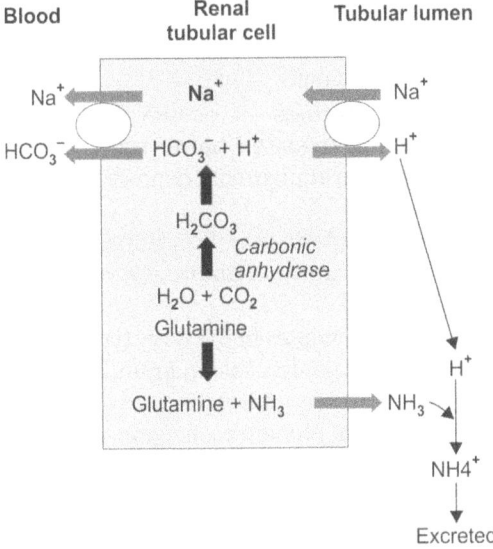

Fig. 10: Excretion of titratable acid as ammonium ions.

3. Describe the sources, daily requirement, absorption, biochemical functions and deficiency manifestations and toxicity of Iron.

Refer 2006 Essay Question 8 and refer 2011 Essay Question 4.

Iron is a trace element needed for human beings.

Sources: Leafy vegetables are a major source of iron followed by jaggery, liver. Pulses and cereals are a low source of iron. Milk is a very poor source of iron.

Daily Requirement: Adults: 20 mg/day, pregnant women: 40 mg/day, children: 20–30 mg/day.

Absorption (Fig. 11)

- Only ferrous form is absorbed
- HCl, vitamin C reduces iron to ferrous form, so increases its absorption. Phytic acid and oxalic acid form salts with iron so inhibits iron absorption
- Calcium and copper inhibits iron absorption
- Duodenum and jejunum are the sites of absorption
- When iron stores in the body are depleted, absorption is enhanced. When iron stores are adequate, absorption is decreased. This is called mucosal block theory

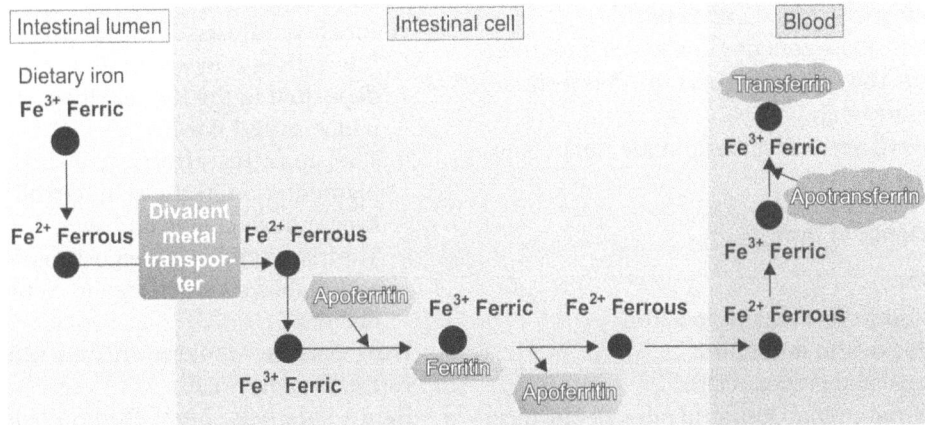

Fig. 11: Absorption and transport of iron.

- Ferrous iron in the intestinal lumen binds to mucosal cell protein called divalent metal transporter (DMT-1). This iron is transported into the mucosal cell. The unabsorbed iron is excreted
- Inside the mucosal cell, iron is incorporated into apoferritin to form ferritin. Whenever there is iron deficiency this ferritin supplies the iron. In iron deficiency erythropoietin is produced in kidney which enhances iron absorption.

Transport of Iron (Fig. 11)

- Transport of iron is done by the transport protein—transferrin
- Ceruloplasmin, the ferro-oxidase enzyme—oxidizes ferrous iron to ferric state
- Iron is taken up by the peripheral cells through transferrin receptors
- Total iron binding capacity (TIBC) is provided by the transferrin. It increases in iron deficiency anemia.

Storage

Iron is stored as ferritin in mucosal cells, liver, spleen, bone marrow.

Biochemical Functions of Iron

- Iron is the integral part of hemoglobin and myoglobin and is required for transport of oxygen
- Cytochromes and nonheme proteins of electron transport chain and oxidative phosphorylation need iron
- Peroxidase contains iron which is required for the phagocytosis of bacteria by neutrophils
- Iron is needed for the immune competence of body.

Deficiency of Iron

Causes

- Indian diet contains less iron
- Hookworm infestation
- Repeated pregnancies
- Chronic blood loss as in piles, peptic ulcer and uterine bleeding
- Nephrosis, subtotal gastrectomy and lead poisoning are other causes of iron deficiency

Clinical Features

- Microcytic hypochromic anemia ensues
- In anemia body cells lack oxygen and the person becomes apathic
- Severe iron deficiency leads to heart failure
- Chronic deficiency leads to achlorhydria, impaired attention, irritability, lower memory, poor scholastic performance.

Toxic Manifestations

- Acute intoxication—diarrhea, nausea, abdominal pain
- **Hemosiderosis**—it occurs in patients receiving repeated blood transfusions. Hemosiderin pigments deposit in spleen and liver
  - Hemosiderin is an iron storage protein which can hold about 35% of iron by weight
  - It accumulates in the body (spleen and liver as golden brown granules) when the supply of iron is in excess, e.g. repeated blood transfusions
  - Hemosiderosis is commonly observed among Bantu tribe in South Africa. This is attributed to a high intake of iron from their staple diet corn which is low in phosphate content and their habit of cooking foods in iron pots.
- **Hemochromatosis:**
  - It is a disease in which iron is directly deposited in the tissues (liver, spleen, pancreas and skin)
  - The manifestations are bronzed pigmentation of the skin, cirrhosis of liver and pancreatic fibrosis
  - The triad of cirrhosis, hemochromatosis, and diabetes are referred to as bronze diabetes.
- **Iron vessels**—cooking in iron utensils causes iron overload
- Bantu siderosis, hemochromatosis are other causes of iron overload.

4. What is polymerase reaction? Write a note on the steps involved in PCR and its applications (Fig. 12).

Refer 2010 Short Note 13 and 2017 Short Note 19.

It is an in vitro DNA amplification procedure in which millions of a particular sequence of DNA can be produced within few hours.
- Two primers of about 20-30 nucleotides with complementary sequence of the flanking region are needed
- Step 1-Separation: DNA strands are separated by heating at 95°C for 15 seconds to 2 minutes
- Step 2-Annealing: The primers are annealed by cooling to 50°C for 0.5-2 minutes. Then they hybridize with their complementary single-stranded DNA separated already
- Step 3-Polymerization: New DNA strands are synthesized by Taq polymerase. This enzyme is derived from bacteria that found in hot springs. The polymerase reaction is allowed to take place at 72°C for 30 seconds in presence of dNTPs of adenine, guanine, cytosine and thymine to duplicate both strands of DNA
- Step 4: Steps 1,2 and 3 are repeated to double up the DNA strands. After 20 cycles one million times amplifications will occur
- These cycles are repeated by automated instrument tempcycler.

Clinical Applications
- **Detection of infectious diseases—** tuberculosis and viral diseases like HIV and hepatitis. PCR detects even one bacillus present in the specimen and PCR is used in the diagnosis of viral infections like hepatitis C and HIV.
- **Medicolegal cases:** PCR allows the DNA in a single cell or in a hair follicle to be analyzed. This is highly useful in forensic medicine to identify the criminal.
- PCR is especially useful for prenatal diagnosis
- **Diagnosis of genetic disorders:** PCR technology has been widely used to amplify the gene segments that contain known mutations for diagnosis of inherited diseases, such as sickle cell anemia, thalassemia, etc.

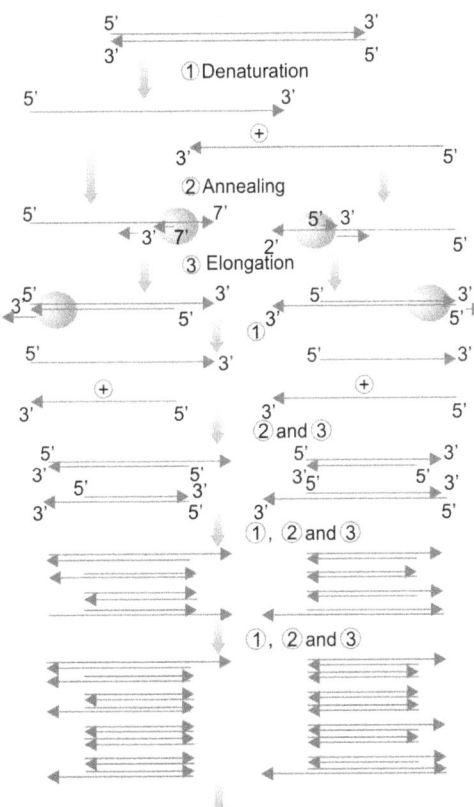

FIG. 12: Polymerase chain reaction.

II. SHORT NOTES

1. Metabolism of LDL (Fig. 13).

Refer 2005 Short Note 30 and 2014 Essay Question 2.
- LDL transports cholesterol from liver to peripheral tissues
- It has only apo B100.

Production of LDL
- Most of the LDL is derived from VLDL but a small part is directly released from the liver

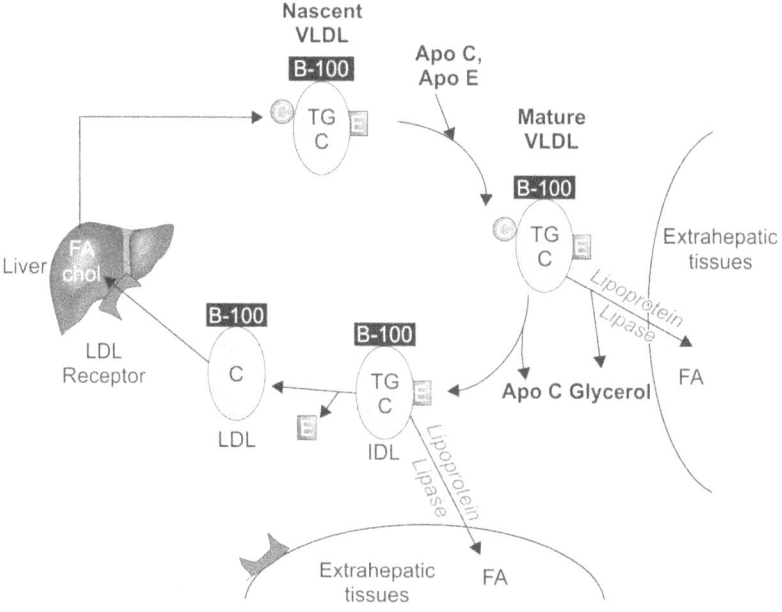

Fig. 13: LDL metabolism.

- LDL is taken by peripheral tissues and by hepatocytes by **receptor mediated** endocytosis—this is a regulated mechanism
- It is also removed by an unregulated independent mechanism by scavenger receptors by forming foam cells. This mechanism is active when blood cholesterol level is very high.

Structure of LDL Receptor (Fig. 14)

LDL receptor also called "apoB, E" receptor, since it is specific for apoB100 and E. It looks like pits and occurs on the cell surface of all cells especially hepatocytes. These pits are coated with a protein called clathrin on the cytosolic side of the cell membrane. The glycoprotein receptor spans the membrane, the B100 binding region being at the exposed amino terminal end.

Metabolc fate of LDL—LDL cholesterol after binding to LDL receptors is taken up by endocytosis. The apoprotein and cholesteryl ester are then hydrolyzed in the lysosomes, and cholesterol is translocated into the cell. The receptors are recycled to the cell surface. This influx of cholesterol inhibits in a coordinated manner HMG-CoA synthase, HMG-CoA reductase, and, therefore, cholesterol synthesis. It stimulates ACAT activity; and down-regulates synthesis of the LDL receptor. Thus, the number of LDL receptors on the cell surface is regulated by the cholesterol requirement for membranes, steroid hormones, or bile acid synthesis.

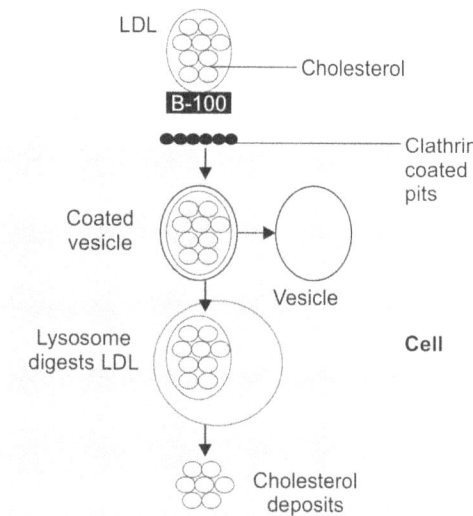

Fig. 14: LDL receptor.

2. Mode of action of enzymes.

Definition: Enzymes are biocatalysts which are proteins in nature (except ribozymes). They are specific in their reaction. They are heat liable and colloidal which are required in small quantities for their action.

Active Site of the Enzyme

- This is the region of the enzyme where the substrate binding and catalysis occurs
- Active site occupies a smaller portion of the enzyme
- It contains specific amino acid residues and possesses three dimensional structure
- Situated in a cleft or crevice of the enzyme molecule
- It is not rigid but flexible in structure and shape to promote proper substrate binding by conformational changes
- Substrate binds to the enzymes at the active site by noncovalent bonds [s]
- Substrate binds to the enzymes [E] at the active site to form enzyme-substrate complex [ES] which is the first step in enzyme catalysis E+S↔ES→E+P
- After the catalysis the product [P] is released and the enzyme becomes free for further use.

Mechanism of Action of Enzymes

- The first step in an enzymatic reaction is the formation of enzyme substrate complex (ES)
  E + S ⇌ ES ⇌ E + P
- An enzyme substrate complex is formed through multiple noncovalent interactions at the active site of the enzyme
- This ES complex is then converted to the product (P) and the enzyme is liberated.

Models to Explain the Mode of Action

- Depending upon the substrate binding to the active site of the enzymes, two models have been proposed to explain the mechanism of enzyme action:
  1. **Lock and key model**: Rigid template model, Fischer's template theory—the active site is rigid and complementary to the substrate. The substrate fits into active site like lock and key. This could not explain the flexibility shown by enzymes
  2. **Koshland's induced fit model**—this model explains that the enzymes are not rigid and preshaped. When the substrate interacts with the enzyme it induces a conformational change to produce the substrate binding site.

3. Write about post-transcriptional processing. Mention about post transcriptional inhibitors.

Refer 2011 Essay Question 3.
- The primary transcripts are longer than the mRNA. They are known as the heterogeneous nuclear mRNA or hnRNA
- They have to undergo certain processing to become mature RNA. This process is called post-transcriptional modifications.

Post-transcriptional Processing (Fig. 15)

Modification in mRNA

Splicing
- The long primary transcripts have coding regions called exons and uncoding regions called introns
- The introns should be removed and the exons should be spliced together. This is done by using small nuclear RNA (snRNA).
- They attach with the terminal portions of introns and cleave at one end forming a lariat
- This lariat is removed and the exons reattached by nucleophilic attack of terminal base of 1st exon to terminal base of 2nd exon.

Formation of Poly A tail:

The 3' end of mRNA is attached with 20–250 adenine nucleotides. This is to protect the 3'end from the attack of 3' exonuclease present in the cytoplasm

5' capping

The 5' end is capped by 7-methylguanosine triphosphate. This will prevent the attack of cytoplasmic 5' exonuclease attack on mRNA.

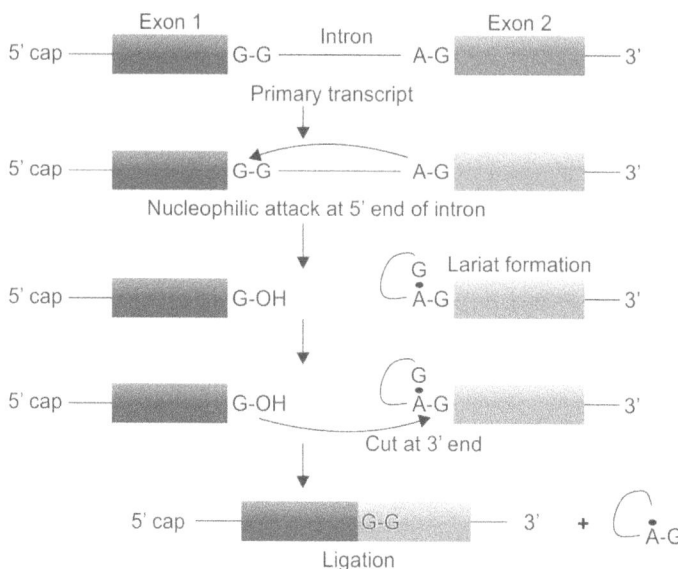

Fig. 15: Post-transcriptional modification of mRNA.

Methylation:

N_6 of adenine molecules and 2' hydroxy group of ribose are methylated.

Modification in tRNA

- Trimming, converting the existing bases into unusual bases
- Addition of CCA nucleotides to 3' terminal end of tRNAs.

Ribosomal RNA

- Pre-ribosomal RNA synthesized originally are converted to ribosomal RNAs by post-transcriptional modifications.

Post-transcriptional Inhibitors

Inhibitors – Prokaryotes

- **Rifampicin**—inhibits initiation by binding to β subunit of RNAP, no PDE bond used in the treatment of TB and leprosy
- **Actinomycin D-chemotherapy**—binds to DNA template and interferes the movement of RNAP

Other Inhibitors

- **Alpha amanitin**—toxin from mushroom—inactivates RNA polymerase II
- **3' deoxyadenosine**—causing chain termination.

4. Describe about the various patterns of diseases in protein electrophoresis.

Refer 2006 Short Note 30.

Principle

The term electrophoresis refers to the movement of charged particles through an electrolyte when subjected to an electric field.

- Cations (positivy charged ions) move towards cathod and anions (negative) to anode.
- When a biological mixture is subjected to electrophoresis, the compounds in the mixture move in relation to their net charge, size, molecular weight and mass and gets separated according to these characteristics so that the desired compound can be identified and isolated.

Clinical Applications

- Separation of serum proteins, lipoproteins and other classes of macromolecules. Electrophoretic pattern of plasma proteins—normal and abnormal **(Fig. 16)**.

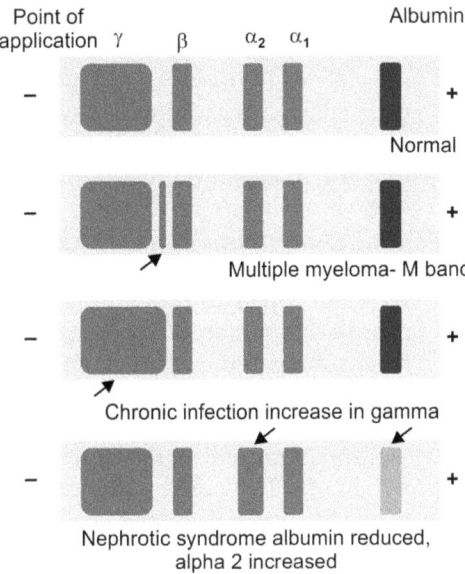

Fig. 16: Serum protein electrophoresis in health and disease.

Normal Bands

- 5 bands—albumin (55-65%), Alpha 1- globulin (2-4%), alpha-2 globulin (6-12%), beta globulin (8-12%) and gamma globulin (12-22%)
- Albumin has maximum and gamma globulin has minimum mobility.

Abnormal Bands

- Nephrotic syndrome—globulin is produced more by liver in compensation of renal loss of albumin. So alpha-2 band is prominent
- Cirrhosis—albumin synthesised in liver is decreased due to cirrhosis and so albumin band is thin and less prominent
- Multiple myeloma—light chain immunoglobulins are produced more so there will be a prominence in gamma globulin region (M band).

Hemoglobin Electrophoresis

- S band is seen in sickle cell anemia
- Various hemoglobinopathies and thalassemias can be diagnosed
- **Immunoelectrophoresis**—to separate various classes of immunoglobulins
- **Blotting techniques**—electrophoresis is an integral part of blotting techniques.

5. **Write about glycated hemoglobin, fructosamines, advanced glycation end products.**

All the three are laboratory investigations performed on cases of diabetes mellitus for diagnosing and monitoring the prognosis and predicting complications

Glycated Hb or Glycosylated Hemoglobin – (HbA1C)

- The best index of long-term control of blood glucose level is measurement of glycated hemoglobin or glycosylated Hb (HbA1c).
- When there is excess glucose in blood, it goes and binds with proteins especially Hb.
- When once attached, glucose is not removed from Hb. Therefore, it remains inside the RBC throughout the lifespan of RBC (120 days).

Interpretation

- It is used for monitoring the response to treatment
- Normal level: 4–7%
- Diabetes: 8–15%
- HbA1c level reveals the mean glucose level over previous 10-12 weeks
- It is not affected by recent food intake or recent changes in sugar level
- Elevated HbA1c indicates poor control of diabetes
- The risk of retinopathy and nephropathy are directly proportional to elevated HbA1c level.

Fructosamine

- In diabetes mellitus (DM) cases apart from Hb albumin is also glycated by the same principle like HbA1c to produce glycated albumin which is called fructosamine albumin
- This reflects the glucose control over a recent past period of 2-3 weeks as the half life of albumin is about 20 days
- This estimation is preferred in cases of gestational DM.

Advanced Glycation End Products: (AGEs, AGEP)

- In DM, glycation can also occur in matrix proteins which is irreversible
- This will lead into the loss of elasticity in collagen, atherosclerosis, microvascular damage, formation of diabetic cataract, etc.
- The concentration of AGE is 4 times greater than normal in vascular tissues in cases of DM
- Aminoguanidins reduce the formation of AGE and it can be given to the cases of DM to reduce the complications.

6. Pyruvate dehydrogenase complex (Fig. 17).

Refer 2014 Short Answer Question 26.
- PDH is a multienzyme complex
- Here pyruvate is oxidatively decarboxylated to acetyl-CoA
- It is a completely irreversible reaction
- This multienzyme catalyzes conversion of pyruvate to acetyl-CoA connecting aerobic glycolysis and TCA cycle. It is an irreversible process

Pyruvate + CoA-SH + TPP + lipoic Acid + NAD + FAD

Pyruvate dehydrogenase ↓

Acetyl-CoA + CO_2 + NADH +H^+ + $FADH_2$

- This multienzyme consists of 3 apo-enzymes –
  - Enzyme 1: Pyruvate dehydrogenase which decarboxylates pyruvate. TPP is its coenzyme
  - Enzyme 2: Dihydrolipoyl transacetylase—lipoamide receives the hydroxyethyl group transferred from TPP as acetyl group
  - Enzyme 3: Dihydrolipoate dehydrogenase—oxidation of lipoamide and regenerating TPP, lipoamide, FAD.
- It needs 5 coenzymes – TPP, lipoic acid, coenzyme A, NAD, FAD
- It is the committed step for complete oxidation of glucose and produces 5 ATP from one molecule of glucose
- This is analogous to alpha-ketoglutarate dehydrogenase multienzyme complex of TCA cycle
- Regulation—allosteric inhibition by the products—acetyl-CoA and NADH.

7. Disorders of tyrosine metabolism.

Tyrosine is an aromatic amino acid. It is synthesized from phenylalanine. It is both glucogenic and ketogenic.

Inborn errors associated with tyrosine metabolism (Fig. 18)

Phenylketonuria (PKU)

- It is an autosomal recessive disease with an incidence of 1:10,000 births. It is due to deficiency of phenylalanine hydroxylase.

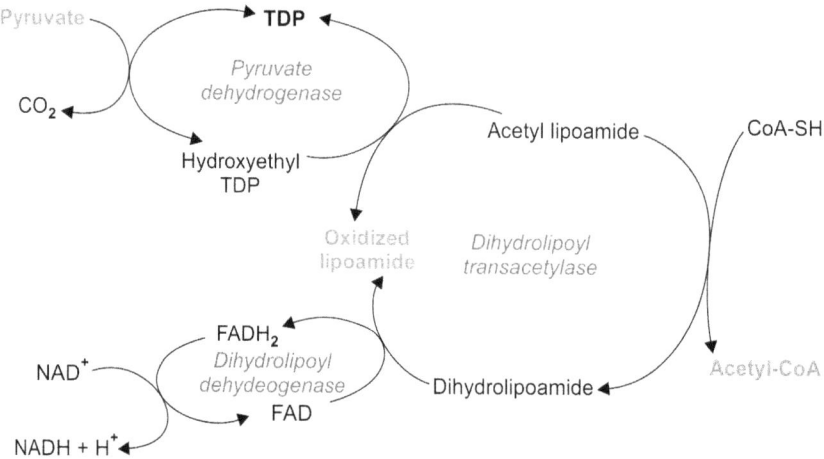

Fig. 17: Reaction of pyruvate dehydrogenase complex.

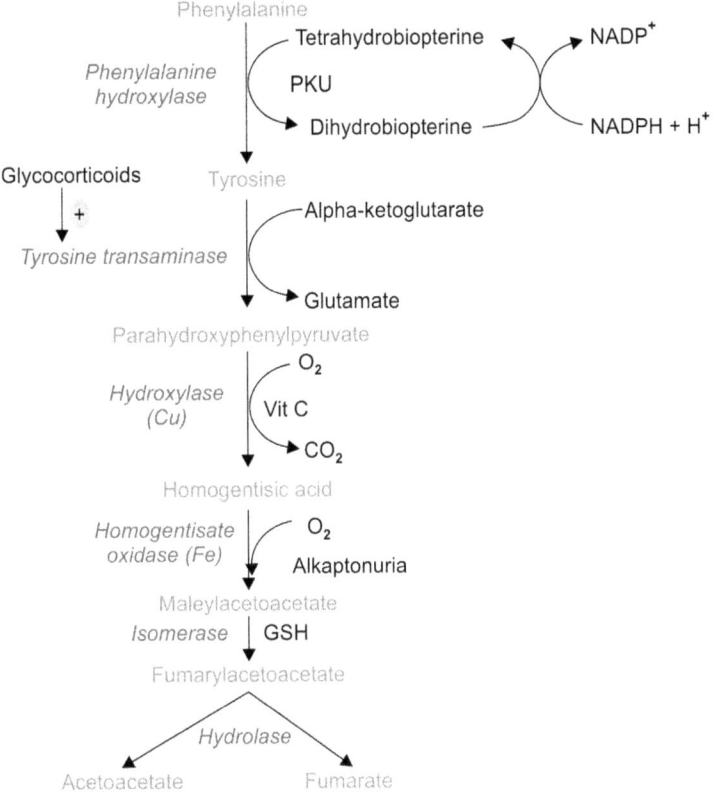

Fig. 18: Metabolism of phenylalanine and tyrosine.

Two Inborn Errors of Tyrosine Metabolism:

Alkaptonuria

- It is an autosomal recessive condition affecting 1:250,000 births
- It is due to the defect in homogentisate oxidase enzyme
- Homogentisate gets accumulated and oxidized to benzoquinone acetate and forms alkaptone bodies
- Alkaptone bodies get deposited in intervertebral discs, cartilages of nose and pinna of ear developing ochronosis. Black pigments get deposited over joint cavities causing arthritis
- Urine turns black on standing. $FeCl_3$ test is positive. Benedict's test is strongly positive since homogentisate is a reducing agent. Generally it is a harmless condition.

Albinism

- It is an autosomal recessive disorder with incidence of 1 in 20,000
- It is due to deficiency of tyrosinase leading to melanin deficiency
- Ocular fundus hypopigmented and color of iris may be red or grey. Patient will have nystagmus, photophobia and decreased visual acuity
- Skin is hypopigmented and sensitive to UV rays. Skin contains nevi and melanomas. Hair is also white.

Hypertyrosinemias

Tyrosinemia type I (Hepatorenal Tyrosinemia):

- It is an autosomal recessive condition affecting 1.5/1000 births
- It is due to fumarylacetoacetate hydrolase deficiency

- In the first 6 months of life—death occurs
- Cabbage-like odor, hypoglycemia and liver failure are seen along with mild mental retardation and it is usually fatal
- Urine contains tyrosine, para-hydroxyphenylpyruvate, hydroxyl-phenyllactate
- Treatment: Diet low in tyrosine and phenylalanine.

Tyrosinemia type II-(Oculocutaneous Tyrosinemia - Richner Hanhart Syndrome):

- It is due to deficiency of tyrosine transaminase
- Mental retardation, palmar keratosis, painful corneal lesions and photophobia are seen
- Urinary tyrosine and tyramine levels elevated
- Treatment: Diet low in proteins

Tyrosinemia type III (Neonatal Tyrosinemia):

- Due to absence of para-hydroxyphenylpyruvate hydroxylase
- Transient increase in tyrosine level in newborn children
- Dietary restriction of proteins.

Hawkinsinuria

- Autosomal dominant type
- Due to deficiency of para-hydroxyphenylpyruvate oxidase
- Excretion of the derivative of p-HPPA - hawkinsin in urine.

8. Southern blot technique and its applications.

Refer 2005 Short Note 38 and 2008 Short Note 40.

Blotting is a technique for transferring DNA, RNA and proteins on to a carrier so they can be separated, and often follows the use of a gel electrophoresis (Fig. 19). The southern blot is used for transferring DNA, the northern blot for RNA and the western blot for protein

- **Southern blot (Fig. 20):** This technique was found out by EM Southern
  - This technique is based on DNA hybridization technique
  - Used to detect specific DNA segment
- **Steps:**
  - DNA is extracted from the tissues.
  - It is fragmented using restriction endonucleases.
  - The cut fragments are separated by electrophoresis in agarose gel.
  - It is then treated with NaOH to convert DNA to single-stranded DNA.
  - The gel is then blotted over a nitrocellulose membrane.
  - An exact replica of the pattern in the gel is reproduced in the membrane. The DNA gets attached to the membrane.
  - The DNA is fixed to the membrane at 80°C.

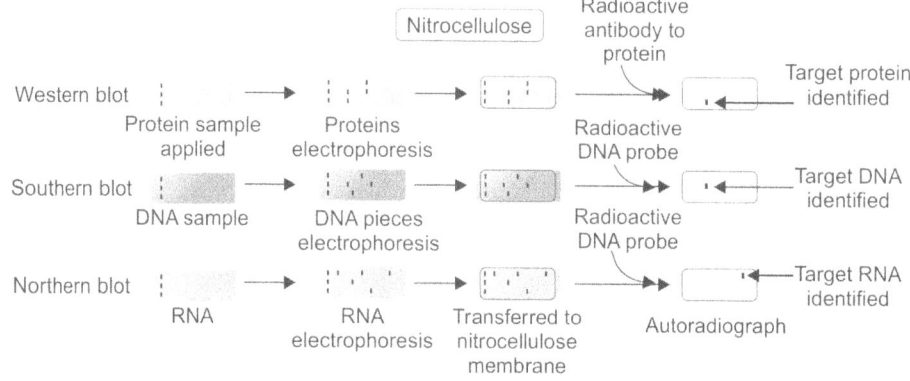

Fig. 19: Southern blot technique.

- A radioactive DNA probe which is complementary to the desired DNA fragment is applied
- This probe gets attached to the desired DNA (DNA hybridization)
- The membrane is washed and a radiographic film is exposed on the membrane
- The X-ray is developed to identify the DNA.

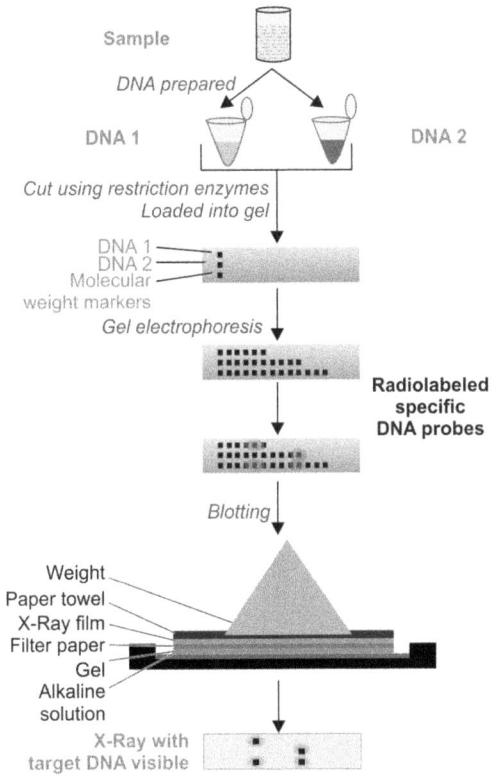

Fig. 20: Southern Technique.

III. SHORT ANSWER QUESTIONS

1. **Inhibition of ATP synthesis (Fig. 21).**

This comprises inhibition of all the complexes of mitochondrial electron transport chain and oxidative phosphorylation at complex 5.

Site Specific Inhibitors

- **Complex I to coenzyme Q (CoQ) specific inhibitors.**
    - Barbiturates—amobarbital
        - Antibiotic—piericidin
        - Rotenone, insecticide, fish poison
        - Alkylguanidines—hypotensive drugs.
- **Complex II to coenzyme Q**
    - Carboxin.
- **Complex III to cytochrome c inhibitors:**
    - Antimycin
    - British anti-Lewisite (BAL)
    - Naphthoquinone.

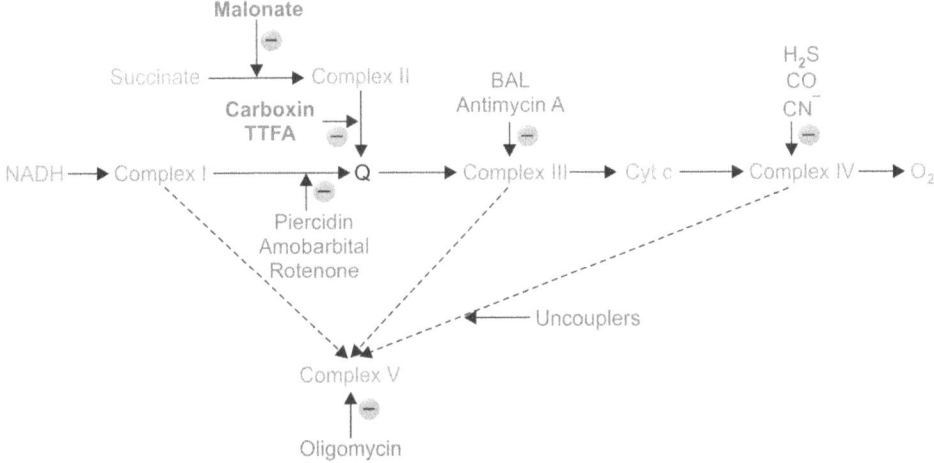

Fig. 21: Inhibitors of electron transport chain.

- **Complex IV—cytochrome oxidase inhibitors:**
  - CO—carbon monoxide
  - CN— cyanide
  - H_2S—Hydrogen sulfide
  - Azide.
- **Site between Succinate dehydrogenase and CoQ:**
  - Carboxin—inhibits transfer of ions from FADH2
  - Malonate—competitively inhibits succinate dehydrogenase.

Inhibitors of Oxidative Phosphorylation
- Atractyloside—inhibits translocase
- Oligomycin—inhibits flow of protons through Fo
- Ionophores—For example, valinomycin mobile ion carriers, allows K to permeate mitochondria; gramicidin—channel former.

Uncouplers of Oxidative Phosphorylation
- 2,4-dinitrophenol (2,4 DNP)
- 2,4-dinitrocresol (2,4 DNC)
- Chlorocarbonyl cyanide phenylhyrdrazone (CCCP).

Physiological Uncouplers
- Thyroxine
- Thermogenin in brown adipose tissue.

2. **Wald's visual cycle (Fig. 22).**

Refer 2008 Short Note 8.
- It is an important cycle to explain how vitamin A helps in vision through the visual pigments
- Rhodopsin plays the pivotal role in vision. It is the membrane protein found in the photoreceptor cells of the retina.
- Rhodopsin is made up of the protein opsin and 11-cis-retinal.
- When light falls on the retina, 11-cis-retinal isomerizes to all-trans-retinal.
- A single photon can excite the rod cell. The photon produces immediate conformational changes.
- The unstable intermediates produced are: Rhodopsin → bathorhodopsin → lumirhodopsin → metarhodopsin → and finally opsin + all-trans-retinal.
- The all-trans-retinal is then released from the protein and transported out of the retinal epithelium by an ABC protein. The all-trans-retinal is isomerized to 11-cis-retinal in the retina itself in the dark by the enzyme retinal isomerase. This reaction takes place in the retinal pigment epithelium.

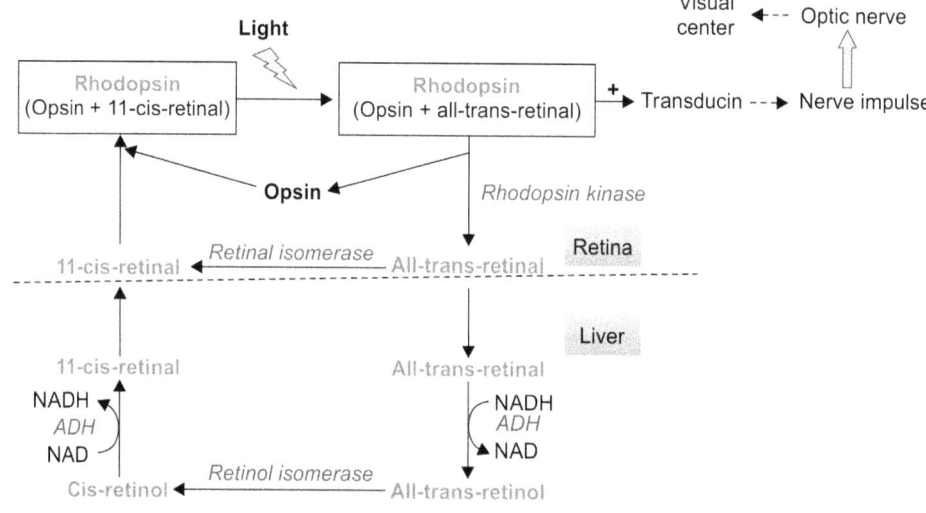

Fig. 22: Wald's visual cycle.

- The 11-cis-retinal combines with opsin to generate **Rhodopsin.** Alternatively the all-trans-retinal is transported to the liver and then reduced to all-trans-retinol by alcohol dehydrogenase (ADH)
- The all-trans-retinol is isomerized to 11cis-retinol and then oxidized to 11-cis-retinal in liver. This is then transported to retina. This completes the Wald's visual cycle
- Visual pigments are G protein coupled receptors. 11-cis-retinal keeps it in an inactive form which gets activated by photoexcitation. Cyclic GMP is also generated at the same time and it acts as a gate for cation specific channels
- G protein of retina is transducin
- Nerve impulse thus generated is transmitted to visual centers in brain.

3. Biochemical functions of vitamin C.

Refer 2005 Essay Question 5 and 2008 Short Note 21.

Vitamin C or ascorbic acid is a water-soluble vitamin. It is also known as Co-hydroxylase.

Biochemical Functions

- **Reversible oxidation and reduction:** Vitamin C can change between ascorbic acid and dehydroascorbic acid
- Vitamin C is the coenzyme for hydroxylase:
  - **Hydroxylation of proline and lysine:** Post-translational hydroxylation of proline and lysine residues are necessary for the formation of cross-links in collagen to give strength to the fibers
  - **Tyrosine metabolism:**
    a. **Dopamine hydroxylase** is a copper containing enzyme involved in the synthesis of the catecholamines— norepinephrine and epinephrine from tyrosine in the adrenal medulla and central nervous system
    b. Vitamin C helps in oxidation of para-hydroxyphenylpyruvate to homogentisic acid
  - **Hydroxylation of tryptophan** to 5-hydroxytryptophan (serotonin) by hydroxylase enzyme needs vitamin C.
  - **Steroid synthesis:** Vitamin C is needed for the hydroxylation reactions in adrenal cortex
  - **Bile acid formation:** Vitamin C is required for the rate-limiting enzyme— 7α-hydroxylase
  - **Carnitine synthesis:** Vitamin C helps in the hydroxylation of gamma-butyrobetaine to form carnitine

Role of Vitamin C in Iron Metabolism

- Vitamin C enhances the absorption of iron from the intestines by reducing ferric iron to ferrous iron.
- **Folic acid metabolism:**

  $$\text{Folic acid} \xrightarrow{\text{Folate reductase} \atop \text{Vitamin C}} \text{Tetrahydrofolate}$$

- **Hb metabolism**
  - $\text{MetHb} \xrightarrow{\text{Vitamin C}} \text{Hb}$

- **Antioxidant property**
  - It prevents cancer formation— especially bladder cancer caused by aniline dye.
- **Immune functions:**
  - Vitamin C stimulates phagocytic action of leukocytes and produces antibodies
- **Prevention of cataract:** Vitamin C reduces the risk of cataract formation.

4. Functions of phosphorus.

Refer 2007 Short Note 29.

- It is an intracellular ion seen mostly in bone and teeth and 10% in muscles
- Daily requirement—500 mg/day and serum concentration is 3–4 mg/dL

Biochemical Functions

- **Formation of bone and teeth**—vitamin D stimulates osteoblasts to produce alkaline phosphatase which leads to the formation of calcium phosphate hydroxyapatite crystals which is deposited on the bone causing mineralization
- **Production of high energy phosphates like:**
  - ATP—energy currency of the cell
  - CTP—needed for phosphatidylcholine and other compound synthesis
  - GTP—is needed for G proteins
  - UTP—bilirubin conjugation and glycogen metabolism.

- Synthesis of coenzymes like NAD and NADP
- DNA and RNA synthesis—phosphodiester bond links the sugar units which forms backbone of nucleic acids
- Esters—formation of G6P, F6P, etc.
- Phospholipids like lecithin formation
- Formation of phosphoproteins like casein
- Activation of enzymes by phosphorylation
- Phosphate buffer system: It is made of Na_2HPO_4/NaH_2PO_4. It has a pK_a of 6.8.

5. Calcitonin.

- Secreted by parafollicular cells of thyroid gland
- It is a polypeptide of 32-34 amino acids and its secretion is stimulated by serum calcium, gastrin, glucagon and biological amines
- It decreases serum calcium level by inhibiting resorption of bone and decreases the activity of osteoclasts and increases the activity of osteoblasts
- Calcitonin and PTH are antagonistic to each other but both together promote growth and remodeling of bone
- In kidney—calcitonin increases excretion of phosphates in urine along with parathyroid hormones.

6. Define BMR and mention the factors affecting it.

Refer 2005 Short Note 26.

Definition: Basal metabolic rate is the energy required by an awake individual during physical, emotional and digestive rest. It is the minimum amount of energy required to perform vital functions, such as circulation, respiration, working of heart, etc. to maintain life.

Normal Value

Men—34-37 kcal/m²/hr (24 kcal/kg body weight/day)
Women—30-35 kcal/m²/hr
Resting metabolic rate: About 3% higher than BMR. It is the energy required to maintain life or vital functions of body
- **Measurement of BMR:**
  - Direct method—by the heat evolved;
  - indirect method—by volume of O_2 consumed and CO_2 evolved.

Factors Affecting BMR
- **Age:** In old age, BMR is lowered
- **Sex:** Males have a higher value
- **Temperature:** BMR increases in cold climate
- **Exercise:** It increases during exercise
- **Fever:** 12% increase during fever
- **Thyroid hormones:** BMR is raised in hyperthyroidism.

7. Consequences of diabetic ketosis.

- Diabetic ketoacidosis (DKA) is common in Type I DM. Combination of hypoglycemia, glycosuria, ketonuria and ketonemia are seen in DKA
- Metabolic acidosis with increased anion gap
- Reduced buffers: Plasma bicarbonate is used for buffering these acids
- Kussmaul's respiration—acidotic breathing due to compensatory hyperventilation
- Breath smells of acetone
- Osmotic diuresis induced by ketonuria leads to dehydration
- Loss of sodium as the ketone bodies are excreted in urine as their sodium salt
- High potassium level due to lowered uptake of K
- Dehydration
- Coma—due to hypokalemia, dehydration and acidosis.

8. Membrane proteins (Fig. 23).

- The bilipid plasma membrane is made up of lipid, proteins and small amount of carbohydrates
- The membrane proteins are 2 types
  1. Peripheral proteins—on the surface of bilayer
  2. Integral proteins—deeply embedded in bilayer
- **Peripheral proteins:** Present on the surfaces of the bilayer. They are attached by ionic and polar bonds to polar heads of lipids. They anchor proteins to lipid bilayer

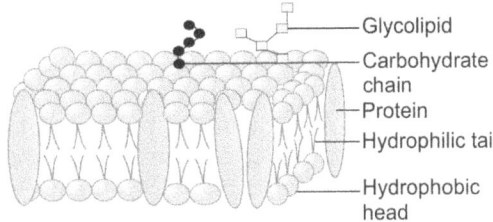

Fig. 23: Structure of cell membrane.

- **Integral membrane proteins:** These proteins are deeply embedded in the bilayer and attached by hydrophobic bonds or van der Waals forces
- **Transmembrane proteins:** They span the whole bilayer. They serve as receptors for hormones, neurotransmitters, ion channels, etc.

9. Coenzyme activity of biotin.

Refer 2004 Short Note 2.
- Biotin is a water-soluble vitamin
- Other name: Egg white injury factor.

Biochemical Functions

- Biotin acts as co enzymes for carboxylation reactions. So known as cocarboxylase
  - CO_2 is attached to the nitrogen of biotin molecule
  - This reaction requires ATP and it occurs in 3 steps.
  - Coenzyme: Biotin gets attached to enzyme carboxylase by amide linkage to ε amino group of lysine
    (i) **Biotin (nonprotein) + carboxylase (apoenzyme) → holocarboxylase**
    ATP + HCO_3 (CO_2) → carbonic phosphoric anhydride (CO_2 + P)
    (ii) **Holocarboxylase + carbonic phosphoric anhydride → P_i + CO_2 biotin enzyme**
    (iii) **CO_2 biotin enzyme + any receptor (X) → XCO_2 + Biotin + Enzyme**
  - Examples of CO_2 fixation reaction:
    - Acetyl-CoA carboxylase: Rate-limiting enzyme of De novo synthesis of fatty acid

    Acetyl-CoA + CO_2 + ATP ⟶ malonyl-CoA + ADP + Pi
  - Propionyl-CoA carboxylase in gluconeogenesis
  - Propionyl-CoA + CO_2 + ATP ⟶ Methylmalonyl-CoA + ADP + Pi
  - Pyruvate carboxylase in gluconeogenesis
  - Pyruvate + CO_2 + ATP ⟶ Oxaloacetate + ADP + Pi
  - Leucine metabolism – β-methylcrotonyl-CoA carboxylase
    β-methylcrotonyl-CoA → β-methylglutaconyl-CoA.

10. Lecithin-cholesterol acyltransferase.

- LCAT is Lecithin-cholesterol acyltransferase enzyme present in plasma
- It is synthesized in liver
- Its activity is associated with HDL and stimulated by apo A1
- Apo A1 of HDL activates LCAT in plasma which is then bound to HDL disc
- It catalyses the transfer of an acyl group from lecithin to cholesterol forming cholesterol ester
  Lecithin + cholesterol $\xrightarrow{LCAT}$ lysolecithin + cholesterol ester
- This reaction is responsible for reverse Cholesterol transport mediated by HDL.

11. Carcinoid syndrome (malignant carcinoid syndrome).

- Serotonin is synthesized by the argentaffin cells of gastrointestinal tract and it is necessary for GI motility
- Carcinoid tumors are malignant tumors of argentaffinomas in the small intestines and appendix
- There will be increased secretion of serotonin from these tumors (>40 mg/dL)
- Oat cell carcinoma of lung also produce increased serotonin secretion
- Flushing, diarrhea, sweating and hypertension will be present as symptoms
- Pellagra may be associated with this condition due to niacin deficiency
- Estimation of urinary 5-HIAA is diagnostic of malignant carcinoid tumor. Normal

level 25 mg/day and in carcinoid tumor the level is increased more than that.

12. Write about urea cycle disorders.

Urea cycle disorders: Due to defect in the enzymes of urea cycle
- Hyperammonemia type I
  - Enzyme deficient is carbamoyl phosphate synthetase I. Incidence is 1 in 100,000
  - It is an autosomal recessive disease
  - Very high level of ammonia in blood, mental retardation
- Hyperammonemia type II
  - Enzyme deficient is ornithine transcarbamoylase.
  - X-linked
  - Ammonia, glutamine increased in blood. Orotic aciduria due to channelling of carbamoyl phosphate to pyrimidine synthesis.
- Citrullinemia:
  - Enzyme deficient is argininosuccinate synthetase.
  - It is autosomal recessive disorder.
  - High blood levels of ammonia and citrulline. Citrullinuria—1–2 g/day
- Argininosuccinic aciduria:
  - Enzyme deficient is argininosuccinate lyase—Incidence 3/200,000
  - Argininosuccinate in blood and urine.
  - Friable brittle tufted hair (trichorrhexis nodosa)
- Hyperargininemia:
  - Enzyme deficient is arginase—incidence 1 in 100,000
  - Arginine increased in blood and CSF.
  - Instead of arginine, cysteine and lysine are lost in urine.
- Hyperornithinemia:
  - Due to defective ornithine transport protein due to defect in *ORNT1* gene
  - Autosomal recessive condition
  - Hyperornithinemia, hyperammonemia and homocitrullinuria are seen (HHH syndrome)
  - Urea level decreased.

13. Write about acute phase and negative acute phase protein.

- Some plasma proteins level get increased 50–100 folds during inflammatory and neoplastic conditions. They are: C-reactive proteins, ceruloplasmin, alpha-1 antitrypsin (AAT) and alpha-2 macroglobulin (AMG)
- During certain inflammatory conditions the level of some proteins get decreased in blood. They are known as negative acute phase proteins. For example, albumin, transthyretin (prealbumin), retinol binding protein and transferrin

14. What are the derivatives of aromatic amino acids? Write about serotonin.

- Aromatic amino acids are those amino acids with benzene (phenyl) ring and heterocyclic ring
- They are:
  - Those with phenyl ring: Phenylalanine, tyrosine
  - Those with indole ring: Tryptophan
  - Those with imidazole ring: Histidine
- **Derivatives of phenylalanine:** Tyrosine
- **Derivatives of tyrosine:** Catecholamines— DOPA, dopamine, adrenaline and noradrenaline, melanin, thyroxine
- **Derivatives of Tryptophan:** Alanine, niacin, NAD, NADP, serotonin, and melatonin, alanine
- **Derivatives of histidine:** Histamine, glutamate

Serotonin (Fig. 24)
This pathway occurs in brain, mast cells, platelets and gastrointestinal tract. 1% of tryptophan is converted to serotonin
- **Step-1 (hydroxylation of tryptophan):** Tryptophan is hydroxylated to 5-hydroxytryptophan by tryptophan hydroxylase which needs a cofactor tetrahydrobiopterin and NADPH
- **Step-2 (Decarboxylation):** 5-hydroxytryptophan is decarboxylated to serotonin which is 5-hydroxytryptamine (5HT). Decarboxylase enzyme requires pyridoxal phosphate as coenzyme

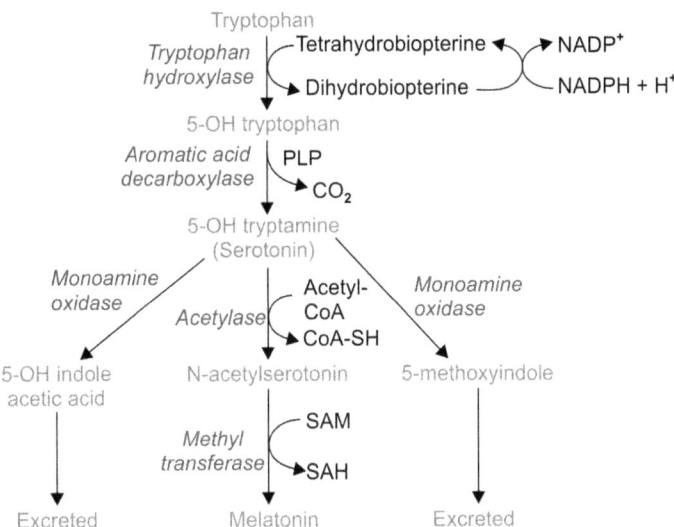

Fig. 24: Serotonin pathway of tryptophan metabolism.

- **Degradation of serotonin:** Serotonin undergoes acetylation by acetyl-CoA and methylation by S-adenosyl methionine to form **melatonin** (N-acetyl 5-methoxy serotonin)
- **Serotonin:** It is also oxidized by monoamine oxidase to form 5-hydroxyindole acetic acid (5HIA) which is excreted in urine.

Melatonin

- It is the acetylated and methylated product of serotonin secreted by pineal gland
- It is involved in diurnal variations, sleep wake cycles and biological rhythm
- It is also a neurotransmitter.

Functions of Serotonin

- Serotonin is synthesized by neurons and by the argentaffin cells of gastrointestinal tract
- It is a neurotransmitter in the brain and an anti-depressant
- It is a vasoconstrictor and induces smooth muscle contraction
- Serotonin level is low in cases of depressive psychosis and it is involved in inducing sleep, appetite, mood and temperature regulation
- It decreases the sensitivity to pain.

15. High anion gap metabolic acidosis.

- The sum of cations and anions in ECF is always equal to maintain the electrical neutrality
- There is always a difference between the measured anions and cations
- **The unmeasured anions constitute the anion gap.** This is due to the presence of protein anions, sulfate, phosphate and organic acids. **The normal value is 12 mmol/L.** It is increased in some forms of metabolic acidosis
- It is calculated as difference between $(Na^+ + K^+)$ and $(HCO_3^- + Cl^-)$.

High Anion Gap Metabolic Acidosis

- In metabolic acidosis, accumulation of acid anions will make the anion gap between 15 and 20
- This anion gap is increased when there is a decrease in cations as in hypokalemia, hypocalcemia. When the cations are increased anion gap is altered as in hypoalbuminemia
- High anion gap metabolic acidosis (HAGMA) is seen in a) renal failure—the excretion of H^+ and generation of bicarbonate both are deficient. b) diabetic ketoacidosis. c) lactic acidosis—lactic acid

is increased in tissue hypoxia, circulatory failure (normal lactic acid is less than 2 mmol/L).

16. Write about alpha-I antitrypsin and diseases associated with it.

- Alpha-1 antitrypsin (AAT)—otherwise called as alpha-antiproteinase or protease inhibitor
- It inhibits all serine proteases having a serine at their active center like plasmin, thrombin, trypsin, chymotrypsin, elastases and cathepsin
- These serine protease inhibitors are abbreviated as serpins
- AAT is synthesized in liver
- AAT is a glycoprotein with a molecular weight of 50KD
- Normal serum concentration is 75–200 mg/dL
- AAT deficiency causes emphysema and it is associated with nephrotic syndrome.
- Emphysema: AAT level is reduced in cases of emphysema. Bacterial infections in ling attract macrophages which release elastases. In AAT deficiency the unopposed action of elastases will cause damage to lung tissues leading to emphysema. About 5% of emphysema are due to AAT deficiency
- Nephrotic syndrome: AAT molecules are lost in urine causing deficiency of AAT.

17. Important functions of serine.

- Serine is an aliphatic OH group containing nonessential glucogenic amino acid
- It is deaminated to pyruvate and transaminated to hydroxypyruvate.

Functions

- Serine donates one carbon group to one-carbon pool. Serine hydroxymethyl transferase enzyme helps in the formation of glycine by the removal of one carbon which will be accepted by H_4F
- Serine is used in methionine metabolism to form cysteine from cystathionine
  Serine + homocysteine ⟶ Cysteine + homoserine
- Serine is converted to alanine by dehydration followed by transamination

- Phospholipid: Phosphatidyl serine is formed from serine + Phosphatidic acid
- Serine analogs are used to inhibit nucleotide synthesis
  For example: Azaserine—anticancer drug; Cycloserine—antituberculous.

18. Types of DNA repair mechanism. Write in detail about any one repair mechanism.

Refer 2003 Short Note 11.
- Synthesis of DNA is known as replication
- The process of replication occurs with high fidelity. Proofreading is done after replication to correct mistakes in arrangement of bases and base pairs
- Inspite of all these things alterations in base arrangements may occur due to various physical and chemical agents causing damage in DNA which can be corrected by the following mechanisms:
  – Mismatch repair
  – Nucleotide excision repair (NER) Base excision repair
  – Double strand break.

Mismatch Repair (Fig. 25)

- This may occur due to copying error
- During replication one to few bases may be unpaired in a DNA strand causing mismatch

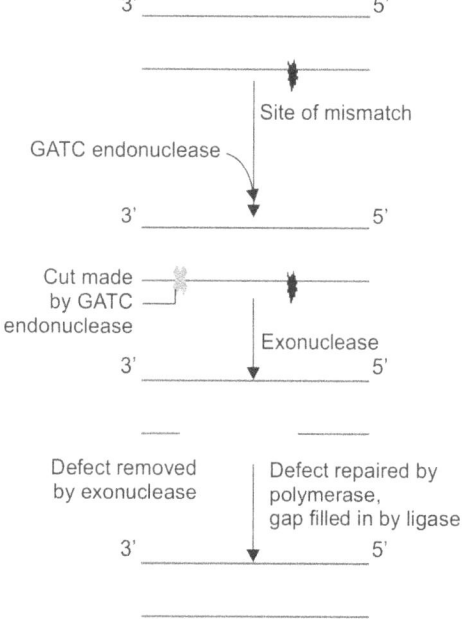

Fig. 25: Mismatch repair.

- Mut proteins identify the mismatched nucleotides based on the degree of methylation
- GATC sequences which are present 1/1000 nucleotides approximately are methylated on the adenine residue on the parent strand (not on the newly synthesized strand)
- GATC endonuclease cuts the strand bearing the mismatch and the mismatched nucleotide(s) is/are removed by an exonuclease
- The gap left is then filled in by DNA polymerase enzyme and the ends are joined to the 5'phosphate of the remaining original strand by DNA ligase enzyme.

19. Oxidative phosphorylation (OXPHOS) diseases.

- The circular mitochondrial DNA is inherited from the mother cytoplasmically
- Mother transmits mtDNA through oocyte
- During cell division mtDNA replicates and segregate to the daughter cells
- If a mutation occurs in mtDNA, the genome will lead to mitochondrial myopathies
- They are known as OXPHOS or oxidative phosphorylation diseases
- OXPHOS syndromes and their features are:
  - Leber's hereditary optic neuropathy (LHON) - Complex I defects: Blindness, cardiac conduction defects
  - Myoclonic epilepsy ragged red fiber disease (MERRF): Myoclonic epilepsy, myopathy, dementia
  - Mitochondrial encephalomyopathy, lactic acidosis, and stroke-like episodes (MELAS)—complex I defect, lactic acidosis, strokes, myopathy, seizures and dementia
  - Leigh's syndrome—complex I.

20. Hybridoma technology and its application (Fig. 26).

- Polyclonal antibodies are commonly produced when an animal is injected with an antigen. In nature monoclonal antibodies can be produced in multiple myeloma. To produce larger amount of monoclonal antibodies in the laboratory hybridoma technique is used
- Hybridoma technique is the production of unlimited amount of monoclonal antibodies (McAb) in the laboratory against a particular epitope of the antigen.

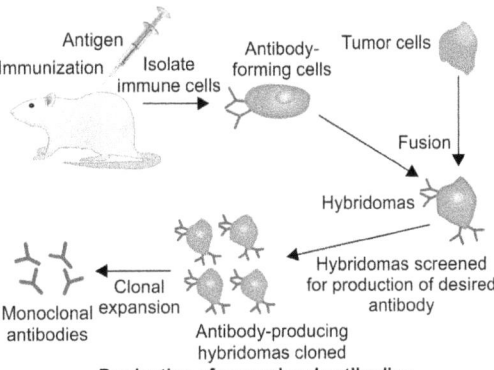

Fig. 26: Hybridoma technique.

Steps

- The antigen is injected into mice. Spleen cells from the immunized mice are fused with mice myeloma cells to produce hybrid cells which contain gene of normal mice and myeloma cells
- As the normal cells do not have multiplication potential. The hybridized normal cells die in normal culture condition within 5–6 days. The myeloma cells lack the enzyme HGPRTase and so there will be no DNA salvage pathways
- When HAT medium containing hypoxanthine, aminopterin and thymidine is used, the aminopterin the folic acid antagonist will inhibit the de novo synthesis of DNA. So both the pathways are blocked leading to the death of nonfused myeloma cells whereas the fusion cells survive. This is because the normal cells provide HGPRTase enzyme and the hypoxanthine and thymidine in the HAT medium together make the DNA synthesis possible
- The normal cellular genes provide the information for the synthesis of specific antibody. The myeloma cancer genes get multiplied and make the hybrid cells immortalized.

Applications

- Monoclonal antibodies produced by hybridoma technique are used for immunosuppresion for treatment of autoimmune diseases, transplantation rejection, rheumatoid arthritis, non-Hodgkin lymphoma and metastatic breast cancer
- It is also used in early detection of pregnancy, detection and treatment of cancer and diagnosis of leprosy.

21. Functions of pyridoxal phosphate.

Refer 2014 Short Note 21.

Pyridoxal phosphate is the coenzyme form of the vitamin pyridoxine (B6)

Biochemical Functions of Pyridoxal Phosphate (PLP)

- **Transamination (Fig. 27):** PLP acts as a coenzyme for transaminase enzymes—AST and ALT forming Schiff base
- PLP acts as a coenzyme for **decarboxylation of amino acids to form biologically important amines**, e.g.
  Glutamate ⟶ GABA + CO_2
  Histidine ⟶ Histamine + CO_2
  Cysteine ⟶ Taurine + CO_2

- PLP plays important role in **methionine and cysteine metabolism** in the reactions catalyzed by cystathionine synthase, cystathionase—desulfhydrases and trans-sulfuration reactions
- **Heme synthesis:** ALA synthetase is a PLP dependent enzyme
- **For the synthesis of niacin:** Kyneurinase needs PLP as coenzyme
- **Glycogen phosphorylase:** This enzyme contains PLP.

Deficiency Manifestations

- Neurological—↓ biological amines—serotonin, GABA, epinephrine
  - Convulsions: Children
  - Demyelination: Low sphingomyelin
  - Peripheral neuritis
  - Carpal tunnel diseases
- Dermatological—low niacin from tryptophan—pellagra
- Hematological—↓ heme synthesis.

22. K_m value.

Refer 2003 Short Note 8.

- K_m is the substrate concentration at which V_i is half the maximal velocity ($V_{max}/2$) attainable at a particular concentration of enzyme. K_m thus has the dimensions of substrate concentration
- According to Michaelis theory, the formation of enzyme substrate complex is a reversible while the breakdown of complex to enzyme and product is irreversible

$$V_i = \frac{V_{max}[S]}{V_m + [S]}$$

- The Michaelis-Menten equation illustrates in mathematical relationship between initial reaction velocity V_i and substrate concentration [S]
- $V_i = V_{max}[S]/K_m + [S]$ where, V_i = initial velocity, [S] = molar substrate concentration, K_m = Michaelis-Menten constant
- It denotes the affinity of enzyme for substrate. The lesser the value of k_m, the affinity of the enzyme for the substrate is more. K_m value is substrate concentration at half maximal velocity—means 50%

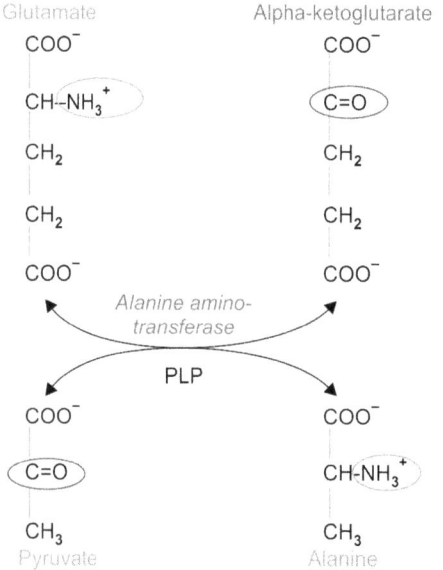

Fig. 27: Transamination.

of enzyme molecules are bound with substrate molecules at that particular substrate concentration
- K_m is independent of enzyme concentration. If enzyme concentration is double, the V_{max} will be double, but ½ V_{max} will remain same. In other words irrespective of enzyme concentration, 50% molecules are bound to substrate at that particular substrate concentration
- K_m is the signature of enzymes and characteristic feature of a particular enzyme for a specific substrate
- K_m is a constant. K_m denotes the affinity of enzyme for substrate and it is inversely related to the dissociation constant.

23. Write about amino sugar with example and its importance.

- Amino sugars are sugars in which OH— group is substituted with amino groups usually in the second carbon of hexoses.
- They do not show reducing property. They do not produce osazones
  For example: Glucosamine—present in hyaluronic acid, heparin and in blood group substances
  - Galactosamine—present in chondroitin sulfate of cartilage, bone and tendons
  - Mannosamine—constituent of glycoproteins
  - Erythromycin, carbomycin contain amino sugar.
- Amino group in amino sugar is further acetylated to produce N-acetylated sugars, such as N-acetylglucosamine and galactosamine which are constituents of glycoproteins, glycosaminoglycans and cell membrane antigens.

24. Lactose intolerance.

Refer 2011 Short Answer Question 8.
- It is due to the absence or deficiency of lactase or beta-galactosidase enzyme
- In lactose intolerance due to the absence of lactase enzyme, lactose remains accumulated and it becomes a substrate for bacterial fermentation. This causes production of H_2 and CO_2 gases. These accumulated gases and osmotically active products draw water from the intestinal lumen causing abdominal discomfort, diarrhea and dehydration
- Cause may be congenital or acquired.
- Acquired lactose intolerance occurs due to sudden change in milk containing diets.
- Treatment: Lactobacillus in curd, yeast. Patient should not be given milk in this condition.

25. Diagnostic uses of enzymes.

- Many of the blood analyte estimations are done by using enzymes
- Example:
  - Glucose oxidase—to estimate glucose
  - Peroxidase—glucose and cholesterol
  - Urease—to estimate urea
  - Uricase—to estimate uric acid
  - Hexokinase—glucose
  - Cholesterol oxidase—cholesterol
  - Lipase—triglycerides.
- Peroxidases are used to identify antibody by fixing them on antigens—in ELISA
- Restriction endonucleases—to cut DNA at specific sites—recombinant DNA technology and in southern blotting techniques.

26. Cahill and Cori cycle.

Refer 2011 Short Note 25.

Cahill Cycle (Glucose Alanine Cycle) (Fig. 28)

- Alanine synthesized in muscle is transported to liver where it is converted to glucose.
- Muscle protein → alanine $\xrightarrow{\text{Transamination}}$ pyruvate $\xrightarrow{\text{Gluconeogenesis}}$ glucose.

Significance

- Liver maintains glucose output by gluconeogenesis of alanine
- It also maintains nitrogen balance.

Cori Cycle (Lactic Acid Cycle) (Fig. 29)

Definition: Transferring lactate from muscle tissues to liver and resynthesis of glucose in liver is known as Cori cycle.

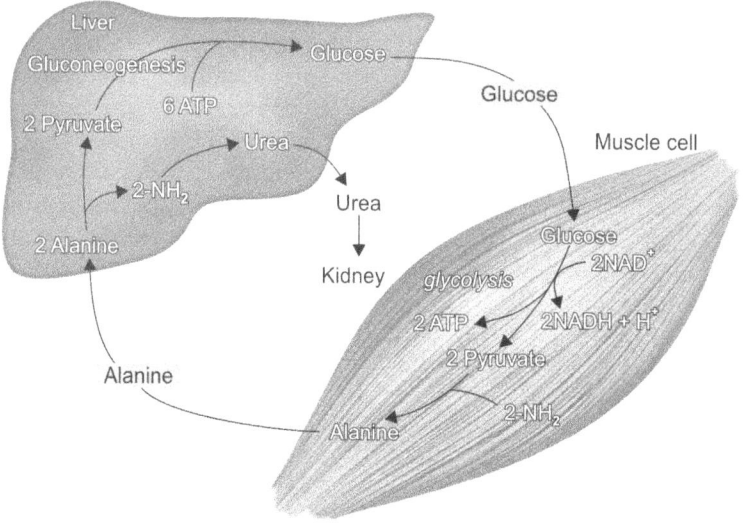

Fig. 28: Glucose alanine cycle.

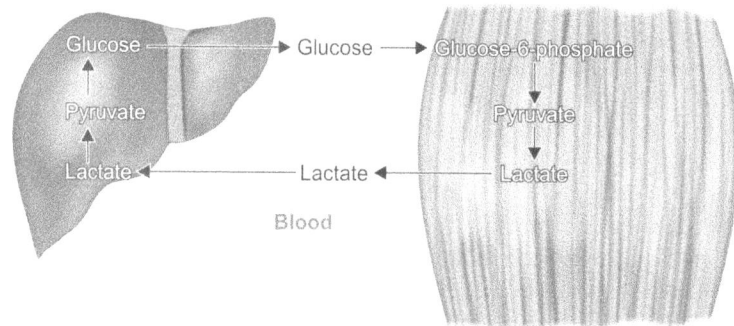

Fig. 29: Cori cycle.

Effects

- In contracting muscle, pyruvate is reduced to lactate which gets accumulated in muscle and may lead to muscular cramps in strenuous muscular exercise.
- It rescues lactate for further use (gluconeogenesis) and counteracts lactic acidosis.
- It is of less importance in starvation but important in more normal situations especially in certain cells, such as matured RBC, medulla, retina which are lacking mitochondria and virtually anaerobic.
- Lactate is carried from skeletal muscle to liver through blood. In the liver lactate is converted to pyruvate and by gluconeogenesis it is converted to glucose which is then transported to muscles for energy supply.

27. Vitamin K cycle.

Refer 2009 Short Answer Question 8.

Common name: Antihemorrhagic vitamin, coagulation vitamin

Metabolism of Vitamin K (Vitamin K Cycle) (Fig. 30)

The vitamin is synthesized by intestinal bacteria and so need not to be taken through diet. Its absorption depends on chylomicrons and bile salts, and it is finally stored in liver.

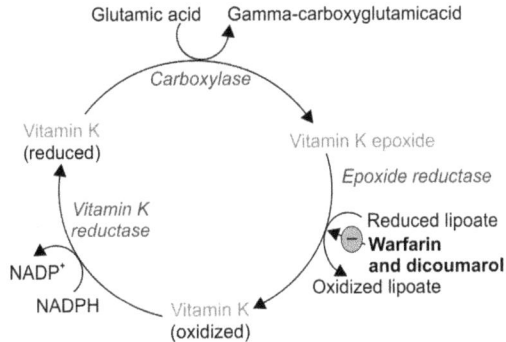

Fig. 30: Vitamin K cycle.

Functions

Vitamin K is involved in post-translational modifications of clotting factors, such as factor II, VII, IX and X which undergo gamma-carboxylation to get active forms.

Carboxylation of Clotting Factors and Significance

- All the pre-translational clotting factors contain glutamic acids at their ends of polypeptide chains which are converted to gamma-carboxyglutamic acid in the presence of carboxylase, O_2, CO_2, vitamin K (quinone form), $NADP^+$ and H^+
- These carboxylated clotting factors now possess two negative charges on their γ-carboxyglutamate which in turn chelate with two positive charges of Ca^{++}. This complex converts prothrombin to thrombin
- Bone protein osteocalcin also gets activated by gamma-carboxylation and also other structural proteins of kidney, lung and spleen
- This gamma-carboxylation is inhibited by warfarin and dicoumarol by competitive inhibition of epoxide reductase enzyme.

28. Functions of copper.

Refer 2015 Short Answer Question 45.
- Copper is a trace element. it is present in all parts of the body, more in liver, kidney and muscles

- It is present in enzymes, such as ceruloplasmin, cytochrome oxidase, superoxide dismutase, etc.
- It helps in absorption and incorporation of iron into Hb
- It is necessary for the action of tyrosinase enzyme in tyrosine metabolism
- It acts a cofactor for hydroxylation reactions done by vitamin C
- Normal requirement is 1.5–3 mg/day for an adult.

29. Chylomicrons.

- Chylomicrons (CM) are one of the lipoproteins.
- These are spherical bodies made up of lipid and proteins. The outer layer has polar heads—phospholipid, apoproteins and free cholesterol and inner core contains nonpolar lipids, such as TAG, tails of PL, cholesteryl esters
- Lipoproteins are classified according to their density into 4 major types:
  1. Chylomicron
  2. Very low density lipoproteins (VLDL)/prebeta lipoproteins
  3. Low density lipoproteins (LDL)/beta lipoproteins.
  4. High density lipoproteins (HDL)—alpha lipoprotein.

Structure and Functions of Chylomicron (Fig. 31)

- Rich in TAG
- The TAG of CM are derived from dietary lipids—exogenous
- These are very larger molecules having lower density than VLDL
- They contain high concentrations of lipid and lower concentrations of proteins
- It is synthesized in intestinal mucosal cells and secreted into the lacteals of lymphatic system
- It contains apo B-48 synthesized from intestinal cells and apo A. Apo C and E are added from HDL.
- **Metabolism of CM**: It occurs in adipose tissues and skeletal muscles

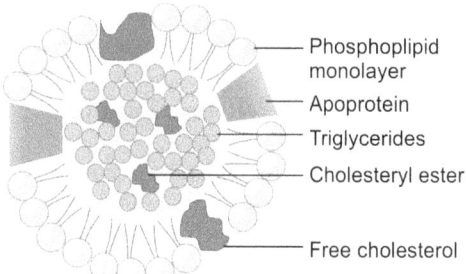

Fig. 31: Structure of chylomicron.

- Lipoprotein lipase present in the endothelial layer of capillaries of adipose tissues, muscles and heart but not in liver hydrolyses TGL in CM into fatty acids and glycerol
- The liberated fatty acids are taken up by muscle cells and adipose tissues
- When the TAG content is getting hydrolyzed the CM shrink in size to form CM remnant
- The CM remnants with apo B-48 and E are taken up by hepatic cells by receptor mediated endocytosis
- Apo E binds hepatic receptors.
- **Function:** They transport dietary TAG from intestines to adipose tissues for storage; and to muscles or heart for their energy need.

30. Nucleosomes.

Nucleosomes and Chromatin

- The double-stranded DNA wraps twice around a histone octamer formed by H2A, H2B, H3, and H4 condensed to 10 nm diameter spherical particles are called nucleosome. Core histones + DNA = **Nucleosome**
  - Long stretch of DNA in association with the nucleoproteins–histones is called chromatin which is further condensed to form chromosomes
  - Histones are nucleoproteins having basic amino acids
  - There are 5 classes of histones—H1, H2A, H2B, H3, and H4
  - H1—histones are loosely attached to DNA present in between the linker DNA
  - Core proteins are composed of 8 molecules of histone octamer—(H2A, H2B, H3, and H4)
  - H2A, H2B—rich in lysine and H3, H4—rich in arginine

31. Definition and importance of creatine clearance test.

- Measurement of clearance is a test for glomerular filtration test (GFR)
- It provides most useful general index for the assessment of the severity of the renal damage
- Normal GFR for young adults is 120–130 mL/min/1.73 m^2
- **Clearance tests:** Done to assess the glomerular filtration and renal blood flow
- Renal clearance of a substance is the volume of plasma from which the substance is completely cleared by the kidney in 1 minute
- **Clearance** = mg of substance excreted per min/mg of substance per mL of plasma; $C = U \times V/P$
  C = Clearance of the substance;
  U = Concentration of the substance in urine;
  P = Concentration of the substance in plasma;
  V = Volume of urine passed per minute.
- Clearance is expressed as milliliter of plasma per unit time
- **Creatinine clearance test:** It is based on the rate of excretion of metabolically produced creatinine which is excreted through urine
- Creatinine is freely filtered by the glomeruli but not reabsorbed by the tubules. A small amount of creatinine is secreted by the tubules
- 24-hours urine is collected and blood is also collected for estimation of creatinine. Urinary volume is measured (V) and the concentration of creatinine in urine (U) and plasma (P) are estimated and by using

the formula C = U × V/P the creatinine clearance is calculated
- Normal range for creatinine clearance is 90 to 120 mL/min
- Reduced creatinine clearance indicates chronic renal damage and reduced blood flow to glomeruli.

32. Hyponatremia.

Decreased sodium level in blood is called hyponatremia. Normal serum concentration of sodium is 140 mEq/L
- **Causes**
  - Vomiting, diarrhea, burns
  - Addison's disease, renal tubular acidosis, chronic renal failure, congestive cardiac failure
- Hyperglycemia
- SIADH, Drugs—ACE inhibitors, lithium, NSAIDs, vasopressin and oxytocin.
- **Pseudo-or dilutional hyponatremia**—hyperproteinemia (myeloma) and mannitol
- **Signs and symptoms**
  - Dehydration
  - Abdominal cramps
  - Oliguria
  - Tremors, and
  - Coma
  - May be asymptomatic.

33. Telomerase.

Refer 2017 Short Answer Question 19.
- There are 23 pairs of chromosomes in human beings
- Chromosomes—supercoiled chromatin fibres are condensed to form chromosomes
- Center of the chromosomes is centromere which is rich in AT with repeated DNA sequences of about 1 million base pairs with specific binding proteins. This region is called Kinetochore which is the anchor for mitotic division
- The 4 end pieces of chromosomes are called as **telomeres**
- Replication will not take place upto these ends—3' or 5' ends
- Telomerases or telomere terminal transferases do the job of replicating at these end pieces of chromosomes.
- Telomerase acts as a reverse transcriptase to synthesize this small DNA strand
- In old age telomerase activity is lost leading to chromosomal instability and cell death
- Drugs which prevent expression of gene for telomerase act as anticancer agents.

34. Primary antioxidant enzymes and their activity.

- In biologic system, the harmful effects of free radicals are inhibited or destroyed by antioxidants
- There are different types of antioxidants available to mitigate the damaging effects
- According to their nature and their action, there are:
  - Enzymatic antioxidants, such as superoxide dismutase (SOD), catalase, glutathione peroxidase and glutathione reductase, etc.
  - Nonenzymatic nutrient antioxidants, such as vitamin C, carotenoids, vitamin E and metabolic antioxidants, such as glutathione, ceruloplasmin, etc.
- Primary antioxidant enzymes are as superoxide dismutase (SOD), catalase, glutathione peroxidase and glutathione reductase, etc.

• Superoxide dismutases: It catalyze rapid dismutation of superoxide radical to hydrogen peroxide and oxygen

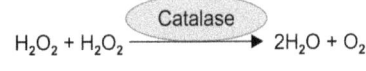

• Catalase: It reduce peroxide (H_2O_2) to water

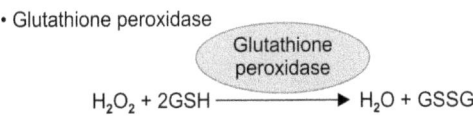

• Glutathione peroxidase

$H_2O_2 + 2GSH \xrightarrow{\text{Glutathione peroxidase}} H_2O + GSSG$

Fig. 32: Primary antioxidant enzymes.

- Actions of enzymatic antioxidant system:
  - Superoxide dismutase converts superoxide radicals to hydrogen peroxide and O_2. This is the first line of defense to protect cells from the damaging effects of superoxide
  - Catalase: Hydrogen peroxide is then metabolized by catalase to produce water and oxygen
  - Glutathione peroxidase: It detoxifies hydrogen peroxide to water while reduced glutathione (G-SH) is converted to oxidized glutathione (GS-SG). The enzyme glutathione reductase regenerates reduced glutathione using NADPH.

35. Metabolic acidosis.

Refer 2004 Short Note 16 and 2011 Short Note 14.

36. Specialized products of glycine (Fig. 33).

- Creatine, creatine phosphate and creatinine (glycine + arginine + S adenosylmethionine)
- Heme (glycine + succinyl-CoA)
- Purine bases and nucleotides—C4, C5 and N7
- Glutathione (Gamma-glutamylcysteinyl-glycine)
- Conjugation for xenobiotics

- Constituent of proteins like collagen. (glycine + proline + hydroxyproline)
- Methylenetetrahydrofolate by glycine cleavage system
- Glucose—it is glucogenic.
- **Creatine production from glycine (Fig. 34)**
  - Creatine and creatinine are the non-protein nitrogenous substances present in normal urine. They are synthesized by 3 amino acids—arginine, glycine and methionine. The synthesis occurs in kidney, liver and muscles
  - Normal serum level of creatinine is 0.7–1.4 mg/dL; serum creatine is 0.2–0.4 mg/dL.

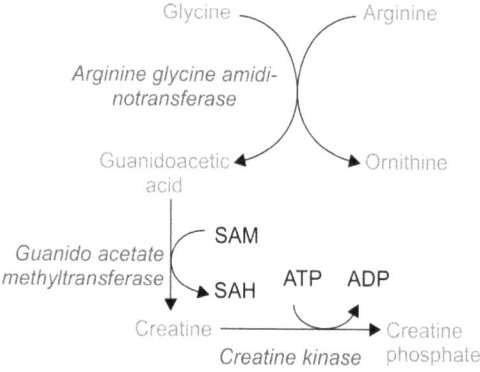

Fig. 34: Synthesis of creatine.

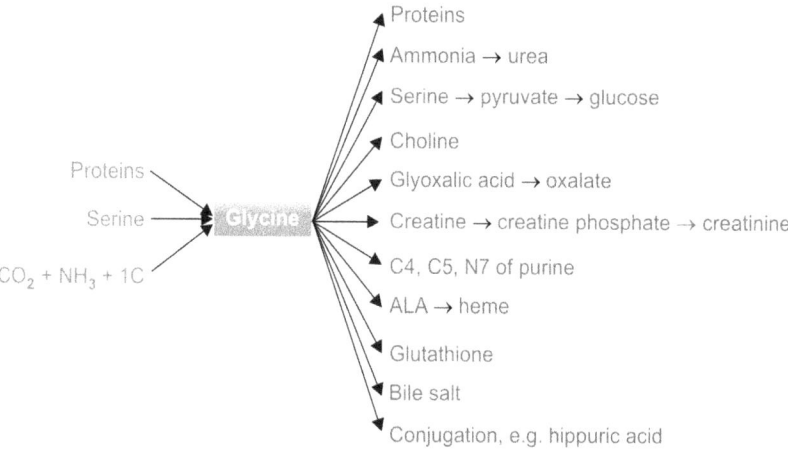

Fig. 33: Fate of glycine.

- Serum creatinine is a marker of renal failure. Creatinine clearance test is used to measure GFR.
- **Production of heme (Fig. 35):** Succinyl-CoA combines with glycine catalyzed by the enzyme ALA synthase in the presence of the coenzyme pyridoxal phosphate in the mitochondria to form alpha-amino-beta-keto-adipic acid which is converted by the same enzyme to delta-aminolevulinic acid. It is the rate-limiting step in heme synthesis.
- **Synthesis of purine (Fig. 36):** Whole molecules of glycine are contributed for the formation of C4, C5 and N7 of purine ring.
- **Conjugating agent**
  Glycine acts as a conjugating agent:
  - It conjugates bile acids to produce conjugated bile acids which are less toxic. Glycocholic acid and glycol-cheno-deoxy-cholic acid are the conjugated primary bile acids
  - In the liver Glycine conjugates benzoic acid and detoxifies it to form hippuric acid which is easily excreted from urine

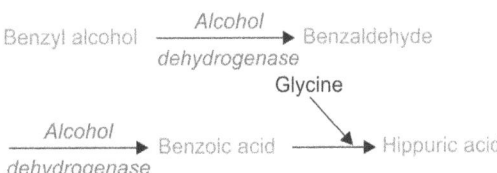

- **Neurotransmitter**
  - Glycine acts as an inhibitory neurotransmitter by opening chloride specific channels. It causes overexcitation in high concentration.
- **Glutathione formation**
  - Glutathione is gamma-glutamyl-cysteinylglycine. It is a tripeptide of biochemical importance. Glutamate combines with cysteine to form gamma-glutamyl-cysteine which combines with glycine to form glutathione. Each step needs one ATP.

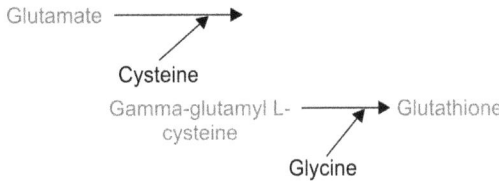

37. Thyroid function tests.

Refer 2003 Short Note 16.
- Thyroid gland synthesize the thyroid hormones—thyroxine (T_3 and T_4) and calcitonin
- Thyroid function tests are useful in assessing the functioning of thyroid gland and to diagnose the hyper- and hypothyroidism.

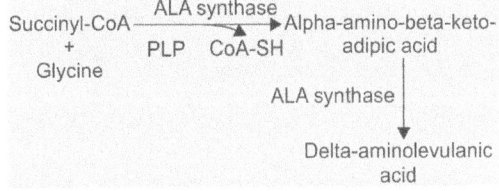

Fig. 35: Role of glycine in heme synthesis.

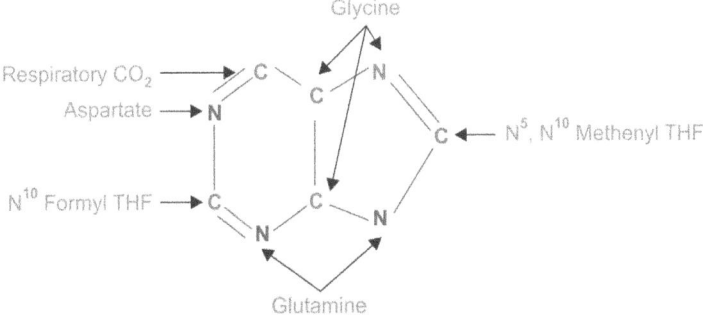

Fig. 36: Contribution of glycine to purine ring.

In Vitro Thyroid Function Test

Assay of Hormones

- **Serum Total T_3 and T_4 by immunoassay—RIA/ELISA**
  - Normal T_3 = 70–200 ng/dL; T_4 = 5–12.5 µg/dL
  - In hyperthyroidism, thyroid hormone levels—both T_3 and T_4 levels are increased but TSH levels decreased
  - In hypothyroidism, T_3 and T_4 are reduced in serum but TSH level is increased.
- **Free T_3 and T_4 (fT_3 and fT_4)**
  - More reliable test
  - Normal value of Free T_4 = 10–27 pmol/L; T_3 = 3 to 9 pmol/L
  - Values increased in hyperthyroidism and thyrotoxicosis and decreased in hypothyroidism
- **Thyroid binding proteins—thyroid-binding globulin (TBG)**
  - Normal level of TBG = 12–28 µg/mL
  - TBG—increased in hypothyroidism, pregnancy and in estrogen therapy
  - Level decreased in hyperthyroidism, nephrotic syndrome.
- **Resin uptake test (T_3RU or T_3U)**
  - Indirect estimate of binding capacity of plasma TBG
  - Radioactive iodine labeled ^{125}I-T_3 is added to the patient's serum which will occupy the free binding sites on TBG. Excess unattached ^{125}I-T_3 is removed and the amount taken up by the resin is estimated
  - Normal value of T_3U is 25–35%
  - Values increased in hyperthyroidism and decreased in hypothyroidism.
- **Plasma TSH (RIA method)**
  - Normal value = 2–6 µU/mL
  - In primary hyperthyroidism TSH level is elevated due to lack of feedback but in secondary hyperthyroidism, TSH and T3 and T4 levels are low.
- **Thyroid antibodies:**
  - To detect autoimmune disorders of thyroid gland caused due to the antibodies against thyroid tissues.

In Vivo tests

- **Thyroid iodine uptake test**—using ^{131}I. Normal value—1–13% absorbed after 2 hours and 15–45 and absorbed after 24 hours
- **TRH stimulation test**
  - An abnormal response is observed in hyperthyroidism and hypopituitrism.
- **TSH stimulation test**
  - IV administration of TSH will increase radioactive iodine thyroid uptake and blood thyroid hormone level
- **Thyroid scanning**—ultrasonogram.

38. Biochemical features of hemolytic jaundice.

Bilirubin is the end product of catabolism of heme. Normal value of total bilirubin is 0.2–0.8 mg/dL; unconjugated bilirubin is 0.2–0.6 mg/dL and conjugated bilirubin is 0–0.2 mg/dL.

- There are 3 types of jaundice—hemolytic (prehepatic) jaundice, hepatocellular (hepatic) jaundice and obstructive (post-hepatic)—due to acquired causes.

Prehepatic (Hemolytic Jaundice)

This is due to increased break down of Hb to bilirubin due to hemolysis and the level of unconjugated bilirubin is high. Urine is normal in color and hence it is called acholuric jaundice.

Causes

- Rh incompatibility—newborn; erythroblastosis fetalis
- Incompatible blood transfusion
- Congenital spherocytosis—sickle cell Hb
- Glucose-6-phosphate dehydrogenase deficiency.

Biochemical Features

- Unconjugated bilirubin—increased in plasma
- Urobilinogen—increased in urine and faeces
- Absence of bilirubin in urine.

39. Modes of gene therapy.

It is an intracellular delivery of genes to generate a therapeutic effect by correcting an existing abnormality. Somatic gene therapy is the insertion of new gene into somatic cell of the patient. Germ cell gene therapy is considered as unethical.

Procedure

- The healthy gene should be isolated
- This gene is incorporated into a vector or carrier like viruses as expression cassette
- The vector is then delivered to the target cells
- There are 3 ways of applying gene carrying vectors which are as follows:
  1. Exvivo strategy—patients cells are cultured in the laboratory, the new genes are infused into the cells and the modified cells are administered back to the patient
  2. In situ strategy—when the vector containing the gene is injected intravenously or directly into the tissue.
  3. In vivo strategy—the vector is injected directly to the target cell itself. For Example, cystic fibrosis gene to the respiratory tract cells.
- The vectors used for gene delivery are:
  - Retroviruses:
    - They are RNA viruses that replicate through DNA intermediate. Moloney Murine leukemia virus is commonly used. The *gag, pol, env* genes are deleted from the virus rendering it incapable of replication inside human body
    - In human cells the reverse transcriptase carried by the vector converts RNA to DNA which is integrated to target cell DNA.
  - Adenoviruses
  - Plasmid liposome complex
  - Gene gun method.

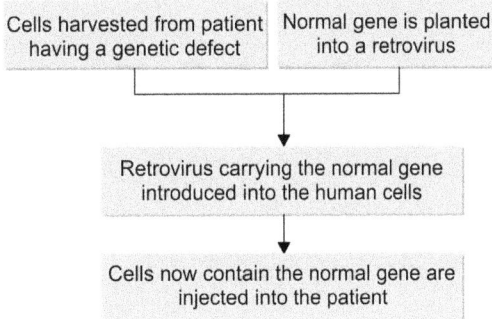

Fig. 37: Gene therapy.

Applications: Gene therapy is effective in inherited disorders caused by single genes. Various diseases like severe combined immunodeficiency (SCID), Duchenne muscular dystrophy, cystic fibrosis, familial hypercholesterolemia are treated by gene therapy.

MBBS Examination 2017

ANSWER ALL QUESTIONS

I. Essay questions   (10/15 Marks each)
1. Write in detail about metabolism and regulation of ketone bodies. Add a note on diabetic ketoacidosis.
2. Write in detail about the metabolism and functions of cysteine. Name the associated inborn errors.
3. A. Write in detail the investigations required to differentiate various types of jaundice. B. Describe the metabolism of bilirubin.
4. Brief about the conversion of phenylalanine to tyrosine. Describe in detail about phenylketonurias.

II. Short notes   (4/5 Marks each)
1. Significance of hexose monophosphate shunt.
2. Galactosemia.
3. Dietary fiber.
4. Reverse cholesterol transport.
5. Iron absorption.
6. Gout.
7. Role of lungs in maintenance of pH of blood (second line of defence).
8. Tests to assess glomerular functions.
9. Southern blot.
10. Post-transcriptional modifications.
11. Obesity.
12. Functions of prostaglandins.
13. HDL metabolism.
14. Significance of citric acid cycle.
15. DNA repair mechanism.
16. Glutathione.
17. Tests to assess renal tubular functions.
18. Polymerase chain reaction.
19. Metabolic acidosis.

III. Short answer questions
                            (2/3/4 Marks each)
1. Uncouplers of electron transport chain.
2. Beriberi.
3. Niemann-Pick disease.
4. Any two mucopolysaccharides—locations and its functions.
5. Rapoport-Luebering shunt.
6. Glycated hemoglobin.
7. Essential fatty acids.
8. Reactions catalysed by biotin.
9. Antioxidant vitamins and minerals.
10. Wilson's disease.
11. Name of any four neurotransmitters.
12. Four functions of albumin.
13. Factors affecting electrophoresis.
14. Hyperkalemia.
15. Functions of phosphate ions.
16. Any two antimetabolites and its uses.
17. Any four uses of polymerase chain reaction.
18. Inhibitor of protein translation.
19. Telomerase.
20. Alkaptonuria.
21. Substrates for gluconeogenesis.
22. Apoproteins and its significance.
23. Two isoenzymes and their clinical significance.
24. Significance of 2,3-bisphosphoglycerate.
25. Importance of HMP pathway.
26. Deficiency manifestations of B12.
27. Competitive inhibition.
28. Inhibitors of ETC.
29. Functions of mucopolysaccharides.
30. Liposomes.
31. Applications of electrophoresis.

32. Lesch-Nyhan syndrome.
33. Products formed from glycine.
34. Maple syrup urinary disease.
35. Inhibitors of transcription.
36. Histamine.
37. Gamma-aminobutyric acid.
38. Phase II reactions of xenobiotics.
39. Functions of parathormone.
40. Nitric oxide.

I. ESSAY QUESTIONS

1. **Write in detail about metabolism and regulation of ketone bodies. Add a note on diabetic ketoacidosis.**

Refer 2013 Essay Question 6.
- The ketone bodies are three in number, namely—**acetoacetate, β-hydroxybutyrate and acetone**. Acetoacetate is primary ketone bodies and the other 2 are secondary ketone bodies
- Acetyl-CoA formed from fatty acids can enter and get oxidized in TCA cycle only when carbohydrates are available. During starvation and in uncontrolled diabetes mellitus, the acetyl-CoA takes the alternate fate of formation of ketone bodies

- Level of KB in blood is **less than 1 mg/dL**
- **Site of formation:** Liver—mitochondrial matrix of liver cells
- **Site of utilization of KB:** Extrahepatic tissues
- **Uses:** During starvation, it is the major fuel for brain, heart and muscles. Brain gets 75% of energy from KB during starvation
- **Precursor:** Acetyl-CoA.

Synthesis of Ketone Bodies (Ketogenesis) (Fig. 1)

Reactions
- **Condensation**: Two molecules of acetyl-CoA condense to form acetoacetyl-CoA, this reaction is catabolized by thiolase
- **Production of HMG-CoA**: Acetoacetyl-CoA condenses with another molecule of acetyl-CoA to produce β-hydroxy β-methylglutaryl-CoA (HMG-CoA) by the enzyme HMG-CoA synthase. This is the key regulatory enzyme of ketogenesis
- **Lyase reaction:** HMG-CoA is cleaved to acetoacetate and acetyl-CoA by the action of HMG-CoA lyase present only in liver
- **Reduction and spontaneous decarboxylation:** Acetoacetate is reduced by

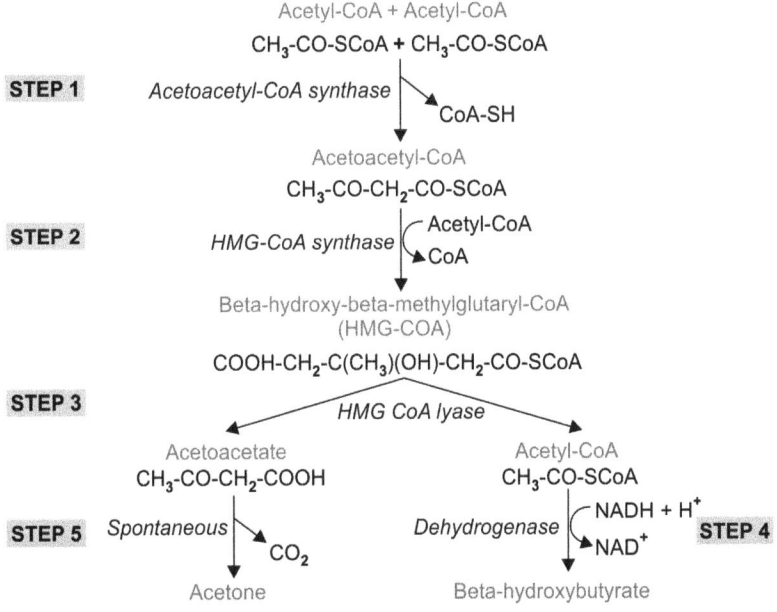

Fig. 1: Ketogenesis.

dehydrogenase to beta-hydroxybutyrate in the presence of NADH **or** it undergoes spontaneous decarboxylation to form acetone.

Utilization of ketone bodies: Ketone body utilization takes place in extrahepatic tissues for energy production. Tissues like heart, renal cortex, prefer ketone bodies than glucose for energy production.

Regulation

- The formation and excess production of ketone bodies depend upon the non-availability of carbohydrates to the body which may be due to excess utilization of fatty acids to meet the energy requirement of the cells
- Glucagon stimulates ketogenesis; insulin inhibits it
- Increased ratio of glucagon/insulin in diabetes mellitus promotes ketogenesis.

Ketolysis Reactions

Acetoacetate is activated to acetoacetyl-CoA by thiophorase enzyme.

1. Acetoacetate + Succinyl-CoA → Acetoacetyl-CoA + Succinate
2. Then acetoacetyl-CoA enters into beta oxidation pathway to produce energy.

Conditions which Lead to Elevated Ketone Bodies (Ketosis)

1. Diabetic ketoacidosis
2. Prolonged fasting
3. Muscle wasting disease.

When the blood level of ketone bodies is more than 1 mg/dL that will lead to ketonemia, ketonuria-excretion of KB in urine and smell of acetone in breath.

Diabetic ketoacidosis: It is one of the metabolic changes in diabetes along with hyperglycemia and hypertriglyceridemia.

Features of Ketosis

1. Metabolic acidosis
2. Kussmaul's respiration—acidotic breathing due to compensatory hyperventilation
3. Breath—smells of acetone
4. Osmotic diuresis
5. Dehydration
6. Sodium loss
7. Coma.

Laboratory Evaluation of Ketoacidosis

Ketone bodies appear in urine under pathological conditions such as uncontrolled diabetes mellitus, persistent vomiting, von-Gierke's disease. The major ketone bodies are three—acetoacetic acid, beta-hydroxybutyric acid and acetone.

Ketone bodies in urine are analyzed by Rothera's test, rapid tests such as ketostix strips and acetest tablets.

Rothera's Test

Principle: Freshly prepared sodium nitroprusside reacts with ketone bodies and form a purple colored ferropentacyanide complex. This test is specific for acetoacetate and beta hydroxybutyrate.

Procedure: 5 mL of urine is saturated with solid ammonium sulphate. Three drops of sodium nitroprusside is added and then strong ammonia is poured along the sides of the tube to get a purple ring.

---

2. **Write in detail about the metabolism and functions of cysteine. Name the associated inborn errors.**

Refer 2008 Essay Question 7.
- Methionine and cysteine are sulphur containing amino acids
- Methionine is an essential amino acid; from methionine, the nonessential amino acid—Cysteine is produced.

Synthesis of Cysteine from Methionine (Fig. 3)

- **Activation of methionine to S-adenosyl methionine (Fig. 2):** Methionine adenosyl transferase enzyme transfers the adenosyl group to the sulphur atom of methionine to form the active methionine S-adenosyl methionine (SAM).

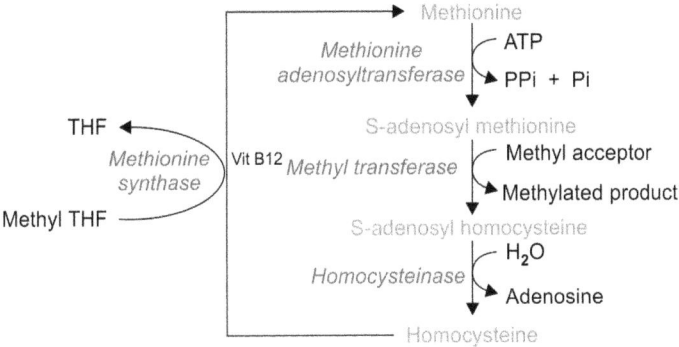

Fig. 2: S-adenosyl methionine cycle.

- **Transfer of methyl group to other acceptors (Transmethylation):** SAM donates methyl group to methyl acceptors by methyl transferases to form S-adenosyl homocysteine (SAH)
- **Formation of homocysteine:** From S-adenosyl homocysteine adenosine group is removed by homocysteinase to form homocysteine
- **Resynthesis of methionine:** Homocysteine forms methionine by homocysteine methyl transferase. This step uses methyl tetrahydrofolate which becomes THFA in the presence of B12
- **Formation of cysteine:** Homocysteine combines with serine to form cystathionine using cystathionine synthase in the presence of PLP. Cystathionine is hydrolyzed to cysteine and homoserine by cystathioninase. PLP acts as a coenzyme for this step also. This is trans-sulphuration reaction
- **Final oxidation of homoserine:** Homoserine is deaminated and decarboxylated to propionyl CoA which is converted to methyl malonyl-CoA and then to succinyl-CoA with the help of deoxyadenosyl cobalamin. Succinyl-CoA enters into

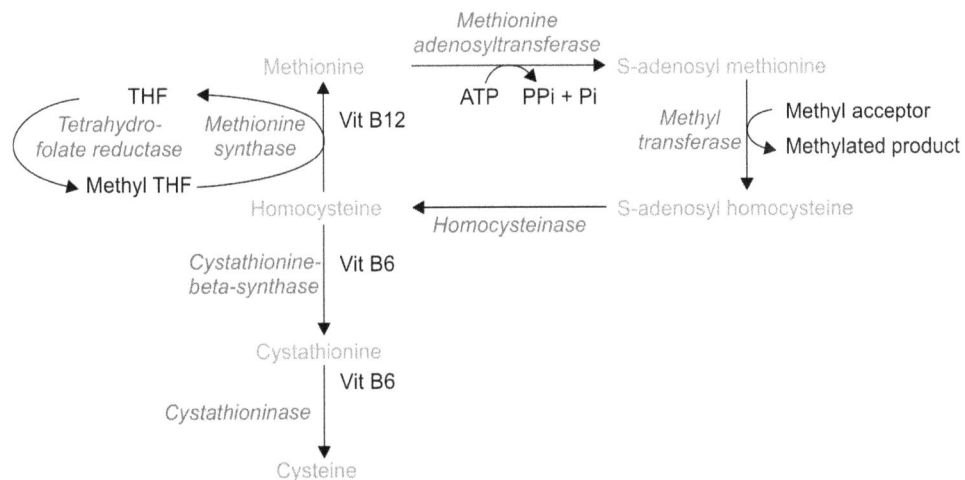

Fig. 3: Metabolism of methionine.

TCA cycle and hence methionine is a glucogenic amino acid.

Degradation of Cysteine

- Cysteine is transaminated to beta-mercaptopyruvic acid and then to pyruvate. Beta mercaptopyruvic acid transfers sulphur to cyanate to form thiocyanate
- Sulfur group is removed and excreted as H_2S or elemental S or sulfite
- Decarboxylation of cysteine gives rise to beta-mercaptoethanolamine which is used for the synthesis of coenzyme A from pantothenic acid.

Metabolic Functions of Cysteine

Formation of Glutathione

- Glutathione is involved in Meister cycle which is needed for amino acid transport.
- Glutathione is needed as a cofactor in maleylacetoacetate isomerase
- Cysteic acid → taurine, iodine to hydrogen iodide
- Glutathione is needed for glutathione peroxidase, glutathione reductase to protect RBCs from free radical induced damage
- Conversion of met Hb to normal Hb
- Glutathione is involved in conjugation reactions in detoxification reactions.

SH Group to Stabilize Protein Structure

Disulphide bridges are formed by cysteine residues in proteins and are needed to stabilize the structure of proteins.

Activation of Enzymes

Cysteine is having SH groups which are involved in the active centers of many enzymes.

Synthesis of Taurine

Cysteine is oxidized to cysteic acid which is then decarboxylated to form taurine. Taurine is a conjugating agent—used to conjugate bile acids. Taurocholic acid is the conjugated form of bile acids.

Synthesis of Cystine

Two molecules of cysteine condense together to form the diamino dicarboxylic acid—**cystine** by synthase enzyme.

Associated Disorders

Synthesis of Cysteine

- **Homocystinurias:**
  - These are autosomal recessive disorders of about 1:200,000 child births in methionine metabolism
  - Homocystinurias are due to the following conditions:
    - Cystathionine beta synthase deficiency
    - Cobalamin deficiency: N^5 methyl THFA homocysteine methyltransferase is dependent on B12
    - Deficient N^5, N^{10} methylene THFA reductase
- **Cystathioninuria (AR):** It is due to **cystathioninase deficiency.**

Disorders of Cysteine Metabolism

Cystinuria (Lysine–Cystinuria)

- Transport disorder of neutral amino acids–Cystine-Ornithine-Arginine-Lysine
- One of Garrod's tetrad
- Autosomal recessive disorder
- Abnormal excretion of cystine along with the excretion of Ornithine, Arginine and Lysine (Cystine-Lysinuria)
- In acidic pH cystine crystalluria is seen
- Stone formation leads to obstructive uropathy and renal failure
- Cyanide nitroprusside test—positive—gives magenta color
- **Treatment:** Increase the urinary volume by increasing fluid intake and alkalinization of urine by sodium bicarbonate.

Cystinosis

- It is an inherited disorder—autosomal recessive
- There is distribution of cystine crystals in lysosomes
- Accumulation of cystine in liver, spleen and bone marrow
- Blood smear shows the presence of cystine crystals in WBC
- **Treatment:** To give adequate fluids to increase the urinary output

- To alkalinize the urine by giving sodium bicarbonate
- Administration of D-pencillamine.

3. A. Write in detail the investigations required to differentiate various types of jaundice. B. Describe the metabolism of Bilirubin.

Refer 2005 Short Note 3 (2009/II/18).

Different types of Jaundice and Investigation of a Case of Jaundice

- Normal value of total bilirubin is 0.2–0.8 mg/dL; unconjugated bilirubin is 0.2–0.6 mg/dL and conjugated bilirubin is 0–0.2 mg/dL
- If the levels are increased the person becomes jaundiced
- There are 3 types **of jaundice**—hemolytic (prehepatic) jaundice, hepatocellular (hepatic) jaundice and obstructive (posthepatic).

Function tests for differential diagnosis of jaundice

No.	Tests	Hemolytic jaundice	Hepatic jaundice	Obstructive jaundice
1.	Serum total bilirubin	Increased	Increased	Increased
2.	Serum conjugated bilirubin Unconjugated bilirubin	Normal High	Increased Increased	Increased Normal
3.	Van den Bergh	Indirect +	Biphasic	Direct +
4.	Alkaline phosphatase	Normal	Increased	Highly increased
5.	Urine–bile salt (Hay's test)	Nil	Nil	Present
6.	Urine—conjugated bilirubin	Nil	Present	Present
7.	Urine–urobilinogen	Increased	Nil	Nil
8.	Fecal stercobilinogen	Increased	Decreased	Absent

- **Indirect van den Bergh test:** Unconjugated bilirubin in blood, (positive in prehepatic and hepatic jaundice)
- **Direct van den Bergh test:** Conjugated bilirubin in blood is positive—helps in detection of posthepatic jaundice
3. **ALP—normal range:** 40–125 U/L increases slightly in hepatic jaundice and more in posthepatic jaundice
4. **Hay's test:** This test is specific for identification of urine bile salts—positive for posthepatic jaundice
5. **Fouchet's test (conjugated bilirubin in urine):** This test gives positive result for both hepatic and posthepatic
6. **Ehrlich test (for urobilinogens):** Positive in prehepatic and positive in early stages of hepatic.

Catabolism of Hb (Synthesis of Bilirubin) (Fig. 4)

- Occurrence: *Endothelial cells of liver, bone marrow, spleen.*
- End product of heme metabolism is bile pigments—bilirubin and biliverdin
- From Hb, globin chains are separated and hydrolyzed and the amino acids are channeled into the amino acid pool
- The iron is re-utilized
- **About 6 g of Hb is broken down per day, from which about 250 mg of bilirubin is formed**
- Normal **plasma free bilirubin level is**—0.2–0.7 mg/dL
- Normal **plasma conjugated bilirubin level is**—0.1–0.4 mg/dL.

Steps

1. This occurs at the microsomal fraction of cells by the microsomal enzyme system—

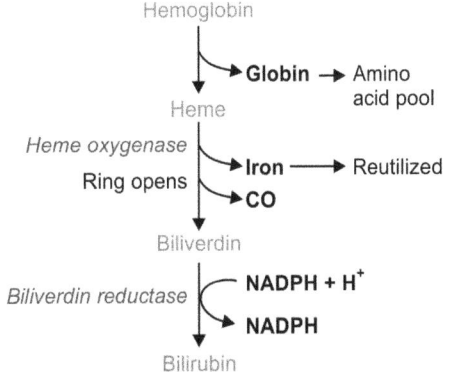

Fig. 4: Synthesis of bilirubin.

heme oxygenase in the presence of NADPH, cytochrome C and O_2
2. Ferric iron (Fe^{3+}) and CO are released with the production of linear tetrapyrrole green pigment biliverdin. Iron is taken up by the protein transferrin. Biliverdin is reduced to red yellow pigment called bilirubin by NADPH dependent reductase. Bilirubin is conjugated and water soluble
3. **Transport of bilirubin to liver**: Bilirubin thus formed is insoluble and toxic and it is in unconjugated form. It is transported in plasma bound to albumin. 1 molecule of albumin can bind with 2 molecules of bilirubin
4. **Uptake of bilirubin by liver parenchymal cells**: Done by carrier mediated active process. In liver cells bilirubin is bound to an intracellular protein called **ligandin.** This binding is inhibited by taking aspirin or penicillin and this will produce kernicterus in newborn babies
5. **Conjugation of bilirubin (Fig. 5)**: Unconjugated toxic bilirubin is conjugated with UDP glucuronic acid by UDP glucuronyl transferase enzyme. Bilirubin monoglucuronide is formed first (20%) which is then converted to diglucuronate (80%). This conjugation process is interfered by drugs like primaquine, novobiocin and pregnenolone, etc.
6. **Excretion of bilirubin to bile**: This is done by an active process against a concentration gradient. This is **the rate-limiting step** for the entire process. This excretion is mediated by multispecific organic anion transporter

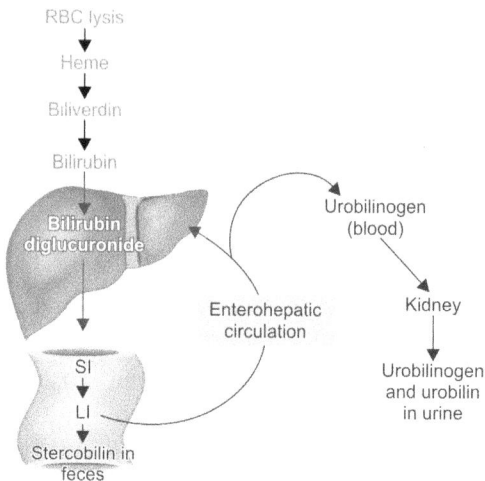

Fig. 6: Fate of bilirubin.

7. **Fate of conjugated bilirubin in intestine (Fig. 6)**:
   – After the secretion of conjugated bilirubin into bile, it passes through hepatic and common bile duct into the intestinal lumen
   – In the intestine, the conjugated bilirubin is hydrolysed by the bacterial beta glucuronidase to get converted to unconjugated bilirubin
   – Free bilirubin thus formed is reduced further into colorless tetrapyrrole urobilinogen, which is oxidized to an orange yellow pigment urobilin
   – Rest of urobilinogen is reduced to stercobilinogen which is oxidized to a brown pigment called stercobilin, which is excreted in feces (250 to 300 mg/day)
   – A part of urobilinogen (20%) enters into enterohepatic circulation to get re-excreted at the liver by portal circulation
   – A small amount of urobilinogen is excreted through the urine (less than 4 mg/day).

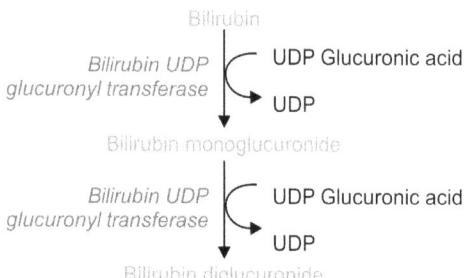

Fig. 5: Conjugation of bilirubin.

4. **Brief about the conversion of phenylalanine to tyrosine. Describe in detail about phenylketonurias.**

Refer 2015 Essay Question 6.

Conversion of Phenylalanine to Tyrosine (Fig. 7)

Synthesis of tyrosine: Tyrosine is hydroxylated phenylalanine

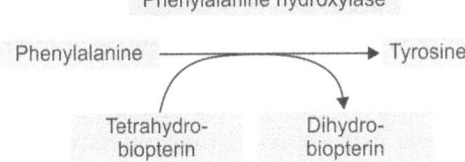

Step 1: Conversion of phenylalanine to tyrosine by hydroxylation: Phenylalanine hydroxylase enzyme hydroxylates phenylalanine to tyrosine in the presence of the cofactor tetrahydrobiopterin, and coenzymes—NADPH and NADH. It is an irreversible reaction. Further tyrosine is catabolized by various steps to form fumarate (glucogenic pathway) and acetoacetate (ketogenic pathway).

- Tyrosine is an aromatic amino acid. It is synthesized from phenylalanine. It is both glucogenic and ketogenic.

Catabolism of Tyrosine (Fig. 7)

Step 2: Transamination: Tyrosine is transaminated by tyrosine transaminase using PLP and alpha ketoglutarate to form p-hydroxy phenylpyruvate and glutamic acid. This step is induced by glucocorticoids.

Step 3: Synthesis of homogentisic acid (dihydroxyphenyl acetate): p-hydroxyphenylpyruvate is converted to homogentisate by hydroxylase enzyme. It is a copper containing enzyme. Ascorbic acid is required for this reaction.

Step 4: Formation of maleylacetoacetate: By the cleavage of aromatic ring homogentisate is converted to maleyl acetoacetate by a dioxygenase called homogentisate oxidase which contains an iron atom at its active site.

Step 5: Isomerization of maleyl to fumaryl acetoacetate: Maleyl acetoacetate is converted to its isomer fumaryl acetoacetate by isomerase using glutathione (GSH) as its cofactor.

Step 6: Hydrolysis of fumarylacetoacetate: Fumaryl acetoacetate is cleaved into fumarate (glucogenic) and acetoacetate (ketogenic) by a hydrolase enzyme.

Other Products Formed from Tyrosine

- Melanin pigments
- Catecholamines
- Thyroxine
- Tyramine.

Phenylketonuria

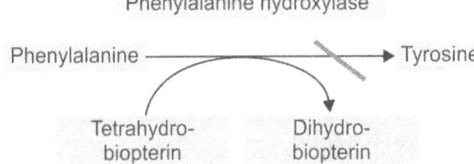

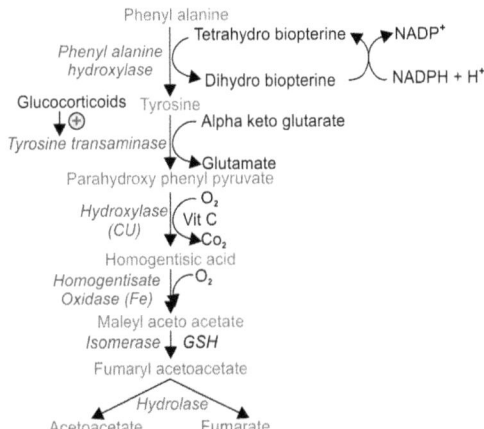

Fig. 7: Metabolism of phenylalanine and tyrosine.

- It is an autosomal recessive disease with an incidence of 1:10,000 births
- It is due to deficiency of phenylalanine hydroxylase
- So phenylalanine is not converted into tyrosine and it accumulates hyperphenylalaninemia
- The excess of phenylalanine is converted to phenyl pyruvate, phenyl lactate, and phenylacetate and phenylacetylglutamine. Phenyl pyruvate, phenyl lactate, phenyl acetate are excreted in urine.

Clinical Manifestations

- The child is mentally retarded
- Convulsions, tremors, agitation, hyperactivity may be present

- The child often has hypopigmentation due to reduced availability of tyrosine for melanin production
- Phenyl lactate in sweat causes mousy body odor
- **Laboratory diagnosis:**
  - Blood level of phenylalanine is elevated—normal level is 1 mg/dL, which is elevated to >20 mg/dL.
  - This is confirmed by Tandem mass spectroscopy
  - Guthrie's test is confirmative
  - Urine ferric chloride test is positive.
  - DNA probes—to diagnose the defects in phenylalanine hydroxylase and dihydrobiopterin reductase.

Treatment

- Early detection
- **Low phenylalanine diet:** Tapioca based diet which has low phenylalanine is the treatment of choice.

Gene therapy is under trial.

II. SHORT NOTES

1. Significance of hexose monophosphate shunt.

Refer 2005 Short Note 2.

2. Galactosemia.

Refer 2005 Short Note 7.

3. Dietary fiber.

Refer 2008 Short Note 10.

4. Reverse cholesterol transport.

High-density lipoprotein (HDL) cycle.
Refer 2010 Short Note 6.

HDL cycle is the main transport form of cholesterol from peripheral tissues to liver for excretion through the bile or for utilization.

Metabolism

- Intestinal cell synthesize HDL which is discoidal in shape
- Lecithin-cholesterol acyltransferase (LCAT) binds to the nascent HDL and converts free cholesterol to cholesterol ester. Thus HDL becomes spherical in shape (HDL 3)
- Free cholesterol derived from peripheral tissue is taken up by HDL 3. It is mediated by ABC protein (ATP binding cassette protein 1)
- The esterified cholesterol moves into the interior of HDL disc
- Mature HDL spheres are taken up by liver cells by apo A I mediated receptor mechanism
- Hepatic lipase hydrolyses HDL phospholipid
- The released cholesterol esters are taken into liver cells to be converted to bile acids and excreted through bile
- Cholesterol ester transfer protein (CETP) transfers cholesterol from HDL to VLDL and LDL in exchange for TG.

Significance

- By this cycle, cellular and lipoprotein cholesterol is delivered back to the liver where excess cholesterol is excreted into bile. **This is known as reverse cholesterol transport**
- Excretion of cholesterol needs esterification with polyunsaturated fatty acid (PUFA). Thus PUFA helps in lowering cholesterol in the body and so cholesterol is an antiatherogenic
- This prevents deposition of cholesterol in the tissues and this cycle is thought to be antiatherogenic and high level of HDL cholesterol confers a decreased risk of coronary heart disease.

Functions

- **Antiatherogenic known as good cholesterol**
- **Involved in reverse cholesterol transport.**
- HDL subfractions–HDL 1 (bad and contains only Apo E), HDL-2
- Good and antiatherogenic-HDL-3 contains Apo A-II and its role is controversial
- Act as a reservoir for apoproteins which can be donated or received from other lipoproteins

- As an antioxidant it prevents the oxidation of LDL.

5. Iron absorption.

Refer 2006 Essay Question 8 and 2011 Essay Question 4.

Iron is a trace element needed for human beings.

Absorption (Fig. 8)
- Only ferrous form is absorbed
- HCl, vitamin C reduces iron to ferrous form, so increases its absorption. Phytic acid and oxalic acid form salts with iron so inhibits iron absorption
- Calcium and copper inhibits iron absorption
- Duodenum and jejunum are the sites of absorption
- When iron stores in the body are depleted, absorption is enhanced. When iron stores are adequate, absorption is decreased. This is called mucosal block theory
- Ferrous iron in the intestinal lumen binds to mucosal cell protein called divalent metal transporter (DMT-1). This iron is transported into the mucosal cell. The unabsorbed iron is excreted
- Inside the mucosal cell, iron is incorporated into apoferritin to form ferritin. Whenever there is iron deficiency this ferritin supplies the iron. In iron deficiency erythropoietin is produced in kidney, which enhances iron absorption.

6. Gout.
Refer 2005 Short Note 17.

7. Role of lungs in maintenance of pH of blood (second line of defence).
Refer 2007 Short Note 32.

8. Tests to assess glomerular function.
Refer 2004 Short Note 18 Clearance tests.

To Assess Glomerular Function
- Glomerulus acts as a sieve in filtering blood but it retains cells and proteins thus forming a glomerular filtrate—normally 170-180 litres/day. Out of this only 1.5 liters of fluid is excreted as urine and the rest are reabsorbed through the tubules
- **Glomerular filtration rate (GFR):** Normal GFR is 120–125 mL/min. This is reduced in renal failure
- **Clearance tests:** Done to assess the glomerular filtration and renal blood flow
- **Renal clearance of a substance is the volume of plasma from which the substance is completely cleared by the kidney in 1 minute**
- **Clearance** = mg of substance excreted/min/mg of substance/mL of plasma; $C = U \times V/P$; C = Clearance of the substance; U = Concentration of the substance in urine; P = Concentration of the substance in plasma; V = Volume of urine passed/minute

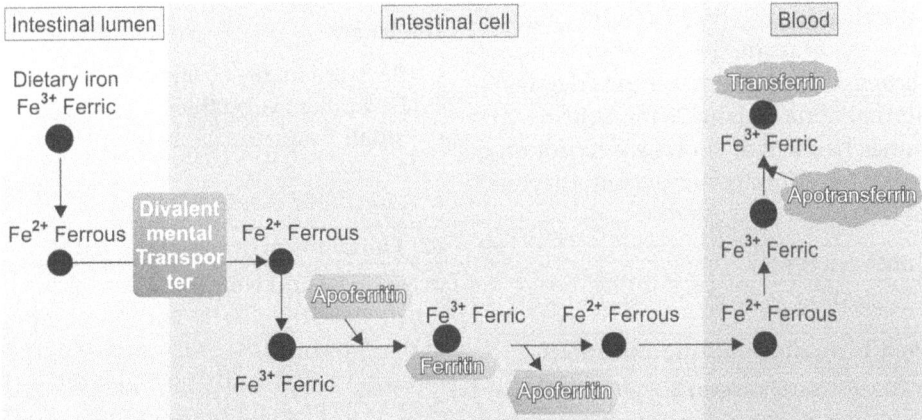

Fig. 8: Absorption and transport of iron.

- Clearance is expressed as milliliter of plasma per unit time
- **Clearance tests:** This test is done by using either endogenous markers such as-urea or creatinine or exogenous markers like inulin, ^{51}Cr-labelled EDTA, ^{99}Tec-labelled EDTA etc. Out of all Creatinine clearance test is the best
- **Creatinine clearance test:** It is based on the rate of excretion of metabolically produced creatinine which is excreted through urine. Creatinine is freely filtered by the glomeruli but not reabsorbed by the tubules. A small amount of creatinine is secreted by the tubules
- 24-hours urine is collected and blood is also collected for estimation of creatinine. Urinary volume is measured (V) and the concentration of creatinine in urine (U) and plasma (P) are estimated and by using the formula $C = U \times V/P$ the creatinine clearance is calculated
- Normal range for creatinine clearance is 90-120 mL/min
- Reduced creatinine clearance indicates chronic renal damage and reduced blood flow to glomeruli
- **Urea clearance** is the mL of blood which is cleared of urea per minute. Patient is asked to empty the bladder and 200 mL of water is given to drink. After one hour the volume of voided urine is measured, blood urea and urine urea are estimated.
- Urea clearance = UV/P (where U = mg of urea/mL of urine, P= mg of urea/mL of plasma, V = volume of urine excreted)
- Normal value is about 75 mL/min
- Values below that shows a deteriorating renal function (progression to renal failure).

9. Southern blot.
Refer 2008 Short Note 40.

10. Post-transcriptional modifications.
Refer 2011 Essay Question 3.

11. Obesity.
Refer 2012 Short Note 4.

- It is the most prevalent nutritional disorder. It is otherwise known as **overnutrition**
- It is a state in which excess fat has accumulated. There is an increase in number and size of adipocytes
- This is due to increased energy intake and decreased energy expenditure.

Obesity Index or BMI Calculation
- $BMI = W/H^2$. (W = weight in kg; H = height in meters)
- It is used to assess obesity.

Major Causes
- Food habits—intake of calorie rich food in excess amounts
- Lack of exercise
- Genetic causes—due to mutation of leptin–hormone secreted by adipocytes
- Effects of neuropeptide-Y, ghrelin and non esterified fatty acids can cause obesity.

Diseases Related to Obesity
- Effects on insulin
  - Sensitivity of peripheral tissues to insulin is decreased
  - No. of insulin receptors are decreased in adipocytes
  - Plasma insulin level is elevated.
- Cardiovascular risk
- Diabetes mellitus
- Hypertension
- Metabolic syndrome
- Reduced life span.

Treatment
- Reduced intake of calories and fat
- Diet rich in vegetables
- Small frequent meals with lots of vegetables
- Controlled exercise.

12. Functions of prostaglandins.
Refer 2013 Short Note 9.
Prostaglandins are 20 carbon compounds derived from prostanoic acid. There are 5 important types of prostaglandins—PGD, PGE, PGF, PGI and thromboxanes which are widely distributed in the body having variable functions.

On CVS

- **PGI2:** It is a powerful vasodilator, hence used in treatment of hypertension. PGI2 inhibits vasodilatation and inhibits platelet aggregation to promote thrombus formation
- **TXA2** produced by platelets are vasoconstrictors and cause platelet aggregation. PGI and TX are having opposite actions.

On Ovary and Uterus

PGF2: It induces termination of pregnancy and induction of labor by stimulating uterine muscles. So it is used in medical termination of pregnancy and to arrest postpartum bleeding.

On Respiratory Tract

- PGE is a potent bronchodilator whereas PGF is bronchoconstrictor
- PGE 1 and 2 are used in treatment of asthma.

On Immunity and Inflammation

PGE2 and D$_2$: These induce inflammation by increasing the permeability of capillaries.

On GIT

PGE: It inhibits gastric secretion so it is used for treating gastric ulcers.

Metabolic Effects

PGE$_2$ stimulates glycogenesis, induces calcium mobilization form bones and inhibits lipolysis.

13. HDL metabolism.

Refer 2010 Short Note 6.

14. Significance of Citric acid cycle.

Refer 2004 Essay Question 1.

The TCA cycle is a series of reactions in mitochondria that oxidize acetyl residues and reduce coenzymes which on re-oxidation are linked to the formation of ATP.

Significance

- Final common oxidative pathway: Carbohydrates, fatty acids, glucogenic amino acids are metabolized to acetyl-CoA and enter into TCA cycle. It is an integration of major metabolic pathways
- There will be complete oxidation of acetyl-CoA
- Fat is burnt on the wicks of carbohydrates and excess carbohydrates are converted to fats but fats will not be produced from carbohydrates
- Carbon atoms of amino acids enter into this cycle through the intermediates
- ATP generation (energetics).

Reactions	Co-enzyme	ATP (old calculation)	ATP (new calculation)
Isocitrate to α-KG	NADH	3	2.5
α-KG to succinyl-CoA	NADH	3	2.5
Succinyl-CoA to succinate	GTP	1	1
Succinate to fumarate	FADH$_2$	2	1.5
Malate to oxaloacetate	NADH	3	2.5
Total ATP		12	10

- Amphibolic pathway (amphi = both)
  - The citric acid cycle is both anabolic and catabolic and so called as amphibolic
  - It is not only a pathway for oxidation of two-carbon units—it is also a major pathway for interconversion of metabolites arising from **transamination** and **deamination** of amino acids
  - It also provides the substrates for **amino acid synthesis** by transamination, as well as for **gluconeogenesis** and **fatty acid synthesis**
  - Anabolic or synthetic reactions of TCA cycle:
    - Oxaloacetate and α-ketoglutarate serve as precursor for aspartate and glutamate respectively. These 2 amino acids are utilized for the synthesis of other amino acids by transamination and also for the synthesis of purines and pyramidines
    - Succinyl-CoA is utilized for the synthesis of heme and porphyria.

- Citrate from mitochondria is transported to cytosol by tricarboxylic acid transporter where it is cleaved to form oxaloacetate and acetyl-CoA by ATP citrate lyase. Acetyl-CoA is utilized for fatty acid synthesis
- **Anaplerosis of TCA cycle (Fig. 9):** Anaplerotic reactions are filling up reactions or influx reactions or replenishing reactions which supply 4 C units to the TCA cycle. By this, the intermediates of TCA cycle can serve as a source of precursors of biosynthetic pathways such as:
  - Succinyl-CoA for heme synthesis
  - Amino acids can be derived from the intermediates, e.g. glutamic acid from alpha ketoglutarate, aspartate from oxaloacetate
  - The anaplerotic reactions are:
    - Conversion of pyruvate and CO_2 to oxaloacetate by pyruvate carboxylase which require biotin, ATP and Mg^{++}
    - Transamination of aspartate to form oxaloacetate and transamination of glutamate to form a ketoglutarate by transaminase enzymes with PLP as the coenzyme
    - A cytoplasmic enzyme: NADP dependent malic enzyme converts pyruvate to malate which can enter into mitochondria as an intermediate of TCA cycle
    - Aromatic amino acids such as phenyl alanine and tyrosine are degraded to form fumarate
    - Deamination of glutamate by glutamate dehydrogenase irreversibly to produce a ketoglutarate
    - Succinyl-CoA can be synthesized from carbon skeletons of amino acids—valine, isoleucine and methionine and also from odd chain fatty acid propionyl-CoA.

15. DNA repair mechanism.

Refer 2003 Short Note 11.

- Synthesis of DNA is known as replication
- The process of replication occurs with high fidelity. Proofreading is done after replication to correct mistakes in arrangement of bases and base pairs
- In spite of all these things alterations in base arrangements may occur due to various physical and chemical agents

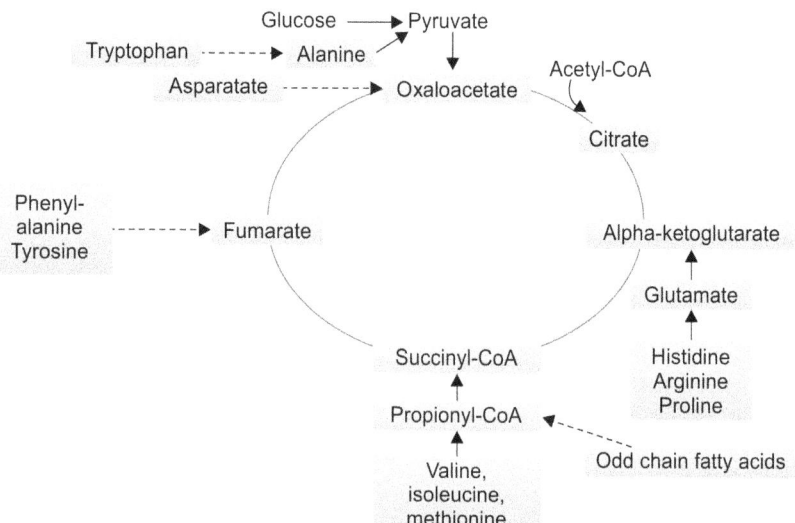

Fig. 9: Influx of intermediates (anaplerotic reactions of TCA cycle).

causing damage in DNA which can be corrected by the following mechanisms.
1. Mismatch repair
2. Base excision repair
3. Nucleotide excision repair (NER)
4. Double strand break.

Mismatch Repair (Fig. 10)

- This may occur due to copying error
- During replication one to few bases may be unpaired in a DNA strand causing mismatch
- Mut proteins identify the mismatched nucleotides based on the degree of methylation.
- GATC sequences which are present 1/1000 nucleotides approximately are methylated on the adenine residue on the parent strand (not on the newly synthesized strand)
- GATC endonuclease cuts the strand bearing the mismatch and the mismatched nucleotide(s) is/are removed by an exonuclease
- The gap left is then filled in by DNA polymerase enzyme and the ends are joined to the 5'phosphate of the remaining original strand by DNA ligase enzyme.

Base Excision Repair (Fig. 11)

- **Depurination of DNA,** which happens spontaneously owing to the thermal lability

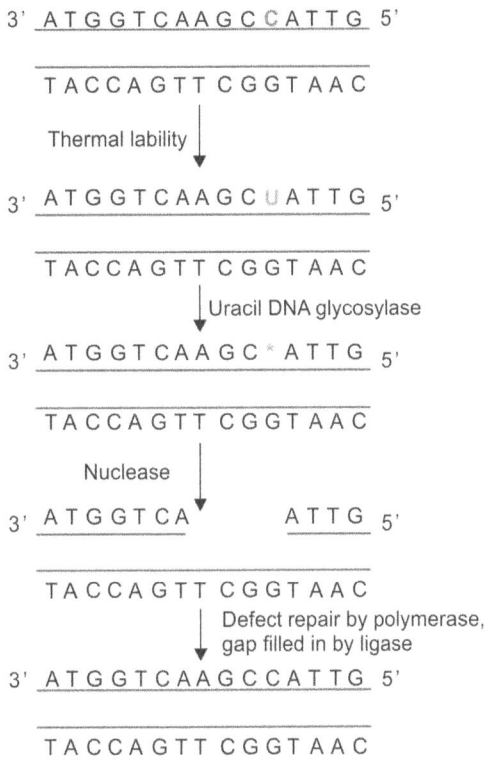

Fig. 11: Base excision repair.

of the purine N glycosidic bond, occurs at a rate of 5000–10,000/cell/d at 37 °C causing base alterations. Spontaneous deamination of cytosine to uracil may occur or by Alkylating or deaminating compounds which will be repaired by this process
- **Specific glycosylases** can recognize these abnormal bases and remove the base from the deoxyribose phosphate backbone of DNA. This will produce an apyrimidinic or apurinic site as per the base removed
- **Specific endonucleases** do the excision and a lyase enzyme removes it. The gap is then filled in by DNA polymerase and ligase enzymes.

Nucleotide Excision Repair (For Thymine-Thymine Dimer) (Fig. 12)

- This mechanism is used to repair and replace regions of damaged DNA up to 30 bases in length due to damage by ultraviolet (UV) light causing joining of adjacent pyrimidines usually thymines producing dimers

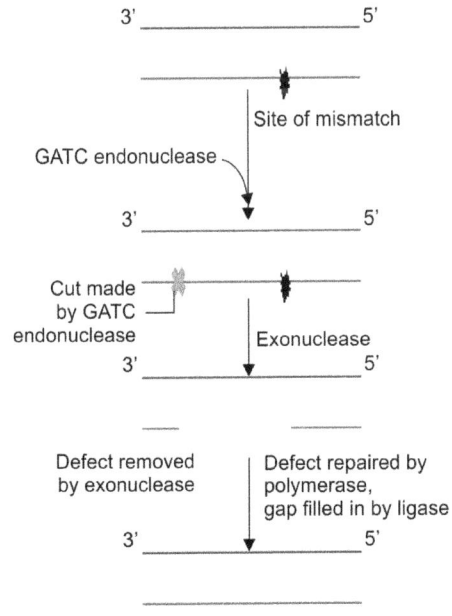

Fig. 10: Mismatch repair.

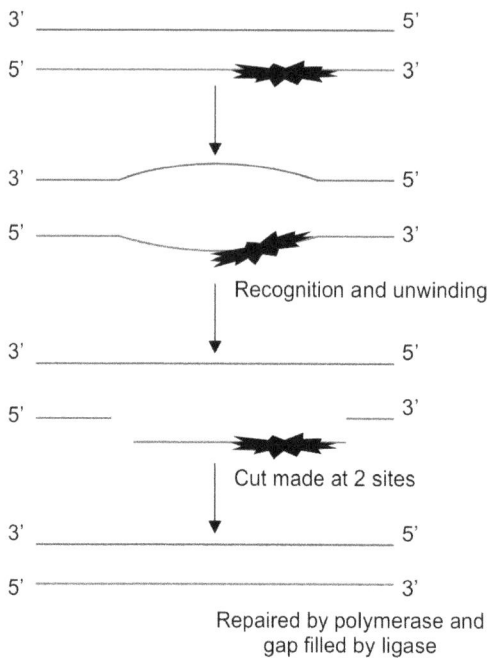

Fig. 12: Nucleotide excision repair.

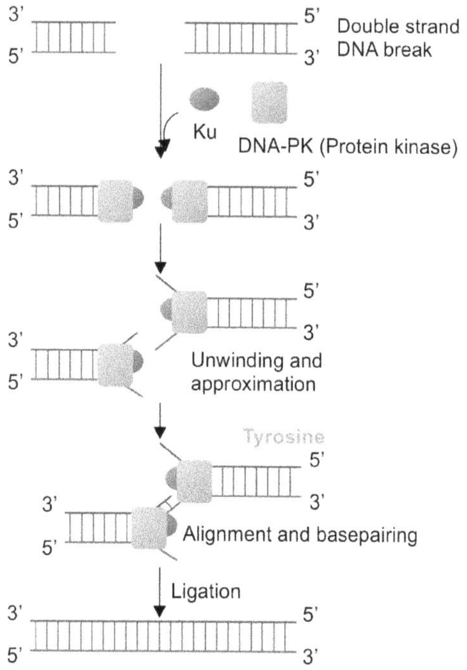

Fig. 13: ds DNA break repair.

- A special UV specific endonuclease (uvr-ABC excinuclease), recognizes the dimer and cleaves the damaged strand on either side of the dimer releasing a short oligonucleotide leaving a gap
- This gap is then filled in by normal cellular enzymes like DNA polymerase and ligase.

dsDNA Repair (Fig. 13)

- Double-strand breaks can occur in DNA as a result of ionizing radiation or oxidative free radical generation. Some chemotherapeutic agents can destroy cells by causing ds breaks or preventing their repair
- DNA PK (protein kinase) has one binding site for the free ends of the DNA and another for dsDNA just inside these ends. It therefore allows for the approximation of these two separated ends
- The unwound, approximated DNA forms base pairs
- The extra nucleotide tails are removed by an exonuclease; and the gaps are filled and closed by DNA ligase.

Biomedical Importance

Xeroderma Pigmentosum

- It is an autosomal recessive condition in which there is defect in nucleotide excision repair mechanism
- Pyrimidine dimers are formed in the skin cells which are exposed to UV light. The patient becomes highly sensitive to UV rays. Sunlight causes blisters in the skin
- Because of the defective repair system, the cells cannot repair the damaged DNA resulting in skin cancer. Death occurs in second decade due to skin cancer
- This is also caused by defects in the genes coding for any of the xeroderma pigmentosum (XP) proteins required for the repair.

Ataxia Telengiectasia

- Autosomal recessive disease due to mutated ATM gene
- It is associated with DNA repair mechanisms
- Caused due to UV sensitivity

- Associated with cerebellar ataxia, telengiectasia in eyes, lymphoreticular neoplasms. It is present in 1:40000 persons.

Other Diseases of Defective DNA Repair

Other diseases of defective DNA repair are Fanconi's anemia, Bloom's syndrome, Lynch syndrome, Cockayne syndrome and hereditary polyposis, colon cancer.

16. Glutathione.

Refer 2012 Short Answer Question 50.
Glutathione is gamma-glutamyl-cysteinyl glycine. It is a tripeptide of biochemical importance. Glutamate combines with cysteine to form gamma-glutamyl-cysteine, which combines with glycine to form glutathione. Each step needs one ATP.

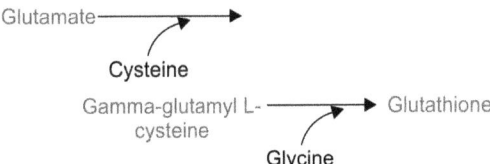

Functions of Glutathione

- **Role in absorption of amino acids in intestines, kidney tubules and in brain:** Glutathione is involved in Meister cycle which is needed for absorption and transport of neutral amino acids in intestines, kidney tubules and brain.
  Meister cycle (role of glutathione in amino acid transport) (Fig. 14)
  - Glutathione is involved in Meister cycle which is needed for absorption and transport of neutral amino acids in intestines, kidney tubules and brain.
  - Glutathione reacts with the amino acid to be transported to form gamma glutamyl amino acid by the enzyme GGT (gamma-glutamyl transferase).
  - Gamma-glutamyl amino acid is then acted by gamma-glutamyl cycle transferase to release the free amino acid and oxoproline. 5-oxoprolinase enzyme converts oxoproline to glutamate. 5-oxoprolinase enzyme deficiency will cause oxoprolinuria.
  - Free amino acid is thus transported across the membrane and glutathione is reformed by combining with cysteine and glycine
- **Coenzyme role:** Glutathione is needed as a cofactor for
  - Maleyl acetoacetate isomerase, converting maleyl acetoacetate to fumaryl acetoacetate
  - Cysteic acid → Taurine.

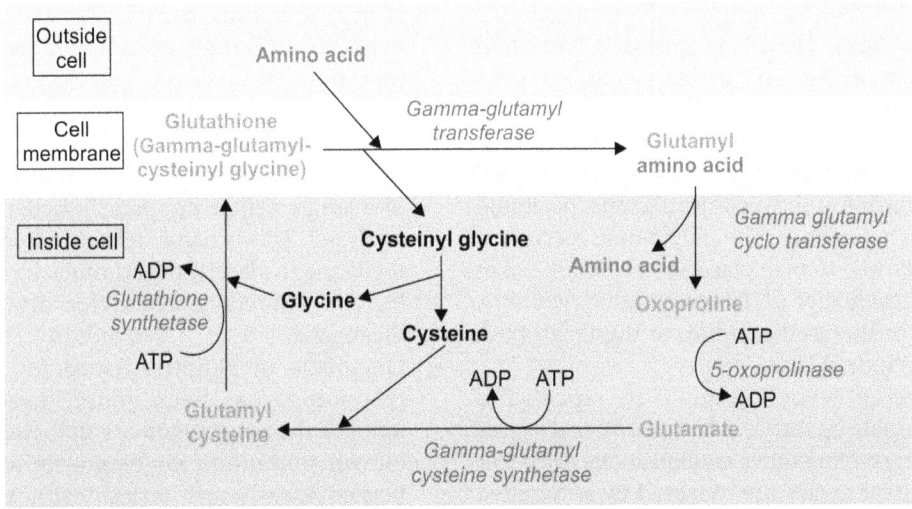

Fig. 14: Meister cycle.

- **To maintain the integrity of RBC membrane:** Glutathione present in the RBC is needed for inactivation of free radicals formed inside. Glutathione peroxidase and glutathione reductase enzymes play important role in keeping glutathione in reduced state
- **Conversion of met-Hb:** Met Hb cannot transfer oxygen. Glutathione helps in the reduction of met-Hb to normal Hb
- **Conjugation reactions:** Glutathione (GSH) acts as a conjugation agent in detoxification reactions
- **Activation of enzymes:** Glutathione keeps certain enzymes with SH groups in their active site in reduced form.

17. Tests to assess renal tubular functions.
Refer 2014 Short Answer Question 34.

18. Polymerase chain reaction (Fig. 15).
Refer 2014 Short Answer Question 40.
It is an in vitro DNA amplification procedure in which millions of a particular sequence of DNA can be produced within few hours.
- Two primers of about 20-30 nucleotides with complementary sequence of the flanking region are needed
- Step 1—Separation: DNA strands are separated by heating at 95°C for 15 sec to 2 min
- Step 2—Annealing: The primers are annealed by cooling to 50°C for 0.5 to 2 minutes. Then they hybridize with their complementary single stranded DNA separated already
- Step 3—Polymerization: New DNA strands are synthesized by Taq polymerase. This enzyme is derived from bacteria that found in hot springs. The polymerase reaction is allowed to take place at 72°C for 30 sec in presence of dNTPs of adenine, guanine, cytosine and thymine to duplicate both strands of DNA
- Step 4: Steps 1, 2 and 3 are repeated to double up the DNA strands. After 20 cycles one million times amplifications will occur
- These cycles are repeated by automated instrument tempcycler.

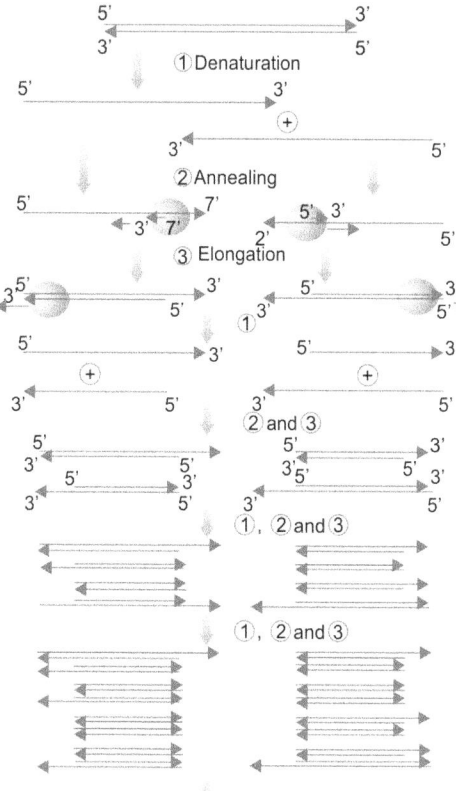

Fig. 15: Polymerase chain reaction.

Clinical Applications
- Detection of infectious diseases: Tuberculosis and viral diseases like HIV and hepatitis. PCR detects even one bacillus present in the specimen and PCR is used in the diagnosis of viral infections like hepatitis C and HIV
- Medicolegal cases: PCR allows the DNA in a single cell or in a hair follicle to be analyzed. This is highly useful in forensic medicine to identify the criminal
- PCR is especially useful for prenatal diagnosis
- Diagnosis of genetic disorders: PCR technology has been widely used to amplify the gene segments that contain known mutations for diagnosis of inherited diseases such as sickle cell anemia, thalassemia, etc.

19. Metabolic acidosis.
Refer 2004 Short Note 16.
- Acidosis is reduction of pH less than 7.38. it is classified into metabolic and respiratory acidosis
- Metabolic acidosis is primarily due to base deficit. The bicarbonate deficit may occur due to excess acid production or depletion of bicarbonate
- **Anion gap:** It is difference between measured cations and measured anions. Usually it shows the unmeasured anions. **The normal value is 12 mmol/L**
- Anion gap is calculated as the difference between $(Na^+ + K^+)$ and $(HCO_3^- + Cl^-)$
- Decreased anion gap is seen in—hypoalbuminemia, multiple myeloma.

Metabolic Acidosis is Classified into

1. **High anion gap metabolic acidosis- (HAGMA)** accumulation of acid anions
   - Due to accumulation of acid anions- Value between 15 and 20
   - **Causes:**
     - Renal failure: H^+ excretion is less
     - Diabetic ketoacidosis
     - Lactic acidosis: Hypoxia, circulatory failure, many drugs, and bacterial metabolism increase lactic acid. Methanol, ethanol also cause lactic acidosis.
2. **Normal anion gap metabolic acidosis- (NAGMA)**
   - Loss of both anions and cations, the anion gap is normal, but acidosis may prevail
   - **Causes**
     - Diarrhea—loss of bicarbonate and cations—Na or K or both from intestinal secretions
     - Hyperchloremic metabolic acidosis—in renal tubular acidosis, acetazolamide therapy and ureteric transplantation into large gut.
   - **Metabolic acidosis is compensated by**
     a. Respiratory compensation: Hyperventilation so that pCO_2 comes down. There will be Kussmaul respiration, low pH, bicarbonate will be low. pCO_2 starts decreasing due to respiratory compensation
     b. Renal compensation: Increased excretion of acid and conservation of base occurs. This sets within 2 to 4 days
     c. Associated hyperkalemia is seen commonly due to distribution of K^+ and H^+.
- **Clinical features**
  - Hyperventilation
  - Kussmaul respiration
  - Depressed myocardial contractility.
- **Treatment**
  - To stop production of acid by giving IV fluids and insulin
  - Oxygen to be given to patients with lactic acidosis
  - Potassium level to be monitored
  - Required bicarbonate amount to be calculated from the base deficit
  - mEq of base needed = Body weight in kg × 0.2–base excess in mEq/L.
- Acidosis is reduction of pH less than 7.38. It is classified into metabolic and respiratory acidosis
- Metabolic acidosis is primarily due to base deficit. The bicarbonate deficit may occur due to excess acid production or depletion of bicarbonate
- **Anion gap:** It is difference between measured cations and measured anions. Usually it shows the unmeasured anions. **The normal value is 12 mmol/L**
- Anion gap is calculated as the difference between $(Na^+ + K^+)$ and $(HCO_3^- + Cl^-)$.
  Decreased anion gap is seen in–hypoalbuminemia, multiple myeloma.

III. SHORT ANSWER QUESTIONS

1. Uncouplers of electron transport chain.
- **Uncouplers of oxidative phosphorylation:**
  - 2,4-dinitrophenol (2,4 DNP)
  - 2,4-dinitrocresol (2,4 DNC)

- 3. Chlorocarbonylcyanidephenyl hydrazone (CCCP).
- **Physiological uncouplers:**
  1. Thyroxine
  2. Thermogenin in brown adipose tissue.

2. Beriberi.

Refer 2009 Short Note 26.

3. Niemann-Pick disease.

Refer 2011 Short Note 23 Sphingolipidoses.
- It is one of the inherited lipid storage diseases—lysosomal storage diseases or sphingolipidoses
- Niemann-Pick disease is due to sphingomyelinase enzyme deficiency and so degradation of sphingomyelin will not occur
- There will be accumulation of sphingomyelin
- This condition is characterized by enlarged liver and spleen, mental retardation, damage to central nerve system, cherry red spot in macula of eye
- Child will die within 2 years of birth.

4. Any two mucopolysaccharides—locations and its functions.

Refer 2012 Short Note 25.
- Glycosaminoglycans or mucopolysaccharides are heteropolysaccharides containing the repeating units of disaccharides made up of uronic acid and amino sugars
- They are the essential components of connective tissue structure.

Common GAG

- Hyaluronic acid
- Chondroitin sulfate
- Dermatan sulfate
- Heparin
- Heparin sulfate
- Keratan sulfate.
- **Hyaluronic acid:** Anionic, non-sulfated glycosaminoglycan
  - **Site of occurrence:** Present in loose connective tissues, tendons, synovial fluid of joints, vitreous humor of eye
  - **Repeating units:** Composed of D-glucuronic acid and N-acetylglucosamine, linked by β-1,4 and β-1,3 glycosidic bonds
  - **Functions:** Acts as lubricant and shock absorber. It helps in migration of cells in reproduction in embryogenesis and in wound healing.
- **Chondroitin sulfate**
  - **Site of occurrence:** It is present in ground substance of connective tissues present in cartilage, bone, tendons, cornea and skin
  - **Repeating units:** It is made up of repeating units of glucuronic acid and N-acetyl galactosamine to which sulfate group is attached.
- **Functions:** It provides an endoskeletal structure to maintain the structure and shape of the tissues like cartilage.
- **Therapeutic uses:** It is used to treat osteoarthritis as anti-inflammatory agent, stimulating the synthesis of proteoglycans.

5. Rapoport-Luebering shunt.

Refer 2007 Short Note 18.

6. Glycated hemoglobin.

Refer 2013 Short Note 49.

7. Essential fatty acids.

Refer 2012 Short Answer Question 4.
Essential fatty acids are those which cannot be synthesized by the body but have to be supplemented in diet. They are polyunsaturated fatty acids. They are
- Linoleic acid (18 C)- ω6
- Linolenic acid (18 C)- ω3
- Arachidonic acid (20 C)-ω6—can be formed, if the dietary supply of linolenic acid is sufficient. So it cannot be strictly categorized under essential fatty acid.

Significance of EFA

- Used for esterification and excretion of cholesterol
- They form the components of biological membranes and increase the fluidity of membranes of cells

- Eicosanoids (prostaglandin, prostacycline and thromboxanes) are derived from arachidonic acid
- They are anti-atherogenic.

Deficiency of essential fatty acid (EFA) causes acanthocytosis, acrodermatitis, hyperkeratosis and hypercholesterolemia. Deficiency of unsaturated fatty acid leads improper synthesis of skin, this is called as phrynoderma or toad skin, it is characterized by horny eruptions on the posterior and lateral parts of limbs, back and on the buttocks, hair loss, poor wound healing.

8. Reactions catalyzed by biotin.

Refer 2004 Short Note 2.
- Biotin is a water soluble vitamin
- Other name: Egg white injury factor.

Biochemical Functions
- Biotin acts as coenzymes for carboxylation reactions. So known as cocarboxylase
  - CO_2 is attached to the nitrogen of biotin molecule
  - This reaction requires ATP and it occurs in 3 steps
  - **Coenzyme:** Biotin gets attached to enzyme carboxylase by amide linkage to ε amino group of lysine
    I. **Biotin (non-protein) + Carboxylase (apo enzyme) holocarboxylase**
       $ATP + HCO_3 (CO_2) \rightarrow$ **Carbonic phosphoric anhydride (CO_2 + P)**
    II. **Holocarboxylase + Carbonic phosphoric anhydride $\rightarrow P_1 + CO_2$ (Biotin enzyme)**
    III. **CO_2 Biotin enzyme + X (any receptor) $\rightarrow XCO_2$ + Biotin + Enzyme**
  - Examples of CO_2 fixation reaction:
    I. Acetyl-CoA carboxylase: Rate limiting enzyme of de novo synthesis of fatty acid
       Acetyl-CoA + CO_2 + ATP $\longrightarrow$ Malonyl-CoA + ADP + Pi
    II. Propionyl-CoA carboxylase in gluconeogenesis
        Propionyl CoA + CO_2 + ATP $\longrightarrow$ Methylmalonyl-CoA + ADP + Pi
    III. Pyruvate carboxylase in gluconeogenesis
         Pyruvate + CO_2 + ATP $\longrightarrow$ Oxaloacetate + ADP + Pi
    IV. Leucine metabolism–β–methylcrotonyl-CoA carboxylase
        β-methylcrotonyl-CoA $\rightarrow$ β methyl-glutaconyl-CoA.

9. Antioxidant vitamins and minerals.

Refer 2011 Short Note 20.
- **Antioxidants** are compounds which prevent lipid peroxidation or rancidity by free radicals or control the oxidation process
- **Naturally occurring antioxidants**
  - **Vitamins** E and C, **Provitamin** β-carotene
  - **Mineral**: Selenium.

Vitamins
- **Vitamin E** is the most effective chain breaking antioxidants. It is the lipid phase antioxidant
- It inhibits the propagative phase
- Vitamin E would intercept the peroxyl free radical and inactivate it
- This oxidative form of vitamin E is converted to vitamin E by ascorbic acid
- **Ascorbic acid** becomes dehydroascorbate by reacting with vitamin E radical. Two molecules of dehydroascorbate combine together to form ascorbate.
- **Vitamin C** is the aqueous phase antioxidant
- **Carotenoids:** Beta-carotenes are natural antioxidant and it reduces the incidence of cancer.

Mineral
- **Selenium:** It acts as non-specific intracellular antioxidant. Its action is complementary to vitamin E. Vitamin E reduces the requirement of selenium
- **Zinc:** Extracellular superoxide dismutase is dependent on zinc for antioxidant action.

10. Wilson's disease.

Refer 2007 Short Note 24.

11. Name of any four neurotransmitters.

- They are chemical substances secreted by the nerve cells to help in communications between neurons
- They are present in the synapses between nerve cells
- As per their actions they are either
  1. Excitatory neurotransmitters like acetylcholine, glutamine, serotonin– which open cation channels
  2. Inhibitory neurotransmitters like GABA or glycine—they open anion channels
- Most of the neurotransmitters are amino acids and their derivatives are amines.

Amino Acids and Their Derivatives

1. Gamma-aminobutyric acid (GABA)
- It is an inhibitory neurotransmitter
- Synthesized from the amino acid glutamate by decarboxylation
- It controls cortical functions, motor control and vision and anxiety
- It is used to treat convulsions in epilepsy and also to induce sleep.

2. Histamine
- Found mainly in hypothalamus
- Synthesized by decarboxylation of histidine by histidine decarboxylase which needs PLP
- There are 3 classes of histamine receptors—H1, H2 and H3
- H1 receptor antagonists like diphenhydramine are used to treat allergic conditions and upper respiratory disorders
- H2 receptor antagonists like Ranitidine or cimetidine are used to treat peptic ulcers.

3. Serotonin—5 hydroxytryptamine
- It is a derivative of tryptophan by hydroxylation and PLP dependent decarboxylation
- It is synthesized in neural tissues and enterochromaffin cells or argenta of gastrointestinal tract
- Serotonin is involved in sleep, appetite, mood elevation and temperature regulation
- The degradation of serotonin gives rise to 5-hydroxyindoleacetic acid (5-HIAA) which is a marker to diagnose malignant carcinoid tumors.

4. Catecholamines: Epinephrine, norepinephrine, dopamine
- They are synthesized from phenylalanine and tyrosine
- Dopamine is a major neurotransmitter in the basal ganglion and it controls voluntary movement. Dopamine content is reduced in cases of Parkinson's disease.

12. Four functions of albumin.

Refer 2015 Short Answer Question 59.
- The total protein content of plasma is 6-8 g/dL
- Plasma proteins consist of albumin, globulins-($\alpha 1$, $\alpha 2$, β and γ) and fibrinogen
- Albumin—3.5 to 5 g/dL; globulins—2.5-3.5 g/dL and fibrinogen—200-400 mg/dL
- Normal albumin: Globulin ratio is 1.2:1-1.5:1
- **Albumin:** It is produced by the liver and of 69,000 D molecular wt. It is a globular protein elliptical in shape and it has 585 amino acids arranged in one polypeptide chain.

Functions of Albumin

- **Transport protein:** It transports various substances like bilirubin, free fatty acid, drugs like aspirin, hormones like thyroxine, steroid hormones, minerals like calcium, copper, etc.
- **Colloid osmotic pressure:** It maintains colloid osmotic pressure in vascular and extravascular compartments. It contributes to plasma oncotic pressure. It cannot pass between intracellular and extracellular compartment. So exerts a net osmotic pressure. The osmotic pressure of plasma is about 278-305 mOsm/kg, which is necessary for movement of water from ECF to ICF in arteriolar end and reverse in venular end of capillaries
- **Buffer:** Albumin has the maximum buffering capacity. Histidine residues are present in albumin which can bind to H^+ and can function as a buffer

- **Nutrition:** Liver takes up amino acids from diet and converts it into albumin. It is then released in blood and taken up by other tissues by pinocytosis. So albumin is a source of amino acids for the cells. PEM is characterized by hypoalbuminemia which results in growth retardation and edema. Human albumin is used in the treatment of liver diseases, hemorrhage, shock and burns.

13. Factors affecting electrophoresis.

Refer 2006 Short Note 30.

Electrophoresis is the process of separation of charged particles in an electrical field. As per the mode of separation it is classified into—a) moving boundary and b) zone electrophoresis

Factors Affecting Electrophoresis

- **Supporting media:** It may be paper, cellulose acetate, agar gel, starch, polyacrylamide gel, etc. The composition of the supporting medium can influence the rate of migration of compounds. Fine resolution is possible with polyacrylamide gel
- **Electrical field:** Rate migration is directly proportional to the voltage, the current and indirectly proportionate to the resistance
- **Buffer:** Composition, concentration and pH of the buffer affect the rate of migration of compounds
  - Buffer should not bind with the compounds to be separated. Barbitone buffer is preferred in separation of proteins
  - Ionic strength is proportionate to the current carried by the buffer. So ionic strength of 0.05 is preferred for protein separation
  - pH determines the extent of ionization and therefore the degree and direction of migration depend on pH.
- **Sample:** The movement of the ions in an electric field depends on the charge, size and shape of the sample molecule.
  - The rate of migration increases with increase in net charge on the compound
  - As size of the molecule increases the rate of migration decreases and vice versa
  - Molecules of same size with different shapes show different migration due to different frictional and electrophoretic forces.

14. Hyperkalemia.

Refer 2013 Short Answer Question 32.

15. Functions of phosphate ions.

Refer 2014 Short Answer Question 49.

16. Any two antimetabolites and its uses.

- Antimetabolites are involved in cancer chemotherapy acting as anticancer drugs
- They are synthetic analogs of cell cyclic specific drugs which act on the synthetic pathways of DNA.

Synthetic Nucleotides and their Importance

- These are structurally similar nucleotides but functionally opposite—mild variation in structural configuration—either in heterocyclic ring or in sugar moiety
- They inhibit enzymes of nucleic acid synthesis
- Disruption of base pairing
- Hence they are used for the treatment for—a) cancer, b) for gout—allopurinol and c) drugs for immunosuppresants to be given in organ transplant cases, e.g. azathioprine.

Folic Acid Analog

Methotroxeate (amethopterin): It inhibits dihydrofolate reductase enzyme and blocks the regeneration of tetrahydrofolate. And so the synthesis of dTMP is inhibited and thereby DNA synthesis is inhibited.

Synthetic Analogues of Purines

- **6 mercaptopurine** (purenethol)
- It inhibits the conversion of IMP to AMP and GMP
- Used for treating acute leukemia, immunosuppresant. It acts by inhibiting protein synthesis.

Side effects—bone marrow depression, nausea, vomiting.

Synthetic Analogues of Pyrimidines

- **5' Flurouracil** (thymidine analogue)
  - ↓ DNA-thymineless death, ↓ thymidylate synthase and prevents protein synthesis
  - **Treatment:** Adenocarcinoma—breast, stomach, colon
  - **Toxicity:** Myelosuppression.
- **5'-iodo 2'-deoxyuridine (5-IUdR)**
  - Antiviral-↓ viral DNA synthesis—Inhibits DNA viral replication-chickenpox and herpes
  - **Local application:** Effective for herpes simplex keratitis.

17. Any four uses of polymerase chain reaction.

Refer 2014 Short Answer Question 40.
It is an in vitro DNA amplification procedure in which millions of a particular sequence of DNA can be produced within few hours.

Clinical Applications/Uses

- **Detection of infectious diseases:** Tuberculosis and viral diseases like HIV and hepatitis. PCR detects even one bacillus present in the specimen and PCR is used in the diagnosis of viral infections like hepatitis C and HIV
- **Medicolegal cases:** PCR allows the DNA in a single cell or in a hair follicle to be analyzed. This is highly useful in forensic medicine to identify the criminal
- **PCR** is especially useful for prenatal diagnosis
- **Diagnosis of genetic disorders:** PCR technology has been widely used to amplify the gene segments that contain known mutations for diagnosis of inherited diseases such as sickle cell anemia, thalassemia, etc.

18. Inhibitor of protein translation.

Refer 2014 Essay Question 8 last part.
Translation is the process of synthesis of proteins in prokaryotes and eukaryotes. They are inhibited by the following drugs. And the inhibition differs in prokaryotes and eukaryotes.

Prokaryotes

Reversible inhibitors in prokaryotes.

Antibiotics: Bacteriostatic

- Tetracyclins—bind to 30S-prevents attachment of aminoacyl tRNA-A site
- Chloromycetin—inhibits peptidyl transferase
- Erythromycin and clindamycin—prevents translocation.

Bactericidal Antibiotics

- Aminoglycosides
  - Streptomycin is irreversible inhibitor of 30S ribosomes
  - Low concentration-misreading mRNA
  - Pharmacological concentration-prevents initiation complex; total inhibition of translation.

Inhibitors: Eukaryotes

- **Cycloheximide:** Inhibits both human and bacterial peptidyl transferase (60S)
- **Diphtheria toxin:** *Corynebacterium diphtheriae*-Inactivates eEF 2 by attaching ADP to eEF2; prevents translocation
- Ricin-castor bean toxin-Inactivates 28 S rRNA.

Inhibitors: Prokaryotes and Eukaryotes

Puromycin: Structural analog of tyrosinyl tRNA—incorporated into the peptide chain causing inhibition of elongation in both prokaryotes and eukaryotes. It acts as a research tool.

19. Telomerase.

Refer 2016 Short Answer Question 34.
- There are 23 pairs of chromosomes in human beings
- **Chromosomes:** Supercoiled chromatin fibers are condensed to form chromosomes
- Center of the chromosomes is centromere which is rich in AT-with repeated DNA sequences of about 1 million base pairs

with specific binding proteins. This region is called kinetochore which is the anchor for mitotic division
- The 4 end pieces of chromosomes are called as **telomeres**
- Replication will not take place upto these ends-3' or 5' ends
- Telomerases or telomere terminal transferases do the job of replicating at these end pieces of chromosomes.
- Telomerase acts as a reverse transcriptase to synthesize this small DNA strand
- In old age telomerase activity is lost leading to chromosomal instability and cell death
- Drugs which prevent expression of gene for telomerase act as anticancer agents.

20. Alkaptonuria.
Refer 2008 Short Note 39.
- **It is an inborn error of metabolism** in the metabolism of tyrosine/phenylalanine
- It is an autosomal recessive condition affecting 1:250,000 births
- It is due to the defect in homogentisate oxidase enzyme

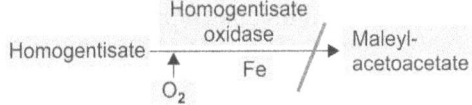

- Homogentisate gets accumulated and oxidized to benzoquinone acetate and forms alkaptone bodies
- Alkaptone bodies get deposited in intervertebral discs, cartilages of nose and pinna of ear developing ochronosis. Black pigments get deposited over joint cavities causing arthritis
- Urine turns black on standing. $FeCl_3$ test is positive. Benedict's test is strongly positive since homogentisate is a reducing agent
- Generally it is a harmless condition.

21. Substrates for gluconeogenesis.
Refer 2012 Short Note 8.

Definition: Synthesis of glucose from non-carbohydrate substrates in liver and kidney (cortex).

Substrates: Pyruvate, lactate, glucogenic amino acids, propionate, glycerol.

22. Apoproteins and its significance.
Refer 2007 Short Note 21.

23. Two isoenzymes and their clinical significance.
Refer 2003 Short Note 5.

Multiple molecular forms of an enzyme catalyzing the same reaction are isoenzymes or isozymes, e.g. lactate dehydrogenase—5 isoenzymes (LDH 1, 2, 3, 4 and 5), creatine kinase—3 isoenzymes (CK-1, 2, 3) and alkaline phosphatase.

Lactate Dehydrogenase
- LDL catalyses the conversion of pyruvate to lactate and vice versa. Normal values ranges from 100–200 U/L
- Elevation of LDH is seen in hemolytic anemia, hepatocellular damage, muscular dystrophy, cancer, etc.
- LDH is tetramer made up of two H (heart) bands and two M (muscle) bands. Both of these are same molecular weight and with minor amino acid variations
- There are 5 isoenzymes. They are LDH1, LDH2, LDH3, LDH4 and LDH5
- With two different polypeptide chains therefore 5 combinations of H and M are possible, namely—H4, H3M, H2M2, M3H, M4. The tissue specificity and diagnostic importance of these 5 isoenzymes is as follows:
  - H4 form found in heart, which is useful for diagnosing heart disease
  - M4 form found in muscle, hence it is useful in diagnosing muscle diseases
  - Isoenzymes of LDH help in the diagnosis of heart and liver diseases
  - Flipped pattern is observed in myocardial infarction (LDH-1 > LDH-2)
  - Increased activity of LDH-5 is an indicator of liver diseases.

Creatine Kinase (CK)
- It catalyzes the synthesis of creatine phosphate from creatine and ATP
- Normal blood ranges from 15-100 IU/L
- It is made up of 2 polypeptides namely M and B. Therefore 3 combinations of

isoenzymes are possible. They are MM found in skeletal muscle, MB found in heart and BB found in brain
- CK subform is highly elevated in muscular dystrophies, acute cerebrovascular injuries. It is most reliable factor in diagnosing AMI
- Three isoenzymes—CK BB(1), CK MB(2), CK MM(3)
- CK BB(1)—present in brain
- CK MB (2) is the earliest reliable marker of myocardial infarction
- CK MM (3) is elevated in muscle diseases.

24. Significance of 2,3 bisphosphoglycerate.
Refer 2007 Short Note 18.

25. Importance of HMP pathway.
Refer 2010 Short Note 30.

26. Deficiency manifestations of B12.
Refer 2011 Essay Question 1.
- **Folate trap:** This also manifests the deficiency manifestations of folic acid like inadequate DNA synthesis with macrocytic anemia
- **Megaloblastic anemia:** Due to premature large RBCs
- **Homocystinuria:** Due to the failure of conversion of homocysteine to methionine. Homocystine level gets elevated in blood leading to homocystinuria which is associated with ischemic heart diseases
- **Methyl malonic aciduria:** Due to the deficiency of B12 there will be no isomerization of L-methylmalonyl-CoA to succinyl-CoA and so there is accumulation of methylmalonic acid in blood which leads to methylmalonic aciduria
- **Demyelination of nerves:** Due to the failure of converting homocysteine to methionine, active methionine level is reduced and so methylation of phosphatidyl choline to phosphatidyl ethanolamine will be inadequate and so demyelination occurs
- **Subacute combined degeneration:** Demyelination of cerebral cortex, dorsal column and pyramidal tract of spinal cord occur causing sensory and motor tracts defective. So it is called combined degeneration. Positive Romberg's sign and Babinski signs are seen
- **Achlorhydria** is associated with B12 deficiency.

27. Competitive inhibition.
Refer 2015 Short Note 9.
Definition: Enzyme inhibitors are organic or inorganic substances which can bind reversibly or irreversibly with the enzymes and alter the catalytic activity of the enzyme, e.g. drugs, toxins, etc.
- **Reversible inhibition:** In this type, the inhibitors bind **non-covalently** with the enzymes and the inhibition will be reversed when the inhibitors are removed. This is further classified into—A. Competitive inhibitors (substrate analogue inhibitors), B. Noncompetitive reversible inhibitors and C. Uncompetitive inhibitors
- **Competitive inhibitors (Substrate analogue inhibitors)**
  - They bind and compete to the substrate binding site of the enzyme forming an enzyme inhibitory complex (EI)
  - K_m value is increased but no change in V_{max}
  - For example, competitive inhibition of succinate dehydrogenase by malonate which resembles succinate (TCA cycle)
  - Many drugs act as competitive inhibitors. For example, sulfonamide is an analogue of PABA and inhibits pteroid synthetase in the folic acid synthesis
  - Allopurinol inhibits xanthine oxidase.

28. Inhibitors of ETC.
Refer 2012 Essay Question 1.

29. Functions of mucopolysaccharides.
Refer 2012 Short Note 25.
- Glycosaminoglycans or mucopolysaccharides are heteropolysaccharides containing the repeating units of disaccharides made up of uronic acid and amino sugars
- They are the essential components of connective tissue structure.

Common GAG

- Hyaluronic acid
- Chondroitin sulfate
- Dermatan sulfate
- Heparin
- Heparan sulfate
- Keratan sulfate.

Functions of Mucopolysaccharides

Hyaluronic Acid

Acts as lubricant and shock absorber. It helps in migration of cells in reproduction in embryogenesis and in wound healing.

Chondroitin Sulfate

It provides an endoskeletal structure to maintain the structure and shape of the tissues like cartilage.

Therapeutic uses: It is used to treat osteoarthritis as anti-inflammatory agent, stimulating the synthesis of proteoglycans.

Dermatan Sulfate

It provides transparency to the cornea and maintains the shape of eye.

Heparin

Produced mainly by mast cells of live. It acts as an anticoagulant, causing release of lipoprotein lipase enzyme to act on the triglycerol.

Heparan Sulfate

It acts as receptors in plasma membrane and mediates cell communications and cell growth. Responsible for charge selectiveness in glomerular filtration.

Keratan Sulfate

It provides transparency of the cornea.

30. Liposomes.

- Liposomes are artificially prepared phospholipid vesicles by sonication of phospholipids and cholesterol
- They are microscopic spherical vesicles
- They may be unilamellar or mutilamellar
- Under specific conditions when mixed in water they arrange to form a bilayer membrane to enclose water in a phospholipid sphere
- They are used to carry certain drugs, proteins, enzymes or genes to target organs where they show superior properties
- They play important roles in cancer chemotherapy, antimicrobial therapy, gene therapy, vaccines and diagnostic imaging.

31. Applications of electrophoresis.

Refer 2006 Short Note 30.

32. Lesch-Nyhan syndrome.

Refer 2012 Short Answer Question 18.

33. Products formed from glycine (Fig. 16).

Refer 2004 Essay Question 3.

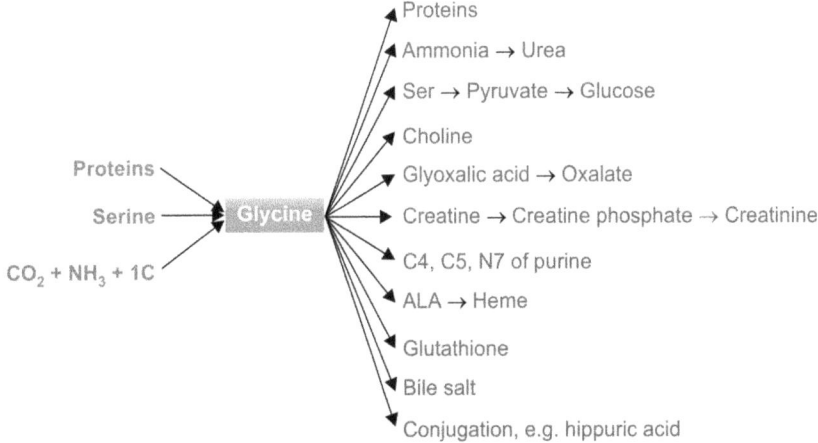

Fig. 16: Products formed from glycine.

- Creatine, creatine phosphate and creatinine (Glycine + Arginine + S-adenosyl methionine)
- Heme (Glycine + Succinyl-CoA)
- Purine bases and nucleotides—C4, C5 and N7
- Glutathione (gamma-glutamyl-cysteinyl glycine)
- Conjugation for xenobiotics
- Constituent of proteins like collagen (Glycine + Proline + Hydroxyproline)
- Methylene tetrahydrofolate by glycine cleavage system.
- Glucose: It is glucogenic.

34. Maple syrup urinary disease.
Refer 2007 Essay Question 10.

35. Inhibitors of transcription.
Refer 2013 Short Answer Question 15.
- Rifampicin: Inhibits initiation by binding to β subunit of RNAP—No Phosphodiester bond—used as antituberculous drug
- Actinomycin D—chemotherapy—binds to DNA template and interferes the movement of RNAP. Actinomycin D and mitomycin block transcription by intercalating with DNA strands
- 3' deoxy adenosine—synthetic analog—causes chain termination
- Alpha amanitin—mushroom poison—inactivates RNA polymerase II.

36. Histamine.
Refer 2014 Short Answer Question 55.
- Histamine is a biological amine—derived from histidine
- It is a decarboxylated product of histidine by histidine decarboxylase which needs PLP
- **Histidine** $\xrightarrow[\text{PLP}]{\text{Histidine decarboxylase}}$ **Histamine +** CO_2
- Histamine is produced in the body from platelet mast cells and basophils
- Effects of histamine are—smooth muscle contraction, enhanced vascular permeability, increased acid secretion
- It causes fall of BP
- Along with slow reacting substances (SRS) it produces allergic reactions against drugs like penicillin. There will be fall of BP and vasodilatation
- Antihistamine drugs block the histamine receptors and control allergic reactions
- Histamine acts on H_2 receptors and stimulates gastric acid secretion. H_2 receptor antagonists are used in the treatment of acid peptic ulcers of stomach.

37. Gamma-aminobutyric acid (Fig. 17).
Refer 2013 Short Answer Question 57.
- Glutamate on decarboxylation produces gamma-aminobutyric acid (GABA)
- It is produced in brain. GABA is an inhibitory neurotransmitter because it opens chloride channels in postsynaptic membranes in CNS
- It inhibits nerve transmission in the brain, calming nervous activity by opening the chloride channel
- Glutamate and GABA are the most abundant neurotransmitters in the central nervous system, and especially in the cerebral cortex. GABA is an inhibitory neurotransmitter because it opens chloride channels in postsynaptic membranes in CNS
- Both formation and catabolism of GABA requires PLP. So in pyridoxine deficiency

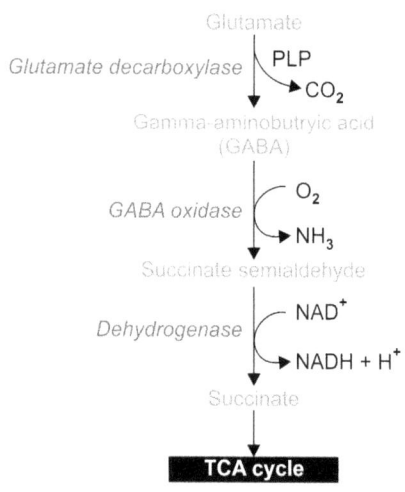

Fig. 17: Synthesis of GABA.

GABA will be deficient leading to convulsions. Sodium valproate inhibits GABA oxidase and is used for epilepsy treatment.

38. Phase II reactions of xenobiotics.

Refer 2011 Short Note 15.
- It is the second phases of detoxification of xenobiotics which is also known as biotransformation
- Here the toxic foreign substances are made to less harmful, water soluble substances and get excreted from the body.

Detoxification by Conjugation

- A xenobiotic which undergoes phase 1 reaction has become a new metabolite which contains chemical groups like hydroxyl (OH), amino (NH_2) and carboxyl (COOH) groups
- Phase 2 reactions are **conjugation reactions**—addition of **conjugating agents** like: Glucuronic acid, glutathione, glutamine, glycine, cysteine, acetylation–CH_3–Acetyl-CoA, methylation–CH_3, S-adenosyl methionine (SAM) and Sulfation–SO_4-PAPS
- **Conjugation by glucuronic acid:** The most common Phase II reaction
- Active glucuronide—UDP glucuronide by UDP glucuronyl transferase in ER
It is induced by barbiturates
- UDP glucuronic acid + R-OH
$$\xrightarrow{\text{UDP-glucuronyl transferase}} UDP + \text{R-glucuronide}$$
Unconjugated bilirubin is conjugated with glucuronic acid to form bilirubin diglucuronide in liver and excreted through bile
- **Conjugation by glutathione (GSH):** Glutathione is a tripeptide containing glycine, cysteine and glutamic acid. It conjugates aliphatic halides, aromatic nitro compounds, halogenated compounds and epoxides formed in Phase I reactions and detoxify them. In the body it is done by the enzyme glutathione S-transferase

$$\text{Xenobiotics + G-SH} \xrightarrow{\text{Glutathione S-transferase}} \text{X-S-G}$$

- **Conjugation with glutamine:** In phenylalanine metabolism, phenylacetic acid is conjugated with glutamine to form phenyl acetyl glutamine which is excreted in urine
- **Conjugation with glycine:** Aromatic carboxylic acids are conjugated with glycine
  - **For example:** Benzoic acid is conjugated with glycine to form hippuric acid
  - **Bile acids:** Cholic acid is conjugated with glycine to form glycocholic acid and deoxycholic acid is conjugated to deoxyglycocholic acid.
- **Conjugation with cysteine:** Cysteine is first acetylated to form acetyl cysteine which gets conjugated with toxic substances like chlorobenzene, bromobenzene, naphthalene and other compounds to nontoxic mercapturic acid
For example: Bromobenzene + Cysteine + Acetic acid ⟶ Bromophenyl mercapturic acid
- **Conjugation with acetic acid (acetylation):** Acetic acid is conjugated to compounds with amino group by the enzyme acetyl transferase
  - Some drugs like sulfanilamide, INH (Isoniazide) and PABA are acetylated before excretion.
- **Conjugation by methylation:**
  - S-adenosyl methionine (SAM) is the active methyl donor
  - The reaction is catalyzed by the enzyme methyl transferase
  - Examples:
    - Nicotinic acid and thyroxine—N-methylated
    - Estrogens—O-methylated
    - Epinephrine and norepinephrine—are methylated at phenolic hydroxyl group.
- **Conjugation by sulfation (with active sulfate)**
  - Phosphoadenosyl phosphosulfate (PAPS)—is the active sulphate formed by the addition of ATP with sulfates

- Sulfotransferase enzyme transfers sulfate group from PAPS to the OH of phenol, cresol, steroids or to NH2 of aliphatic amines to form etheral sulfate.

39. Functions of parathormone.

Refer 2011 Short Note 37.
- Parathormone (PTH) is secreted by the chief cells of parathyroid glands
- It binds with a receptor protein on the surface of target cells. This activates adenyl cyclase
- PTH has 3 major sites of action—intestine, bone and kidney
- All these 3 actions of PTH increase the serum calcium level
    1. **In intestines:** Stimulates production of 1-alpha hydroxylation of 25 hydroxycalciferol to produce the biologically-active form of vitamin D (calcitriol) in the kidney which increases the absorption of calcium from the intestine
    2. **In bone:** Facilitates mobilization of calcium from bone by increasing the number of osteoclasts and activating pyrophosphatase in osteoclasts. It stimulates secretion of collagenase from osteoclasts causing loss of matrix and bone resorption
    3. **In kidney:** Maximizes tubular reabsorption of calcium within the kidney thus resulting in minimal losses of calcium and increased excretion of phosphate.

40. Nitric oxide.

Refer 2011 Short Note 11.

MBBS Examination 2018

ANSWER ALL QUESTIONS

I. Essay questions (10/15 Marks each)
1. Explain the site, steps and energetics of β-oxidation of even chain fatty acids. Add a note on its regulation.
2. What is the normal blood glucose level? Discuss the factors regulating blood glucose in the fasting and postprandial states. Write the diagnostic criteria for diabetes mellitus.
3. Write in detail about ammonia production, transport and disposal. Add a note on disorders of urea cycle.
4. Write briefly the mechanisms by which the pH of the body fluids is regulated. Add a note on acid base disturbances with examples.

II. Short notes (4/5 Marks each)
1. Biochemical functions of vitamin B12.
2. Functions of calcium.
3. Glucose transporters.
4. Von Gierke disease.
5. Metabolism in adipose tissue during starvation.
6. Classify membrane transport mechanism. Add a note on active transport.
7. Fatty liver.
8. Types of enzyme inhibition with suitable examples.
9. Functions of vitamin B6 and its deficiency manifestations.
10. Biochemical changes in atherosclerosis.
11. Tests done to assess synthetic functions of liver.
12. Properties of genetic code.
13. Respiratory acidosis.
14. Importance and applications of recombinant DNA technology.
15. Proteinuria.
16. Post-translational modifications with examples.
17. Blotting techniques.
18. Classify jaundice based on liver function tests.
19. Structure of collagen.
20. Classes of Immunoglobulins

III. Short answer questions (2/3 Marks each)
1. Functions of endoplasmic reticulum.
2. Dietary fiber.
3. Physiological importance of glycogenolysis.
4. Define bengal Basal metabolic rate (BMR) Give its value.
5. Antiatherogenic role of high density lipoprotein cholesterol.
6. IUBMB classification of enzymes.
7. Cori cycle.
8. Suicide inhibition of enzymes.
9. Importance of brown fat.
10. Importance of sphingomyelin.
11. What are metalloenzymes? Give two examples.
12. What is glycemic index? Mention two examples of high glycemic index food.
13. Limiting amino acid with examples.
14. Mechanism of action of methotrexate and dicoumarol.
15. Fluorosis.
16. Hemochromatosis.
17. Serum lipid profile.

18. Refsum disease.
19. Essential pentosuria.
20. Lecithin sphingomyelin ratio.
21. Importance of transamination reaction.
22. Causes of secondary gout.
23. Enzymes as tumor markers.
24. Point mutation.
25. Denaturation reactions of proteins.
26. Cystinosis.
27. Melatonin.
28. Normal value of plasma osmolality and urine osmolality.
29. Orotic aciduria.
30. Cell cycle.
31. Structure of tRNA.
32. Lead poisoning.
33. Secondary hyperuricemias.
34. Draw normal protein electrophoretic pattern.
35. Secondary structure of proteins.
36. Classification of amino acids based on metabolic fate.
37. Hartnup's disease.
38. Microalbuminuria and its importance.
39. Reactive oxygen species.
40. DNA fingerprinting.

I. ESSAY QUESTIONS

1. Explain the site, steps and energetics of β-oxidation of even chain fatty acids. Add a note on its regulation.

Refer 2006 Essay Question 5.

2. What is the normal blood glucose level? Discuss the factors regulating blood glucose in the fasting and postprandial states. Write the diagnostic criteria for diabetes mellitus.

Refer 2005 Essay Question 6.

Diagnostic criteria for diabetes mellitus (WHO)—Refer 2012 Short Answer Question 39.

3. Write in detail about ammonia production, transport and disposal. Add a note on disorders of urea cycle.

Refer 2005 Essay Question 7.

4. Write briefly the mechanisms by which the pH of the body fluids is regulated. Add a note on acid-base disturbances with examples.

Refer 2003 Essay Question 4

II. SHORT NOTES

1. Biochemical functions of vitamin B12.

Refer 2006 Short Note 8

2. Functions of calcium.

Refer 2007 Essay Question 6 (Functions of calcium)

- Activation of enzymes:
  - Through calmodulin—calcium binding regulatory protein of molecular weight —17,000 daltons.
  - Calcium + calmodulin → calcium bound calmodulin
  - Calcium bound calmodulin activates kinases to phosphorylated enzymes for active biological effects, adenyl cyclase
- Activation of enzymes directly by calcium without calmodulin. Example: Pancreatic lipase, enzymes of coagulation pathway, rennin—to clot milk
- Muscle contraction and excitation:
  - Mediated by calcium—calcium channels
  - Calcium released from sarcoplasmic reticulum activates ATPase and increases the action of actin and myosin and facilitates excitation—contraction coupling
  - Interaction of calcium + Troponin C triggers muscle contraction
  - Active transport system uses calcium binding protein called calsequestrin
  - Calcium decreases neuromuscular irritability.
- Nerve conduction: Transmit nerve impulses from presynaptic to postsynaptic region.
- Hormone secretion: Secretion of hormones like Insulin, PTH, calcitonin, vasopressin are mediated by calcium

- Second messenger:
  - Ca and cyclic AMP are the second messengers in hormone action, e.g. glucagon
  - It acts as a second messenger in mechanisms involving G proteins and inositol triphosphate
- Vascular permeability: Ca—decreases passage of serum through capillaries and so used to reduce allergic exudates
- Myocardium: Calcium prolongs systole and so in hypercalcemia—cardiac arrest occurs in systole
- Bone and teeth:
  - Calcium is used in bone and teeth formation; bones act as reservoir of calcium
  - Osteoblasts—induce bone deposition and osteoclasts induce bone demineralization.

3. Glucose transporters.
Refer 2004 Short Note 7 (Absorption of carbohydrates from intestines).

4. Von Gierke disease.
Refer 2003 Short Note 6.

5. Metabolism in adipose tissue during starvation.
Refer 2015 Short Note 2.

6. Classify membrane transport mechanism. Add a note on active transport.
Refer 2013 Short Note 6.

7. Fatty liver.
Refer 2009 Short Answer Question 2.

8. Types of enzyme inhibition with suitable examples.
Refer 2005 Essay Question 1.

9. Functions of vitamin B6 and its deficiency manifestations.
Refer 2014 Short Note 21.

10. Biochemical changes in atherosclerosis.
Lipids play the major role in atherosclerosis. The biochemical changes that occur during this process can be described in four stages which are as follows:

Stage 1:
- Increased levels of cholesterol over time, affects subintimal region of arteries especially in aorta, coronaries and cerebral arteries.
- Oxidized LDL cholesterol particles are first deposited in the arterial walls.
- Though plasma LDL is mainly catabolized through apoB LDL receptor pathway, a small portion of LDL is degraded via uptake by macrophages. This process is accelerated by oxidative damage of LDL caused by free radical. Because of this complications, LDL cholesterol is known as **'bad cholesterol'**
- When macrophages become loaded with cholesterol, they are called foam cells and form the basis of atherosclerosis. Atheromatous plaques are formed from the foam cells deposited on the walls causing increased thrombosis and coronary artery disease.

Stage 2: If the LDL cholesterol level goes on increasing, the lesion progresses fast and the changes become irreversible.

Stage 3 : It is called fibrous proliferation stage which occurs due to release of growth factors from macrophages and platelets. Collagen gets accumulated and can lead to increased C reactive protein.

Stage 4: It consists of narrowing of the arteries due to the proliferation of the plaques leading to narrowing of the vessel and clot formation.
- Atheromatous plaques are formed from the foam cells deposited on the walls causing increased thrombosis and coronary artery diseases
- Insulin and thyroxine increase the binding of LDL to liver cells. This is the cause for hypercholesterolemia in diabetes and hypothyroidism.

11. Tests done to assess synthetic functions of liver.

The tests used to diagnose liver disease are called liver function tests. They are:
- **Tests based on synthetic function:** (synthesis of plasma proteins)—estimation of:
  - Total plasma proteins, serum albumin, globulin, A/G ratio
  - Prothrombin time
- Almost all plasma proteins with exception of immunoglobulins are synthesized by liver. Normal total serum proteins level is 6–8 g/dL
- Albumin is quantitatively the most important protein synthesized by the liver, and reflects the extent of functioning liver cell mass. Normal albumin level is 2.5-3.5 g/dL.
- In hepatocellular diseases hypoalbuminemia occurs.
- Normal serum globulin level is 2–3.5 g/dL. In chronic inflammatory disorders such as hepatitis and in cirrhosis of liver hyperglobulinemia will be present.
- A/G ratio—since albumin has a half life of 20 days, in all chronic diseases of liver, the albumin level is decreased. A reversal of A/G ratio is seen in cirrhosis of liver.

Prothrombin Time (PT)
- Since prothrombin is synthesized by the liver, it is a useful indicator of liver function.
- The half life of prothrombin is 6 hours only. Therefore PT indicates the recent function of liver.
- PT is prolonged only when more than 80% of liver function is lost.
- In vitamin K deficiency PT is prolonged. To differentiate liver dysfunction from that of vitamin K deficiency, vitamin K is given to the patient and PT is measured. Elevated PT even after administration of vitamin K indicates liver dysfunction.

12. Properties of genetic code.
Refer 2005 Short Note 19.

13. Respiratory acidosis.
Refer 2014 Short Answer Question 16.

14. Importance and applications of recombinant DNA technology.
Refer 2003 Short Note 19.

15. Proteinuria.
- The amount of protein excreted normally in 24-hours urine is insignificant and in healthy adults it is usually less than 150 mg/day. When increased proteins appear in urine, it is called proteinuria.
- Normal glomeruli do not permit molecules with molecular weight more than 60,000 to pass through. But when the glomeruli are damaged, they become more permeable and allow the leakage of proteins in urine. Hence proteinuria is indicative of kidney diseases.

Types of proteinuria and their causes
- Functional proteinuria (Transient)—prolonged standing, violent exercise, pregnancy
- Organic proteinuria
  - Overflow proteinuria: Hemolysis, rhabdomyolysis, multiple myeloma
  - Tubular proteinuria: Tubular injury
  - Glomerular proteinuria: Glomerular diseases, pre-eclampsia
- Postrenal proteinuria: Infection of urinary tract, kidney stones.

Tests for Proteins
- **Heat coagulation test:** 3/4 of the test tube is filled with urine and the top portion of the tube is heated by holding the tube at the bottom. A turbidity is seen on the heated portion only. 2 drops of 1% acetic acid is added. A cloudy white precipitate is seen at the top portion. Acetic acid is added to dissolve the phosphates.
- **Sulfosalicylic acid test:** In 2 mL of urine, few drops of 25% sulfosalicylic acid are added to give white precipitate. Sulfosalicylic acid is an alkaloidal reagent and so it neutralzes the positively charged protein to produce precipitation.

16. Post-translational modifications with examples.
Refer 2006 Short Note 27.

17. Blotting techniques.
Refer 2014 Short Note 27.

18. Classify jaundice based on liver function tests.
Refer 2017 Essay Question 3(a).

19. Structure of collagen.
Refer 2009 Short Note 6.

20. Classes of Immunoglobulins.
Refer 2008 Short Note 11.

III. SHORT ANSWER QUESTIONS

1. Functions of endoplasmic reticulum.

It is a network of membrane-enclosed spaces present in the cytoplasm connecting plasma membrane and nuclear envelope.
- Large portion of endoplasmic reticulum is studded with ribosomes giving a granular appearance called rough endoplasmic reticulum (RER). Ribosomes are involved in protein synthesis.
- Smooth endoplasmic reticulum does not contain ribosomes and it is involved in synthesis of lipids and in drug metabolism.

2. Dietary fiber.
Refer 2008 Short Note 10.

3. Physiological importance of glycogenolysis.
- Glycogen is the storage form of glucose in liver and in skeletal muscles
- The normal concentration of blood glucose level is 80–120 mg/dL
- During fasting stage or starvation, or in between meals, when there is no dietary source of glucose, body gets glucose by glycogenolysis mainly from hepatic glycogen
- Muscle glycogen cannot be converted to glucose because of the lack of the enzyme glucose-6-phosphatase
- Gluconeogenesis comes to act next to supply the needed glucose
- Glycogenolysis is very important to supply glucose whenever there is hypoglycemia to regulate normal blood glucose level.

4. Define basal metabolic rate (BMR) Give its value.
Refer 2005 Short Note 26.

5. Antiatherogenic role of high density lipoprotein cholesterol.
Refer 2010 Short Notes 6.

6. IUBMB classification of enzymes.
Refer 2006 Short Notes 22.

7. Cori cycle.
Refer 2009, Short Answer Question 30.

8. Suicide inhibition of enzymes.
Refer 2015 Short Answer Question 7.

9. Importance of brown fat.
- It is made up of polygonal cells and present more in cytoplasm
- It is brown in color due to the presence of many mitochondria and it also has cytochromes.
- Activity of ATP synthase is low and this fat is responsible for diet induced thermogenesis
- It is involved in thermogenesis and important in newborn and in hibernating animals
- Metabolically very active but there is less stored fat in this type
- There is no coupling of oxidation and phosphorylation which is mainly due to the presence of a protein called thermogenin in the inner mitochondrial membrane. There will be production of more heat and less ATP
- Individuals with active brown fat will not be obese.

10. Importance of sphingomyelin.
It is a sphingophospholipid.
- It contains the amino alcohol sphingosine + fatty acid (to form ceramide) + phosphorylcholine.
- It is the only sphingolipid with phosphate group

```
Sphingosine group                              O           CH₃
CH₃–(CH₂)₁₂–CH=CH–CHOH–CH–CH₂–O–P–O–CH₂–CH₂–N⁺–CH₃
                              |              |            |
                              NH             O⁻           CH₃
                              |                    Choline group
                              C=O
              Fatty acid group |
                              R
```

- Sphingomyelin is an important constituent of myelin sheath. It is present more in brain and nervous tissues.

11. What are metalloenzymes? Give two examples.

Refer 2011 Short Answer Question 24.

12. What is glycemic index? Mention two examples of high glycemic index food.

Refer 2013 Short Answer Question 49.
Two examples of high glycemic index are—potato chips and bread.

13. Limiting amino acid with examples.

Refer 2009 Short Answer Questions 9.

14. Mechanism of action of methotrexate and dicoumarol.

Methotroxeate

- It is a folic acid analogue having structural similarity to folic acid.
- It competitively inhibits the enzyme folate reductase
- So tetrahydrofolate (H4F)—the coenzyme of folic acid is not synthesized
- H4F is needed for incorporation of C5 methyl group in thymidine and C2 and C8 of purine ring. So there will be inhibition of DNA synthesis. Cell division is also affected
- Methotroxeate is an anticancer drug useful in the treatment of choriocarcinoma and leukemia.

Dicoumarol

- It is also a competitive inhibitor
- It has structural similarity to vitamin K
- It acts as an anticoagulant by inhibiting vitamin K activity in gamma carboxylation cycle.

15. Fluorosis.

Refer 2008 Short Answer Question 10.

16. Hemochromatosis.

Refer 2006 Essay Question 8 (Toxic manifestations of iron).

17. Serum lipid profile.

Refer 2013 Short Answer Question 8.

18. Refsum disease.

Refer 2013 Short Answer Question 3.

19. Essential pentosuria.

- It is due to the deficiency of the enzyme xylulose reductase and xylitol dehydrogenase in uronic acid pathway
- It is one of the members of Garrod's tetrad of inherited disorders
- It is a harmless condition
- There will be pentosuria—excretion of L-xylulose which gives positive Benedict's test.

20. Lecithin sphingomyelin ratio.

- It is an indicator of fetal maturity analyzed in amniotic fluid during pregnancy
- Upto 28th week of fetal life, the fetal lung synthesizes more sphingomyelin and afterwards there will be increased synthesis of lecithin
- In a full-term healthy newborn, the ratio between lecithin and sphingomyelin will be above 2 in the amniotic fluid. Lecithin sphingomyelin ratio (L/S ratio) above 2 indicates complete lung maturity.
- In respiratory distress syndrome (RDS) the ratio will be less than one and this will be a cause for neonatal morbidity
- It is treated by administration of surfactants.

21. Importance of transamination reaction.
Refer 2008 Short Note 14.

22. Causes of secondary gout.
- Increased diet intake, alcohol consumption
- Increased production of uric acid due to increased turnover of cells as in malignancy, lymphomas, leukemia, polycythemia, psoriasis, after treatment of cancer, trauma and starvation
- Reduced excretion of uric acid—renal failure, thiazide diuretics, lactic acidosis and ketoacidosis.

23. Enzymes as tumor markers.
- Enzymes are present in high concentration inside the cells and released into circulation due to tumor necrosis
- This also leads to tumor metastasis.
- **Examples:**
  - Alkaline phosphatase—bone secondaries, liver secondaries
  - Prostatic acid phosphatase—prostate cancer
  - Prostate specific antigen—prostate cancer
  - Neuron specific enolase—nervous system tumors

24. Point mutation.
Refer 2008 Short Note 34.

25. Denaturation reactions of proteins.
Refer 2009 Short Notes 31.

26. Cystinosis.
- It is a familial storage disorder in which cysteine crystals are accumulated in lysosomes of liver, spleen, bone marrow, WBC, kidney and cornea
- This is an autosomal recessive disorder due to abnormal transport of cystine
- Microscopic picture shows cystine crystals in WBCs
- **Treatment**—to give adequate fluids, alkalinise urine by giving sodium bicarbonate and pencillamine.

27. Melatonin.
- It is the acetylated and methylated product of serotonin secreted by pineal gland
- It is involved in diurnal variations, sleep wake cycles and biological rhythms
- It blocks the secretions of MSH and ACTH
- It is a neurotransmitter.

28. Normal value of plasma osmolality and urine osmolality.
Measurement of urine and plasma osmolality is done by using osmometer.
- Normal plasma osmolality is 285-300 mOsm/kg
- Normal urinary osmolality ranges from 60-1200 mOsm/kg.

29. Orotic aciduria.
It is an autosomal recessive disorder in pyrimidine metabolism.

There are 2 types—type I and II:
- Type I orotic aciduria: The condition results from absence of either or both of the enzymes Orotate phosphoribosyl transferase (ORPTase) and OMP decarboxylase—the enzymes of pyrimidine synthesis
- Type II orotic aciduria: The condition results from absence of the enzyme OMP decarboxylase.

Clinical features
- Growth is retarded and megaloblastic anemia present. Bone marrow cells are affected leading to anemia.
- Orotic acid crystalluria—orotate crystals are excreted in urine which may cause urinary tract obstruction in type I. Type II will have orotidinuria also
- Treatment is by feeding cytidine or uridine. They are converted into UTP which can act as feedback inhibitor. Remission may occur with oral uridine
- Orotic aciduria also occurs in urea cycle defect due to ornithine transcarbamoylase deficiency. Here carbamoyl phosphate gets accumulated and diverted to pyrimidine pathway.

30. Cell cycle.
Refer 2011 Short Note 36.

31. Structure of tRNA.
Refer 2004 Short Note 12.

32. Lead poisoning.
Refer 2003 Short Note 13 (point i).

33. Secondary hyperuricemias.
Refer 2008 Short Note 18.
Secondary causes—secondary to other diseases.

34. Draw normal protein electrophoretic pattern.
Refer 2006 Short Notes 30 (Normal bands).

35. Secondary structure of proteins.
Refer 2007 Short Note 25.

36. Classification of amino acids based on metabolic fate.
Classification of amino acids based on metabolic end products:
- Glucogenic—they end in glucogenic pathway in any one of the intermediates of TCA cycle, e.g. alanine, valine, methionine
- Glucogenic and ketogenic—partly glucogenic and partly ketogenic, e.g. tyrosine, tryptophan, lysine
- Purely ketogenic—converted to ketone bodies, e.g. leucine.

37. Hartnup's disease.
Refer 2010 Short Answer Question 36.

38. Microalbuminuria and its importance.
- It is also called minimal albuminuria or pauci-albuminuria
- When very minimal quantity of albumin (30–300 mg/day) is seen in urine it is known as microalbuminuria
- Early morning midstream sample is preferred for estimation of microalbuminuria
- This is an early indication of diabetic nephropathy and hypertensive nephropathy
- It can be expressed as albumin: creatinine ratio. Normal ratio in males is <23mg/g of creatinine and in females <32 mg/g of creatinine
- It is measured by radial immunediffusion or by ELISA.

39. Reactive oxygen species.
- Reactive oxygen species (ROS)
- They are oxygen free radicals
- Free radicals are molecules or molecular species that contain one or more unpaired electrons and are capable of independent existence
- ROS are the products of partial reduction of oxygen
- They are highly reactive and cause damage in living systems
- The members of ROS include—superoxide anion radical (O_2^-), hydroperoxyl radical (HOO·), lipid peroxide radical (ROO·).

40. DNA fingerprinting.
- Normal chromosomes have tandem repeats which are short sequences of DNA found in scattered sites
- The number of these tandem repeats differs from one person to another and for an individual the sequences are unique in number and in pattern except in identical twins
- This is similar to normal fingerprinting patterns. Hence it is known as DNA fingerprinting. It is also called as DNA profile
- Based on this, the DNA fingerprinting technique is developed and it is an analysis of the DNA sequences of an individual
- The amount of DNA needed for this procedure is very small and minute drops of blood stains, body fluids especially semen, hair or skin fragments are analyzed by this method
- This analyzed DNA is then amplified by using polymerase chain reaction and then compared to other normal samples of the individual.
- Applications:
  - To identify rape criminals and victims
  - To identify the parents and children
  - Used in disputes of immigration.

MBBS Examination 2019

ANSWER ALL QUESTIONS

I. **Essay questions:** (10/15 Marks each)

1. Explain the glycogen metabolism and its regulation. Add a note on associated disorders.
2. Iron: Dietary sources, factors affecting dietary iron absorption, transport and storage, causes and clinical features of iron deficiency anemia.
3. Explain the biochemical basis of clinical features of porphyrias.
4. Describe the primary, secondary, tertiary and quatenary structure of proteins.

II. **Write notes on:** (5/4 Marks each)

1. Lactic acidosis.
2. Explain why B12 deficiency causes macrocytic anemia.
3. How are dietary lipids distributed after digestion and absorption?
4. Phospholipids.
5. Types, functions, tissue specificity and physiological relevance of glucose transporters relevant to insulin secretion and action.
6. Diagnostic criteria for diabetes mellitus and laboratory investigation in diabetes mellitus.
7. Functions of prostaglandins.
8. Absorption of lipids.
9. Mucopolysaccharides with examples.
10. Metabolism of LDL with clinical importance.
11. Mutation.
12. Types, properties and functions of different classes of immunoglobulins.
13. Congenital jaundice.
14. Genomic library.
15. Products formed from tryptophan
16. Renal function tests.
17. Metabolism of catecholamines.
18. Metabolic alterations induced by alcohol metabolism.
19. Functions of proteins and enzymes involved in DNA replication.
20. Tests done to assess biosynthetic functions of liver.

III. **Short answers on:** (2/3 Marks each)

1. Importance of HbA1c testing.
2. Wernicke-Korsakoff syndrome.
3. What is the effect of non-competitive inhibition of Km and Vmax?
4. Schematic representation of the electron transport chain.
5. Carnitine transport.
6. Vitamin K cycle.
7. Metabolic basis of role of aspirin as an anti-platelet agent.
8. How will you interpret following conditions?
    a. Elevated alkaline phosphatase.
    b. Elevated acid phosphatase.
9. Proteasome.
10. How do enzymes reduce the activation energy of a reaction?
11. Biochemical manifestations in protein energy malnutrition.
12. Steatorrhea.
13. Ionophores—types with example.
14. Therapeutic uses of enzymes.
15. Lactose intolerance—cause and treatment.
16. Classes of enzymes with one example each.

17. Formation of vitamin D and the formation of its active form.
18. Lung surfactants and their significance.
19. Name two lipid storage diseases (spingolipidoses) and their enzyme defect.
20. Role of brown adipose tissue in heat generation.
21. Tests to assess biosynthetic function of liver.
22. Splicing of hnRNA (heteronuclear RNA).
23. Give the normal values (reference interval) for the following parameters in blood/serum.
    a) Creatinine; b) Potassium; c) TSH; d) pH
24. Compare promoter with enhancer.
25. Role of anti-diuretic hormone in the regulation of osmolality.
26. Role of different types of RNA in protein synthesis.
27. Hemoglobin electrophoresis of 2 year old boy with severe anemia showed elevated levels of HbF and HbA2 without any HbA. How will you interpret this?
28. Name four conditions in which Albumin: Globulin ratio is reversed and state the reason for the reversal.
29. What are the laboratory tests done for diagnosis of adrenal hypofunction and hyperfunction?
30. Give two examples for xenobiotic metabolism acting on endogenous substance.
31. Cystinuria.
32. Transamination.
33. Principle of electrophoresis technique.
34. Four synthetic analogues of purine and pyrimidine bases used as therapeutic agent.
35. DNA finger printing.
36. Oxygen dissociation curve of hemoglobin.
37. Markers of cholestasis.
38. Henderson–Hasselbalch equation.
39. Laboratory diagnosis of multiple myeloma.
40. Mechanism of action of allopurinol.

I. ESSAY QUESTIONS

1. **Explain the glycogen metabolism and its regulation. Add a note on associated disorders.**

Refer 2006 Essay Question 1 and Disorders Refer 2008 Short Notes 9.

2. **Iron: Dietary sources, factors affecting dietary iron absorption, transport and storage, causes and clinical features of Iron deficiency anemia.**

Refer 2016 Essay 3.
Iron deficiency anaemia: Refer 2013 Short Note 47.

3. **Explain the biochemical basis of clinical features of porphyrias.**

Refer 2009 Essay 5 and 2008 Essay 4.

4. **Describe the primary, secondary, tertiary and quatenary structure of proteins**

Refer 2003 Essay 3 and Refer 2009 Short Note Q-9.

II. WRITE NOTES ON

1. **Lactic acidosis.**

- Lactic acidosis is an important cause for metabolic acidosis with high anion gap (HAGMA).
- In normal state, the plasma lactic acid level is less than 2 mmol/L.
- This lactate level may increase when its production exceed the rate of utilization in the body, or the cells are not able to use the oxygen. Hence glucose is metabolised by anaerobic glycolysis leading to formation of pyruvate and then onto lactate, which accumulates in the tissue.
- There are two types of lactic acidosis namely Type A and Type B based on the causative factors.
- **Type A lactic acidosis:** The basic mechanism here is tissue hypoxia. When oxygen supply to the tissue is not adequate, lactic acid accumulates in the

tissues causing Type A lactic acidosis. The causes for this type of lactic acidosis are, hypovolemia, septic shock and cardiac failure where there is basically defective oxygen delivery.
- **Type B lactic acidosis:** Here there is no deficiency of oxygen supply, but the tissues are unable to use oxygen or require excess oxygen. The common causes for this type of lactic acidosis are liver failure, malignancy, thiamine deficiency and drugs like metformin.

2. **Explain why B12 deficiency causes macrocytic anemia?**

B12-vitamin cobalamin has two important coenzymes: Deoxyadenosylcobalamin and methylcobalamin.

Methyl Cobalamin
- It acts as the coenzyme in the conversion of homocysteine to methionine.
- Folic acid also plays important role in it. In the folic acid metabolism H_4F is reversibly converted to N_5N_{10} methylene tetrahydrofolate by serine hydroxymethyltransferase enzyme which is then irreversibly reduced to N_5 methyl tetra hydro folate.
- This methyl THF donates its methyl group to cobalamin which is converted to methyl cobalamin.
- This methyl B12 then supplies the methyl group to homocysteine to form methionine.
- In the case of B12 deficiency this transfer of methyl group is not possible and so methyl THF is trapped inside the cells and there is no formation of methionine from homocysteine. This is called **folate trap (Fig. 1)**.
- This leads to folic acid deficiency manifestations like inadequate DNA synthesis which causes megaloblastic macrocytic anemia.
- Because of folate trap, the synthesis of purines and pyrimidine are deficient. Thymidylate (TMP) synthesis will not occur which will end in impaired DNA replication.

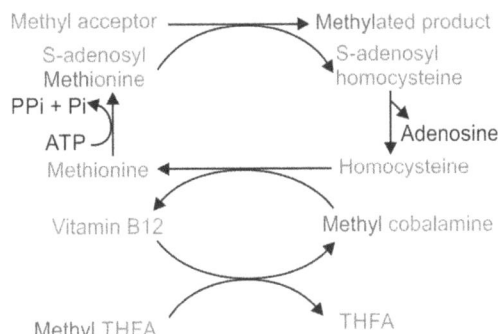

Fig. 1: Folate trap.

- Impaired DNA synthesis prevents cell division and formation of nucleus in new RBCs. Normal erythropoietic process gets disturbed and instead of normoblasts, the size of the red cells remain enlarged to form megaloblasts.
- These megaloblasts get accumulated in the bone marrow which will end in megaloblastic macrocytic anemia.

3. **How are dietary lipids distributed after digestion and absorption?**

Refer 2008 Short Note 22 Distribution–by forming Chylomicron.

4. **Phospholipids.**

Refer 2004 Short Note 1.

5. **Types, functions, tissue specificity and physiological relevance of glucose transporters relevant to insulin secretion and action.**

Refer 2004 Short Note 7 - Absorption of Carbohydrates -b. Facilitated bidirectional transport (GLUT) and 2013-Short Answer Question: 28.

6. **Diagnostic criteria for diabetes mellitus and laboratory investigation in diabetes mellitus.**

Refer Essay 7–2014 and 2013–SAQ-27.

7. **Functions of prostaglandins.**

Refer 2005 Short Note Question 13.

8. **Absorption of lipids.**

Refer 2003 Short Note Question 2.

9. Mucopolysaccharides with examples.

Refer 2012 Short Note Question 30.

10. Metabolism of LDL with clinical importance.

Refer 2003 Short Note Question 7 and 2005 Short Note Question 30.

11. Mutation.

Refer 2008 Short Note Question 34.

12. Types, properties and functions of different classes of immunoglobulins.

Refer 2008 Short Note Question 11.

13. Congenital jaundice.

Refer 2007 Short Note 2.

14. Genomic library.

- Collection of cloned restriction fragments of DNA which represent the entire genome is called DNA library.
- DNA library may be—1. Genomic DNA Library and 2. Complementary DNA (cDNA) library.
- Genomic DNA library: Here both the introns (non-coding sequences) and exons (coding sequences) are represented.
- Complementary DNA library represent only exons and it is synthesised from mRNA by reverse transcription.
- Preparation of Genomic DNA library:
  1. The entire genomic DNA is cut into small pieces by the enzyme restriction endonucleases.
  2. These cut pieces are then introduced into suitable vectors and amplified in bacterial cells to form recombinant DNA.
  3. Collection of these different recombinant clones are called genomic DNA Library
  4. Common vectors used are plasmids, cosmids, BAC, YAC etc.

15. Products formed from tryptophan.

Refer 2006-ESSAY-3
- Tryptophan is an essential amino acid containing indole group.
- It is both glucogenic and ketogenic amino acid.

Products Formed from Tryptophan

1. Vitamin Niacin and its coenzymes–NAD, NADP
2. Serotonin
3. Melatonin
4. Alanine
5. Formyl group (one carbon unit)
6. 5–HIAA
7. Indican

1. **Niacin and its coenzymes–NAD and NADP—kynurenine-Anthranilate pathway)—97% (Fig. 2).**
   - Tryptophan is oxidised by tryptophan pyrrolase—a dioxygenase enzyme to form N-formylkynurenine (NFK). This enzyme is a heme containing enzyme induced by glucocorticoids
   - Formylkynurenine is converted to kynurenine by the enzyme kynurenine formylase
   - Kynurenine is then hydroxylated to 3-hydroxykynurenine by a hydroxylase enzyme
   - 3-hydroxykynurenine is converted to 3-hydroxyanthranilate and alanine by a PLP dependent enzyme kynureninase. Alanine enters into glucogenic pathway after converted to pyruvate
   - In B6 deficiency hydroxykynurenine is converted to xanthurenic acid which gets excreted in urine

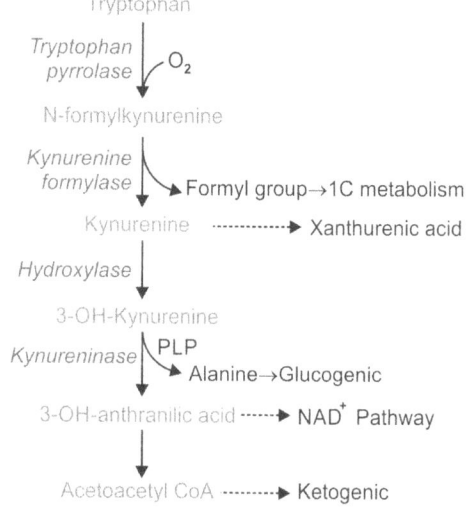

Fig. 2: Kynurenine-Anthranilate pathway.

- 3-hydroxyanthranilate undergoes either decarboxylation to form niacin or it is catabolised to ketoadipic acid and decarboxylated to acetoacetyl-CoA which enter to the ketogenic pathway
- Niacin pathway—3%
- 3-hydroxyanthranilate undergoes decarboxylation to form nicotinic acid by the action of the rate limiting enzyme QPRT-ase (Quinolinate Phospho Ribosyl Transferase) NAD and NADP are formed
- 60 mg of tryptophan will give rise to 1 mg of niacin (Fig. 3)

2. **Serotonin pathway: 1%**
   This pathway occurs in brain, mast cells, platelets and gastrointestinal tract (Fig. 4):
   - *Step-1 (hydroxylation of tryptophan):* Tryptophan is hydroxylated to 5-hydroxytryptophan by tryptophan hydroxylase which needs a co-factor tetrahydrobiopterin and NADPH
   - *Step-2 (decarboxylation):* 5-hydroxy tryptophan is decarboxylated to Serotonin which is (5HT) 5-hydroxytryptamine. Decarboxylase enzyme requires Pyridoxal phosphate as coenzyme.
   - *Degradation of serotonin:* Serotonin undergoes acetylation by acetyl CoA and methylation by S-adenosyl methionine to form melatonin (N-acetyl 5-methoxy serotonin).

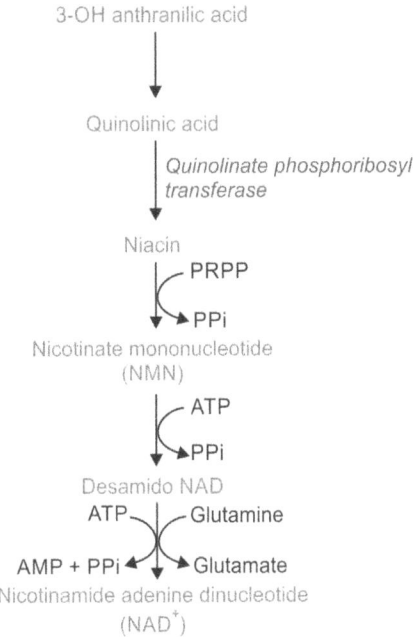

Fig. 3: Niacin pathway.

- Serotonin—also is oxidised by mono amine oxidase to form 5-hydroxy indoleacetic acid (5-HIAA) which is excreted in urine.
- **Melatonin:**
   - It is the acetylated and methylated product of serotonin secreted by Pineal gland

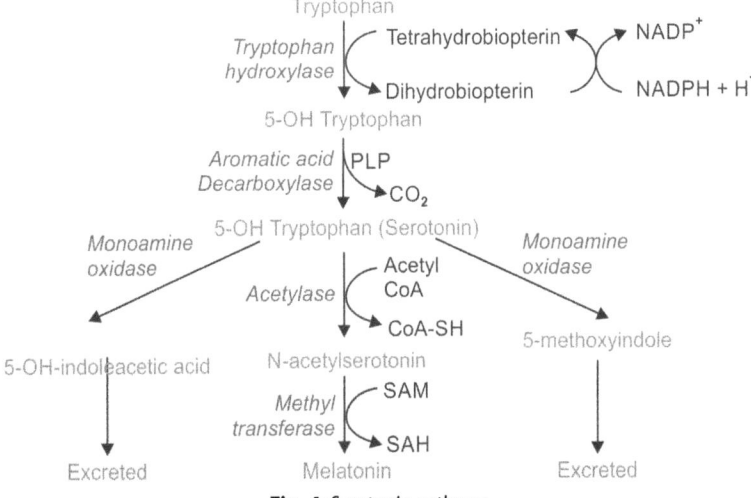

Fig. 4: Serotonin pathway.

- It is involved in diurnal variations, sleep wake cycles and biological rhythm. It is also a neurotransmitter.
- **Serotonin:**
  - Serotonin is synthesised by neurons and by the argentaffin cells of gastro-intestinal tract.
  - It is a neurotransmitter in the brain and an anti-depressant.
  - It is a vasoconstrictor and induces smooth muscle contraction.
  - Serotonin level is low in cases of depressive psychosis and it is involved in inducing sleep, appetite, mood and temperature regulation.
  - It decreases the sensitivity to pain.

16. Renal function tests.

Refer 2017 Short Note 8: Glomerular function tests and 2012 Short Note 18: Renal tubular function tests.

Classification of RFT

1. **To screen for kidney diseases:**
   - **Urine analysis:** Physical, chemical and microscopic examination
     a. *Physical examination:*
        - Volume (24 hours urinary output): Normal—1.5 to 2L/day
        - Appearance: Color
        - pH—N -6.0
        - Specific gravity—N-1.015 to 1.025
        - Osmolality
        - Smell
     b. *Chemical examination:*
        - Qualitative analysis for abnormal constituents of urine—mainly glucose, protein and blood
     c. Microscopic examination of the centrifuged sediment of urine:
        - For RBC,WBC, pus cells, crystals-to rule out urinary stones and casts
   - **Plasma urea, creatinine and electrolytes**
     - **Blood urea (N–15–40 mg/dL):** Blood urea is elevated in renal conditions like acute glomerular nephritis, early stages of nephrosis, malignant hypertension, and pyelonephritis. Elevation of blood urea is known as uremia.
     - **Serum creatinine (0.6 to 1.2 mg/dL):** This is a better marker of renal function than blood urea. It is elevated in renal failure cases.

2. **To assess glomerular function:**
   - Glomerulus acts as a sieve in filtering blood but it retains cells and proteins thus forming a glomerular filtrate- normally 170 to 180 L/day. Out of this only 1.5 liters of fluid is excreted as urine and the rest are reabsorbed through the tubules.
   - **Glomerular filtration rate (GFR):** Normal GFR is 120-125 mL/min. This is reduced in renal failure.
   - **Clearance tests:** Done to assess the glomerular filtration and renal blood flow.
   - Renal clearance of a substance is the volume of plasma from which the substance is completely cleared by the kidney in 1 minute.
   - **Clearance** = mg of substance excreted per min/mg of substance per mL of plasma;
     $C = U \times V/P$ C = Clearance of the substance; U = Concentration of the substance in urine; P = Concentration of the substance in plasma; V= Volume of urine passed per minute.
   - Clearance is expressed as millilitre of plasma per unit time
   - **Clearance tests:** This test is done by using either endogenous markers such as: Urea or creatinine or Exogenous markers like Inulin, ^{51}Cr- labelled EDTA, ^{99}Tec- labelled EDTA etc. Out of all creatinine clearance test is the best.
   - **Creatinine clearance test**: It is based on the rate of excretion of metabolically produced creatinine which is excreted thro' urine. Creatinine is freely filtered by the glomeruli but not reabsorbed by the tubules. A small amount of creatinine is secreted by the tubules.
   - 24 hours urine is collected and blood is also collected for estimation of

creatinine. Urinary volume is measured (V) and the concentration of creatinine in urine (U) and plasma (P) are estimated and by using the formula C = U x V/P the creatinine clearance is calculated.
- **Normal range for creatinine Clearance is 90 to 129 mL/min**
- Reduced creatinine clearance indicates chronic renal damage and reduced blood flow to glomeruli

3. **To assess tubular functions:**
   - Renal tubules reabsorb or secrete certain substances, concentrate the urine and acidify the urine. So it is important for maintaining specific gravity and osmolality of urine.
   - **The following are the tubular function tests:**
     a. **Specific gravity (SG) of urine:** Simplest test. Specific gravity of urine depends on the concentration of the solutes. In early stages of renal failure SG may be low due to kidney's inability to excrete solutes.
     b. Urine concentration test (fluid deprivation test):
        * Fluid intake is restricted for 15 hours. The first urine sample in the morning is collected and SG and osmolality measured.
        * If the SG is more than 1.025 or the osmolality exceeds 850 mOsmol/kg the renal concentration capacity is said to be normal.
        * Renal concentration ability is impaired due to tubular defect or in diabetes insipidus where there is decreased secretion of antidiuretic hormone.
     c. **Measurement of osmolality:** Measurement of urine and plasma osmolality is done by using osmometer. **Normal urinary osmolality ranges from 60 to 1200 mOsm/kg. Normal plasma osmolality is 285 to 300 mOsm/kg**. The ratio between urine/plasma osmolality is calculated. Normal ratio is around 3-4.5. Urinary osmolality is decreased in diabetes insipidus
     d. **Dilution tests:** This is done to check whether kidneys can excrete an excess water load. After emptying the bladder 1000 to 1200 mL of water is given to the patient. Hourly urine is collected for next 4 hours. In each sample volume, specific gravity and osmolality are measured. A normal person will excrete all the water load within 4 hours. It is a more sensitive test.
     e. **Urinary acidification Test** (acid load test—ammonium chloride loading test):
        * This is used to diagnose renal tubular acidosis
        * Ammonium chloride is given orally in gelatin capsule (100 mg/kg body weight) to induce metabolic acidosis. HCl produced is excreted as acidified urine.
        * Hourly urine collected for 2 to 8 hours and pH and acid excretion of each sample noted.
        * At least one sample should have pH lesser than 5.5. pH is not decreased in cases of renal tubular acidosis.
     f. **Fractional excretion of bicarbonate, sodium and phosphate in urine:** Also help in assessing renal tubular functions.

17. Metabolism of catecholamines.

Refer 2012 Short Note 38 and 2015 Essay 6 – Products formed from Tyrosine.
- **Catecholamines:** Catecholamines are derived from tyrosine. They include— epinephrine, norepinephrine, DOPA and dopamine
- Tyrosine is first hydroxylated to DOPA by tyrosine hydroxylase. It requires tetrahydrobiopterin and NADPH.
- DOPA is decarboxylated to form Dopamine by DOPA decarboxylase, a PLP dependent enzyme. Dopamine is a catecholamine which is a neurotransmitter. In Parkinsonism dopamine level is reduced. L-DOPA is used as a drug in Parkinsonism.
- Dopamine is hydroxylated to norepinephrine by dopamine hydroxylase.

- Norepinephrine is methylated to epinephrine by methyl transferase which needs S-adenosyl methionine as the methyl donor.
- Epinephrine is methylated to metanephrine and oxidised to vanillylmandelic acid (VMA) and excreted in urine. Level of VMA is elevated in pheochromocytoma and in neuroblastoma.

18. Metabolic alterations induced by alcohol metabolism.

Refer 2012 SN -28.

19. Functions of proteins and enzymes involved in DNA replication.

Enzymes and Proteins Refer 2012 Short answer questions 21.
1. DNA dependent DNA polymerase—different in bacteria and mammals
    i. Bacterial (prokaryotic) DNA polymerase
        - DNAP-I (Pol I) (Kornberg enzyme): Repair enzyme
        - DNAP- II (Pol II): Proof reading and repair
        - DNAP- III (Pol III): synthesizing leading and lagging strands
    ii. Mammalian (eukaryotic) DNA polymerase (5 types—α, β, γ, δ and ε: Alpha—gap filling, beta—DNA repair, gamma—mitochondrial DNA synthesis, delta—synthesis of leading and lagging strand and epsilon—proof reading and DNA repair
2. Primase
3. DNA topoisomerase—type I and II
4. Helicase
5. DNA gyrase—type II topoisomerases

Functions of Topoisomerases and Gyrases

- There are two topoisomerases: Type - I and II. Type II is called as gyrases
- Both relieve torsional strain generated by DNA unwinding in replication, transcription and recombination
- Type I—catalysing relaxation of supercoiled DNA by breaking a single strand
- **Type II—topoisomerase (gyrase in prokaryotes) cleaves both strands of** DNA and introduces negative supercoils to DNA using ATP.

Other Proteins

Prokaryotes:
- DnaA protein: Initiation of replication at OriC (AT rich)—ATP
- DnaB protein: Helicase of *E. coli* - component of primosome—separation of strands—ATP
- Single strand binding protein - ssb: Helix-stabilising proteins—binds to ss DNA—enhances activity of helicase—protects ss-DNA from degradation by nuclease—prevents premature annealing of double stranded DNA.

20. Tests done to assess biosynthetic functions of liver.

Refer 2018 Short Note 11.

III. SHORT ANSWERS ON

1. Importance of HbA1c testing.

Refer 2007 Short Note 15.

2. Wernicke-Korsakoff syndrome.

Refer 2003 Essay 1: Deficiency of B1 –Cerebral Beriberi

It is due to vitamin B1 deficiency mostly in chronic alcoholics. It is also known as cerebral beri-beri. It is presented with symptoms of encephalopathy which includes ophthalmoplegia, nystagmus and cerebellar ataxia.

3. What is the effect of non-competitive inhibition of K_m and V_{max}?

- In this type, the inhibitors are structurally different from the substrate. So they bind on the enzyme molecule other than the substrate binding site. There is no competition between inhibitor and substrate.
- V_{max} is reduced. K_m is not altered.
- The enzyme reaction is slowed but not stopped e.g., heavy metal poisoning inhibiting enzyme.

4. **Schematic representation of the electron transport chain.**

Refer 2003 Short Note 4 Fig. 18/2007 Essay 7 Figs. 12 and 13.

5. **Carnitine transport (Fig. 5).**

Refer 2012 Short Answer Question 34 and 2006 Essay 5–Preparatory Step 2.

6. **Vitamin K cycle.**

Refer 2016 Short Answer Question 27

7. **Metabolic basis of role of aspirin as an anti-platelet agent.**

Refer 2013 Short Note 9, Fig. 14.
- Cyclooxygenase pathway: In this pathway all the prostaglandins, prostacyclins and Thromboxanes are produced except LTs.
- Phospholipids in the membranes are acted by phospholipases to release Arachidonic acid. Arachidonic acid is acted by cyclo-oxygenase enzyme to produce PGG2, H2 which are converted to PGD2, E2, F2. It is also diverted to synthesise PGI2 by prostacycline synthase and TXA2 by thromboxane synthase.
- There are 2 cyclooxygenase enzymes COX-1 and COX-2.
- Cyclo-oxygenase is activated by catecholamines and inhibited by NSAIDS—non steroidal anti-inflammatory drugs and aspirin.
- Aspirin inhibits cyclooxygenase enzyme -1 irreversibly by acetylation of serine residue present in the active site.
- Regular use of aspirin can prevent heart attack by inhibiting COX-1, thereby preventing the synthesis of TXA2 which is a thrombotic agent. As platelets have no nucleus they cannot produce COX -1. So the inhibitory action of aspirin on COX-1 persist the lifespan of platelets (7-10 days).
- Thus aspirin helps to prevent thrombus formation in the area of atheroscleroyic plaque sites and prevent myocardial infarction.

8. **How will you interpret following conditions?**

a. **Elevated Alkaline phosphatas e.**
Ans: Six isoenzymes of alkaline phosphatase (ALP).
- Alpha-1 ALP, alpha-2 heat labile ALP, alpha-2 heat stable ALP, pre-beta ALP, gamma-ALP, leukocyte ALP(LAP).
- Increase in alpha-1 ALP—obstructive jaundice; alpha-2 ALP indicates hepatitis and pre-beta ALP indicates bone diseases, gamma-ALP—ulcerative colitis; LAP—increased in lymphomas.
- General increase in ALP is seen in obstructive jaundice and bone diseases.

b. **Elevated acid phosphatase (ACP).**
Ans: Normal value in serum is 2.5 to 12U/L.
- Secreted by prostate cells, RBCs, WBCs and platelets.
- The value of ACP is increased in prostate cancer and it is an important tumor marker for prostate cancer.

9. **Proteasome.**

Ans:
- Intracellular proteins are degraded according to their half life which varies in each protein. **Key enzymes have half life of 10 minutes only.**

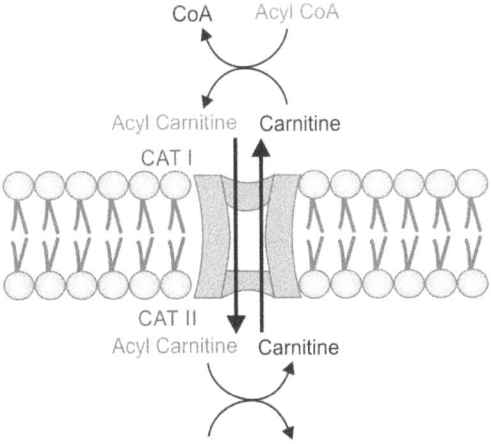

Fig. 5: Carnitine transport.

Types of IC digestion

1. **Lysosomal digestion:**
   - Extracellular proteins are taken by endocytosis and fused with lysosomes and then broken down by them
   - KFERQ (Lys, Phe, Glu, Arg, Gln)—quick disposal by lysosomes
   - ATP independent
2. **Cathepsins:** They are 18 in number. They are the enzymes to digest IC proteases inside phagolysosomes.
3. **Ubiquitin:** Intracellular (IC) protein breakdown involves a small protein called ubiquitin(UB) by a non-lysosomal ATP dependent process by **Ubiquitin proteasome pathway.**

   Proteasome pathway:
   - Ubiquitin attached proteins are targeted for degradation which takes place inside a macromolecule called Proteasome which is present in eukaryotic cells.
   - It has a central cylindrical hollow core formed from stacked rings of pores which has the active sites of proteolytic enzymes. There are two regulatory outer rings on either sides to recognise the ubiquitinated proteins.
   - UB mediated protein degradation produces the digestive products of small oligopeptides of 5-6 amino acids length.
   - Defects in the genes encoding ubiquitin and the related enzymes will result in neurodegenerative disorders—Angelman syndrome, Alzheimer's, Huntington's, Parkinson's, lateral sclerosis, etc.

10. How do enzymes reduce the activation energy of a reaction (Fig. 6)?

- Activation energy is the energy needed to convert the molecules of reacting substances from the ground state to transition site. In this state substrates are placed at a higher energy level.

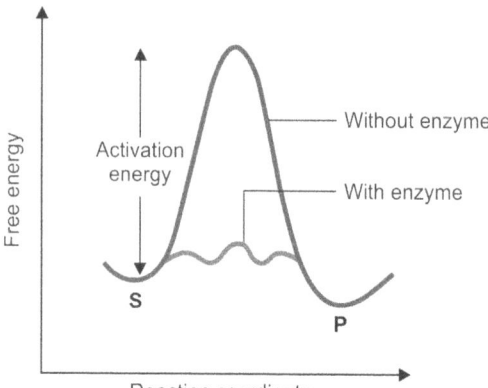

Fig. 6: Activation energy.

(Example—adding of little kerosene before litting fire to wood)
- Enzymes reduce the magnitude of the activation energy.
- Weak interactions between enzyme and substrate are more effective during enzyme substrate binding. This weak interaction is the main driving force for enzyme catalysis.
- Enzyme hydrolysis reduces the magnitude of this activation energy. For example: Acid hydrolysis of sucrose needs very high energy when comparing with hydrolysis by sucrase enzyme.

11. Biochemical manifestations in protein energy malnutrition.

Refer 2004 Short Note 4.

12. Steatorrhea.

Refer 2013 Short Answer Question 25.

13. Ionophores—types with example.

Refer 2014 Short Answer Question 27.

14. Therapeutic uses of enzymes.

Some enzymes are used as therapeutic agents to treat certain diseases. Examples are:
- Streptokinase and urokinase: Myocardial infarction (to lyse the intravascular clot).
- Pepsin and trypsin: Indigestion
- Asparaginase: Acute lymphoblastic leukemia
- Alpha-1 antitrypsin: Emphysema

15. Lactose intolerance—cause and treatment.

Refer 2011 Short Answer Question 08.

16. Classes of enzymes with one example each.

Refer 2006 Short Note 22.

17. Formation of Vitamin D and the formation of its active form.

Refer 2003 Short Note 1.

18. Lung surfactants and their significance.

Refer 2011 Short Answer Question 25.

19. Name two lipid storage diseases (spingolipidoses) and their enzyme defect.

Refer 2009 Short Note 33 Any 2.

20. Role of brown adipose tissue in heat generation.

Refer 2018 Short Answer Question 9.

21. Tests to assess biosynthetic function of liver.

Refer 2018 Short Note 11.

22. Splicing of hnRNA (hetero nuclear RNA).

Ans:
- Splicing of hnRNA is the first step in post transcriptional processing (**Fig. 7**).
- mRNA formed and released from DNA template is known as primary transcript.
- The primary transcripts are longer than the mRNA. They are known as the Heterogenous nuclear mRNA or hnRNA
- They have to undergo certain processing to become mature RNA. This process is called post-transcriptional modifications.
- The long primary transcripts have coding regions called exons and uncoding regions called introns.
- The introns should be removed and the exons should be spliced together. This is called Splicing. This is done by using snRNA.

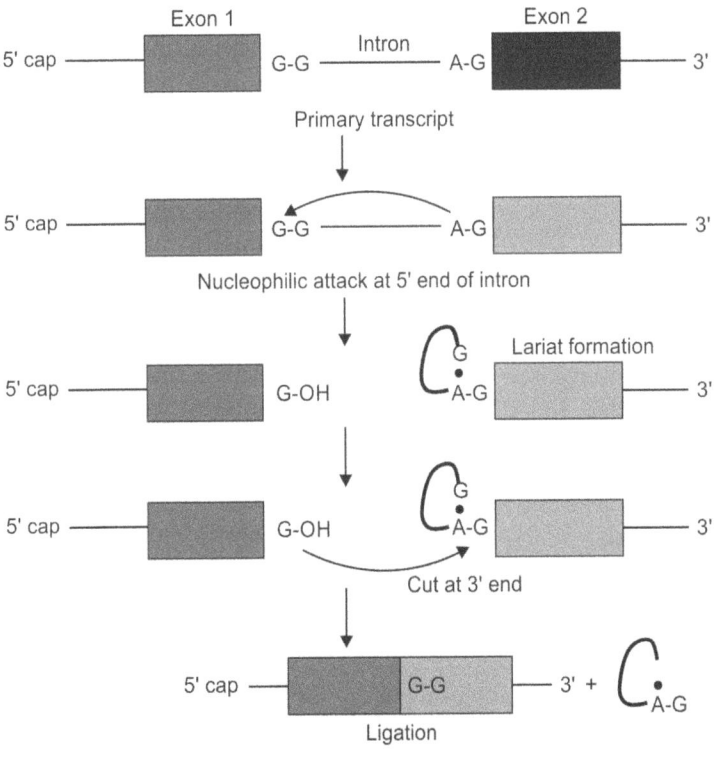

Fig. 7: Splicing.

- They attach with the terminal portions of introns and cleave at one end forming a lariat.
- This lariat is removed and the exons reattached by nucleophilic attack of terminal base of 1st exon on terminal base of 2nd exon.

23. Give the normal values (reference interval) for the following parameters in blood/serum.

a. Creatinine—0.7 to 1.4 mg/dL
b. Potassium—3.5 to 5.0 mEq/L
c. TSH—10 µU/L
d. pH—7.38 to 7.42

24. Compare promoter with enhancer.

Ans:
- **Promoters**: Specific areas on DNA which acts as starting signals for initiation of transcription.
- RNAP attaches itself to the promoter region: It is TATA Box or Pribnow box in prokaryotes; Goldberg-Hogness box in eukaryotes
- **Eukaryotic promoters**—decide where transcription is to commence and how frequently this event is to occur

```
DNA
5'  [Enhancer] ------ P [ Gene ] 3'
```

Enhancer sequence is usually upstream from promoter region. They are separated by 2000bp

Enhancers

- Increase rate of transcription
- Upstream—to 5' side
- Downstream—3'
- Activators: Enhancers with DNA sequences—response elements that bind specific transcription factors.

25. Role of anti diuretic hormone in the regulation of osmolality.

Ans:
- Plasma osmolality is sensed by osmoreceptors in the hypothalamus and they respond by secretion of antidiuretic hormone appropriately.
- When the plasma osmolality is low, secretion of ADH from osmoreceptors is suppressed. Low ADH leads to reduced water reabsorption in the collecting duct-leading to excretion of dilute urine, and thereby restoring plasma osmolality to normal.
- If plasma osmolality is increased, the receptors respond by secreting increased ADH which then causes increased water reabsorption by insertion of aquaporin in the renal tubule—thus reabsorbing solute free water back into the blood thereby correcting plasma osmolality to normal.

26. Role of different types of RNA in protein synthesis.

Ans:
The types of RNA involved in protein synthesis are:
 a. mRNA to be translated
 b. tRNAs—adopter molecules
- **Activation of amino acid and charging**
  - 2 steps reaction of attachment of carboxyl group of amino acid to 3'end of tRNA by aminoacyl-tRNA synthetase enzyme. Each enzyme recognises a specific amino acid. One ATP needed
- **Initiation:**
  - EUK—40S ribosome—binds to cap structure at 5' end of mRNA
  - Initiator sequence: Marker sequence—Kozak consensus sequence
  - Initiator codon: Eukaryotes—AUG—methionine—initiation
  - Factors (Pro): EUK—10 factors—eIF 1 to eIF 10
  - **Steps of Initiation:**
    1. Ribosomal dissociation—80S to 40 S and 60S subunits
    2. Formation of 43S pre-initiation complex: 40S + ternary complex with
- **Elongation—three steps:**
  1. Binding of aminoacyl t-RNA to A site

2. Peptide bond formation—peptidyl transferase—28S RNA of 60S unit (ribozyme)—needs 2 ATP and 2 GTP
3. Process of translocation—movement of growing peptide chain from A to P site—then to E—exit site or empty site
   - Factors—eEF-1 and eEF-2
   - Translocation—needs eEF-2 and GTP
   - 6 amino acids/second are synthesised (prokaryotes—many in 18 seconds)

- **Termination:**
  - Simple process
  - Stop/nonsense codon—UAG, UAA, UGA—recognised by releasing factors - eRF
  - GTP, peptidyl transferase promotes hydrolysis of bond between peptide and tRNA—P site
  - Dissociation of 80S ribosome
  - Release—mRNA

27. Hemoglobin electrophoresis of 2 year old boy with severe anemia showed elevated levels of HbF and HbA2 without any HbA. How will you interpret this?

Ans:
Hemoglobin electrophoresis in a child with anemia showing elevated levels of HbF and HbA2 with absent HbA is diagnostic of **thalassemia major.**

28. Name four conditions in which albumin: globulin ratio is reversed and state the reason for the reversal.

Ans:
- Normal plasma protein levels are :
- Total proteins—6 to 8 g/dL; albumin-3.5 to 5 g/dL and globulin—2.5 to 3.5 g/dL
- Normal A:G ratio is **1.2 to 1.5 : 1**
- It is lowered due to decrease in albumin or increase in globulin which are due to:
  1. Decreased synthesis of albumin in liver—due to liver diseases and in malnutrition
  2. Increased excretion of albumin thro' urine due to renal disorders
  3. Increased synthesis of globulin due to chronic infection,
  4. Multiple myeloma—plasmacytoma where there is paraproteinemia.

29. What are the laboratory tests done for diagnosis of adrenal hypofunction and hyperfunction?

Ans:
Laboratory tests for adrenal function:
- **Adrenal hypofunction:**
  - Urinary free cortisol is low
  - Plasma ACTH level is high
- **Adrenal hyperfunction:**
  - Urinary free cortisol is high
  - Plasma ACTH level is low.

30. Give two examples for xenobiotic metabolism acting on endogenous substance.

Ans:
Xenobiotics are strange or foreign compounds which may be:
a. Exogenous—accidentally ingested or taken as drugs
b. Endogenous—compounds produced in the body during metabolism or by bacterial metabolism.

For example:
- Endogenous compounds which has to be eliminated by body like bilirubin, steroids
- Compounds produced by bacterial metabolism. For example—amines produced by decarboxylation of amino acids like histamine from histidine; cadaverine from lysine; putrescine from ornithine; tyramine from tyrosine and tryptamine from tryptophan.
  1. **Conjugation of bilirubin by Glucuronides:** Unconjugated toxic bilirubin is conjugated with UDP glucuronic acid by UDP Glucuronyl transferase enzyme. Bilirubin

monoglucuronide is formed first (20%) which is then converted to diglucuronide (80%).This conjugation process is interfered by drugs like primaquine, novobiocin and pregnenolone, etc.

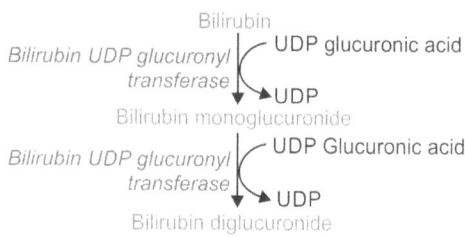

2. **Conjugation by glutathione (GSH):** Glutathione is a tripeptide containing glycine, cysteine and glutamic acid. It conjugates aliphatic halides, aromatic nitro compounds, halogenated compounds and epoxides formed in phase I reactions and detoxify them. In the body it is done by the enzyme Glutathione S-transferase.

Glutathione S-transferase
Xenobiotics + G-SH ⟶ X-S-G

31. Cystinuria.

Ans:
- Cystinuria is one of Garrod's tetrad of inborn errors of metabolism in cysteine
- It is due to defect in the transport of amino acids—cysteine, ornithine, arginine and lysine
- It is an autosomal recessive disorder with crystalluria and calculi formation leading to renal failure
- Amino acids excreted are cysteine, ornithine, arginine and lysine (COAL).

32. Transamination.

Refer 2008 Short Note 14 **(Fig. 8)**.
- Transamination is the exchange of the alpha amino group between one alpha amino acid and another alpha keto acid forming a new alpha amino acid (II) and a new keto acid (II). This is catalysed by a group of enzymes known as transferases or aminotransferases with pyridoxal phosphate (PLP) as its coenzyme.
- It is a reversible reaction.

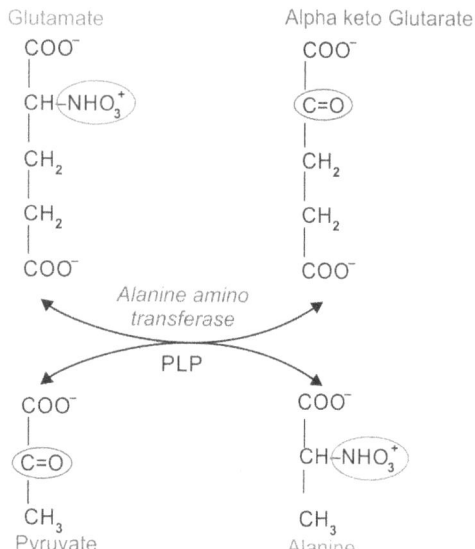

Fig. 8: Transamination.

Reaction sequence/mechanism of transamination:

Amino acid 1 + Keto acid 1 → Amino acid 2 + Keto acid 2

For example: Alanine + Alpha ketoglutarate → Glutamate + Pyruvate (alanine amino transferase, PLP)

(1AA) + (1KA) ----------▶ (IIAA) + (IIKA)

PLP acts as an acceptor of amino group, forming a Schiff's base. In the above example, first the amino group from alanine (amino acid 1) is removed to form pyruvate (keto acid 2). Then this amino group is taken up by alpha ketoglutarate (keto acid 1) to form glutamate (amino acid 2)

Exception: Transamination will not occur in lysine, threonine, proline and hydroxyproline

33. Principle of electrophoresis technique.

Refer 2006 Short Notes 30.

Principle: The term electrophoresis refers to the movement of charged particles through an electrolyte when subjected to an electric field.
- Cations (positively charged ions) move towards cathode and anions (negative) to anode.

- When a biological mixture is subjected to electrophoresis, the compounds in the mixture move in relation to their net charge, size, molecular weight and mass and gets separated according to these characteristics, so that the desired compound can be identified and isolated.

34. Four synthetic analogues of purine and pyrimidine bases used as therapeutic agent.

Refer 2005 Short Note 31 Any 4 in each.

35. DNA finger printing.

Refer 2018 Short Answer Question 40.

36. Oxygen dissociation curve of hemoglobin (Fig. 9).

- Oxygen dissociation curve (ODC)— shows the ability of Hb to load and unload oxygen at physiological partial pressure of oxygen(pO_2)
- It correlates the relationship between partial pressure of arterial oxygen in the x axis and the saturation of haemoglobin in the y axis. It depicts the ability of haemoglobin to take up and give up oxygen depending on partial pressure of oxygen.
- As the oxygen partial pressure rises, more of it binds to haemoglobin. But after maximum limit is reached, the curve flattens as Hb is saturated with oxygen- getting the sigmoid shape curve.
- Conditions that shift the curve to the left increase the oxygen affinity and therefore decrease the diffusion to the tissues. The disease states include, Foetal Hb, methemoglobinemia and high pH. Conditions which shift the curve to the right decrease the oxygen affinity to Hb and therefore delivers more oxygen to the tissues. The conditions include low affinity variants of Hb, High 2, 3 DPG, and low pH.

37. Markers of cholestasis.

Ans:
Name the enzymes of cholestasis
- Alkaline phosphatase

Markers of obstructive jaundice/cholestasis
- Increased conjugated bilirubin in serum
- Clay coloured stools
- Alkaline phosphatase enzyme—increased in serum
- Fecal stercobilinogen—absent
- Urinary Urobilinogen-absent

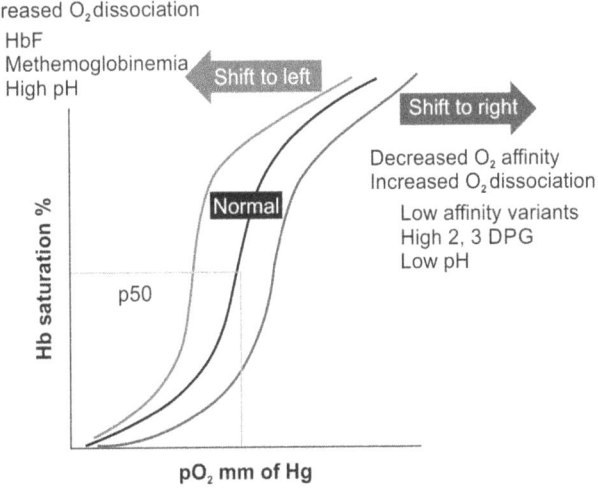

Fig. 9: Oxygen dissociation curve.

38. Henderson - Hasselbalch equation.

Ans:
- This equation expresses the relationship between pH, pKa, concentration of acid and conjugate base
- pH = pKa + log [base]/[acid].

39. Laboratory diagnosis of multiple myeloma.

Refer 2013 Short Answer Question 39 and 51.

40. Mechanism of action of allopurinol.

Synthesis of uric acid **(Fig. 10)**:
- The purine nucleotides are degraded to form uric acid. In the last step xanthine is oxidised to uric acid by the enzyme xanthine oxidase. This enzyme is competitively inhibited by allopurinol.
- Allopurinol is a structural analogue of the substrate xanthine.
- It binds and competes to the substrate binding site of the enzyme forming an enzyme inhibitory (EI) complex.
- K_m value is increased but no change in V_{max}.
- Allopurinol inhibits xanthine oxidase and prevents the synthesis of uric acid. And so allopurinol acts as the drug of choice to treat gouty arthritis.

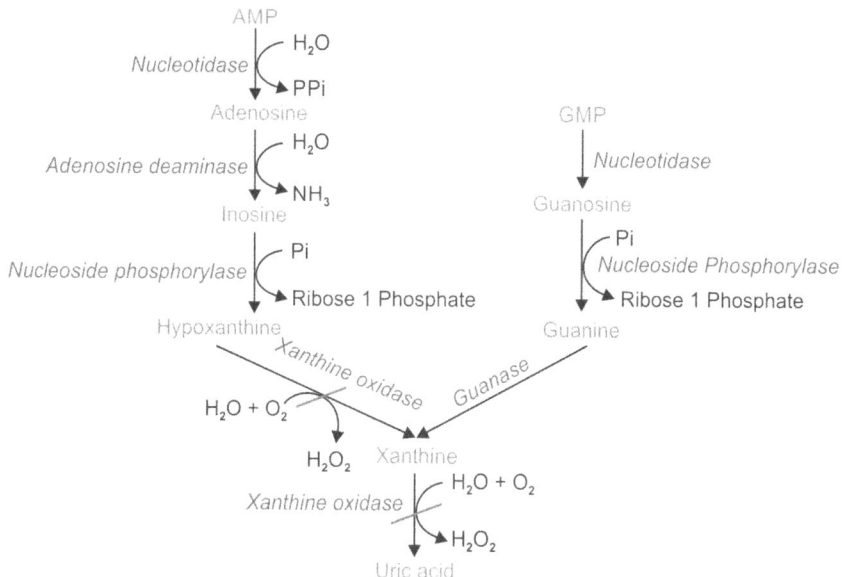

Fig. 10: Synthesis of uric acid.

MBBS Examination 2020

ANSWER ALL QUESTIONS

I. Essay questions: (10/15 Marks each)
1. Write in detail about the galactose metabolism and its applied aspects.
2. Explain the regulation of blood glucose in starvation and well fed state.
3. Write in details about the importance, applications and steps of polymerase chain reaction.
4. Name the plasma proteins. Explain the role of albumin and other transport proteins.

II. Write notes on: (4/5 Marks each)
1. Fatty liver—causes including role of lipotropic factors.
2. Vitamin C—sources, RDA, functions and deficiency manifestations.
3. PDH.
4. Dyslipidemias.
5. Passive transport mechanisms.
6. Reverse cholesterol transport and antiatherogenic effect of HDL.
7. Wald's visual cycle and deficiency manifestation of vitamin A.
8. Isoenzymes—definition and examples.
9. Active transport with examples.
10. Metabolism of ketone bodies.
11. Collagen.
12. ABG and interpretation of results
13. Genetic code
14. a. Name the Enzyme defect in Classical phenylketonuria.
    b. Clinical features of PKU.
    c. Name two test to detect PKU.
15. Cytochrome P450 enzyme systems—functions and properties like induction by drugs.
16. DNA repair mechanisms.
17. Normal level of sodium and potassium and add a note on causes and clinical features of hyponatremia.
18. Balanced diet and glycemic index.
19. Proteinuria—types and characteristic protein present in urine in each type.
20. Gene therapy.

III. Short answers on: (2/3 Marks each)
1. Define active site of enzymes.
2. Glycosidic bond and clinically important glycosides.
3. Name two functions of endoplasmic reticulum.
4. Name three essential fatty acids.
5. Name the enzyme require for glucuronidation of bilirubin.
6. Daily requirement of vitamin A for an adult.
7. Name the defect in Menke's disease.
8. Name the enzyme defect in Von-Gierke's disease.
9. Name one role of phospholipase A.
10. Name three vitamins involved in PDH complex.
11. Name of difference between coenzyme and cofactor.
12. Insulin and its clinical importance.
13. Name
    a. Vth complex of ETC.
    b. One inhibitor of complex III.
    c. Chylomicrons are rich in _____.
14. Apoprotein of chylomicrons are _____.
15. Write two important differences between rickets and osteomalacia.
16. What is the role of gamma-carboxylation in coagulations.

17. Name the enzyme defect in: 1) Niemann-Pick disease 2) Gaucher disease.
18. Name two components of metabolic syndrome.
19. Name the enzyme defect in pentosuria.
20. Name of the defect in Refsum's disease.
21. Name two lab test to detect sickle cell disease.
22. Name two differences of B form and A form DNA.
23. a. Normal creatinine clearance value in adult.
    b. One condition associated with increased creatinine clearance.
24. Form of folic acid involved in purine synthesis.
25. Normal reference range of:
    a. Blood urea
    b. Serum creatinine
    c. Urea/creatinine ratio
    d. 24 hours urinary excretion of creatinine in adult.
26. a. Expand RFLP.
    b. Clinical uses of RFLP
27. Name two markers of obstructive of jaundice.
28. Name two post-translational modification.
29. Name two antioxidant enzymes.
30. a. Mineral required for DNA polymerase activity.
    b. Rifampicin blocks _____ of transcription process.
31. Name one disease related to point Mutations.
32. Name two enzymes of pancreatic injury.
33. Uric acid levels in: a) Male b) Female.
34. Write formula to calculate anion gap.
35. BMI value in: a. Normal individual. b. Obesity.
36. Restriction endonuclease sticky— Meaning.
37. Name the defect Dubin-Johnson syndrome.
38. Name the amino acids involved in polyamines.
39. Name two antioxidant vitamins, one antioxidant mineral.
40. Role of poly 'A' tail.

I. ESSAY QUESTIONS

1. **Write in detail about the galactose metabolism and its applied aspects.**

GALACTOSE METABOLISM (FIG. 1)

- Galactose is a reducing monosaccharide —an aldohexose derived from the disaccharide/milk sugar lactose by hydrolysis by lactase enzyme
- Lactose $\xrightarrow{\text{Lactase (β Galactosidase)}}$ Galactose + Glucose
- Galactose and glucose are linked by β 1 → 4 glycosidic linkage to form lactose
- Galactose is essential for the synthesis of lactose, proteoglycans, glycolipids and glycoproteins
- Metabolism:
- *Step 1:* In liver galactose is pphosphorylated to galactose 1- phosphate by the enzyme galactokinase in the presence of ATP which is the phosphate donor and Mg^{++}.
- *Step 2:* Galactose 1-P reacts with UDP glucose to form UDP galactose and glucose 1-P by the enzyme galactose 1-P uridyl transferase (GALT).

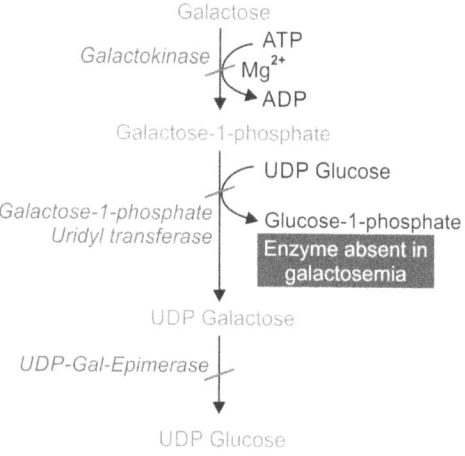

Fig. 1: Galactose metabolism.

- *Step 3:* Epimerisation: The enzyme UDP galactose-4-epimerase converts UDP galactose to UDP glucose. These oxidation and reduction reaction need NAD as coenzyme.
- *Step 4:* Glucose is liberated from UDP glucose after converted to Glu-1-P via the formation of glycogen by glycogenesis and subsequently glycogenolysis.

Disorder of galactose metabolism (Galactosemia)

- It is an inborn error of metabolism in galactose metabolism
- **Incidence:** 1 in 35,000 births
- **Defect:** Deficiency of galactose 1 phosphate uridyl transferase enzyme. Inherited defects of galactokinase, uridyl transferase, or 4-epimerase can also cause galactosemia
- **Features:**
  a. Hypoglycemia—due to accumulation of galactose 1 P which inhibits galactokinase and glycogen phosphorylase.
  b. Unconjugated bilirubin is increased due to reduced conjugation of bilirubin.
  c. Enlargement of liver (jaundice).
  d. Severe mental retardation.
  e. *Congenital cataract:* Due to enzyme deficiency, Galactose is reduced to dulcitol which gets accumulated in lens causing cataract due to its osmotic effect.
  f. Aminoaciduria: Due to renal tubular damage due to deposition of galactose 1-P in renal tubules.
  g. *Galactosemia*—Due to accumulation of galactose in blood and galactosuria.
- **Diagnosis:** Presence of galactose in urine (galactosuria),
- Congenital cataract
- Amniocentesis—for prenatal diagnosis
- **Treatment:**
  Lactose free diet. Mental retardation cannot be corrected

2. **Explain the regulation of blood glucose in starvation and well fed state.**

Refer 2003 Essay 2 and 2005 Essay 6.

3. **Write in details about the importance, applications and steps of polymerase chain reaction.**

Refer 2010 Short Note 13 and 2017 Short Note 18.

4. **Name the plasma proteins. Explain the role of albumin and other transport proteins.**

Refer 2006 Short Note 13 and 2009 Short Note 19.

II. WRITE NOTES ON

1. **Fatty liver-causes including role of lipotropic factors.**

Refer 2009 Short Answer Question 2.

2. **Vitamin C—sources, RDA, functions and deficiency manifestations.**

Refer 2005 Essay 5.

3. **PDH.**

Refer 2012 Short Note 27 (**Fig. 6**) 2014 Short Answer Question 26/2016 Short Note 27.

4. **Dyslipidemias.**

Refer 2011 Short Note 22.

Dyslipidemia may be of two types:

a. Hypolipoproteinemia: Primary (congenital) and secondary (acquired) (**Table 1**)
b. Hyperlipoproteinemia (congenital and secondary) (**Table 2**)

Hypolipoproteinemia

a. Familial hypobetalipoproteinemia

Table 1: Hypolipoproteinemia.

Hypolipoproteinemia	1. Hypoalphalipoproteinemia	Decreased HDL –AD	Increased risk of IHD
	2. Abetalipoproteinemia	Defect in loading of apo-B with lipid	TAG low Accumulation of TAG in intestine Accumulation of cholesterol esters
	3. Tangier disease	Absence of ATP binding cassette transporter-1 (ABC-1)	Low HDL Orange yellow tonsil, muscle atrophy, peripheral neuropathies, atherosclerosis

b. **Secondary hypolipoproteinemia:**
Seen in Kwashiorkor, malabsorption, and in chronic liver diseases.

Hyperlipoproteinemia:

a. **Classification of hyperlipidemias and their clinical importance.**
   - Frederickson's classification of hyperlipoproteinemias are also called as dyslipoproteinemias.
   - They are five types **(Table 2)**.
   - **Importance of hyperlipoproteinemias:**
     1. Elevation of lipids in plasma leads to the deposition of cholesterol on the arterial walls leading to atherosclerosis, affecting commonly the coronary and cerebral vessels. This will lead to ischemic heart disease and cerebrovascular accidents.
     2. Deposition of lipids in subcutaneous tissues leads to xanthomas of various types.
     3. Eruptive xanthomas—small yellow nodules with deposition of TG.
     4. Tuberous xanthomas—yellow plaques containing cholesterol and TG- found over the elbows and knees
     5. Xanthelasma—lipid deposits under the periorbital skin- made up of cholesterol
     6. Tendinous xanthomata—found over tendons.
     7. Deposition of lipids around the cornea leads to corneal arcus indicating hypercholesterolemia.
   - **Management:**
     * Restriction of fat intake
     * Supplementation of diet with PUFA and lipid lowering drugs
     * For example: Statin group of drugs to decrease cholesterol
     * Restriction of body weight
     * Regular exercise
b. Secondary hyperlipoproteinemias: Seen in
   - Hypercholesterolemia: Nephrotic syndrome, hypothyroidism
   - Hypertriglyceridaemia: Chronic renal failure, diabetes mellitus oestrogen therapy.

Table 2: Hyperlipoproteinemia.

Type	Name	Defect	Clinical features
Type I	Familial LP lipase deficiency Apo C II deficiency	LP lipase deficiency	Chylomicrons, TAG increased. Eruptive xanthomas, hepatomegaly, Creamy layer over clear plasma
Type II a	Familial hypercholesterolemia	LDL receptor defect, apo B increased	LDL, cholesterol increased. TAG normal, clear plasma. Atherosclerosis, tuberous xanthoma
Type II b		Apo B, apo C II increased	LDL, VLDL, cholesterol increased. Corneal arcus Slightly cloudy plasma
Type III	Familial dysbetalipoproteinemia Broad β disease or remnant removal disease	Apo E, apo C II increased	VLDL, chylomicron, Cholesterol increased Palmar xanthoma, cloudy plasma Risk of vascular disease
Type IV	Familial hypertriacylglycerolemia	Overproduction of VLDL, Apo C II	VLDL, TAG, cholesterol increased. Associated with diabetes, obesity. Cloudy or milky plasma
Type V	Familial lipoprotein excess	Secondary to other causes	VLDL, chylomicron, TAG increased. Cholesterol level normal. Risk of heart diseases. Creamy layer over milky plasma

5. Passive transport mechanisms.

Ans:
- This is the simple process of passive transport of a particular substance across the membrane which depends upon concentration gradient. This does not require energy. For example, passage of water and gases across membrane.
- The direction is from a region of higher concentration to lower concentration.
- Two types: Simple diffusion and facilitated diffusion
  a. Simple diffusion
     - It occurs from higher to lower concentration
     - Very slow process
     - Does not require energy
     - For example: Diffusion of gases and transport of lipophilic molecules
  b. Facilitated diffusion (Aug 2015)
     - This is a type of passive transport.
     - It is a carrier mediated process which can operate bidirectionally.
     - This mechanism is similar to the V_{max} of enzymes.
     - The entry of the solutes will be competitively inhibited by similar solutes
     - No energy is needed
     - The rate of transport is more rapid than simple diffusion process
     - The carrier molecules exist in the form of 'ping' and 'pong' states
     - For example: Glucose transporter.

6. Reverse cholesterol transport and anti-atherogenic effect of HDL.

Refer 2010 Short Note 6 and 2017 Short Note 4.

7. Wald's visual cycle and deficiency manifestation of vitamin A.

Refer 2006 Essay-Wald's Visual Cycle and Def. Manifestations and 2008 Short Note 8.

8. Isoenzymes—definition and examples.

Refer 2003 Short Note 5.

9. Active transport with examples.

Refer 2009 Short Note 2.

10. Metabolism of ketone bodies.

Refer 2005 Essay 2 and Short Note 14.

11. Collagen

Refer 2009 Short Note 6.

12. ABG and interpretation of results.

Ans:
- To understand the acid base disturbances, one should assess the biochemical parameters like pH, PCO_2, PO_2, bicarbonate and serum electrolytes.
- These parameters of blood gases like pH, PCO_2, PO_2, and bicarbonate levels can be quickly estimated by an instrument called blood gas analyzer (**Fig. 2**).
- These are highly automated instruments consisting of ion-sensitive electrodes and potentiometers and greatly help the clinician to identify the acid base disease state, so that corrective measures can be taken suitably and swiftly.

Sampling
- A heparinised arterial blood sample is collected from an artery, to determine arterial blood gases by trained persons.
- During the procedure, radial artery can be punctured without using a tourniquet and let the arterial pressure push the plunger and fill the syringe. This is to avoid mixing of air in the sample which will interfere with the estimation of ABG.
- The syringe should be capped quickly to prevent contact between the arterial blood sample and the air, and to prevent leaking during transport to the laboratory.
- Firm pressure should be applied firmly to the puncture site to prevent bleeding and hematoma formation.
- The sample for ABG testing should be quickly transported to the laboratory for analysis of various parameters. Some of the components of ABG are measured directly and some are derived by calculations.

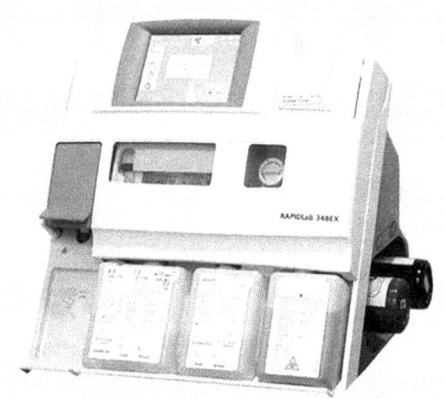

Fig. 2: Blood gas analyzer.

Parameters Measured Directly

pH

pH is measured with a glass electrode and a reference electrode suspended in the blood sample.

pCO_2

pCO_2 is measured by a modified glass electrode. This electrode is bathed in a solution containing sodium bicarbonate (weak bicarbonate buffer). The CO_2 from the blood sample diffuses across a semipermeable membrane into the bicarbonate solution.

pO_2

pO_2 level in arterial blood is assessed by electrochemical measurement of diffusion of O_2 through a permeable membrane into an electrode. This Clark's electrode consists of a silver anode and a platinum cathode which are immersed in an electrolyte buffer solution consisting of KCl and phosphate buffer.

Electrolytes

Serum electrolytes including sodium, potassium, calcium and chloride are determined by ion selective electrode techniques

Diagnosis of Acid-Base Disturbances by ABG

Based on the parameters received from the blood analyser, we can find out the possible acid base disturbance that is present in the patient. If the pH is lower than normal it suggests acidosis and if higher it denotes alkalosis. When this is because of alteration in HCO_3, the reason is metabolic. If the change in pH is due to change in PCO_2, it denotes respiratory disorder. The diagnostic criteria is summed up in **Table 3**.

Detection of Compensation

Primary metabolic disturbances elicit compensatory respiratory responses to maintain normal pH. In an acid base disturbance, the compensatory response is in the same direction. For example, decreased HCO_3 leads to decreased PCO_2 and this is known as the **same direction rule (Table 4)**.

Table 3: Diagnostic criteria - acid base disturbances.

Blood pH	HCO_3	pCO_2	Conditions	Causes
Less than 7.4	Low	Low	Metabolic acidosis	Kidney failure Diabetic ketoacidosis
More than 7.4	High	High	Metabolic alkalosis	Prolonged vomiting Gastric aspiration
Less than 7.4	High	High	Respiratory acidosis	Lung diseases Stroke
More than 7.4	Low	Low	Respiratory alkalosis	Liver failure Hysterical causes

Table 4: Detection of compensation.

Acid base disorder	Primary response	Expected compensation
Metabolic acidosis	Fall of HCO_3	Fall of PCO_2
Metabolic alkalosis	Rise of HCO_3	Rise of PCO_2
Respiratory acidosis	Rise of PCO_2	Rise of HCO_3
Respiratory alkalosis	Fall of PCO_2	Fall of HCO_3

13. Genetic code.

Refer 2005 Short Note 19.

14. a. Name the enzyme defect in classical phenylketonuria (Fig. 3).

Phenylalanine hydroxylase

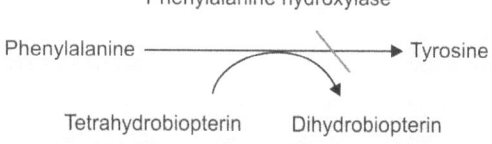

Fig. 3: Phenylketonuria.

b. Clinical features of PKU.

- The child is mentally retarded
- Convulsions, tremors, agitation, hyperactivity may be present.
- The child often has hypopigmentation due to reduced availability of tyrosine for melanin production.
- Phenyl lactate in sweat causes mousy body odor.

c. Name two test to detect PKU.

1. Blood level of phenylalanine is elevated: Normal level is 1mg/dL, which is elevated to >20mg/dL. This is confirmed by Tandem mass spectroscopy
2. Guthrie's test is confirmative
3. Urine ferric chloride test is positive.
4. DNA probes—to diagnose the defects in phenylalanine hydroxylase and dihydrobiopterin reductase

Refer 2017 Essay 4.

15. Cytochrome P450 enzyme systems—functions and properties like Induction by drugs.

Refer 2004 Short Note 20 Drug metabolism – last point.

16. DNA repair mechanisms.

Refer 2003 Short Note 11 and 2017 Short Note 15.

17. Normal level of sodium and potassium and add a note on causes and clinical features of hyponatremia.

Ans:
- Normal level of serum sodium is—136 to 145 mEq/L
- Normal level of serum Potassium is - 3.5 to 5.0 mEq/L.

Hyponatremia: Refer-2016—causes and clinical features.

18. Balanced Diet and Glycemic Index.

Refer: Balanced diet –2007 Short Note 14 and Glycemic index - 2013 Short Answer Question 49.

19. Proteinuria—types and characteristic. Protein present in urine in each type.

Refer 2018 Short Note 15.

20. Gene therapy.

Refer 2010 Short Note 15.

III. SHORT ANSWERS ON

1. Define active site of enzymes (Fig. 4).

Ans:

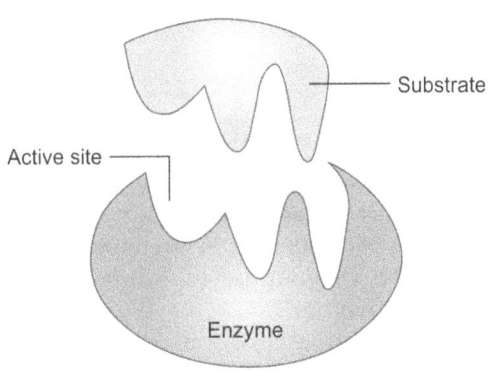

Fig. 4: Active site of enzyme.

- This is the region of the enzyme where the substrate binding and catalyses occurs.
- Active site occupies a smaller portion of the enzyme.
- It contains specific amino acid residues and posses three dimensional structure
- Situated in a cleft of the molecule.
- It is not rigid but flexible in structure and shape to promote proper substrate binding by conformational changes.
- Substrate binds to the enzymes at the active site by non-covalent bonds[s].
- Substrate binds to the enzymes[E] at the active site to form enzyme-substrate complex[ES] which is the first step in enzyme catalysis.

$$E + S \leftrightarrow ES \rightarrow E + P$$

2. Glycosidic bond and clinically important glycosides.

Ans:
Glycosidic bond
- Bond or linkage between 2 sugars or between a sugar and a non-carbohydrate alcohol—aglycone.
- This is formed when the hemiacetal or hemiketal group of a carbohydrate reacts with the OH group of another sugar or an alcohol

Glycosides
Refer 2007 Short Note 20 and 2013 SAQ 5.

3. Name two functions of endoplasmic recticulum.

Refer 2018 SAQ 1.

4. Name three essential fatty acids.

Refer 2005 Short Note 10
- Essential fatty acids cannot be synthesized by the body but have to be supplemented in diet. They are polyunsaturated fatty acids. They are:
  1. Linoleic acid (18 C)-ω6
  2. Linolenic acid (18 C)-ω3
  3. Arachidonic acid (20 C) - ω6 - can be formed, if the dietary supply of linolenic acid is sufficient. So it cannot be strictly categorised under essential fatty acid.

5. Name the enzyme require for glucuronidation of bilirubin.

Ans: UDP-glucuronosyltransferase
- **Conjugation of bilirubin (Fig. 5):** Unconjugated toxic bilirubin is conjugated with UDP glucuronic acid by UDP-glucuronosyltransferase enzyme. Bilirubin monoglucuronide is formed first (20%) which is then converted to diglucuronate (80%). This conjugation process is interfered by drugs like primaquine, novobiocin and pregnenolone, etc.

6. Daily requirement of vitamin A for an adult.

Ans:
- RDA of vitamin A in adult men—750 to 1000 µg/day
  - Adult women—750 µg/day
  - Pregnancy—1000 µg/day

7. Name the defect in Menke's disease.

Ans:
- It is due to a defect in the intestinal absorption of copper.
- Copper may be trapped by metallothein in the intestinal cells.
- The manifestations of Menke's disease include decreased copper in plasma and urine, anemia, and depigmentation of hair.

8. Name the enzyme defect in Von-Gierke's disease.

Ans:
It is also called as glycogen storage disease. Type I

Cause: Glucose 6-phosphatase enzyme is deficient which converts glucose 6 P to glucose.

Glucose 6 P ⟶ Glucose
Glucose 6 phosphatase

9. Name one role of phospholipase A.

Ans:
- Phospholipases are enzymes involved in the hydrolysis of phospholipids (Fig. 6).
- They are phospholipase A2, A1, C and D. Each type specifically acts on a particular site.
- Phospholipases A2 – acts on Phospholipids having unsaturated fatty acids in position-2 to give unsaturated fatty acid + lysolecithin.
- Lecithin ⟶ Lysolecithin + Fatty acid
  PHOSPHOLIPASE A2

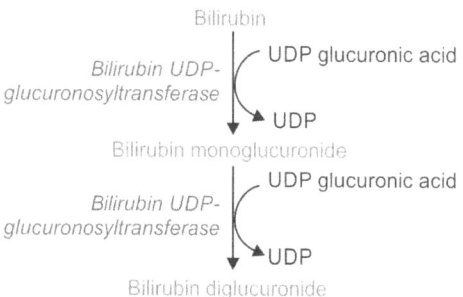

Fig. 5: Conjugation of bilirubin.

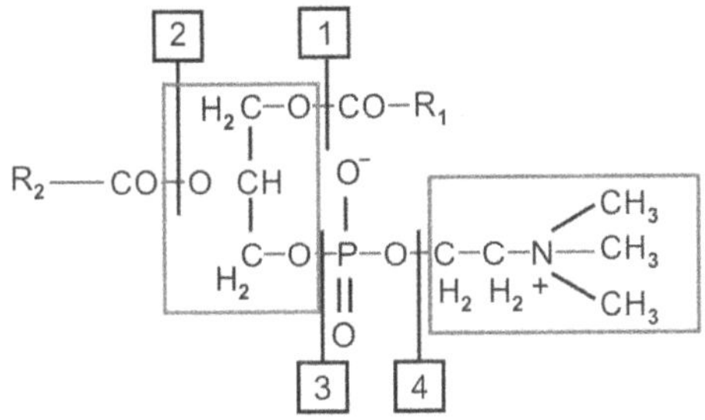

1 = Site of action of phospholipase A_1
2 = Action of phospholipase A_2
3 = Site of phospholipase C
4 = Phospholipase D

Fig. 6: Action of phospholipases.

- Lysolecithin is a detergent and hemolytic agent. This is present in snake venom and causes hemolysis and renal failure in snake bite.

10. Name three vitamins involved in PDH complex.

Refer 2016 Short Note 6.
- Three vitamins involved are: Thiamine (B1), niacin, riboflavin
- It needs five coenzymes: TPP from thiamine, lipoic acid, coenzyme A from pantothenic acid, NAD from niacin, FAD from riboflavin.

11. Name of difference between coenzyme and cofactor.

Ans:

Co-enzymes: The non-protein, organic, low molecular weight and dialysable substance associated with enzyme function. Prosthetic group is known as coenzyme. Otherwise called second substrate or co-substrate. They are tightly and stably incorporated into enzymes.
For example: NAD^+ (nicotinamide adenine dinucleotide).

There are two groups:

First group: Transfer hydrogen, e.g., NAD^+.

Second group: Transfer groups other than hydrogen, e.g., ATP.

Co-factors:
- They are additional non-protein chemical component required for the optimal activity of the enzyme.
- Cofactors include coenzymes and activators like metal ions. They are the metalloenzymes.
- They may be ion activated enzymes, e.g., pancreatic lipase activated by calcium ions.
- The metas may be tightly bound with the enzyme, e.g., copper in tyrosine kinase
- Non-metal ions can be enzyme activators, e.g., amylase activated by chloride ions.

12. Insulin and its clinical importance.

Refer 2006 Short Note 20 Actions.

13. Name
  a. Vth complex of ETC.
  b. One inhibitor of complex III
  c. Chylomicrons are rich in _____.

a. Vth complex of ETC. **Complex V-ATP Synthase:**
  - It is a proton assembly in the inner mitochondrial membrane
  - It has two functional subunits—F_1 and F_0 and looks like a lollipop. F_0 is embedded in the membrane and water insoluble Both F_0 and F_1 are connected by a protein stalk. Protons enter through' F_0 subunit and it acts as a proton channel. F_1 unit projects into the matrix and catalyses ATP synthesis.

b. One inhibitor of complex III—**antimycin, BAL, naphthoquinone.**

c. Chylomicrons are rich in **triacylglycerol.**

14. Apoprotein of chylomicron are ....

Apoprotein of chylomicron are ***A, B-48, C-II and E.***

15. Write two important difference between rickets and osteomalacia.

Ans:
- Both are vitamin D deficiencies
- Rickets occur in children and osteomalacia occur in adults
- **Rickets:** There will be the poor mineralization of bones, they become soft and pliable
- Main features are—bossing of frontal bones, pigeon chest, knock knees, bow legs and rickety rosary—enlargement of epiphysis

at the lower end of ribs and costochondral junction causing beading of ribs. Harrison's sulcus—a transverse depression from the costal cartilage to axilla due to indentation of lower ribs to diaphragm.

Osteomalacia:
- There will be softening of bones due to poor mineralization and increased osteoporosis which leads to fractures
- Calcium and phosphorus values are low in blood
- Serum alkaline phosphatase level is increased.

16. What is the role of gamma-carboxylation in coagulations.

Ans:
Vitamin K is involved in post-translational modifications of clotting factors such as factor II, VII, IX and X which undergo gamma carboxylation to get active forms.

Carboxylation of clotting factors and significance:
- All the pre-translational clotting factors contain glutamic acids at their ends of polypeptide chains, which are converted to gamma carboxyglutamic acid in the presence of carboxylase, O_2, CO_2, vitamin K (quinone form), $NADP^+$ and H^+. These carboxylated clotting factors now possess two negative charges on their γ-carboxyglutamate, which in turn chelate with two positive charges of Ca^{++}; This complex converts prothrombin to thrombin.
- This gamma-carboxylation is inhibited by warfarin and dicoumarol by competitive inhibition of epoxide reductase enzyme.

17. Name the enzyme defect in: 1) Niemann Pick disease; 2) Gaucher disease.

Ans:
1. **Niemann-Pick disease (Sphingomyelinase deficiency):** Accumulation of sphingomyelin. It is characterized by enlarged liver and spleen, mental retardation; fatal in early life.
2. **Gaucher's disease (β Glucosidase deficiency):** Accumulation of Glucosylceramide. It is characterized by enlarged liver and spleen, erosion of long bones, mental retardation in infants.

18. Name two components of metabolic syndrome.

Ans: 1. Adbdominai obesity
2. Insulin resistance or decreased glucose tolerance

19. Name the enzyme defect in Pentosuria.

Ans:
- It is due to the deficiency of the enzyme **xylulose reductase** in uronic acid pathway
- It is one of the members of Garrod's tetrad of inherited disorders
- It is a harmless condition which gives positive Benedict's test.

20. Name of the defect in Refsum's disease.

Ans:
- **Refsum's disease:** This is due to defect in the alpha oxidation due to the deficiency of the enzyme phytanic acid alpha oxidase.
- So phytanic acid is not degraded and gets accumulated in the nervous tissue.
- It is a rare neurological disorder characterised by cerebral ataxia and peripheral neuropathy, retinitis pigmentosa, and nerve deafness.
- Symptoms get regressed with restricted intake of phytanic acid.
Milk contains more phytanic acid and it has to be avoided.

21. Name two lab test to detect sickle cell disease.

Ans:
- **Electrophoresis:** Electrophoresis at alkaline pH shows a slower moving band than HbA. At this pH carboxyl group of glutamic acid is negatively charged. But lack of this charge on HbS makes it less negatively charged, and decreases the mobility towards positive pole. In acidic pH HbS moves faster than HbA.
- **Sickling test:** Blood smear is prepared and reducing agent such as sodium dithionite is added. Blood smear examined under light microscope shows sickled RBC.

22. Name two differences of B form and A form DNA (any 2) (Table 5).

Ans:

Table 5: Differences of A and B forms of DNA.

S. No.	Property	A- DNA	B - DNA
1.	Shape	Broadest	Medium
2.	Type of helix	Right handed	Right handed
3.	Base pairs per turn	11	10
4	Helix diameter	25.5 Å	23.7 Å
5.	Pitch per turn of helix	25.3 Å	35.4 Å
6.	Major groove	Narrow	Wide
7.	Minor groove	Very broad	Narrow

23. a. Normal creatinine clearance value in adult.

Ans:
Normal range for creatinine clearance is 90 to 129 mL/min.

b. One condition associated with increased creatinine clearance.

Pregnancy, early diabetic nephropathy.

24. Form of folic acid involved in purine synthesis (Table 6).

Ans:

Table 6: Folic acid derivative.

S. No.	Folic acid derivative	One carbon group transferred	Compounds produced – involved in purine synthesis
1	$N^5 N^{10}$ Methenyl THF	Methenyl (=CH)	C8 of purine ring
2	Formyl THF	Formyl	C2 of purine ring
3	$N^5 N^{10}$ Methylene THF	Methylene (CH2)	dTMP in DNA

25. Normal reference range of:
a. Blood urea
b. Serum creatinine
c. Urea/creatinine ratio
d. 24 hours urinary excretion of creatinine in adult.

Ans:
a. Blood urea—**20 - 40 mg/dL**
b. Serum creatinine—**0.7 to 1.4 mg/dL**
c. Urea/creatinine ratio—**40-100:1**
d. 24 hours urinary excretion of creatinine in adult—**1-2 g/day**

26. a. Expand RFLP; b. Clinical uses of RFLP.

Ans:
a. RFLP—technique by which organisms may be differentiated by analysis of patterns derived from cleavage of their DNA
b. Clinical uses of RFLP
   - Disputed parenthood
   - human population genetics
   - Geographical isolates
   - Comparison of genitic make UP

27. Name two markers of obstructive of jaundice.

Ans:
1. Conjugated bilirubin is increased in blood
2. Increased level of serum alkaline phosphatase enzyme
   - Absence of urobilinogen in urine
   - Absence of stercobilinogen in feces—clay colored stools
   - Presence of bile salts and bilirubin in urine

28. Name two post-translational modification (any 2).

Ans:
1. Trimming
2. Covalent modifications like—a) phosphorylation, b) glycosylation c) hydroxylation, d) carboxylation and e) addition of groups—methyl, acetyl, farnesyl, amide
3. Subunit aggregation
4. Protein folding

29. Name two antioxidant enzymes.

Ans:
a. **Preventive antioxidants:** They will inhibit the initial production of free radicals. They are catalase, glutathione peroxidase.
b. **Chain breaking antioxidants:** They inhibit the propagative phase. They include-superoxide dismutase

30.
a. Mineral required for DNA polymerase activity ....
b. Rifampicin blocks .... of transcription process.

Ans:
a. Mineral required for DNA polymerase activity.
Ans: Mg^{++}
b. Rifampicin blocks **initiation** of transcription process.

31. Name one disease related to point mutations.

Ans: Sickle cell hemoglobin.

32. Name two enzymes of pancreatic injury.

Ans. Amylase and lipase.

33. Uric acid levels in: a) Male b) Female.

Ans: a. Male—3.5 to 7 mg/dL
b. Female—3.0 to 6 mg/dL

34. Write formula to calculate anion gap.

Ans:
Anion gap (A^-) = $Na^+ + K^+ = Cl^- + HCO_3^-$
= 136 + 4 = 100 + 25
= 15 mEq/L

35. BMI value in: a) Normal Individual; b) Obesity.

Ans:
- Body mass index (BMI) (kg/m^2) = Weight (kg) , [Height (m^2)] (W/H)
- a) Normal individual—18.5 to 24
- b) Obesity —>30

36. Restriction endonuclease sticky—meaning.

Ans:
- Restriction endonuclease enzymes cut DNA of any source into short pieces in a sequence-specific manner.
- These DNA cuts result in blunt ends (e.g., HpaI) or overlapping (sticky) ends (e.g., BamHI).
- Sticky ends are particularly useful in constructing hybrid or chimeric DNA molecules.

37. Name the defect in Dubin–Johnson syndrome.

Ans:
- Congenital conjugated hyperbilirubinemia.
- Dubin-Johnson syndrome—autosomal recessive trait.
- Defect: Defective ATP dependent anion transport in bile canaliculi due to mutation in MRP-2 protein which is responsible for the transport of conjugated bilirubin.
- Defective excretion of conjugated bilirubin and so its level increased in blood. Bilirubin gets deposited in the liver and the liver appears black, and is called Black Liver Jaundice

38. Name the amino acids involved in polyamines.

Ans: Ornithine from arginine in urea cycle and methionine (SAM).

39. Name two antioxidant vitamins, one antioxidant mineral.

Ans:
- Naturally occurring antioxidants—vitamin E and C,
- Mineral—selenium.

40. Role of poly 'A' tail.

Ans:
- Poly A tail formation is one of the post-transcriptional modifications in processing hnRNA to mRNA.
- The 3' end of mRNA is attached with 20-250 adenine nucleotides. This is to protect the 3'end from the attack of 3' exonuclease present in the cytoplasm.

MBBS Examination 2021

ANSWER ALL QUESTIONS

I. Essay questions:
  (2 × 15 = 30 Marks each)
1. Describe the structure of biological membranes. Discuss the various transport mechanisms across membranes with suitable examples.
2. How are dietary lipids digested and absorbed? Write about the transport of lipids in plasma.
3. What is the normal pH of blood? Discuss how the pH of blood is maintained.
4. Discuss the metabolism of phenylalanine. Write a note on the inborn error associated with phenylalanine.
5. Explain the mode of action of enzymes and describe the factors affecting Enzyme activity? Brief the analytical uses of enzymes with example.
6. Describe the reactions of krebs cycle and its regulation? Add a note on its anaplerotic role.
7. Describe the process of replication in prokaryotes? Add a note on inhibitors of DNA replication?
8. Explain the catabolic pathways of tyrosine and disorders associated with tyrosine metabolism?

II. Write notes on:
  (10 × 5 = 50 Marks each)
1. Competitive inhibition of enzyme activity.
2. Biochemical features seen in blood and urine of a patient with hemolytic anemia.
3. Functions of vitamin – C
4. Anaplerotic role of citric acid cycle.
5. Define gluconeogenesis and explain the various steps.
6. Formation and fate of pyruvate.
7. Biological value of proteins.
8. Enumerate the compounds derived from cholesterol and mention their biochemical functions.
9. Synthesis and regulation of porphyrins.
10. Structure and functions of mitochondria.
11. Compounds derived from glycine and their functions.
12. Hyperammonemias.
13. Copper metabolism and its applied aspects.
14. Telomerase and its application.
15. Lesch-Nyhan syndrome.
16. Inhibitors of purine nucleotide biosynthesis.
17. Metabolic acidosis
18. Absorption of dietary iron.
19. Biochemical features of cancer cells.
20. Conjugation reactions in xenobiotics.
21. Fluid mosaic model of cell.
22. State the differences between.
    a. Starch and glycogen.
    b. Dextrin and dextran.
23. Beta oxidation of palmitic acid.
24. Mention the recommended dietary allowance, biochemical functions and deficiency manifestations of vitamin-E
25. Chemiosmotic theory and mechanism of ATP synthesis.
26. Brief the risk factors of cardiovascular disease and its preventive methods.
27. What is nitrogen balance? Enumerate the factors affecting nitrogen balance.

28. List the inborn errors associated with heme metabolism and their features.
29. Oral glucose tolerance test: Indications, method and interpretation.
30. Regulation and significance of HMP shunt.
31. Brief the functions and diagnostic importance of plasma proteins present in the beta region of electrophoretic pattern?
32. Mention the causes, signs, symptoms and treatment of hypokalemia.
33. Explain the precipitation reactions of protein.
34. Describe the DNA repair mechanisms with suitable clinical examples.
35. Explain the role of kidney in regulation of pH.
36. Mention the sources, recommended dietary allowance, function and deficiency manifestation of copper.
37. Brief the causes, symptoms and treatment of cout?
38. Applications of DNA recombinant technology.
39. Brief the in vitro thyroid function tests.
40. Explain the cellular signalling and defense mechanism of free radicals?

I. ESSAY QUESTIONS

1. **Describe the structure of biological membranes. Discuss the various transport mechanisms across membranes with suitable examples.**

Refer biological membrane 2008 SN 5 and transport mechanisms 2013 SN-6.

2. **How are dietary lipids digested and absorbed? Write about the transport of lipids in plasma.**

Refer Digestion and absorption 2008 SN 22 and Transport of lipids – Lipoproteins.
- Lipoproteins help in transporting the lipids in the form of chylomicrons, very low density lipoproteins(VLDL), low density lipoproteins(LDL) and high density lipoproteins (HDL)

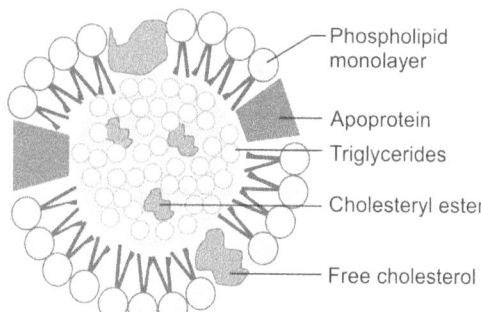

Fig. 1: Structure of lipoprotein.

- Lipoproteins are conjugated proteins. These are spherical bodies made up of lipid and proteins.
- The outer layer has polar heads phospholipid, apoproteins and free cholesterol and inner core contains non-polar lipids such as TAG, tails of PL, cholesteryl esters (**Fig. 1**).

Transport of Lipids (Fig. 2)

A. Metabolism of Chylomicrons:
- It is synthesised in intestine and it contains apoB-48 and apo A. It transports dietary TAG from intestines to adipose tissues.
- It is secreted into the lymphatic system and reach blood stream via thoracic duct.
- Apo C and E are added from HDL in the circulation.
- Apo C-II activates lipoprotein lipase and TAG is removed from CM. Lipoprotein lipase hydrolyses TAG to fatty acid and glycerol. The resulting CM is called Chylomicron remnant – rich in cholesterol esters and cholesterol. CM remnant is taken up by receptors in liver

B. VLDL metabolism:
- TAG synthesised from liver (endogenous) is converted to form nascent VLDL by combining with cholesterol.
- VLDL also contains apoB-100, apo-E and small amounts of apo- C.
- Nascent VLDL is hydrolysed by lipoprotein lipase in peripheral tissues and releases FA and glycerol. Apo–C is transferred back to HDL
- **Metabolism of chylomicrons and VLDL**

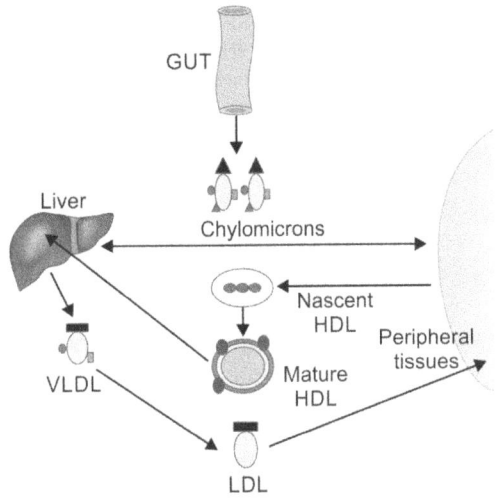

Fig. 2: Metabolism of lipoproteins.

- There will be exchange of TAG from VLDL to HDL and cholesterol ester from HDL to VLDL by cholesterol ester transfer protein.
- Following this there will be formation of VLDL remnant or Intermediate density lipoprotein which will be taken up by liver via LDL receptors or by removal of TAG by further hydrolysis.

C. **LDL metabolism**
- LDL transports cholesterol from liver to peripheral tissues.
- It has only apo-B100.
- Most of the LDL is derived from VLDL but a small part is directly released from the liver.
- LDL is taken by peripheral tissues and by hepatocytes by **receptor mediated endocytosis**—this is a regulated mechanism.
- LDL is also removed by an unregulated independent mechanism by scavenger receptors by forming foam cells. This mechanism is active when blood cholesterol level is very high.

D. **Metabolism and functions of HDL**
- Main transport form of cholesterol from peripheral tissues to liver.
- Anti-atherogenic known as good cholesterol.
- Involved in reverse cholesterol transport.
- HDL sub-fractions- HDL-I (bad and contains only Apo E), HDL-2.
- Good and anti-atherogenic, HDL-3 contains Apo A-II and its role is controversial.
- Acts as a reservoir for apoproteins which can be donated to or received from other lipoproteins.
- As an anti-oxidant it prevents the oxidation of LDL

Metabolism:
- Intestinal cells synthesise HDL which is discoidal in shape.
- Free cholesterol derived from peripheral tissue is taken up by HDL. It is mediated by ABC protein which is a cholesterol efflux regulator protein (CETP).
- The esterified cholesterol moves into the interior of HDL disc.
- Mature HDL is sphere in shape and loaded with cholesterol esters – HDL-3
- These spheres are taken up by liver cells by apo A I mediated receptor mechanism.
- Hepatic lipase hydrolyses HDL phospholipid and TAG, and CE is released into liver cells.
- CETP transfers cholesterol from HDL to VLDL and LDL in exchange for TAG to form HDL -2.

3. **What is the normal pH of blood? Discuss how the pH of blood is maintained.**

Refer 2003 Essay 47 2005 Essay 4.

4. **Discuss the metabolism of phenylalanine. Write a note on the inborn error associated with phenylalanine.**

Refer 2005 Essay 3.

5. **Explain the mode of action of enzymes and describe the factors affecting enzyme activity? Brief the analytical uses of enzymes with example.**

Ans:
- **Mode of action of enzymes: Refer 2016 Short Note 2.**

- **Factors affecting enzyme activity:** Refer 2013 Essay 5-b
- **Analytical uses of enzymes (Diagnostic)** 2016 Short Answer Question 25.

6. **Describe the reactions of Krebs cycle and its regulation? Add a note on its anaplerotic role.**

Ans:
Refer 2004 Essay 1
Anaplerotic role: They are filling up reactions or influx reactions or replenishing reactions which supply 4 C units to the TCA cycle. By this, the intermediates of TCA cycle can serve as a source of precursors of biosynthetic pathways such as **(Fig. 3):**
- Succinyl-CoA for heme synthesis
- Amino acids can be derived from the intermediates. For example: Glutamic acid from alpha-ketoglutarate, aspartate from oxaloacetate.

To make all these intermediates available continuously, anaplerotic reactions will fill up the supply. The anaplerotic reactions are:

- Conversion of pyruvate and CO_2 to oxaloacetate by pyruvate carboxylase which require biotin, ATP and Mg^{++}.
- Transamination of aspartate to form oxaloacetate and transamination of glutamate to form α-ketoglutarate by transaminase enzymes with PLP as the coenzyme.
- Deamination of glutamate by glutamate dehydrogenase irreversibly to produce α-ketoglutarate.
- Succinyl-CoA can be synthesized from carbon skeletons of amino acids— valine, isoleucine and methionine and also from odd chain fatty acid propionyl-CoA.
- A cytoplasmic enzyme—NADP dependent malic enzyme converts pyruvate to malate which can enter into mitochondria as an intermediate of TCA cycle.
- Aromatic amino acids such as phenyl alanine and tyrosine are degraded to form fumarate.

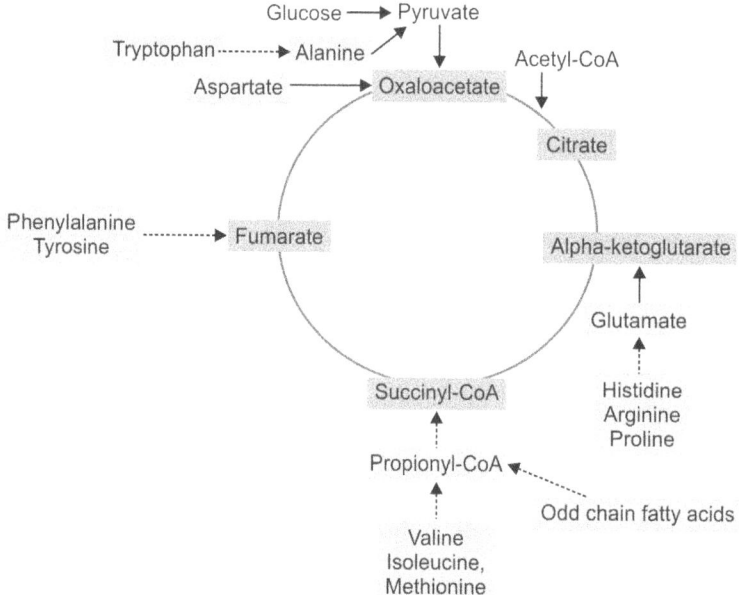

Fig. 3: Influx of intermediates (anaplerotic reactions).

7. **Describe the process of replication in prokaryotes. Add a note on inhibitors of DNA replication.**

Refer 2007 Essay 9.

8. **Explain the catabolic pathways of tyrosine and disorders associated with tyrosine metabolism.**

Refer 2015 Essay 6 and 2012 Short Note 38.

II. WRITE NOTES ON

1. **Competitive inhibition of enzyme activity.**

Refer 2015 Short Note 9.

2. **Biochemical features seen in blood and urine of a patient with hemolytic anemia.**

Ans: Biochemical features of hemolytic anemia: Hemolytic anemia occurs with premature destruction of RBCs and the bone marrow is not able to compensate for the loss leading to anemia and related symptoms.
- **The causes** include sickle cell anemia, G6PD deficiency, infections, toxins and some drugs.
- **Blood findings:**
  - Serum lactate dehydrogenase (LDH) is elevated, especially isoenzymes 1 and 2
  - Serum haptoglobin is low and serves as a diagnostic criterion for hemolysis
  - Elevated unconjugated bilirubin in indicative of hemolysis (though not specific)
- **Urine findings:**
  - Hemoglobinuria
  - Hemosiderin in urine.

3. **Functions of vitamin C.**

Refer 2005 ESSAY 5 Biochemical functions of Vitamin C.

4. **Anaplerotic role of citric acid cycle.**

Refer Essay 6 **(Fig. 3)**.

They are filling up reactions or influx reactions or replenishing reactions which supply 4 C units to the TCA cycle. By this, the intermediates of TCA cycle can serve as a source of precursors of biosynthetic pathways such as:
- Succinyl-CoA for heme synthesis.
- Amino acids can be derived from the intermediates, e.g.: Glutamic acid from alpha-ketoglutarate, aspartate from oxaloacetate.

To make all these intermediates available continuously, anaplerotic reactions will fill up the supply. The anaplerotic reactions are:
- Conversion of pyruvate and CO_2 to oxaloacetate by pyruvate carboxylase which require biotin, ATP and Mg^{++}.
- Transamination of aspartate to form oxaloacetate and transamination of glutamate to form α-ketoglutarate by transaminase enzymes with PLP as the coenzyme.
- Deamination of glutamate by glutamate dehydrogenase irreversibly to produce α-ketoglutarate.
- Succinyl-CoA can be synthesized from carbon skeletons of amino acids—valine, isoleucine and methionine and also from odd chain fatty acid propionyl CoA.
- A cytoplasmic enzyme—NADP dependent malic enzyme converts pyruvate to malate which can enter into mitochondria as an intermediate of TCA cycle.
- Aromatic amino acids such as phenylalanine and tyrosine are degraded to form fumarate.

5. **Define gluconeogenesis and explain the various steps.**

Refer 2007 Essay 1.

6. **Formation and fate of pyruvate.**

Ans:
Formation of Pyruvate: Pyruvate is derived from aerobic glycolysis and then oxidatively decarboxylated to acetyl-CoA by pyruvate dehydrogenase –in mitochondria and finally enters into TCA cycle.

Formation of pyruvate by aerobic Glycolysis: (Emden Meyerhof Pathway): Glycolysis is the primary and very important metabolism for energy source by oxidation of glucose during both aerobic and anaerobic conditions. The pathway takes place in cytosol of all cells.

Reactions of the Pathway: The reactions involved in glycolysis may be divided in three phases (**Fig. 4**):
1. Energy investment phase
2. Splitting phase
3. Energy generation phase

I. Energy investment phase:
1. Glucose is phosphorylated to glucose-6-phosphate in the presence of glucokinase/hexokinase. It is an irreversible step. The two enzymes are having different Km values for their substrate. Hexokinase has high affinity for glucose than glucokinase. Glucokinase is specific for glucose only but hexokinase acts on glucose, fructose and mannose:

   Glucose $\xrightarrow[\text{ATP/Mg+ ADP}]{\text{Glucokinase/hexokinase}}$ Glucose-6-phosphate

2. Glucose-6-phosphate is isomerised to fructose-6-phoshpate in the presence of phosphohexose isomerase. It is a reversible step.

   Glucose-6-phosphate $\xrightleftharpoons{\text{Phosphohexose isomerase}}$ Fructose-6-phosphate

3. Fructose-6-phosphate takes up one more phosphate at 1st carbon and converted to fructose 1, 6-bisphosphate in the presence of phosphofructokinase (PFK). It is an irreversible step.

   Fructose-6-phosphate $\xrightarrow{\text{Phosphofructo-kinase (PFK)}}$ Fructose 1, 6-bisphosphate

   PFK is the rate limiting or key enzyme of this pathway. It is also allosteric and inducible.

II. Splitting Phase:
4. Six carboned fructose 1, 6-bisphosphate is split into 2 molecules of 3 carbon units namely dihydroxyacetone phosphate (DHAP) and glyceraldehydes-3-phosphate in the presence of aldolase-I. These two molecules are interconvertable in the presence of triose phosphate isomerase.

   Fructose 1, 6-bisphosphate $\xrightarrow{\text{Aldolase-I}}$ DHAP +Glyceraldehyde-3-phosphate

   DHAP $\xrightleftharpoons{\text{Triose phosphate isomerase}}$ Glyceraldehyde-3-phosphate

III. Energy generation phase:
5. Glyceraldehyde-3-phosphate is converted into high energy intermediate called 1,3 bisphosphoglyceric acid in the presence of glyceraldehyde-3-phosphate dehydrogenase. This is a reversible reaction. During this process NAD is reduced to NADH which enters into ETC to produce ATP. This is an example for oxidative phosphorylation.

   Glyceraldehydes-3-phosphate

   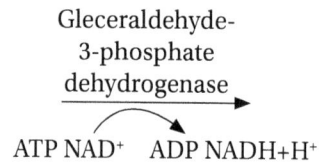

   1,3-bisphosphoglycerate

   1,3- bisphosphoglycerate contains high energy bond

6. **1st substrate level phosphorylation:** 1, 3-bisphosphoglycerate is converted to 3-phosphoglycerate by phosphoglycerate kinase to generate one molecule of ATP.

   1, 3-bisphosphoglycerate

   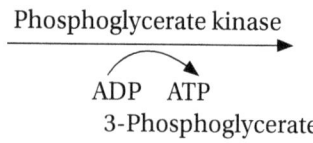

   3-Phosphoglycerate

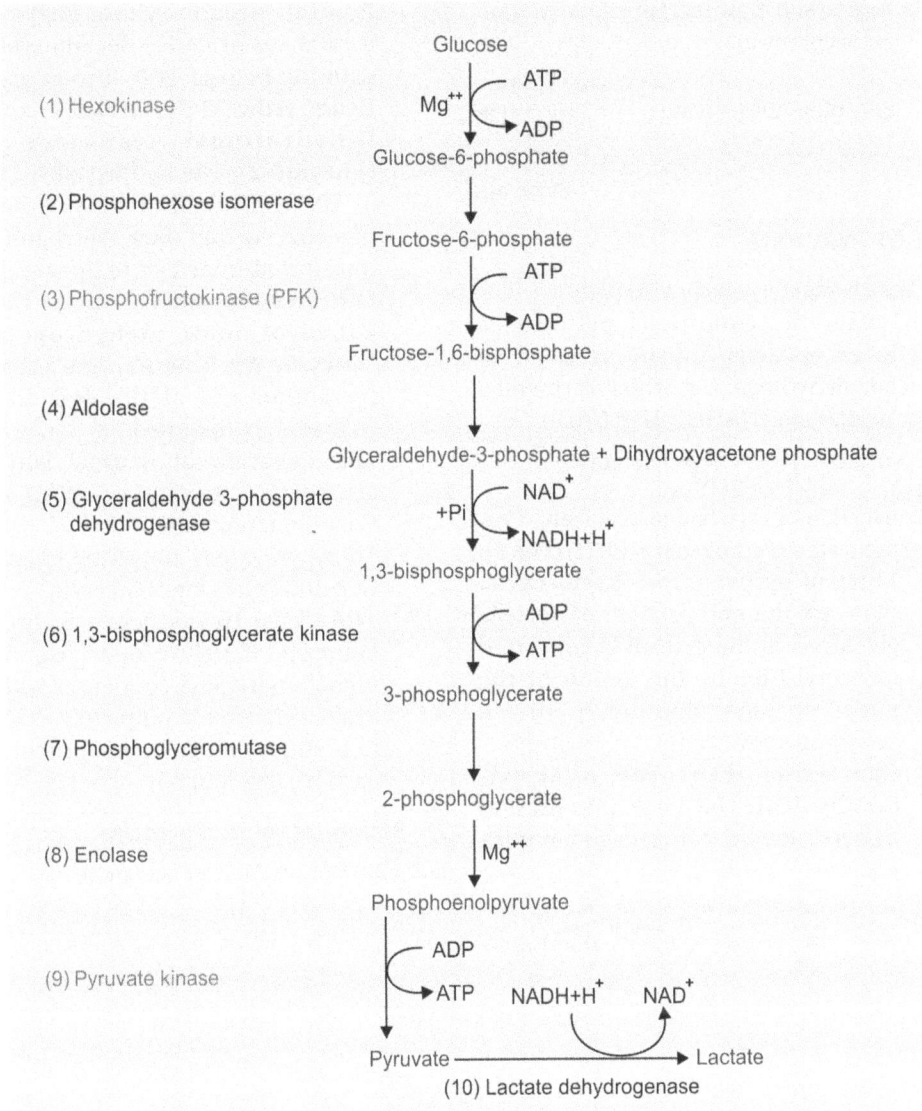

Fig. 4: Glycolysis.

7. 3-phosphoglycerate is converted to 2-phosphoglycerate catalysed by phosphoglycerate mutase.

    3-phosphoglycerate $\xrightarrow{\text{Phosphoglycerate mutase}}$ 2-phosphoglycerate

8. 2-phosphoglycerate is converted to high-energy compound called phosphoenolpyruvate (PEP) in the presence of enolase. This enzyme is inhibited by fluoride to stop glycolysis. Fluoride is added to the sample for estimation of blood glucose.

    2-phosphoglycerate $\xrightarrow{\text{Enolase}}$ Phosphoenolpyruvate ($Mg + H_2O$)

9. **2nd substrate level phosphorylation:** Phosphoenolpyruvate is converted to pyruvate with generation ATP; it is the

second substrate level phosphorylation in this pathway.

$$\text{Phosphoenolpyruvate} \xrightarrow[\text{ADP} \quad \text{ATP}]{\text{Pyruvate kinase}} \text{Pyruvate}$$

FATE OF PYRUVATE

1. *Conversion of pyruvate to lactate:*
   In anaerobic conditions pyruvate is reduced to lactate in the presence of lactate dehydrogenase, which is essential for oxidation of NADH + H to NAD^+.

   $$\text{Pyruvate} \xrightarrow[\text{LDH/NADH}]{} \text{Lactate}$$

2. Conversion of pyruvate to acetacetyl-CoA by pyruvate dehydrogenase (PDH) **(Fig. 5)**:
   - **Entry of pyruvate into Krebs cycle:** Pyruvate the end product of aerobic glycolysis in the cytosol is converted to acetyl-CoA by the action of the multi enzyme complex pyruvate dehydrogenase (PDH).
   - **Conversion of pyruvate to acetyl-CoA by PDH:** The 3 enzymes present in pyruvate dehydrogenase complex are:

- **Pyruvate decarboxylase (Enzyme I):** It catalyses oxidative decarboxylation with the help of TPP—its coenzyme. Hydroxyethyl-TPP is formed.
- **Dihydrolipoyl transacetylase (Enzyme-2):** The hydroxyethyl group of TPP is oxidised to acetyl group by this enzyme and then acetyl group is transferred from TPP to lipoamide to form acetyl lipoamide.
- **Dihydrolipoate dehydrogenase (Enzyme 3):** This enzyme oxidises lipoamide and at the end all the cofactors are reformed.
- The coenzymes of pyruvate dehydrogenase are 5 co-enzymes—NAD, FAD, CoA, lipoic acid and TPP
- Thus pyruvate is converted to acetyl-CoA and enters into TCA cycle
- **TCA Cycle:** Two carboned acetyl-CoA enter into the citric acid cycle in the mitochondria and condenses with 4C oxaloacetate and completely oxidized to produce energy in the form of ATP and CO_2 and water.

7. **Biological value of proteins.**

Refer 2015 Short Answer Question 10.

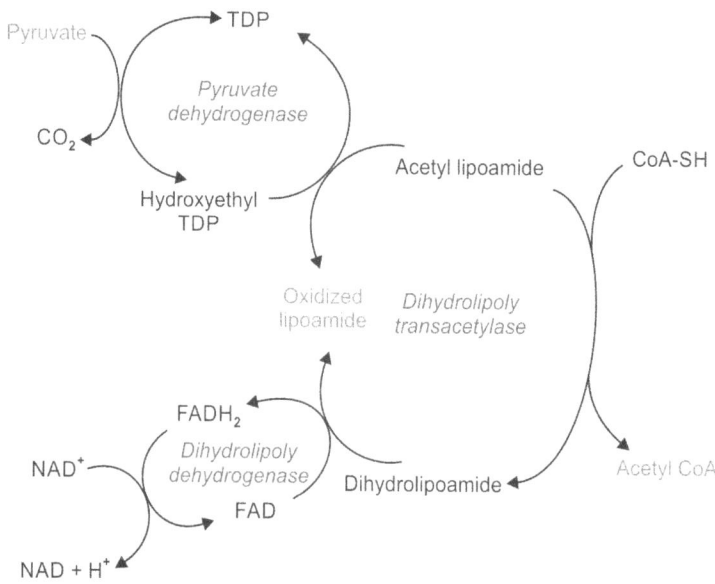

Fig. 5: Reactions of pyruvate dehydrogenase.

8. **Enumerate the compounds derived from cholesterol and mention their biochemical functions.**

Refer 2010 Short Note 29.

9. **Synthesis and regulation of porphyrins.**

Refer 2008 ESSAY 2. Synthesis of Heme and Regulation.

10. **Structure and functions of mitochondria.**

Refer 2013 SAQ 43 (**Fig. 6**).
- Mitochondria is a sub-cellular organelle present in the cytoplasm.
- It is rod like or spherical double membrane structure.
- The inner membrane is folded inside to form cristae, which increase the surface area. Cristae are flat form for ETC cycle enzymes.
- Between two membranes space is present called as intra-mitochondrial space, which contain enzymes like:
  a. Inner mitochondrial membrane contains enzymes of ETC
  b. Fluid matrix contains enzymes of citric acid cycle, urea cycle, heme synthesis, beta oxidation of fatty acids.
- Mitochondrion is major factory for synthesis of ATP, hence called as power house of cell.
- Mitochondria contain its own DNA and RNA for synthesis of proteins (enzymes).

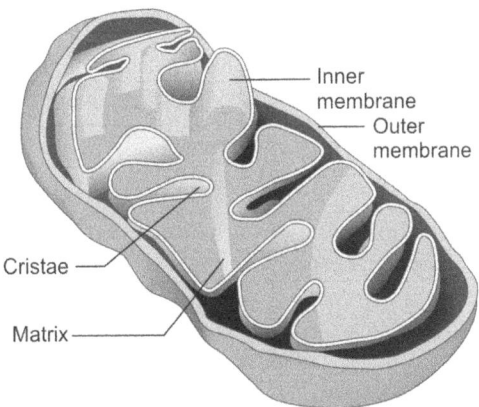

Fig. 6: Mitochondria.

Functions of Mitochondria

1. It helps in oxidative phosphorylation It is called **power house of cell** because it synthesizes ATP through electron transport chain. Energy released from oxidation foodstuffs is trapped as chemical energy in the form of ATP. Inner mitochondrial membrane has the ETC which has got 4 complexes through which electrons are transferred from metabolic reactions to synthesize ATP at the 5th complex by oxidative phosphorylation.
2. Important metabolic pathways occur only in the mitochondria and the enzymes of those pathways and located in various parts of the mitochondria, e.g., TCA cycle, beta oxidation of fatty acids, ketone bodies.
3. Some of the metabolic pathways occur partly in mitochondria and partly in cytosol, e.g., urea cycle, gluconeogenesis, heme synthesis and pyrimidine synthesis.
4. **Cytochrome P450** enzyme systems present in inner mitochondrial membrane is involved in steroidogenesis.
5. **Mitochondrial DNA:** Mitochondria have specific DNA. Message from the DNA can synthesize mitochondrial proteins by the ribosome of mitochondria. Hence mitochondria are considered as the evolutionary remnant of parasites.

11. **Compounds derived from glycine and their functions.**

Refer 2004 Essay 3.

12. **Hyperammonemias.**

Refer 2005 Essay 7 Hyperammonemia.

13. **Copper metabolism and its applied aspects.**

Ans:
- Copper is a trace element present in muscles, liver, bone marrow, brain, kidney, hair and heart.
- It is present in enzymes such as ceruloplasmin, cytochrome oxidase, superoxide dismutase, ALA synthase, tyrosinase and lysyl oxidase.

- The non-enzymatic proteins which contain copper are the storage form in liver such as hepato-cuprein. Others are cerebrocupein in brain, hemocupreine in RBC and erythrocuprein in bone marrow.
- **Normal Requirement of copper:** Adults—1.5 to 3 mg/day.
- **Dietary sources:** Cereals, meat, liver, green vegetables and nuts.
- **Absorption:** Only 10% of dietary copper is absorbed.
- **Excretion:** Mainly through bile.

Functions

- It helps in absorption and incorporation of iron into Hb.
- It is necessary for the action of tyrosinase enzyme in tyrosine metabolism.
- It acts a co-factor for hydroxylation reactions done by vitamin C.
- It increases HDL and so protects the heart.

Abnormal Metabolism of Copper

1. Wilson's disease:
   - It is an inherited autosomal recessive disease. Incidence is 1 in 50,000
   - The basic defect is a mutation in a gene encoding a copper binding ATPase in cells, required for excretion of copper from cells. Hence Cu gets accumulated to produce Cu toxicity.
   - Increased copper content in hepatocytes inhibits the incorporation of copper to apo-ceruloplasmin.
2. Menke's Kinky hair syndrome:
   - It is due to a defect in the intestinal absorption of copper.
   - Copper may be trapped by metallothionein in the intestinal cells.
   - The manifestations of Menke's disease include decreased copper in plasma and urine, anemia, and depigmentation of hair.
3. Copper deficiency anemia;
   - Copper deficiency results in microcytic normochromic anemia.
4. Copper toxicity:
   - This may be due to increased intake of copper which causes toxic manifestations. It enhances the production of free radicals and metallothionein (MT) which binds with copper and makes it non-toxic.
   - Chronic toxicity produces diarrhea and blue-green discoloration of saliva.
   - Copper poisoning produces hemolysis, hemoglobinuria, proteinuria and kidney damage.

14. Telomerase and its application.

Refer 2016 Short Answer Question 33 and 2017 Short Answer Question 19.
- There are 23 pairs of chromosomes in human beings.
- Chromosomes—supercoiled chromatin fibres are condensed to form chromosomes.
- Center of the chromosomes is centromere which is rich in Adenine and Thymine- with repeated DNA sequences of about 1 million base pairs with specific binding proteins. This region is called kinetochore which is the anchor for mitotic division.
- The 4 end pieces of chromosomes are called as **telomeres.**
- Replication will not take place upto these ends—3' or 5' ends
- Telomerases or telomere terminal transferases do the job of replicating at these end pieces of chromosomes.
- Telomerase acts as a reverse transcriptase to synthesise this small DNA strand.

Applications

- In old age telomerase activity is lost leading to chromosomal instability and cell death.
- Drugs which prevent expression of gene for telomerase act as anticancer agents.

15. Lesch-Nyhan syndrome.

Refer 2012 Short Answer Question 18.

16. Inhibitors of Purine nucleotide biosynthesis.

- Certain structural analogs act as competitive inhibitors in purine nucleotide synthesis. They in turn bring about functionally inactive DNA affecting the normal cell division. Hence they are also used a anticancer drugs.

- Inhibitors:
  1. Mercaptopurine (synthetic purine analog): It inhibits conversion of IMP to GMP and AMP.
  2. Methotrexate (folate antagonists—PABA analog): It affects the reactions involving transfer of one carbon group. It inhibits formyl transferase.
  3. Azaserine (glutamine antagonist—Diazo-acetyl L-Serine): It inhibits reactions involving transfer of amino group from glutamine—Step 1 and 4
  4. 6-Thioguanine
  5. 8-Azaguanine } used as anticancer drugs inhibits enzymes of purine nucleotide pathway.
- The steps of purine nucleotide synthesis and the sites of inhibition are shown in **Figure 7**.

17. Metabolic acidosis.
Refer 2004 Short Note 16.

18. Absorption of dietary Iron.
Refer 2006 Essay 8 Absorption.

19. Biochemical features of cancer cells.
- Abnormal new growth of tissues in the body is known as neoplasm. It is classified into benign (harmless) and malignant.
- The term cancer denotes malignant tumors which can occur in any part of the body. Cells of benign tumors also have diminished growth control but they do not invade or spread metastasis
- Cancer cells have certain characteristic features by which they differ from normal cells.

Biochemical Features of Cancer Cells
- Cancer cells proliferate rapidly (**Fig. 8**).

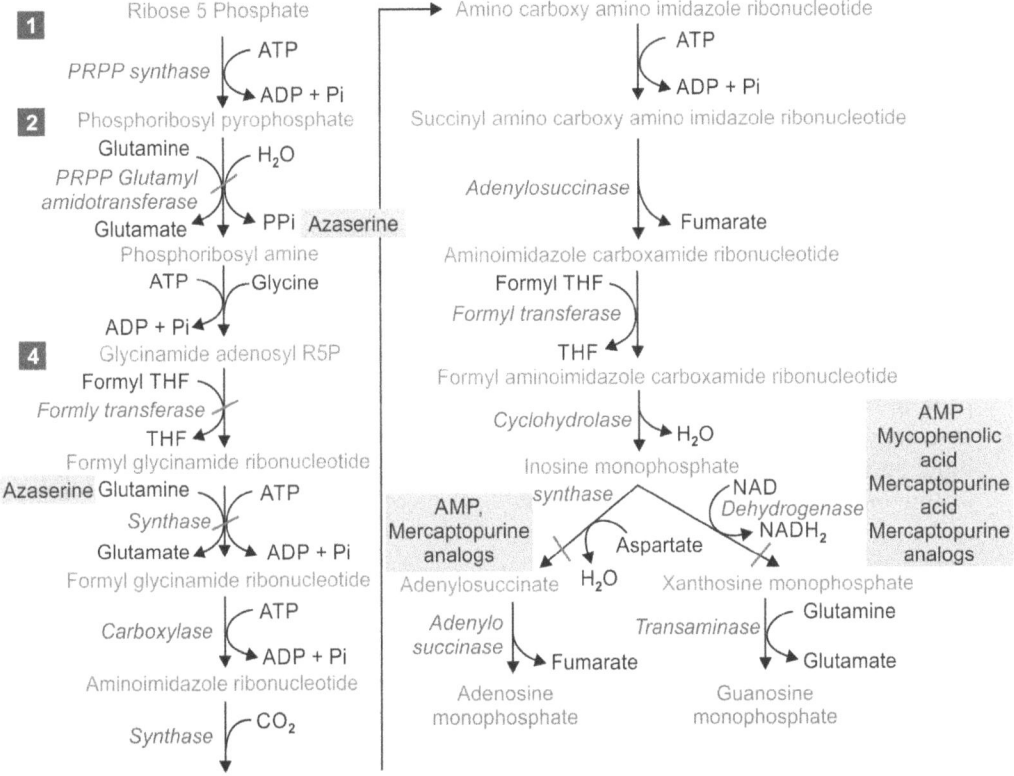

Fig. 7: Steps of purine nucleotide synthesis and the sites of inhibition.

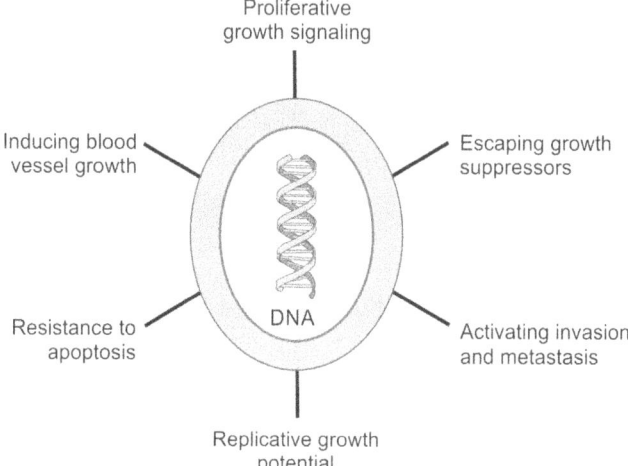

Fig. 8: Features of cancer cells.

- **The doubling time** is the time taken by a tumor to double its size. It is a constant and varies between 10 days to 450 days in human beings.
- They are self sufficient in growth signalling.
- They have diminished growth control.
- They display increased genomic mutation at the level of nucleotide by insertion or deletion or by chromosomal rearrangements.
- They display loss of contact inhibition in culture in vitro.
- They invade local tissues and spread to other parts of the body hich is known as **metastasis.**
- They stimulate local angiogenesis and they are not sensitive to antigrowth signals.
- They are able to evade **apoptosis or programmed cell death.**
- **Oncology** is the study of cancer including biochemical and genetic mechanisms of uncontrolled growth of cancer cells and their ablity to metastasize and the treatment for destroying cancer cells.
- **Cancer** cells become round in shape. There is loss of contact inhibition of movement.

20. Conjugation reactions in xenobiotics.

Refer 2004 Short Note 14.

21. Fluid mosaic model of cell.

Refer 2008 Short Note 5 (Structure of cell membrane).

22. State the differences between:
   a. Starch and glycogen
   b. Dextrin and dextran

Ans:

a. **Starch and glycogen.**
   Both are homopolysaccharides—containing glucose:
   i. **Starch**: It is a plant polysaccharide made up of glucose:
      - It is a linear polysaccharides.
      - It is composed of amylose and amylopectin.
      - Amylose is made up of glucose units with alpha 1,4 glycosidic linkages to form an unbranched long chain.
      - Amylopectin is the insoluble part made up of highly branched glucose units made by alpha 1,6 glycosidic linkage.
      - Alpha-amylase (α-amylase) enzyme acts on $\alpha1,4$ glycosidic bonds to split starch into dextrins and to α-maltose.
      - Beta-amylase (β-amylase) enzyme acts on $\alpha1,6$ glycosidic bonds to split amylopectin into limit dextrin or residual dextrin.
   ii. **Glycogen:** Animal polysaccharide
      - It is a branched polysaccharide.
      - Reserve carbohydrate in animals stored in liver and skeletal muscles.

- It is made up of glucose units linked by α1,4 glycosidic bonds in straight chain and α1,6 glycosidic bonds at branching points.
- It is more branched and more compact.

b. **Dextrin and dextran.**
Both are homopolysaccharides containing glucose.
  i. **Dextrin:**
     - It is a hydrolytic poduct of starch.
     - Alpha-amylase (α-amylase) enzyme acts on α1,4 glycosidic bonds of starch to split into dextrins and α-maltose
     - Beta-amylase (β-amylase) enzyme acts on α1,6 glycosidic bonds to split amylopectin into limit dextrin or residual dextrin.
  ii. **Dextran:**
     - Branched polymer of glucose with 1-6, 1-4 and 1-3 glycosidic bonds.
     - Used for intravenous infusion for treatment of hypovolemic shock as plasma expander.

23. Beta oxidation of palmitic acid.

Refer 2006 Essay 5.

24. Mention the recommended dietary allowance, biochemical functions and deficiency manifestations of vitamin-E

Refer 2004 Short Note 10.

25. Chemiosmotic theory and mechanism of ATP synthesis.

Refer 2006 Short Note 5.

26. Brief the risk factors of cardiovascular disease and its preventive methods.

Refer 2018 Short Note 10 (Changes in atherosclerosis) and 2014 Short Note 45 (Prevention of atherosclerosis)

Risk Factors of Cardiovascular Diseases
- Lipid profile
- **Hyprcholesteriemia:** Normal concen-tration of total serum cholesterol is 150 to 200 mg/dL. If the level is increased it is called hypercholesterolemia
- Lipoproteins
    - Elevated LDL cholesterol level and low HDL cholesterol (less than 60 mg/dL). High apoB: ApoA ratio more than 1.4— high risk
    - Lp(a)—levels more than 30 mg/dL
    - Increased triacylglycerol—more than 175 mg/dL (normal—50 -175 mg/dL)
- Cigarette smoking: High risk factor—modifiable—depends upon age
- Risk factors affecting plasma cholesterol level:
  1. Genetic factors
  2. **Sex:** Cholesterol level is high in males. Females have reduced level due to the protective actions of female sex hormones
  3. **Age:** Level rises with age. Rate of LDL receptor synthesis is decreased in old age
  4. **Diet:**
     - Saturated fatty acids increase blood cholesterol due to down regulation of LDL receptors.
     - Polyunsaturated fatty acids stimulate excretion of cholesterol and increase catabolic rate of LDL due to up regulation of LDL receptors
     - Dietary fibers can lower blood cholesterol level
  5. **Exercise:** Regular exercise will increase HDL level and make the total cholesterol level low.
  6. **Body weight:** Obesity may be due to sedentary life which is accompanied by increased level of FFA which is incorporated into VLDL which is converted to LDL which causes hypercholesterolemia.
  7. **Stress:** Can stimulate secretion of Catecholamines which in turn synthesise VLDL and LDL to cause high level of cholesterol.
  8. **Other diseases:** Diabetes mellitus, hypertension, hypothyroidism. Nephrotic syndrome can cause hypercholesterolemia.

27. What is nitrogen balance? Enumerate the factors affecting nitrogen balance.

Ans:
- A normal healthy adult is said to be in nitrogen balance which means the dietary intake of N_2 equals the daily loss through urine feces and skin.
- When excretion exceeds intake, it is negative nitrogen balance, when intake exceeds excretion, it is positive nitrogen balance.
- Positive nitrogen balance—in growth and pregnancy.
- Negative nitrogen balance—in acute illness—after trauma, surgery, burns and in protein deficiency.

Factors Affecting Nitrogen Balance
- Growth—+ve nitrogen balance during growing period
- Hormones—growth hormones insulin, androgen, +ve nitrogen balance
- Pregnancy—positive nitrogen balance
- Convalescence—positive nitrogen balance
- Acute illness—after trauma, surgery, burns, negative nitrogen balance
- Protein deficiency—negative nitrogen balance.

28. List the inborn errors associated with heme metabolism and their features.

Ans:
A. Disorders connected with heme synthesis—porphyrias: Refer 2009 Short Note 5.
B. Disorders connected with catabolism of heme. Congenital hyperbilirubinemia—Refer 2007 Short Note 2.

29. Oral glucose tolerance test: Indications, method and interpretation.

Refer 2008 Short Note 30.
Abnormal GTT: Refer 2015 Short Answer Question 8.

30. Regulation and significance of HMP shunt.

Refer 2007 Short Note 5 and 2010 Essay 2.

31. Brief the functions and diagnostic importance of plasma proteins present in the beta region of electrophoretic pattern (Fig. 9).

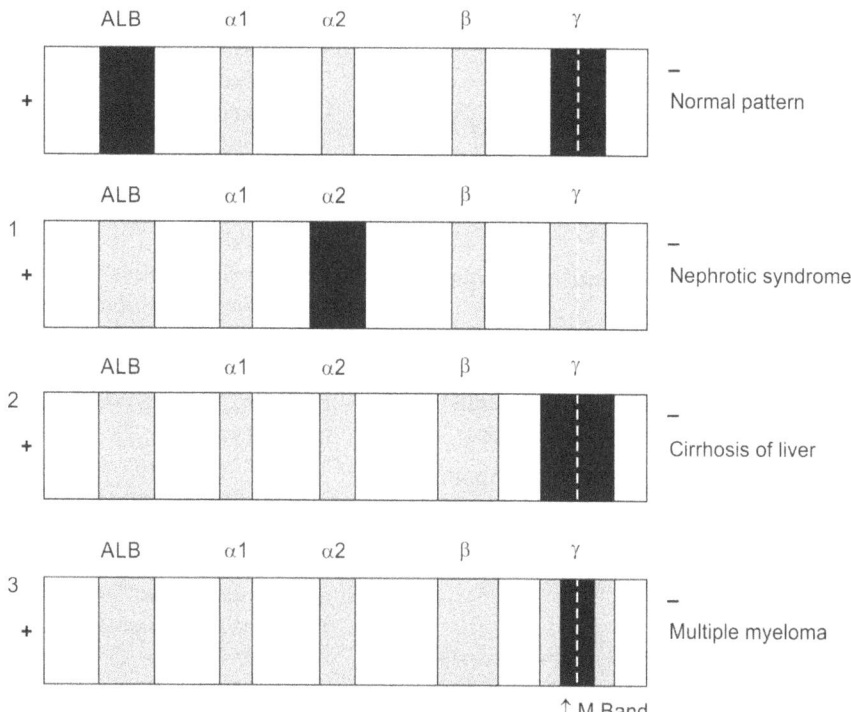

Fig. 9: Electrophoretic pattern of plasma proteins.

Table 1: Plasma proteins—in Beta band of EPP.

S. No.	Names of proteins—β band	Normal level in plasma—mg/dL	Compounds carried and functions	Clinical importance
1.	Hemopexin	50–100	Heme Loss of heme and iron	↑ - Diabetes mellitus, pregnancy, hematological malignancy ↓ - hemolysis and liver dysfunction
2.	Transferrin	200–300	Iron	↑ - Pregnancy, iron deficiency anemia, ↓ - Chronic infection, malnutrition, hemolysis and liver dysfunction
2.	Fibrinogen	200—400	Helps in coagulation. Acute phase protein	↑ - Acute inflammation—pneumonia, TB, rheumatic diseases, nephrotic syndrome ↓ - Complications during delivery – DIVC, antepartum hemorrhage, eclampsia
3.	C- reactive protein	Less than 10 mg/L	Acute phase protein, stimulate complement activity and phagocytosis	↑ - coronary artery disease, inflammation
4.	LDL	80–130	Transports cholesterol from liver to peripheral tissues carries cholesterol, phospholipids and TGL. Contains ApoB -100	↑ - Myocardial infarction

Ans:
- Electrophoresis refers to the migration of charged particles in an electric field. It is used for the separation of serum proteins
- Bands of plasma protein electrophoresis Refer 2006 Short Note 30.

Norma bands

Five bands:
1. Albumin (55–65%),
2. Alpha-1 globulin (2–4%),
3. Alpha-2 globulin (6–12%),
4. Beta globulin (8–12%)
5. Gamma globulin (12–22%).

Albumin has maximum and gamma globulin has maximum mobility.

Proteins in beta region of electrophoretic pattern and their importance:

β-globulin: They include **(Table 1)**:

Hemopexin, transferrin, $β_2$, fibrinogen, C-reactive protein (CRP), low density lipoprotein(LDL).

---

32. Mention the causes, signs, symptoms and treatment of hypokalemia.

- Potassium is the major intracellular cation and maintains intracellular osmotic pressure.
- Normal potassium level → 3.5 – 5.2 mEq/L.
- **Hypokalemia**: Plasma potassium level below 3 mEq/L is hypokalemia.
- **Causes:**
  1. Increased renal excretion: Cushing's syndrome, hyperaldosteronism, hyperreninism, hypomagnesemia, renal tubular acidosis.
  2. Shift/redistribution of potassium: alkalosis, Insulin therapy, thyrotoxic periodic paralysis, hypokalemic periodic paralysis.
  3. Gastrointestinal loss: Diarrhea, vomiting, aspiration, deficient intake, malabsorption
  4. Intravenous saline infusion in excess.
  5. Drugs: Insulin, salbutamide, osmotic diuretics, thiazides, corticosteroids.
- **Signs and symptoms:** Muscular weakness, fatigue, muscle cramps, hypotension, decreased reflexes, palpitation, cardiac arrhythmias, and cardiac arrest. ECG waves are flattened, T wave is inverted. This may be corrected by oral feeding of orange juice.
- **Treatment:** Adequate supplementation of potassium. About 100 mmol KCl per day in 3-4 divided doses.

33. **Explain the precipitation reactions of protein.**

Refer 2012 Short Note 17.

34. **Describe the DNA repair mechanisms with suitable clinical examples.**

Refer 2003 Short Note 11 and 2007 Essay 9.

35. **Explain the role of kidney in regulation of pH.**

Refer 2005 ESSAY 4 and 2003 Essay 4. (Renal regulation/II line of defense).

36. **Mention the sources, recommended dietary allowance, function and deficiency manifestation of copper.**

Refer 2021 Short Note 13 Copper metabolism.

37. **Brief the causes, symptoms and treatment of gout?**

Refer 2005 Short Note 17.

38. **Applications of DNA recombinant technology.**

Refer 2006 Short Note 31.

39. **Brief the in vitro thyroid function tests.**

Refer 2003 Short Note 16.

40. **Explain the cellular signalling and defense mechanism of free radicals.**

Refer 2010 SAQ 21, 2018 SAQ 39.

Free radicals are molecules or molecular species that contain one or more unpaired electrons and are capable of independent existence.

Reactive Oxygen Species-(ROS)

- They are oxygen free radicals
- The products of partial reduction of oxygen are highly reactive and cause damage in living systems.
- The members of ROS include—superoxide anion radical (O_2^-), hydroperoxyl radical (HOO·), lipid peroxide radical (ROO·), nitric oxide (NO^+) etc.
- ROS have short life span and generate new ROS by chain reaction
- They are extremely reactive and damage all tissues.

LIPID PEROXIDATION

It is auto-oxidation of lipids exposed to toxic oxygen radicals to cause damage to tissues in vivo.

It is a chain reaction to get continuous supply of free radicals to initiate and elongate peroxidation.

Antioxidants are the substances which can prevent lipid peroxidation, e.g., vitamin E, selenium.

PUFA present in cell membrane are easily destroyed by peroxidation.

Phases of lipid peroxidation: There are three phases of lipid peroxidation:

1. Initiation; 2. Propagation; 3. Termination phases.

1. **Initiation phase:**
   - Primary event is the production of R' (carbon centered radical) or ROO' (lipid peroxide radical) by the interaction of PUFA with free radicals
   - Reaction 1-A: $RH + OH' \longrightarrow R' + H_2O$
   - Reaction 1-B: $ROOH \longrightarrow ROO' + H^+$
   The R' and ROO' are degraded to malondialdehyde which can be estimated to measure the lipid peroxidation.

2. **Propagative phase:**
   - R' reacts with molecular oxygen forming peroxyl radical which can attack another PUFA.
   - Reaction 2: $R' + O_2 \longrightarrow ROO'$
   - Reaction 3: $ROO' + RH \longrightarrow ROOH + R'$
   - The net result is the formation of ROOH—hydroperoxide
   - This occurs as a chain reaction or propagation
   - Accumulation of this lipid damages lead to the destruction of membranes.

3. **Termination phase:**
   - The above reaction proceeds until one peroxyl radical combines with another peroxyl radical to form inactive products
   - Reaction - 4A: $ROO' + ROO' \longrightarrow ROOR + O_2$
   - Reaction - 4B: $R' + R' \longrightarrow R-R$
   - Reaction - 4C: $ROO' + R' \longrightarrow RO-RO$

PREVENTION AND DEFENSE MECHANISMS OF PEROXIDATION

Role of antioxidants:

- Antioxidants are compounds which prevents lipid peroxidation or rancidity by free radicals or control the oxidation process.
  Types: I. As per the nature
- **Naturally occurring antioxidants**, e.g., vitamin E and C, selenium, β-carotene
- **Chemicals:** Butylated hydroxyanisole (BHA), butylated hydroxytoluene (BHT)
  As per their action: Two types—a) Preventive and b) Chain breaking antioxidants
  a. **Preventive antioxidants:** They will inhibit the initial production of free radicals. They are catalase, glutathione peroxidase and ethylenediaminetetraacetic acid (EDTA)
     - Catalase: $2H_2O_2 \longrightarrow O_2 + H_2O$
     - Glutathione peroxidase: $2H_2O_2 \longrightarrow 2H_2O$
     - EDTA
  b. **Chain breaking antioxidants:**
     - They inhibit the propagative phase
     - $O_2^- + O_2^- + 2H^+ \longrightarrow H_2O_2 + O_2$
     - They include: Superoxide dismutase, uric acid and Vit E
     - Vit E would intercept the peroxyl free radical and inactivate it before a PUFA can be attacked.
     - $T\text{-}OH + ROO' \longrightarrow TO' + ROOH$
     - The phenolic hydrogen of alpha tocopherol reacts with the peroxyl radical converting it to a hydroperoxide product.
     - The tocoperoxyl radical thus formed is stable and will not propagate the cycle any further.
     - This oxidative form of vit E is converted to vit E by ascorbic acid. Ascorbic acid becomes dehydroascorbate by reacting with vit E radical. Two molecules of Ddehydroascorbate combine together to form ascorbate.
     - Other antioxidants are ceruloplasmin, caffeine and beta-carotene.
  - Some antioxidants used in therapy are vitamin C, vitamin E, dimethylthiourea (DMTU), dimethyl sulfoxide, allopurinol.

MULTIPLE CHOICE QUESTIONS

1. **The marker enzyme of lysosome is:**
   A. Lactate dehydrogenase.
   B. Cathepsin
   C. Galactosyl transferase
   D. Glucose - 6 - phosphatase
   Ans: B. Cathepsin

2. **One of the following is a lysosomal disorder:**
   A. Inclusion cell disease
   B. Cystic fibrosis
   C. Alport's syndrome
   D. Prions disease
   Ans: A. Inclusion cell disease

3. **What is the biochemical basis for using sodium fluoride while collecting sample for glucose estimation?**
   A. For inhibiting glycolysis
   B. For better separation of serum
   C. For better separation of plasma
   D. For better estimation of cholesterol
   Ans: A. For inhibiting glycolysis

4. **A three-month-old child exclusively on breastfeeds presented with incessant crying, poor weight gain. Clinical examination revealed enlarged liver, cataract and positive Benedict's test of the urine. The most likely condition is:**
   A. Von Gierke's disease
   B. McArdle's disease
   C. Galactosemia
   D. Lactose intolerance
   Ans: C. Galactosemia (cataract)

5. **Which of the following is derived lipid?**
   A. Triacyl glycerol
   B. Plasmalogen
   C. Prostaglandin
   D. Ganglioside
   Ans: C. Prostaglandins

6. The major apolipoprotein seen in chylomicron is.
   A. Apo B48.
   B. Apo B100
   C. Apo AI
   D. Apo AII
   Ans: A. Apo B48

7. One of the following enzyme is not a protein:
   A. Lactase
   B. Hydrolase
   C. Ribozyme
   D. Ligase
   Ans: C. Ribozyme

8. To which class of enzymes is aldolase classified:
   A. Oxidoreductase
   B. Isomerase
   C. Lyase
   D. Ligase
   Ans: C. Lyase

9. Which vitamin is excreted as oxalic acid?
   A. Retinoic acid
   B. Ascorbic acid
   C. Folic acid
   D. Pantothenic acid
   Ans: B. Ascorbic acid (vitamin C)

10. The vitamin required for the synthesis of catecholamines is:
    A. Vitamin K
    B. Vitamin B12
    C. Vitamin C
    D. Vitamin B6
    Ans: D. Vitamin B6: Its Coenzyme PLP acts as a coenzyme for decarboxylation by dopamine carboxylase.

11. Which of the following is an uncoupler of oxidative phosphorylation?
    A. Carbon monoxide
    B. Cyanide
    C. Oligomycin
    D. 2,4 Dinitrophenol
    Ans: D. 2,4 Dinitrophenol

12. Physiological uncoupler of oxidative phosphorylation is one of the following.
    A. Thyroxine
    B. Tyrosine
    C. Valinomycin
    D. Carboxin
    Ans: A. Thyroxine

13. Citric acid cycle is otherwise called as amphibolic cycle because it has both:
    A. Anabolic and catabolic
    B. Mitochondrial and cytoplasmic
    C. Reversible and irreversible
    D. Protein and lipid substrates
    Ans: A. Anabolic and catabolic (amphibolic)

14. Total number of ATP's generated in one cycle of citric acid cycle is.
    A. 8
    B. 10
    C. 16
    D. 14
    Ans: B. 10 (Ten)

15. Which of the following causes negative nitrogen balance?
    A. Growth hormone
    B. Insulin
    C. Corticosteroid
    D. Androgen
    Ans: C. Corticosteroids

16. Factors affecting basal metabolic rate are all of the following except:
    A. Temperature
    B. Exercise
    C. Fever
    D. Glucagon
    Ans: D. Glucagon

17. Which of the following amino acid is required for synthesis of heme?
    A. Lysine
    B. Cysteine
    C. Phenylalanine
    D. Glycine
    Ans: D. Glycine (first step of heme synthesis –by ALA synthase)

18. Sickle cell anemia is characterized by the following except:
    A. Homozygous recessive inheritance
    B. Chronic hemolytic anemia, episodes of pain hyperbilirubinemia
    C. Polymerization of deoxyhemoglobin and under hypoxia
    D. Valine in position six of beta chain replaced by glutamate.

Ans: D. Valine in position six of beta chain is replaced by glutamate:
- This is a wrong statement.
- Correct answer is glutamic acid in the sixth position of beta chain of HbA is changed to valine in HbS.

19. Factors affecting the fluidity of the cell membrane are all of the following except:
    A. Trans fatty acids
    B. Cholesterol
    C. Tight junction
    D. Transition temperature

Ans: C. Tight junction

20. Impaired functions of aquaporins leads to:
    A. Diabetes mellitus
    B. Cirrhosis
    C. Nephrogenic diabetes insipidus
    D. Hartnup's disease

Ans: C. Nephrogenic diabetes insipidus

21. Which amino acid hydroxylation requires iron?
    A. Proline
    B. Tyrosine
    C. Cysteine
    D. Leucine

Ans: A. Proline

22. Which of the following analyte analysis require fasting specimen?
    A. Serum uric acid
    B. Serum alkaline phosphatase
    C. Serum triglycerides
    D. Serum protein

Ans: C. Serum triglycerides

23. The following ions can be quantitatively analyzed using flame photometer except:
    A. Sodium
    B. Lithium
    C. Calcium
    D. Cadmium

Ans: D. Cadmium

24. Which of the following hormones uses cAMP as second messenger?
    A. Glucagon
    B. Atrial natriuretic peptide
    C. Insulin
    D. Estrogen

Ans: A. Glucagon
(ANP—cyclic GMP; Insulin—tyrosin kinase and oestrogen—intracellular receptors)

25. Which of the following syndrome has primary hyperaldosteronism?
    A. Down syndrome
    B. Gilbert syndrome
    C. Conn's syndrome
    D. Cushing syndrome

Ans: C. Conn's syndrome—aldosterone secreting tumor
(Down's—Chromosomal disorder; Gilbert—congenital unconjugated hyperbilirubinemia, Cushing's—adrenal hyperfunction)

26. Which of the following enzymes uses selenium as cofactor?
    A. Hexokinase
    B. Transaminase
    C. Ferrochelatase
    D. 5' Deiodinase

Ans: D. 5' Deiodinase
(A. Hexokinase—Mg^{++}, C. Ferrochelatase—Fe)

27. Which of the following is non-heme iron containing protein?
    A. Cytochrome C1
    B. Catalase
    C. Nitric oxide synthase
    D. Transferrin

Ans: C. Nitric oxide synthase
(All the other three are iron containing proteins)

28. The following antioxidants are used commercially in food industry except:
    A. Butylated hydroxytoluene (BHT)
    B. Butylated hydroxyanisole (BHA)
    C. Vitamin E
    D. Vitamin A
Ans: D. Vitamin A
(All the other three are anti-oxidants used in food industry)

29. In which organelle does the aldehyde dehydrogenase produces the toxic acetaldehyde?
    A. Cytosol
    B. Endoplasmic reticulum
    C. Mitochondria
    D. Membrane of the cell
Ans: C. Mitochondria
(Cytosol—alcohol dehydrogenase)

30. Care should be taken while correcting metabolic acidosis to prevent sudden.
    A. Hyperkalemia
    B. Hypokalemia
    C. Hyponatremia
    D. Hypernatremia
Ans: B. Hypokalemia

31. High anion gap metabolic acidosis occurs in all of the following conditions except:
    A. Lactic acidosis
    B. Diabetic ketoacidosis
    C. Renal tubular acidosis
    D. Salicylate poisoning
Ans: C. Renal tubular acidosis
(All the other three conditions – A,B,D-can cause HAGMA)

32. Diagnostic criteria for [SIADH—syndrome of inappropriate antidiuretic hormone secretion] include all, except:
    A. Hyponatremia (<135mmol/L)
    B. Urine sodium (>20 mmol/L)
    C. Urine osmolality (>100 mOsm/kg)
    D. Increased plasma osmolality
Ans: D. Increased plasma osmolality
(A,B,C – are the characteristic features of SIADH)

33. Post-transcriptional processing of primary transcript mRNA does not include:
    A. Poly A tailing
    B. 5' capping
    C. Removal of introns
    D. Proof reading
Ans: D. Proof reading
(A,B,C are the post-transcriptional modifications of hnRNA – mRNA)

34. Mushroom toxin amanitin blocks the enzyme
    A. DNA polymerase
    B. RNA polymerase - II
    C. RNA polymerase- I
    D. RNA polymerase - III
Ans: B. RNA polymerase II
(A – Enzyme of DNA Replication; C and D are also for the synthesis of RNA transcription- but not affected by amanitin)

35. Anticancer agent methotrexate inhibits the enzyme:
    A. Thioredoxin reductase
    B. Dihydrofolate reductase
    C. Ribonucleotide reductase
    D. Thimydylate synthase
Ans: B. Dihydrofolate reductase
(Methotroxeate has structural similarity to folic acid and so it competitively inhibits DHF reductase enzyme)

36. Enzyme involved in the purine salvage pathway is:
    A. Adenine phosphoribosyltransferase
    B. Amidophosphoribosyltransferase
    C. Glycinamide ribonucleotide synthetase
    D. Phosphoribosyl synthase.
Ans: A. Adenine phosphoribosyltransferase

37. HHH syndrome includes the following except:
    A. Homocitrullinuria
    B. Hyperornithinemia
    C. Hypouricemia
    D. Hyperammonemia
Ans: B. Hyperornithinemia

38. **The first line of defense for trapping ammonia is conversion of:**
    A. Glutamate to glutamine
    B. Urea synthesis
    C. Glycine to glutathione
    D. Serine to glycine
    Ans: A. Glutamate to glutamine
    (B- Urea synthesis – II line of defense; C and D – not connected)

39. **Factors causing decreased absorption of calcium include the following except:**
    A. Parathyroid hormone
    B. Phytic acid
    C. Oxalates
    D. Phosphates
    Ans: A. Parathyroid hormone—increases absorption of calcium.

40. **Which of the following is a ferroxidase?**
    A. Hemosiderin
    B. Ferritin
    C. C-reactive protein
    D. Ceruloplasmin
    Ans: D. Ceruloplasmin

41. **Cystic fibrosis is due to the defect in the transport of:**
    A. Copper ions
    B. Chloride ions
    C. Cysteine
    D. Potassium ions
    Ans: B. Chloride ion

42. **The predominant cation of intracellular fluid compartment is:**
    A. Potassium
    B. Sodium
    C. Calcium
    D. Magnesium
    Ans: A. Potassium

43. **Which of the following is not a reducing sugar?**
    A. Glucose
    B. Fructose
    C. Lactose
    D. Sucrose
    Ans: D. Sucrose: It has no free aldehyde or keto group and so it is a non- reducing sugar.

44. **Anderson glycogen storage disease is caused by deficiency of:**
    A. Branching enzyme
    B. Debranching enzyme
    C. Muscle phosphorylase
    D. Liver phosphorylase
    Ans: A. Branching enzyme (All the four are glycogen storage diseases)

45. **The following are lipotropic factor except:**
    A. Choline
    B. Lecithin
    C. Methionine
    D. Sphingomyelin
    Ans: D. Sphingomyelin: It is a sphingophospholipid.

46. **The regulatory synthesis of cholesterol is:**
    A. HMG-Co-A synthase
    B. Acetoacetyl Co-A synthase
    C. HMG-Co-A reductase
    D. Mevalonate kinase
    Ans: C. HMG-CoA reductase
    It is the rate limiting enzyme of cholesterol synthesis; A,B,D are other enzymes of cholesterol synthesis.

47. **Following are the factors affecting enzyme activity except:**
    A. Temperature
    B. pH
    C. Substrate concentration
    D. Active site of the enzyme
    Ans: D. Active site of the enzyme—substrate binding site in the enzyme and it is not a factor for the activity of the enzyme.

48. **Which metalloenzyme contains copper?**
    A. Alcohol dehydrogenase
    B. Hexokinase
    C. Tyrosinase
    D. Lipase
    Ans: C. Tyrosinase

(A. Alcohol dehydrogenase—Zn; B. Hexokinase—Mg^{++}; D. Lipase—calcium)

49. Which hypervitaminosis causes histmine release and itching?
A. Thiamine
B. Riboflavin
C. Niacin
D. Biotin

Ans: C. Niacin
(Other vitamins will not produce toxic reactions in increased doses)

50. Which vitamin plays a role in regulation of gene expression and tissue differentiation?
A. Vitamin E
B. Vitamin K
C. Vitamin D
D. Vitamin A

Ans: D. Vitamin A (retinoic acid)

51. All of the following diseases are transmitted maternally except:
A. Mitochondrial encephalopathy, lactic acidosis stroke like episodes (MELAS)
B. Leber's hereditary optic neuropathy
C. Myoclonic epilepsy
D. Hemophilia

Ans: D. Hemophilia
(A, B, C are due to mutation in mitochondrial DNA and transmitted maternally)

52. Iron-sulfur proteins are found in:
A. Complex IV and V
B. Mitochondrial outer membrane
C. Complex I and II
D. Ubiquinone

Ans: C. Complex I and II

53. The biologic effect of glucagon over metabolism include all of the following except:
A. Increased Glycogenolysis
B. Increased Ketogenesis
C. Increased Glycogenesis

Ans: C. Increased glycogenesis
(A and B - are the effect of glucagon where there is hyperglycemia)

54. Which of the following enzyme is inhibited by fluoroacetate?
A. Fumerase
B. Succinate thiokinase
C. Aconitase
D. Citrate synthase

Ans: C. Aconitase: It is a non-competitive inhibitor.

55. Value of specific dynamic action of carbohydrate is:
A. 25%
B. 5%
C. 30%
D. 15%

Ans: B. 5%

56. Negative nitrogen balance is associated with following situations except:
A. Lack of an essential amino acid
B. Inadequate dietary protein
C. Burns
D. Recovery from acute illness

Ans: A. Lack of an essential amino acid

57. The following are congenital hyperbilirubemias except:
A. Dubin-Johnson syndrome
B. Turner's syndrome
C. Gilbert's syndrome
D. Rotor syndrome

Ans: B. Turner's syndrome—chromosomal disorder with one X chromosome.
(A and D are congenital conjugated hyperbilirubinemia and C - congenital unconjugated hyperbilirubinemia)

58. Which of the following intermediate of citric acid cycle is the precursor of heme synthesis?
A. Acetyl-CoA
B. Glutaryl-CoA
C. Succinyl-CoA
D. Isocitrate

Ans: C. Succinyl-CoA: First step of heme synthesis—Glycine + Succinyl-CoA—to give rise to ALA by ALA synthase enzyme.

59. In porphyria cutanea tarda, the enzyme that is affected is:

A. Uroporphyrinogen III cosynthase
B. Uroporphyrinogen decarboxylase
C. Uroporphyrinogen- I synthase
D. Coproporphyrinogen oxidase

Ans: B. UPG decarboxylase

60. Which vitamin deficiency causes homocysteinemia?

A. Thiamin
B. Niacin
C. Folate
D. Biotin

Ans: C. Folate
(Other three vitamins have no role over homocysteine metabolism/folate trap)

61. Which hormone acts by binding to intracellular receptors?

A. Glucagon
B. Calcitonin
C. Estrogen
D. Oxytocin

Ans: C. Estrogen
(A,B - Cyclic AMP; D - Calcium)

62. The protein responsible for the transport of iron across the mucosal cell is:

A. Hepcidin
B. Transferrin
C. Ferroportin
D. Hemoglobin

Ans: B. Transferrin

63. Which of the following instrument used the property of absorption for measuring the analytic concentration?

A. Flame photometer
B. pH meter
C. Colorimeter
D. Luminometer

Ans: A. Flame photometer

64. Amino acids are visualized by staining with which of the following agent in paper chromatography:

A. Ninhydrin
B. Sulfuric acid
C. Diphenylamine
D. Oil-Red-O

Ans: A. Ninhydrin

65. Which of the flowing hormone acts through cell surface receptor B by activating tyrosine kinase?

A. Somatostatin
B. Adrenaline
C. Nitric oxide
D. Insulin

Ans: D. Insulin

66. Which of the following causes hypouricemia?

A. Deficiency of phosphoribosyl amidotransferase
B. Deficiency of glucose 6 phosphatase
C. Deficiency of adenosine deaminase
D. Deficiency of adenosine phosphorribosyl transferase

Ans: C. Deficiency of adenosine deaminase

67. Which of the following pituitary hormone is a glycoprotein?

A. Growth hormone
B. Follicle stimulating hormone
C. Adrenocorticotropic hormone
D. Protein

Ans: B. Follicle stimulating hormone
(A and C are - Polypeptide; D - Protein)

68. Which of the following mineral deficiency causes acrodermatitis enteropathica?

A. Copper
B. Chromium
C. Zinc
D. Manganese

Ans: C. Zinc

69. Which of the following is involved in detoxication process?
    A. Transaminases
    B. Dehydrogenases
    C. Cytochrome P450 enzymes
    D. Decarboxylases
    Ans: C. Cytochrome P450 enzyme

70. Which amino acid produces putrescine by bacterial metabolism in intestine?
    A. Histidine
    B. Ornithine
    C. Tryptophan
    D. Lysine
    Ans: B. Ornithine

71. Which of the following is not a feature of Conn's syndrome?
    A. Elevated plasma aldosterone
    B. Decreased plasma rennin
    C. Hypernatremia
    D. Decreased plasma pH
    Ans: Decreased plasma pH

72. The constituents for calculating the osmolal gap include the following except:
    A. Sodium
    B. Potassium
    C. Glucose
    D. Urea
    Ans: B. Potassium

73. Which among the following is not a phase two detoxification reaction?
    A. Methylation
    B. Acetylation
    C. Conjugation
    D. Hydrolysis
    Ans: D. Hydrolysis: This is a phase one reaction.

74. Inhibitors of renin-angiotensin system include all of the following except:
    A. Increased blood pressure
    B. Decreased blood pressure
    C. Salt in-take
    D. Angiotensin-II
    Ans: B. Decreased blood pressure

75. Southern blot technique is used to identify:
    A. Specific sequences of DNA
    B. Specific sequences of RNA
    C. Specific sequences of protein
    D. Specific RNA-protein interaction
    Ans: A. Specific sequences of DNA

76. Transcription is catalyzed by:
    A. DNA dependent RNA polymerase.
    B. RNA dependent DNA polymerase.
    C. Reverse transcriptase.
    D. DNA ligases.
    Ans: A. DNA dependent RNA polymerase

77. Orotic aciduria is due to the deficiency of the enzyme:
    A. Dihydroorotase
    B. Dihydroorotase dehydrogenase
    C. Orotidine monophosphate decarboxylase
    D. Uridine monophosphate kinase
    Ans: C. OMP Decarboxylase

78. Secondary hyperuricemia is due to:
    A. Abnormal PRPP synthetase
    B. Glucose 6-phosphatase deficiency
    C. Glutathione reductase variant
    D. Rapidly growing malignant tissues like—leukemia, lymphoma
    Ans: D. Rapidly growing malignant tissues like—leukemia, lymphoma.

79. Hartnup's disease is associated to:
    A. Carcinoid tumors
    B. Defective replete of bilirubin
    C. Defective absorption of aromatic amino acids
    D. Defective absorption of minerals
    Ans: C. Defective absorption of aromatic amino acids

80. Maple syrup urine disease (MSUD) is due to which defect in the branched chain amino acid metabolism?
    A. Acetylation
    B. Decarboxylation
    C. Methylation
    D. Hydroxylation
    Ans: B. Decarboxylation

Topic-wise University Questions

From 2003 to 2021

1. **Subcellular organelles and cell membrane**
   - Structure of cell membrane (2008, 08, 10,14)
   - **Structure of cell membrane and transport mechanisms (2021)**
   - Fluid mosaic model/structure of cell membrane (Feb 2008)
   - Sub-cellular organelles (2010)
   - Functions of mitochondria (2012, 13) and **structure (2021)**
   - Comparison between prokaryotic and eukaryotic cell (2006, 13)
   - Active transport (2009)
   - **Passive transport (2019)**
   - Symport (2010I)
   - Ionophores (2014) and **types (2019)**
   - Transport across membrane (2013)
   - Lysosomes (2009)
   - Apoptosis (2008)
   - Membrane proteins (2016)
   - Endoplasmic reticulum (2018, 2 functions -**2020**)

2. **Enzymes**
   - Difference between coenzymes and cofactors (2020)
   - Zymogens (2013, 2009)
   - Active site of enzyme (2020)
   - Significance of multienzyme complex (2014)
   - Lineweaver–Burk plot (Aug 12)
   - Effects of different factors on rate of enzyme catalyzed reactions (2013) and mode of enzyme action and analytical use of enzyme with example (2021)
   - Classification of enzymes (2006, 2019)
   - IUBMB classification of enzymes (2006, 18)
   - Factors regulating enzyme activity (2010).
   - Name four clinically important enzymes and their importance (2010)
   - Km value and its significance (2003, 2016)
   - Covalent modification of enzymes in regulation of enzyme activity (2013)
   - Isoenzymes (2003, 04, 05, 08, 2005, 07)
   - Isoenzymes of LDH (2012)
   - Two isoenzymes and their clinical significance (2017)
   - Enzyme inhibition (2005, 11)
   - Competitive inhibition (2015, 2017, 2018, 2021)
   - **Effect of non-competitive inhibition of K_m and V_{max} (2019)**
   - Allosteric inhibition (2012)
   - Allosteric enzymes and its regulation (2005, 2014)
   - Suicidal inhibition (2013, 2015)
   - Drugs acting as enzyme inhibitors (2013, 14)
   - Factors regulating enzyme activity (2006, 2010)
   - Enzymes in AMI (2008)
   - Enzyme poisons (2009)
   - Enzymes in diseases (2014)
   - Liver enzymes (2015)
   - Metal co-factors of enzyme (2013)
   - Define, classify enzymes and explain concept of active site (2010)
   - Cardiac troponins (2009)
   - Effect of temperature on enzyme activity (2009)
   - Mode of action of enzymes (2016)
   - Metalloenzymes (2011)

- Diagnostic uses of enzymes (2016) **(2021)**
- Therapeutic uses of enzymes (2019)
- How enzymes reduce the activation energy of a reaction (2019)
- Interpret: a) Elevated alkaline phosphatase b) Elevated acid phosphatase (2019)

3. Carbohydrate chemistry

- Mutarotation (2006)
- Define and classify polysaccharides with examples (2006)
- Mucopolysaccharides **(with example 2019)**. Notes on hyaluronic acid (2012)
- Heteropolysaccharides and functions (2012)
- Functions of mucopolysaccharides (2017)
- Chondroitin sulphate (2007)
- Glycosides (2007, 2013)
- **Glycosidic bond and clinically important glycosides (2020)**
- **Differences between: a) Starch and Glycogen; b) Dextrin and dextran (2021)**
- Glycosaminoglycans (2009)
- Isomerism in carbohydrates (2011)
- Epimers (2009)
- Anomerism (2012)
- Stereoisomerism (2015)
- Benedict's test (2009)
- Ribose and deoxyribose (2009)
- Amino sugar with example and importance (2016)

4. Carbohydrate metabolism

- Describe biochemical actions of insulin in carbohydrate, lipid and protein metabolism. Name the disorder associated with insulin deficiency. How do you confirm the diagnosis (2006, 07)
- Regulation of blood glucose (2005, 2008, 2011, 2013, **2020**)
- Structure and functions of insulin (2009)
- Absorption of carbohydrates (2004, 2008)
- Insulin dependent glucose transporters and their tissue distribution (2013, **2019 – types and functions**)
- **Glucose transporters (2018)**
- Glycolysis. Describe Substrate level phosphorylation and its importance in this pathway (2009,10)
- Key enzymes of glycolysis (2009)
- Two differences between glucokinase and hexokinase (2014)
- Energetics of complete oxidation of 1 mole of glucose to CO_2 and H_2O in aerobic condition (2013)
- Substrate level phosphorylation (2010)
- Rapoport-Luebering shunt (2007, 10)
- Significance of 2,3 bisphosphoglycerate cycle (2017)
- 2, 3 BPG formation and its role (2) Aug 2013, glycolysis in RBC (2012, 13, 14, 15)
- Pyruvate dehydrogenase complex (2016, **2020**)
- **Three vitamins involved in PDH complex**
- Glycogen metabolism and GSD (2006,11, **2019**)
- Glycogenolysis (2011)
- von Gierke's disease (2003, 14, 13)
- GSD (20 08)
- HMP shunt pathway—significance (2005) HMP shunt (2007, 10, 12, 13)
- Significance of HMP shunt (2013)
- Importance of HMP shunt pathway (2012)
- HMP shunt—significance, disorders (2010)
- Importance of glucose six phosphate dehydrogenase deficiency (2009)
- Metabolism of glucose 6P (2015)
- Glucose 6P dehydrogenase enzyme (2013)
- Synthesis of glucose from alanine and regulation (2014)
- Gluconeogenesis, regulation, glucose-alanine cycle (2007, 08,10,12, **2020**)
- Substrates for gluconeogenesis (2017)
- Cori's cycle and glucose-alanine cycle (2011)
- Cahill and Cori cycle (2016)
- Uronic acid pathway (2009)
- **Galactose metabolism and its applied aspect (2020)**
- Galactosemia (2005, 08, 13, 2017)
- **Essential pentosuria (2018, 2020)**
- Fructose intolerance (2011)
- Lactose intolerance (2013, 16)

- Fate of oxaloacetate (2015)
- Metabolism of propionyl-CoA (2009)
- Laboratory criteria for diagnosis of diabetes mellitus (2013)
- Biochemical basis of development of cataract in DM (2013)
- HbA_{1C} (2007, 11, 12)
- Glycated Hb, fructosamine, advanced glycation end products (2016)
- Metabolic changes, complications and investigations of DM (2014)
- WHO criteria of diagnosis of DM/lab criteria for diagnosis of DM (2013)
- Renal glycosuria (2007, 09, 10)
- Causes of hypoglycemia (2012)
- Oral GTT (2008, 14, **2021**)
- Abnormal GTT (2015)
- GTT (2008)
- Digestion and absorption of carbohydrates. Write the metabolic fate of pyruvate (2016)
- Consequences of diabetic ketosis (2016)
- **Formation and fate of pyruvate (2021)**
- **Two components of metabolic syndrome (2020)**

5. **TCA cycle**
- TCA cycle (2004, 06, 09, 10, 11, **2021**)
- Significance of citric acid cycle (2017)
- Explain how pyruvate enters Krebs cycle. How many ATPs are produced (2009)
- Anapleurotic reactions (2006, **2021**)
- Sources of acetyl-CoA (2005)
- Fate of acetyl-CoA (2005)

6. **Integration of metabolism**
- Compare the metabolic changes in well fed state and starvation (2012, 2015)
- Role of liver in integration of metabolism during postprandial state (2003)
- Metabolic adaptations in fed state (2012)
- Metabolic adaptations in fasting state (2015)

7. **Lipid chemistry**
- Essential FA (2005, 12, **2020**)
- Phospholipids (2004, 05, 07, 12, 15, **2019**)
- Functions of phospholipids (2012, 15)
- **Role of phospholipase A**
- **Metabolic basis of role of aspirin as an anti-platelet agent (2019)**
- Eicosanoids (2005)
- Prostaglandins (2005, 13, 15)
- Functions of prostaglandins (2017)
- PUFA (2007)
- Cholesterol structure and function (2009)
- Amphipathic lipids (2015)
- Cardiolipin (2012)
- Phosphatidyl inositol (2009)
- Pulmonary surfactants/**lung surfactant** (2011, 2013, **2021**)
- Lipid peroxidation (2009)

8. **Lipid metabolism**
- Lipases (2014)
- Function of lipoprotein lipase (2015)
- Liposomes (2017)
- Lipid profile (2013)
- Absorption of lipids (2003, 2019)
- Obesity (2017)
- **Digestion and absorption of lipids/TAG and transport of lipids** (2008, 10, 2011, **2021**)
- Steatorrhoea (2013)
- Fatty acid synthase complex (2011)
- FA synthesis (2005)
- Multienzyme complex (2014)
- Beta-oxidation of fatty; acids under the following heading: a. Definition; b. Site; c. Steps; D. Energetic (2008, 2018, 2021)
- Beta oxidation, carnitine, energetics (2008)
- Carnitine shuttle (2013)/**carnitine transport (2019)**
- Oxidation of palmitic acid (2014)
- Types of fatty acid oxidation (2012)
- Zellweger syndrome (2012, 13)
- Refsum's disease (2013)/**defect in Refsum's disease (2020)**
- Sources and fate of acetyl-CoA (2005, 09)
- Ketone bodies (2005, 2020)
- Tests to identify ketone bodies in urine (2002)
- Rothera's test (2010)
- Synthesis and utilization of ketone bodies (2005, 07, 08)

- What are ketone bodies? Describe the formation of ketone bodies (2006, 07, 08, 11)
- Name the ketone bodies. How are they formed and utilised in the body. Add a note on the metabolic changes in diabetic ketoacidosis (2013)
- Define ketosis and its causes (2014)
- Products of arachidonic acid (2012)
- Prostaglandins (2005)
- Classification and functions of lipoproteins. Metabolism of LDL (2005, 2016)
- Lipoproteins (2005)
- Chylomicrons (2016)
- **Chylomicrons are rich in -------- and apoprotein of chylomicron are ------ (2020)**
- **LDL metabolim and clinical importance (2019)**
- LDL metabolism (2005, 16)
- Role of LDL receptors and diseases caused its defects (2003)
- Apo lipoproteins (2007, 15)
- Apo-proteins and its significance (2017)
- HDL functions and metabolism (2010)
- HDL cycle (2011)
- Reverse cholesterol transport (2017) **and anti-atherogenic effect of HDL (2020)**
- HDL metabolism (2017)
- Role of HDL as scavenger of cholesterol (2010)
- Hyperlipidemias—classification and importance (2011, 12)
- Frederickson's classification of hyper-lipidemia (2011, 12)
- **Dyslipidemia (2020)**
- Cholesterol synthesis, regulation and products obtained from it (2004, 10, 06, 11)
- Cholesterol synthesis and regulation. Sources and fate of acetyl-CoA (2009)
- Catabolism of cholesterol (2008)
- Important derivatives of cholesterol (2010, 2021)
- Cholesterol lowering action of fibrates (2015)
- Mechanism of actions of statins (2013)
- Bile salts (2004), BS-synthesis and biological role (2013)
- **Risk factors of cardiovascular disease and its preventive methods (2021)**
- Sphingolipidoses (2009)
- **Two lipid storage diseases (2019)**
- Niemann Pick's disease (2017)
- **Enzyme defeci in Niemann-Pick disease and Gaucher's disease (2020)**
- Fatty liver and lipotropic factors (2009, 13, 14, 2018, 2020)
- Lipotropic factors (2013, 15)
- Alcohol metabolism (2012, 2019)
- Prevention of atherosclerosis (2014)
- Metabolism of adipose tissue in starvation (2015)
- Lecithin cholesterol acyl transferase(LCAT) (2016, 2018)
- Importance of brown fat (2018, 2019)
- Biochemical changes in atherosclerosis (2018)

9. **ETC and oxidative phosphorylation**
- Chemiosmotic hypothesis (2006, 07, 08, 09, 10, 11)
- **Schematic representation of ETC (2019)**
- **Name: a) V complex of ETC; b) One inhibitor of Complex III (2020)**
- **Chemiosmotic theory and mechanism of ATP synthesis (2021)**
- Inhibitors of ETC (2005, 10, 2017)
- Uncouplers (2004)
- Two examples of substrate level phosphorylation (2014)
- Coupling of oxidative phosphorylation, uncouplers (2002, 08, 09, 11)
- Role of cytochromes in ETC (2006)
- Oxidative phosphorylation (2007, 08, 09, 1, 14)
- Biological oxidation—definition, ETC, oxidative phosphorylation (2007, 13)
- Components and chemiosmotic theory of ETC (2011)
- Components, reactions and inhibitors of ETC (2012)
- Mechanism of cyanide poisoning (2013, 14, 15)

- ATP synthesis–Essay (2013)
- Mechanism of ATP synthesis (2013)
- Inhibition of ATP synthesis (2016)
- Compounds affect ETC and oxidative phosphorylation (2014)
- Shuttle pathways across the membrane (2015)
- OXPHOS (oxidative phosphorylation disease) (2016)

10. VITAMINS

A. Fat Soluble Vitamins

- Vitamin A (2006, 10)
- Wald's visual cycle (2008, 09, 16) **and deficiency manifestations (2020)**
- **Daily requirement of vitamin A for adults (2020)**
- Functions and deficiency of vitamin A (2014)
- Ocular changes in vitamin A deficiency (2015)
- Role of vitamin D in calcium metabolism (2005)
- Active form of vitamin D and its role (2011)
- **Formation of vitamin D and its active form (2019)**
- **Two differences between rickets and osteomalacia (2020)**
- Chemistry, sources, RDA and role of vitamin D (2003)
- Justify the statement that vitamin D is an hormone (2003)
- Rickets (2009)
- Deficiency of vitamin D (2014)
- Metabolism of vitamin D (2015)
- Vitamin K (2009, 11)
- Vitamin K cycle (2016, 2019)
- Vitamin E—**RDA, biochemical functions and deficiency manifestations** (2004, 10, 2021)
- **Role of gamma-carboxylation in coagulation (2020)**

B. Water Soluble Vitamins

- Thiamine (2003, 07, 12, 13, 15)
- Active form of thiamine and riboflavin (2012)
- Beriberi (2009, 2013)
- **Wernicke's Korsakoff syndrome (2019)**
- Role of niacin as coenzyme (2011)
- Biotin (2004, 08)
- Coenzyme activity of biotin (2016)
- Coenzyme role of pyridoxine (2014)
- Functions of pyridoxal phosphate (2016)
- Functions and RDA of B6 (2014)
- Folic acid (2010)
- Folate trap (2013, 14)
- FIGLU (2013)
- One carbon compound (2015)
- Histidine load test. (2011)
- Biochemical functions of B12 (2011, 13, 18)
- Deficiency manifestation of vitamin B12 (2017)
- **Why B12 deficiency causes macrocytic anemia? – Explain (2019)**
- Methylmalonic aciduria (2006)
- Vitamin C (2005, 12, 2021)
- Vitamin C functions (2008, 09, 11, 13, 2016)
- Vitamin C—dietary source, functions and **deficiency manifestations** (2013, 2021)
- Role of vitamins in TCA cycle (2013)
- Antioxidant vitamins and minerals (2017)

11. Energy and Nutrition

- SDA (2013)
- Calculate daily calorie requirement (2003)
- Biological value of protein (2010)
- PEM (2004, 06, 09, 08, 11, 2019)
- Kwashiorkor (2005)
- Disorders of kwashiorkor (2014)
- Differences between kwashiorkor and marasmus (2013, 14)
- RDA (2005)
- BMR (2005, 08, 07, 2018)
- Define BMR and mention the factors affecting it (2016)
- Balanced diet (2007, 11, 12, 2020)
- Fiber diet (2008, 10, 13, 14, 15)
- Nutritional importance of protein (2010)
- **Nitrogen balance and factors affecting (2021)**
- **BMI value in: a) Normal individual; b) Obesity (2020)**

- Total parenteral nutrition (2010)
- Obesity (2012)
- Limiting amino acids (2009, 13)
- Glycemic index (2018 2020)
- Respiratory quotient (2011)
- Biologic values of proteins (2015, **2021**)

12. Hemoglobin

- Structure of Hb (2004)
- Abnormal Hb (2010)
- Binding of Hb to oxygen (2012)
- **Oxygen dissociation curve of Hb (2019)**
- **Hemoglobin electrophoresis in thalassemia (2019)**
- **Biochemical features seen in blood and urine of a patient with hemolytic anaemia (2021)**
- Hemoglobinopathies (2008)
- Sickle cell disease/Sickle cell Hb (2008, **2020**)
- HbS (2008, 2010 –II)
- Thalassemia (2012)
- Glycosylated Hb (2007)
- Methemoglobin (2009)

13. Heme synthesis and break down

- Heme synthesis and porphyrias (2008, 09)
- Regulation of heme synthesis (2014)
- Porphyrias (2009, 2019, **2021**)
- Porphyrias. Any three in detail (2009, 10)
- **Inborn errors of heme metabolism and their features (2021)**
- Acute intermittent porphyria (AIP) (2006)
- Hemoglobin catabolism (2011), heme catabolism/degradation (2005, 11)
- Synthesis and conjugation of bilirubin (2005, 11)
- Excretion of bilirubin and clinical importance of bilirubin estimations (2010)
- Formation of bilirubin (2009)
- Transport of bilirubin (2010)
- Vandenbergh reaction (2008, 10, 12)
- Why cholelithiasis patient passes clay coloured stools (2014)
- Congenital hyperbilirubinemias (2007)
- Classification of jaundice based on LFT (2018)
- **Congenital jaundice (2019)**
- **Markers of cholestasis (2019)**
- **Two markers of obstructive jaundice (2020)**
- **Defect in Dubin-Johnson syndrome (2020)**
- Obstructive jaundice (2004)
- Physiological jaundice (2006)
- Investigations of jaundice (2013)
- Investigations required to differentiate various types of jaundice. Describe the metabolism of bilirubin (2017)

14. Chemistry of Amino acids: Structure and properties

- Essential amino acids (2005, 2014)
- Isoelectric pH (06, 2015)
- Basic amino acids (2012)
- Classification of amino acids based on metabolic fate (2018)

15. Proteins—chemistry: Structure and function

- Structure of proteins (2003, 06, 07, 11, 10, 2019)
- Levels of organization of proteins (2009)
- Methods of elucidation of protein structure (2003)
- Primary structure (2015)
- Alpha helix (2006, 07, 08, 11)
- Secondary structure of proteins (2008, 06, 07, 11, 12)
- Forces stabilizing secondary structure (2012)
- Quaternary structure of proteins with examples (2012)
- Denaturation (2009, 2013)
- Precipitation reactions of proteins (2012, **2021**)
- Collagen (2009, 2018, 2020)
- Glycoproteins (2010)
- Biologically important peptides (2015)
- Protein targeting and disorders connected with that (2014)
- Proteasome (2019)

16. Protein and amino acid metabolism

- Sources and metabolism of ammonia (2014)

- Ammonia metabolism and urea cycle (2015)
- Transamination (2008, 10, 2019)
- Urea cycle (2005, 06, 09, 08)
- Urea cycle and its disorders (2012)
- Urea cycle disorders (2016)
- **Hyperammonemias (2021)**
- Differences between CPS I and CPS II (2010)
- Urea cycle disorder causes orotic aciduria. Explain (2011)
- Causes of increase in urea level (2012)
- Metabolism of glycine (2004, 09, 11)
- Glutathione (2009, 2017)
- Functions of glutathione (2012)
- Role of glutathione in amino acid transport (2005)
- Formation of specialized products from glycine (2009, 10, 2016, 2017, 2021)
- Compounds from glycine (2011)
- Functions of glycine (2014)
- Formation of creatine (2008)
- Clinical relevance of creatine (2012)
- Important functions of serine (2016)
- Mention the AA which take part of one carbon pool (2011)
- Metabolic role of methionine (2007, 08, 09)
- Transmethylation (2008, 10, 15)
- Active methionine (2013)
- Functions of methionine and cysteine (2008)
- Metabolism and functions of cysteine. Name the associated inborn errors (2017)
- Homocystinuria (2014)
- Cystinosis (2018)
- Cystinuria (2019)
- Steps of SAM cycle. Transmethylation with five examples (2010)
- Products from methionine (2008)
- Derivatives of aromatic amino acids. Write about serotonin (2016)
- Name the inherited disorder in tyrosine metabolism with the enzyme deficiency (2005, 12)
- Disorders of tyrosine metabolism (2016)
- Name aromatic amino acids and write about metabolism of phenylalanine (2003, 05, 13, 2021)
- Write about the conversion of phenylalanine to tyrosine. Describe phenylketonurias (2017)
- PKU (2010, 11, 13, 14, 15, **2021**)
- Alkaptonuria (2004, 08, 10, 12, 17)
- Formation of epinephrine (2010)
- **Metabolism of catecholamines (2019)**
- **Catabolism of tyrosine and disorders (2021)**
- Synthesis of tyrosine and its products (2015)
- Products of tyrosine (2013)
- Functions of tyrosine in the body (2012)
- Tryptophan metabolism and IEMs associated with it (2006)
- Hartnup's disease (2010)
- Malignant carcinoid syndrome (2016)
- Derivatives of tryptophan (2012, **2019**)
- GABA (2010, 2013)/Gamma aminobutyric acid (2017)
- Metabolism of branched chain amino acids (2007)
- MSUD (2009, 12, 13/Maple syrup urinary disease (2017)
- Polyamines (2007, 14, 2020)
- Histidine load test. (2011)
- Histamine (2014, 2017)
- Synthesis and mechanism of action of NO. (2011)
- Nitric oxide (2011, 14, 2017)
- Any four neurotransmitters (2017)

17. Plasma proteins

- Functions of plasma proteins (2006, 09)
- **Functions and importance of plasma proteins in beta region of electrophoresis (2021)**
- **Name plasma proteins. Role of albumin and other transport proteins (2020)**
- **Conditions in which A:G ratio is reversed and the reason for it (2019)**
- Functions of albumin and four functions (Aug 09, Feb 12, Nov 15, Aug 17)
- Acute phase and negative acute phase proteins (Aug 2016)
- Alpha I antitrypsin and the diseases associated with it (Aug 2016)

18. Immune chemistry

- Structure and functions of immunoglobulins (Feb 08, 11, 12, 14, 2019)
- Types of Ig (2013, 14)
- Classes of immunoglobulins (2018)
- Bence Jones protein (2009)
- Bence Jones proteinuria (2012)
- Multiple myeloma (2013, 2014)
- **Laboratory diagnosis of multiple myeloma (2019)**
- Hybridoma technology and its application (2016)

19. Minerals

- Calcium normal blood levels and factors regulation it (2004, 05,14)
- Write in detail about calcium metabolism (2004, 07, 12)
- Calcium homeostasis (2009, 13)
- Hormonal regulation of calcium (2015)
- Functions of calcium (2014)
- What are the different forms of calcium in the blood?
- Functions of phosphorus (2007, 2016)
- Functions of phosphates (2024)
- Functions of phosphate ions (2017)
- Iron (2005, 06)
- Storage and transport of iron in the body (2008, 11, 06)
- Ferritin (2011)
- Biochemical functions of iron (2014)
- Digestion, absorption and transport of iron (2006, 08,11)
- **Absorption of dietary iron (2021)**
- Sources, RDA, absorption, biochemical functions and deficiency manifestations and toxicity of iron (2016) and **clinical features of Iron deficiency anemia (2019)**
- Iron deficiency and manifestations (2013)
- Bronze diabetes (2012)
- Trace elements (2003)
- Biochemical functions of zinc (2015)
- Metabolism of zinc (2004, 2006)
- Zinc and selenium (2008)
- Functions of selenium (2009)
- Mention the enzymes which require selenium as cofactor (2011)
- Iodine (2013)
- Functions and sources of iodine (2013)
- Wilson's disease (2007, 15)
- Functions of copper (2015, 2016)
- **Copper metabolism and its applied aspects (2021)**
- **Sources, RDA, function and deficiency manifestation of copper (2021)**
- Fluorosis (2011, 09, 2010)
- Metabolic role of Mg (2010)/functions of Mg (2015)

20. Xenobiotics

- Detoxification of xenobiotics (2005, 07, 11)
- Detoxification by hydroxylation (2005)
- **Two examples for xenobiotic metabolism acting on endogenous substance (2019)**
- Phase II detoxification (2011)/phase II reactions of xenobiotics (2017)
- Conjugation (2012, 13, 15, 2021)
- Conjugating agents (2013)
- What are xenobiotics? (2008)
- Cytochrome-P 450 (2004, 2013, 2015) - **functions and properties like induction by drugs (2020)**

21. Pollution and heavy metal poisons

- Describe any two heavy metal poisoning (Feb 2014)
- Carbon monoxide (2009)
- Lead poisoning (2018)

22. Free radicals and antioxidants

- Cytochrome P450 (2004, 10, 2015, 2014)
- Functions of cytochrome 450 (2013, 14)
- Free radicals (2010)
- Antioxidants (2011)
- Primary antioxidant enzymes and their activity (2016)
- Antioxidant-vitamins (2017)
- **Two antioxidant vitamins, one antioxidant mineral (2020)**
- **Two antioxidant enzymes (2020)**

23. Acid-base balance

- What is the normal pH of blood? Describe the various mechanisms which maintain it. Mention the acid base disorders (2003, 2013, 2015, 2021)

- How acid-base balance is maintained in the body (2003, 05, 07, 09, 10, 11)
- Blood buffers (2008, 15)
- Buffer systems in the body (2006, 07, 03, 05, 09, 08, 10, 11, 15)
- Bicarbonate buffer (2014)
- Chloride shift (2015)
- **Henderson-Hasselbalch equation (2019)**
- Name the important buffer system in the body. Describe the role of lungs and kidney in acid-base maintenance (2016)
- Role of plasma and renal buffers in maintaining acid base homeostasis (2011, 15)
- Role of lungs in acidbase balance (2003, 05, 07, 10, 11, 12, 17)
- Role of kidneys in acid-base balance (2003, 05, 07, 09, 12, 10, 11, 13, 15)
- Anion gap (2005, 2010, 2021)
- Metabolic acidosis (2004, 07, 06, 09, 11, 2016, 2017, 2021)
- High anion gap metabolic acidosis (2016)
- Metabolic alkalosis (2014)
- Causes of respiratory acidosis (2012, 13)
- Compensatory changes in respiratory acidosis (2014)
- Causes of metabolic acidosis (2008)
- Acidosis causes hyperkalemia why? (2011)
- Alkali reserve (2009)
- **Lactic acidosis (2019)**

24. Electrolyte and water balance

- Explain the metabolic interrelationships between sodium concentration and water volume. (2011)
- Name the major intracellular and extracellular anions. (2011)
- Water distribution and its balance in the body. (2010)
- Dehydration (2010)
- Water toxicity (2010
- **Normal serum Na and K levels and add a note on causes and clinical features of hyponatremia (2020)**
- Write the normal serum Na and K levels (2011)
- Hyponatremia (2016)
- Sodium homeostasis (2012)
- Normal serum electrolytes (2014)
- Hyperkalemia (2013, 14, 17)
- **Hypokalemia (2021)**
- Disorders of potassium homeostasis (2014)
- Chloride shift (2015)

25. Hormones

- Mechanism of hormone action. (2013)
- Write about cAMP mediated signal transduction (2003)
- Mechanism of action of thyroid hormones (2005)
- G proteins (2006)
- Mechanism of action of steroid hormones (2012)
- Functions of adrenocortical hormones (2009)
- **Laboratory tests done for diagnosis of adrenal hypofunction and hyperfunction (2010**
- **Metabolism of catecholamines (2019)**
- Role of parathormone in Ca, p homeostasis (2011)
- Functions of parathormone (2017)
- cAMP (2005, 11, 13)
- Functions of glucocorticoids (2012)
- Action of insulin (2007, 09, 15)
- Action of glucagon (2014)
- Hyperglycemic hormones (2015)
- Hypothyroidism presents with hypercholesterolemia why? (2011)
- Mention two second messengers (2010)
- Oxytocin (2010)
- Calcitonin (2016)
- Addison's disease (2010)

26. Nucleotide chemistry and metabolism

- What are nucleotides and name three important nucleotides and their importance (2010, 13, 14)
- Synthetic nucleotides (2005)
- Functions of nucleotides (2013, 14)
- Any two antimetabolites and its use (Aug 2017)
- **Four synthetic analogs of purine and pyrimidine bases used as therapeutic agent (2019)**

- Mechanism of action of allopurinol (2019)
- Form of folic acid involved in purine synthesis (2020)
- Inhibitors of purine nucleotide biosynthesis (2021)
- Deoxyribonucleotides from ribonucleotides (2014)
- Sources of carbon and nitrogen in purine ring (2008)
- Denovo synthesis of purine nucleotides (2006, 2008)
- Differences between CPS-I and CPS-II (2010)
- Synthesis of uric acid (2009)
- Gout (2005, 07, 08, 09, 15, 17)
- **Causes, symptoms and treatment of gout (2021)**
- Hyperuricemia (2008, 11, 09)
- Salvage pathway (2004, 05, 07, 10, 11, 12, 15)
- Purine salvage pathway (2012, 15)
- Orotic aciduria (2010, 15)
- Lesch-Nyhan syndrome (2012, 2017)
- Lesch-Nyhan syndrome presents with hyperuricemia. Explain. (2011)
- Write the enzyme defect in: A. Lesch-Nyhan syndrome, b. Orotic aciduria—2008, 2012, 2013

27. Structure of nucleic acids and replication-II

- Types, functions, components of nucleic acids, Chargaff's rule, types of DNA double helix and differences between DNA and RNA (2006, 10)
- Nucleosome (2016)
- Telomerase (2016, 2017, 2021) and application (2021)
- Structure of DNA (2006)
- **Two differences of B and A forms of DNA (2020)**
- Bases in nucleic acids (2012)
- Replication (2007, 12)
- Enzymes of Replication (2012)
- **Mineral required for DNA polymerase activity (2020)**
- Proteins and enzymes involved in DNA replication (2019)
- DNA replication in prokaryotes and inhibitors of DNA replication (2021)
- Okasaki fragments (2013, 15)
- DNA repair mechanism (2003, 07, 12, 15, 2017, **2020**)
- Types of DNA repair mechanism. Write in detail about any one repair mechanism (2016)
- Point mutation (2018, 2020)
- Mutation (2008, 11)
- Types of mutation (2013, 15)
- Mutagens (2012)
- Differences between DNA and RNA (2008)
- Cell cycle (2011)
- Classify RNA and its functions (2009)
- tRNA (2004, 10, 06, 10, 14, 2015)
- mRNA (2015)

28. Transcription and translation

- **Compare promoter with enhancer (2019)**
- Post transcriptional modifications (2008, 11, 2013, 2017)
- Post-transcriptional processing and post transcriptional inhibitors (2013, 17)
- **Splicing of hnRNA (heteronuclear RNA) (2019)**
- **Role of poly-A tail (2020)**
- Reverse transcription (2009)
- Transcription and post-transcriptional processing (2011, 13, 15)
- Rifampicin blocks ------- of transcription process (2020)
- Inhibitors of transcription (2017)
- Reverse transcriptase (2013)
- Genetic code (2005, 07, 10)
- Degeneracy of the code (2005)
- Wobble hypothesis (2008)
- **Role of different types of RNA in protein synthesis (2019)**
- Translation (2013, 14)
- Protein synthesis, post-translational modification (2013, 14)
- Inhibitors of protein synthesis (2013)/ Inhibitors of protein translation (2017)

- Post-translational modification (2006, 07, 10, 12, 14, **2020**)

29. Regulation of gene expression-II
- Lac operon (2004, 06, 10, 13, 14)

30. Applications of molecular biology
- Restriction enzymes (2007, 12, 14, 13)
- **Restriction endonuclease (2020)**
- Use of plasmids (2009)
- Applications of recombinant DNA technology, (2003, 06, 07, 2014, **2021**)
- Describe recombinant DNA technology and explain different techniques with its applications (2013, 14, **2021**)
- PCR (2010, 12, 14, 2017, **2020**)
- Any four uses of PCR (2017)
- Blotting techniques (2014)
- Southern blotting (2005, 2016, 2017)
- Gene therapy (2010, 15, 19)
- Modes of gene therapy (2016}
- Cloning. Steps of recombinant DNA technology (2011)
- Hybridoma technology and its application (2016)
- DNA fingerprinting (2018, 20**19**)
- **Genetic library (2019)**
- **Expand RFLP and its clinical uses (2020)**

31. Aids and cancer
- Oncogenes (Feb 2007, 08, 2012)
- Protooncogenes and oncogenes (2008)
- **Biochemical features of cancer cells (2021)**
- Tumor suppressor genes (2 examples) (2014, 2009)
- Applications of tumor markers (2003, 04, 05, 09, 13)
- Carcinogenic virus (2009)
- Anti-neoplastic effect of methotrexate (2014)
- Enzymes as tumor marker (2018)

32. Isotopes
- What are isotopes? Applications of isotopes in biochemistry. (2010)

33. Special techniques
- Chromatography (2009)
- **ABG and interpretation of results (2020)**
- Paper chromatography (2015)
- Affinity chromatography—principle (2012)
- TLC (2006)
- Colorimeter (2009)
- Beer Lambert's law (2013)
- Principle and applications of electrophoresis (2006, 2007, 11, 12, 13, 2017, 2019)
- Factors affecting electrophoresis (2017)
- Separation of serum proteins by paper electrophoresis. Patterns of electrophoresis in multiple myeloma and nephrotic syndrome (2010)
- Serum protein electrophoresis (2011, 12)
- Various patterns of diseases in protein electrophoresis (2016)
- **Hb electrophoresis—interpretation (2019)**
- Blotting techniques (2005)
- Southern blot technique (2008)
- RIA (2013)
- ELISA (2013)
- Flurometry (2008)

34. Function tests
- **Renal function tests (2019)**
- Tests to assess glomerular functions (2017)
- Tubular function tests (2012, 14)
- Tests to assess renal tubular functions (2017)
- Clearance tests (2004)
- Creatinine clearance test (2002) **and normal value in adult – (2020)**
- Definition and importance of creatine clearance test (2016)
- Renal threshold substances (2009)
- Tests for thyroid function (2003, 13)
- **In vitro thyroid function tests (2021)**
- Assessment of hypothyroidism (2011)
- Biochemical investigations in cirrhosis (2003)
- LFT (2005, 09, 12)

- Classify jaundice based on liver function test (2018)
- Tests done to assess synthetic functions of liver (2018, 2019)
- Proteinuria (2018, **2020**)
- **Microalbuminuria and its importance (2018)**

35. Normal values—(Reference values)

- Normal values in blood/serum (2019, 2020)
  a. Creatinine
  b. Potassium
  c. TSH
  d. pH
  e. Urea
  f. Urea/creatinine ratio
  g. 24 hours urinary excretion of creatinine in adults
  h. Uric acid levels in male/female
- Formula to calculate anion gap

EU GSPR Authorised Reprsentative
Logos Europe, 9 rue Nicolas Poussin
1700, La Rochelle, France
Phone: +33 (0) 6 67 93 73 78
E-mail: contact@logoseurope.eu

www.ingramcontent.com/pod-product-compliance
Ingram Content Group UK Ltd.
Pitfield, Milton Keynes, MK11 3LW, UK
UKHW050455150426
5217IPUK00025B/1703